Neoconstructivism

Neoconstructivism

THE NEW SCIENCE OF COGNITIVE DEVELOPMENT

Edited by

SCOTT P. JOHNSON

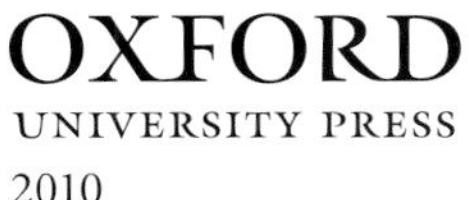

2010

OXFORD
UNIVERSITY PRESS

Oxford University Press, Inc., publishes works that further
Oxford University's objective of excellence
in research, scholarship, and education.

Oxford New York
Auckland Cape Town Dar es Salaam Hong Kong Karachi
Kuala Lumpur Madrid Melbourne Mexico City Nairobi
New Delhi Shanghai Taipei Toronto

With offices in
Argentina Austria Brazil Chile Czech Republic France Greece
Guatemala Hungary Italy Japan Poland Portugal Singapore
South Korea Switzerland Thailand Turkey Ukraine Vietnam

Published by Oxford University Press, Inc.
198 Madison Avenue, New York, New York 10016
www.oup.com

Library of Congress Cataloging-in-Publication Data

Neoconstructivism : the new science of cognitive development / edited by Scott P. Johnson.
p. cm.
Includes bibliographical references and index.
ISBN 978-0-19-533105-9
1. Cognition in infants. 2. Attention in infants. 3. Perception in infants.
I. Johnson, Scott P., 1959–
BF720.C63N46 2009
155.4′13—dc22 2009007210

9 8 7 6 5 4 3 2 1

Printed in China
on acid-free paper.

FOREWORD

What is Neoconstructivism?

Nora S. Newcombe
Temple University

Piaget was supposed to have solved the problem of the origins of knowledge, to have bridged the nativist–empiricist split. This goal was one of his aims in beginning to study children's cognitive development, and, at the end of his life, he regarded this goal as accomplished (Chapman, 1988). Yet, even before his death, criticisms of Piaget were mounting (Gelman & Baillargeon, 1983). They now form a familiar litany: no clear evidence for stages and structuralism, insufficient attention to the gradualisms and localisms of cognitive progress, excessive emphasis on verbal justifications of judgments. Among these limitations, two issues stand out: an overly lean delineation of the starting points for cognitive development, and a description of the mechanism of cognitive change that was little more than a re-naming of the phenomenon as accommodation.

So, how do we characterize starting points and developmental change? These two questions were addressed in a bold way by the resurgence of nativism, which came roaring back on the intellectual scene in the 1950s with Chomsky's (1959) critique of Skinner and which had become the dominant paradigm for thinking about the origins of knowledge by 1980 or so. Nativism solves the first of Piaget's problems by definition—by postulating the richest starting points imaginable, ones that encompass all the "core knowledge" required to understand the world. An important addition to this philosophically classic position, appearing in force in Fodor (1983), was the idea that the mind/brain is organized into *modules* that are not only neurally specialized and present from the beginning but that do not accept information from each other. Indeed, nativists have argued that evolution could not work to create human intelligence without such modular organization—there must be some *thing* for evolution to select or weed out (Cosmides & Tooby, 1994). And nativism solved the second of Piaget's main problems (one that had shrunk to minuscule size by the hypothesized existence of so much innate knowledge) essentially by fiat—by postulating simple "triggers" that led children to select parameters or fill content into slots. More recently, they have added the hypothesis that change occurs when human language bridges the gap across modules of core knowledge (Spelke, 2003).

None of these postulates of nativism are, however, supported by the evidence. Starting points are strong, but infants are not tiny adults with insufficient control over their arms and legs. There is much more conceptual change than nativists envision and strong evidence that environmental input is integral to cognitive development in complex ways that go far beyond triggering (Newcombe, 2002). There is also good reason to think that language, while helpful to human thought, is not the sine qua non of cognitive flexibility (Newcombe & Ratliff, 2007). So, what's the alternative to nativism? Information-processing theorists of the 1970s and 1980s retained lean starting points and used production system modeling to address the problem of change (Klahr & Wallace, 1976). However, there seems to be more initial competence than most such modelers were willing to contemplate. In addition, these modeling efforts, like the connectionist modeling that succeeded production systems, have often failed to use empirical information about the kind and sequence of environmental information to constrain the models (Newcombe, 1998). Vygotsky has sometimes been presented as an alternative to Piaget, but his work concentrates too exclusively on social and cultural interaction to seem to provide a satisfying overall framework for many aspects of cognitive development (Newcombe & Huttenlocher, 2000).

The need for new approaches to cognitive development became increasingly evident by 1990, and several books began to fill the need for nonnativist approaches to cognitive development: Elman et al. (1996); Gopnik and Meltzoff (1997); Karmiloff-Smith (1992); Siegler (1996); Thelen and Smith (1994). However, each of these approaches also has some limitations, for example, of scope or specificity. In addition, they competed with each other, so that, for example, connectionism and dynamic systems theorists spent much time debating whether their efforts were similar or different (Spencer, Thomas & McClelland, in press). The end result is that there is not, as yet, a dominant theoretical framework within which to situate the large volume of exciting recent empirical work on cognitive development—research that sometimes seems to define theory better than debate that is self-consciously theoretical (Oakes, Newcombe, & Plumert, in press). Research on cognitive development has gained steadily in interest for several reasons—better techniques and methods, established phenomena with richly detailed data that allow for finely tuned competing explanations to be pitted against each other, and better and better contact with insights and methods from cognitive science, neuroscience, computer science, and comparative psychology. But it is missing an "ism" to define it.

Into this healthy and hopeful intellectual ferment comes this book. It is forthrightly titled *Neoconstructivism*, returning us to consider Piaget in a new light. Perhaps his life work did after all come close to his goal of reconciling nativism and empiricism. He was wrong about many things—the viability of structuralism, the leanness of starting points, the lack of a need for close study of input and mechanism. He was also living at a time when he could not follow up thoroughly on his nods to social interaction, or to what might have been his fascination with the architecture and processes in the physical substrate (the brain that is the mind). Nevertheless, his fundamental idea seems now to have been absolutely right: that a biologically prepared mind interacts in biologically evolved ways with an expectable environment that nevertheless includes significant variation. The chapters in this book collectively show us the promise of neoconstructivism.

Here are some tenets that I think unite the neoconstructivist approach.

- Everyone is a Darwinist. That is, all theorizing in cognitive development is situated in a context in which we must consider the adaptive value of thinking, and how it developed over evolutionary as well as developmental time. There is no need to cede the Darwinian high ground to the modularity theorists or to the nativists in general.
- Experience expectancy is a key concept. Keeping this valuable concept (delineated by Greenough, Black, & Wallace, 1987) firmly in mind, we can see how nature's solution to the problem of the construction of knowledge could as easily—arguably more easily—have been the selection of neural abilities that will inevitably learn from their expectable input what needs to be learned. There is no a priori need for specific content to be wired in—although of course some may be.
- The world is richly structured and well equipped with perceptual redundancies and correlations that support experience-expectant learning. This idea is a fundamentally Gibsonian one, although it acquires new resonance in contemporary theorizing, in which we can specify how the information is "picked up" rather than simply asserting that it is.

- Humans (and perhaps other species as well) bring to the task of learning about their world a rich endowment in computing probabilities, lying at the heart of the work on statistical learning discussed in this book, as well as of Bayesian approaches to cognition and its development. These abilities go a long way to solve the problem of profligate association that nativism is fond of using to attack more balanced approaches that include empiricist elements.
- A richly structured world and a strong capacity for probabilistic reasoning interact, within the experience-expectancy framework, to select among and/or to integrate the multiple cues typically available to draw conclusions about causality, to remember spatial location, and so forth.
- Action plays a key role in learning and development, just as Piaget thought, not only because it creates the occasion for experiment but also because it allows for situations that are more replete with information than observation.
- Development and learning are closely intertwined concepts but not quite the same. Development is learning as the learner changes. For example, the learner acquires a shape bias or the idea that words are reliable cues to categories. As another and different example, perceptual tuning, especially in the first year of life, works by pruning capacities not by adding to capacity, to create a fundamentally altered learner.
- Developmental change can be quantitative, qualitative, or both at the same time, depending on the granularity of observation. The oft-cited dichotomy between quantitative and qualitative change that is supposed to distinguish theories of developments should be consigned to the dustbin of history; see Thelen and Smith's (1994) elegant discussion of the "view from above" and the "view from below."
- Analyses of the causes and mechanisms of developmental change need to proceed on all four of Aristotle's fronts—looking for formal, material, final, and efficient causes. Formal cause is analogous to developmental description (and "thick" description [see Geertz, 1973] comes close to being a cause); material cause is analogous to the neural substrate; final cause is analogous to putting development in an evolutionary and adaptive context; efficient cause is analogous to an analysis of the interactions of input with the neural substrate and the current cognitive state of the learner.

The chapters in this book cover many domains (although not all) and more important, they agree in many ways, subscribing either explicitly or implicitly to the list of key ideas listed above. But within the species of neoconstructivists, there are also dimensions of variation, just as cats differ in their markings, eye color, or even in the possession versus absence of a tail. The two most important differences among the chapter authors are the following:

- How strongly domain-general is human cognition and cognitive development? Some investigators in the neoconstructivist tradition embrace domain generality while others clearly work within a domain-specific framework. Note, however, that, importantly, domain specificity does not entail either nativism or modularity.
- How bottom-up versus top-down is human cognition and cognitive development? Some chapter authors seem to think that bottom-up approaches are necessary to avoid the extremes of nativism while others are more comfortable with top-down influences—recognizing that those influences may themselves be constructed.

Going back to the issue of a new "ism" to replace nativism as the framework for thinking about cognitive development—is neoconstructivism just one more "ism" that can be added to the list of contenders for a contemporary alternative? Does it vie with connectionism, or dynamic systems thinking, or emergentism, or overlapping wave theory, or small-p piagetianism, or other terms or schools of thought? Very importantly, I think the simple answer is No. The eight tenets listed above establish a neoconstructivist big tent that can cover all of the specific schools of thought mentioned above and more. What can then ensue is the sorting out of the specific issues in empirical description, theory making and modeling that are the normal business of a mature science. Piaget's biggest idea, if not his many smaller ones, has turned out to be right after all.

References

Chapman, M. (1988). *Constructive evolution: Origins and development of Piaget's thought.* New York, NY: Cambridge University Press.

Chomsky, N. (1959). A review of B. F. Skinner's *Verbal Behavior. Language, 35*, 26–58.

Cosmides, L., & Tooby, J. (1994). Origins of domain specificity: The evolution of functional organization. In L. A. Hirschfeld & S. A. Gelman (Eds), *Mapping the mind: Domain specificity in cognition and culture.* (pp. 85–116). New York: Cambridge University Press.

Elman, J. L., Bates, E. A., Johnson, M. H., Karmiloff-Smith, A., Parisi, D., & Plunkett, K. (1996). *Rethinking innateness: A connectionist perspective on development.* Cambridge, MA: MIT Press.

Fodor, J. A. (1983). *The modularity of mind.* Cambridge, MA: MIT Press.

Geertz, C. (1973). Thick description: Toward an interpretive theory of culture. In *The Interpretation of Cultures: Selected Essays* (pp. 3–30). New York: Basic Books.

Gelman, R., & Baillargeon, R. (1983). A review of some Piagetian concepts. In J. H. Flavell and E. Markman (Eds.), *Cognitive development: Vol. 3, Handbook of child development* (pp. 167–230). New York: Wiley.

Gopnik, A., & Meltzoff, A. (1997). Words, thoughts and theories. Cambridge, MA: MIT Press.

Greenough, W. T., Black, J. E., &Wallace, C. S. (1987). Experience and brain development. *Child Development, 58*, 539–559.

Karmiloff-Smith, A. (1992). Beyond modularity: A developmental perspective on cognitive science. Cambridge, MA: MIT Press.

Klahr, D., & Wallace, J. G. (1976). Cognitive development: An information-processing view. Oxford: Lawrence Erlbaum.

Newcombe, N. S. (1998). Defining the radical middle. (Essay review of J. Elman et al., *Rethinking Innateness*). *Human Development, 41*, 210–214.

Newcombe, N. S. (2002). The nativist-empiricist controversy in the context of recent research on spatial and quantitative development. *Psychological Science, 13*, 395–401.

Newcombe, N. S., & Huttenlocher, J. (2000). *Making space: The development of spatial representation and reasoning.* Cambridge, MA: MIT Press.

Newcombe, N. S., & Ratliff, K. R. (2007). Explaining the development of spatial reorientation: Modularity-plus-language versus the emergence of adaptive combination. In J. Plumert & J. Spencer (Eds.), *The emerging spatial mind* (pp. 53–76). Oxford University Press.

Oakes, L. M., Newcombe, N. S., & Plumert, J. M. (2009). Are dynamic systems and connectionist approaches an alternative to "good old-fashioned cognitive development"? In J.P. Spencer, M. Thomas & J. McClelland (Eds.), *Toward a new grand theory of development? Connectionism and dynamic systems theory re-considered* (pp. 268–284). Oxford: Oxford University Press.

Siegler, R. S. (1996). *Emerging minds: The process of change in children's thinking.* New York: Oxford University Press.

Spelke, E. S. (2003). What makes us smart? Core knowledge and natural language. In D. Gentner and S. Goldin-Meadow (Eds.), *Language in mind: Advances in the investigation of language and thought.* Cambridge, MA: MIT Press.

Spencer, J. P., Thomas, M., & McClelland, J. (Eds.) (in press). *Toward a new grand theory of development? Connectionism and dynamic systems theory re-considered.* Oxford: Oxford University Press.

Thelen, E., & Smith, L.B. (1994). *A dynamic systems approach to the development of cognition and action.* Cambridge, MA: MIT Press.

CONTENTS

III. LEARNING MECHANISMS

IV. INDUCTION

V. FOUNDATIONS OF SOCIAL COGNITION

VI. THE BIG PICTURE

CONTRIBUTORS

Morten H. Christiansen
Department of Psychology
Cornell University

Jessica B. Cicchino
Department of Psychology
Carnegie Mellon University

Leslie B. Cohen
Department of Psychology
University of Texas at Austin

Rick Dale
Department of Psychology
University of Memphis

Sarah Gerson
Department of Psychology
University of Maryland, College Park

Rebecca Gómez
Department of Psychology
University of Arizona

Erin E. Hannon
Department of Psychology
University of Nevada, Las Vegas

Scott P. Johnson
Department of Psychology
University of California, Los Angeles

Natasha Kirkham
Centre for Brain and Cognitive Development
Birkbeck College, University of London

Irene Leo
Department of Psychology
University of Padova

Denis Mareschal
Centre for Brain and Cognitive Development
Birkbeck College, University of London

Andrew N. Meltzoff
Institute for Learning and Brain Sciences
University of Washington

M. Keith Moore
Institute for Learning and Brain Sciences
University of Washington

Nora S. Newcombe
Department of Psychology
Temple University

Alfredo F. Pereira
Department of Psychological and Brain Sciences
Indiana University—Bloomington

Paul C. Quinn
Department of Psychology
University of Delaware

David H. Rakison
Department of Psychology
Carnegie Mellon University

Florencia Reali
Department of Psychology
University of California, Berkeley

John E. Richards
Department of Psychology
University of South Carolina

Jenny R. Saffran
Department of Psychology
University of Wisconsin—Madison

Francesca Simion
Department of Psychology
University of Padova

Vladimir M. Sloutsky
Center for Cognitive Science
Ohio State University

Linda B. Smith
Department of Psychological and Brain Sciences
Indiana University—Bloomington

David M. Sobel
Department of Cognitive and Linguistic Sciences
Brown University

Gert Westermann
Department of Psychology
Oxford Brookes University

Amanda Woodward
Department of Psychology
University of Maryland, College Park

Introduction

The term *neoconstructivism* was generated by combining *neo*, taken from the Greek *neos*, meaning "new," and *constructivism*, taken from (among other sources) the pioneering theorist and researcher Jean Piaget. Piaget's constructivist theory holds that cognitive development is a continual process of building knowledge on previous skills (e.g., perception, memory, and action repertoires) and existing knowledge structures, from a foundation at birth consisting largely of reflexes and sensory impressions. It seems to me a first principle of any theory of development that *development happens*—every human being that ever existed or ever will started out as a fertilized egg and grew from there. This is hardly an insightful observation, yet it is rarely mentioned in the literature, and consequently our understanding of the "growth" of cognition is woefully incomplete. Piaget's constructivism, and now neoconstructivism, represent attempts to address this problem.

The origins of this book are rooted in an idea that came to me in 2003. The idea was motivated by the following observations. Research on cognitive development, particularly in infancy, consists largely of demonstration studies—experiments designed to show some cognitive skill at a particular age, often with little or no consideration of limitations characteristic of young infants' perceptual skills and cortical immaturity, and often with little or no consideration of development. Demonstration studies can be contrasted with process studies—experiments designed to examine mechanisms underlying performance or development that support the skill in question or bring it about.

Back in 2003, I thought that the balance of the field was weighted heavily toward demonstration studies, which tend to grab attention and headlines ("Infants Are Smarter Than You Think" and such). These studies have an important place in the literature, and my colleagues and I have produced a few ourselves. Yet progress in the field relies also on an understanding of process, in particular developmental mechanisms, because an understanding of development is required for a complete characterization of any psychological phenomenon. My idea in 2003 was to organize a symposium focusing on process studies as a theme for a major developmental conference. I began attending conferences in 1992 (the International Conference on Infant Studies, or ICIS, in Miami), and was not aware of any such symposium having been organized previously. So I asked around, got agreements from four principal researchers in the area (most of whom are represented by chapters in this book), and submitted it to ICIS for the 2004 meeting in Chicago under the title "The Big Questions in Infant Cognition: Trenchant Debate, Tentative Answers." Talks were presented on object perception, categorization, word learning, and dorsal/ventral visual processing.

The reviewers accepted the symposium, and the reception at the conference itself far exceeded any of our expectations. The room was packed and overflowing; some audience members sat on the floor, stood at the back, and stacked up deep outside the doors. At that time, I thought either

(a) we got lucky in terms of the conference schedule, (b) this is a fluke, or (c) there is pent-up demand for discussion of developmental mechanisms at our conferences. To find out, I tried it a second time, submitting a symposium titled "Origins and Ontogenesis of Human Cognition" (all of whose contributors have chapters in this book) to the 2007 meeting of the Society for Research in Child Development in Boston. This time, the talks centered on memory development, grammar learning, and social cognition. Again, the room, though substantially larger than the 2003 symposium, was full to overflowing.

Finally, I organized a smaller meeting, held in November 2006 in New York City and generously funded by the National Science Foundation, bringing together 12 of the 24 authors who appear in this book. Participants in the meeting and authors in this book are all active researchers in cognitive development whose work, though involving a wide range of methods and approaches, coheres in a common framework: an explicit focus on developmental mechanisms of human cognition. The meeting was productive, enlightening, and encouraging, and suggested to me (and, I think, the other participants) that we are really onto something worthwhile.

I think the fields of developmental and cognitive science need this book and others like it. The range of methods and approaches is not necessarily representative of relevant research as a whole, but it is representative of some of the questions that are being asked and of some of the important findings that have been yielded in the past several decades. I hope you find it useful.

I would like to thank the authors for their hard work; Catharine Carlin at Oxford University Press for her enthusiasm and patience; the National Science Foundation for funding the meeting in 2006; the NSF, National Institute of Child Health and Human Development, Economic and Social Research Council, and Nuffield Foundation for supporting my own work, and my family, in particular Kerri Johnson.

Scott P. Johnson
Los Angeles

PART I

Objects and Space

CHAPTER 1
Attention in the Brain and Early Infancy

John E. Richards

Hypothesis: Infant Attention Development Is Controlled by Infant Brain Development

Attention shows dramatic changes over the period of infancy. At birth, there is little intrinsic control of behavior and attention is affected mainly by salient physical characteristics of the infant's environment. By the age of 2 years, the infants' executive control systems are functioning and infants voluntarily direct information processing flow by allocating attention on the basis of well-defined goals and tasks. These changes in attention affect a wide range of cognitive, social-emotional, and physiological processes.

The attention changes in young infants occur simultaneously with substantial changes in the brain. At birth, the structure, myelination, connectivity, and functional specialization of the brain are relatively primitive. Much of the brain's structural development occurs between birth and 2 years. Many brain areas showing these changes are closely linked in adult participants to cognitive processes such as attention. A natural inclination is to hypothesize that the changes in attention development are caused by the changes in these brain areas.

One example of the brain changes is the axonal myelination of neurons. Myelin is a fatty substance that in adult brains covers the axons of many neurons. Figure 1.1 shows a "typical" neuron with an unmyelinated portion (cell body, dendrites) and whose axon is completely covered by the myelin sheath. Myelin appears as "white" when viewed in the brain (fatty tissue reflects light). Thus, in autopsied brains, there are large areas called "white matter" that consist of long myelinated axons. Myelination is seen in magnetic resonance imaging (MRI) T1-weighted scans as long channels of white matter surrounded on the edges by gray matter. Figure 1.1 shows MRIs from a newborn, 6-month-old infant, 15-month-old infant, 10-year-old child, and an adult. The changes in the myelination appear to be rapid from birth to the 15-month MRI scan, then slower afterwards. Myelination of the axon results in less noisy and quicker transmission, making the communication between neurons more efficient. It often is used an explanatory mechanism for how changes in the brain affect cognitive development (e.g., Klingberg, 2008; Yakolev & Lecours, 19672008). The changes in myelin have been documented in several publications, most notably in the work of Yakolev and Lecours (1967), Kinney and colleagues (Kinney, Brody, Kloman, & Gilles, 1988; Kinney, Karthigasan, Borenshteyn, Flax, & Kirschner, 1994), and Conel (1939 to 1967). (also see Johnson, 1997; Klingberg, 2008; Sampaio & Truwit, 2001).

The relationship between brain development and attention development has been hypothesized by several models. I recently reviewed my own view of the relationship between brain centers controlling eye movement, brain development in these areas, and developmental changes

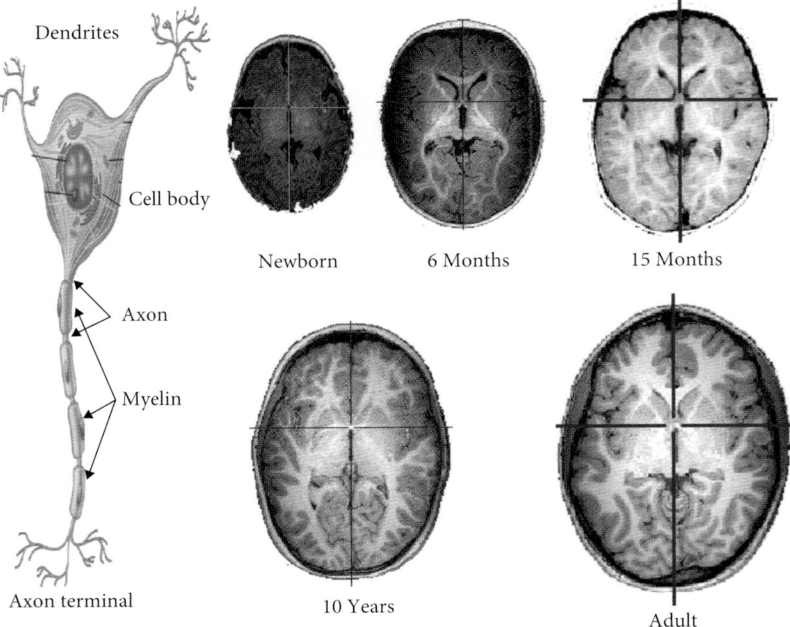

Figure 1.1 **The left figure is a cartoon drawing of a "typical" neuron with unmyelinated dendrites, cell body, and axon terminal, and the myelin sheath covering the axon. The MRIs are T1-weighted slices taken at the same anatomical level (anterior commisure) from participants from birth to adult. The myelination of the long axons in the brain is seen as "white" matter in the adults and there are large changes from the newborn to the adult period.**

in attention (Richards, 2008). I will briefly summarize my observations here.

There are three types of eye movements used to track visual stimuli and each eye movement type is controlled by areas of the brain that show different developmental trajectories. "Reflexive saccadic" eye movements occur in response to the sudden onset of a peripheral stimulus, are controlled largely by subcortical brain areas, and are largely intact by 3 months of age. "Voluntary saccadic" eye movements are under voluntary or planned control, involve several parts of the cortex (occipital, fusiform gyrus, parietal cortex, frontal eye fields), and show rapid development from 3 to 9 months of age. "Smooth pursuit" eye movements occur either voluntarily or involuntarily toward smoothly moving objects, involve several cortical areas of the brain involved in voluntary saccadic eye movements and some areas not involved in voluntary saccadic eye movements (medial temporal, parietal), and show changes beginning at 3 months and lasting throughout the period of infancy.

There have been several models theorizing how the areas of the brain controlling the eye movement develop, and how these changes affect attention-controlled eye movements, including models by Bronson (1974, 1997), Maurer and Lewis (1979, 1991, 1998), Johnson and colleagues (Johnson, 1990, 1995; Johnson et al., 1991, 1998, 2003, 2007), Hood (Hood, 1995; Hood, Atkinson, & Braddick, 1998), and Richards (Richards, 2002, 2008; Richards & Casey, 1992; Richards & Hunter, 1998). Iliescu and Dannemiller (2008) review several pertinent "neurodevelopmental" models. These models hypothesize that change in the brain areas controlling the eye movements result in the overt changes in the eye movements. With respect to attention-directed eye movements, particularly in the first few months, the voluntary saccadic system is most relevant. It has been hypothesized that connections within primarily visual areas of the cortex (e.g., primary and secondary visual cortex) and myelination/connectivity to other areas of the cortex (e.g., parietal area PG) show growth spurts in about 3 to 6 months. These brain changes are accompanied by changes in the voluntary tracking of objects in the visual field (Richards & Holley, 1999), changes in the attention-directed eye movements toward peripheral visual targets (Hunter & Richards, 2003, submitted; Richards & Hunter, 1997), and changes in the ability to shift attention "covertly" without making an eye movement (Richards, 2000a, 2000b, 2001, 2005, 2007b; also see Richards, 2004b, and the section "Brain and Attention: Spatial Orienting").

What's inside a baby's head?

The previous section presented the hypothesis that brain changes in young infants are responsible for the changes seen in psychological processes, with an emphasis on attention-directed eye movements. There are many aspects of infant cognitive development that have been explained as a function of brain development; the field of "developmental cognitive neuroscience" uses this as a basic explanatory mechanism (Johnson, 1997; Nelson & Luciana, 2008). However, these models are severely limited in their description of what the actual brain is like for infants at a specific age or a specific infant at a specific age. They also are limited in their measurement of brain function (see the section "How to Measure Brain Activity in Infants"). I will review two ways in which brain development has been modeled in past research. Then, I will assert that structural MRI techniques should be used for this purpose.

The primary information about brain development in infants comes from nonhuman animal models of brain development, primarily primates. For example, our knowledge of the patterns of myelination, synaptogenesis, and neurochemical development comes primarily from study of normally developing nonhuman animals. Nonhuman animals may be studied by sacrificing the animal at a specific age and performing a brain dissection, or with invasive neuroscientific techniques such as direct neural recording or lesions. These techniques may be applied to individuals who also participate in tasks measuring behavioral performance and psychological processes. An example of this approach is work on infant memory by Bachevalier (2008). She has shown that changes in memory in young monkeys are closely related to the development of the brain areas that are the basis for this type of memory in adults. Lesioning these areas in the infant monkey disrupts the onset or occurrence of this type of memory. Bachevalier makes the parallel between the age-related monkey performance and human infant performance on analog versions of the visual preference procedure and visual discrimination tasks. She concludes that her experiment suggests that the basic neural systems underlying these memory tasks in monkeys and humans are parallel, and that studies of infant monkeys inform us about comparable memory development in infant humans.

There are several assumptions necessary for the study of the study of infant nonhuman animal to be relevant to human infants. First, this study requires that a correlation can be made between ages of the nonhuman animals and human infants. For example, in a study of changes in synaptogenesis in visual areas, Bourgeois (1997) showed changes in rat, cat, macaque monkeys, and humans. Figure 1.2 shows comparable changes in the primary visual cortices of four different species. These changes show some similarity in the overall pattern of change. However, the pattern of changes often is not isomorphic across species (e.g., compare the prolonged decay in synaptic density in humans in Figure 1.2), and a comparison of development between species in one brain area might not be the same for other brain areas. Second, one can relate the changes in the brain in the nonhuman animals, the importance of these brain areas for a specific psychological process, and the changes in these psychological processes in human infants. This analysis presumes that there is an unequivocal relationship between the psychological process and the brain area in development, which is a questionable assumption.

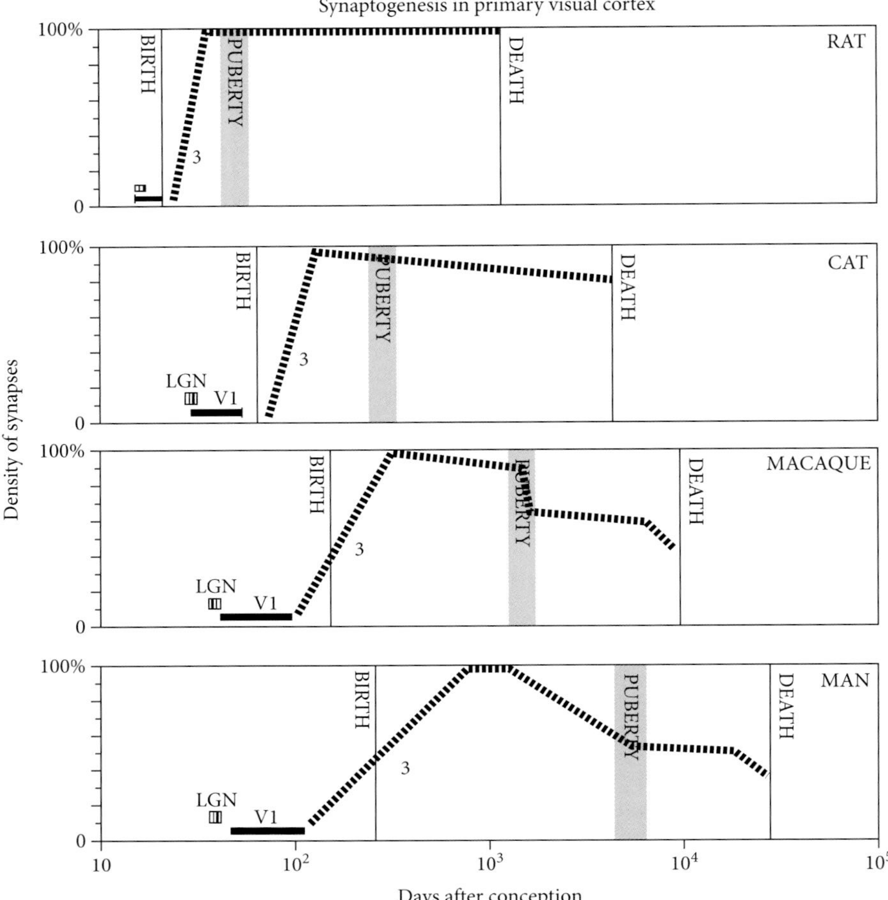

Figure 1.2 Changes in the relative density of synapses in the primary visual cortex for four species. The increase in synaptic density indicates synaptogenesis occurring, and the decline represents synaptic pruning. Note the differences in the pattern of development relative to specific developmental events (birth, puberty, death) in the four species. From Bourgeois (1997).

This type of analysis does not take into account different developmental patterns for other brain areas and the influence of these brain areas on human infant psychological activity. Third, this type of study assumes that brain–behavior relations in nonhuman animals are comparable to those in humans. This assumption is doubtful due to the complexity of human behavior relative to animals, the extremely large changes in brain size between nonhuman animals and humans, and the relative size of brain areas in humans and nonhuman animals (e.g., prefrontal cortex; occipital cortex). Finally, these types of studies use analogical reasoning as a basis for nonhuman animal models being relevant for human infants. They cannot apply the invasive methods directly to human participants and cannot inform us about the developmental status of the brain of individual infants.

A second way in which information about human brain development has been obtained is from postmortem studies of young infants. Infants who die of neural-related causes and/or other causes have been studied for a wide range of neuroanatomical, neurochemical, and cytoarchitectural processes (synaptogenesis

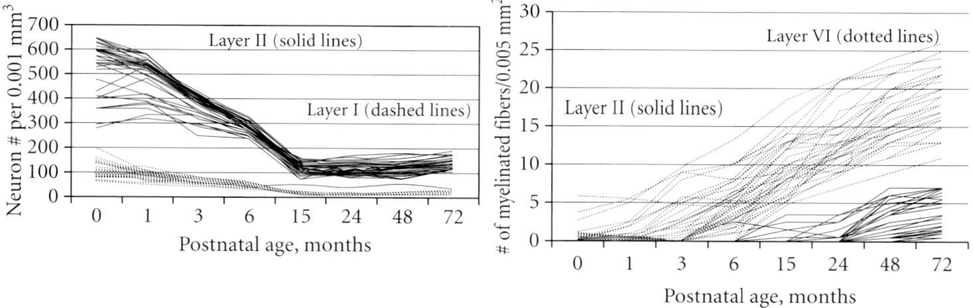

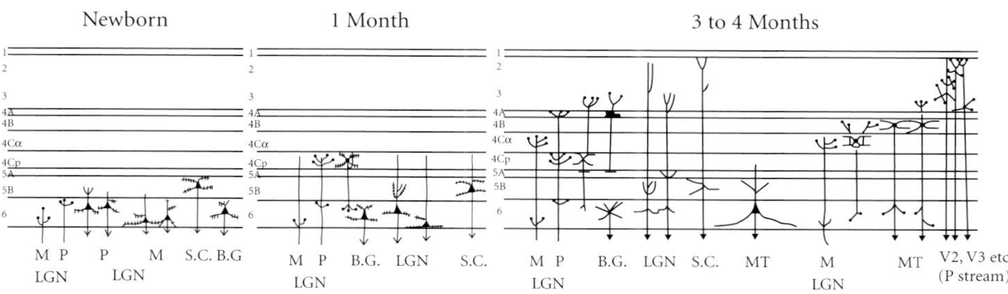

Figure 1.3 Work from Conel's postmortem neuroanatomical studies (Conel, 1939 to 1967). The top graphs show neural density in layers I and II (left figure) and the myelinated fiber density in layers II and VI (right figure), both shown as a function of postnatal age (from Shankle et al., 1998). The bottom figures show innervations of the layers in the primary visual cortex by different cell types at birth, 1 month, and 3 to 4 months of age.

in Huttenlocher, 1990, 1994; myelination in Kinney et al., 1988, 1994). The most well-known version of this kind of study is a series of studies by Conel (1939–1967). Conel studied the neuroanatomical and cytoarchitecture of the layers of the human cerebral cortex in autopsied individuals. He measured six anatomical features, including cortical layer thickness, cell density, numbers of cell types, and myelinated fiber density (Shankle, Romney, Landing, & Hara, 1998). Figure 1.3 shows two types of results from these studies. The top figures display neuron density and number of myelinated fibers in two cortical layers as a function of age. Notice that the myelination of the layer 6, which receives input from noncortical areas and is involved in simple cortical functioning, shows myelination changes very early. Alternatively, layer 2, which has communications within layers and with other cortical areas and is involved in more complex cortical functioning, shows an extended time course for myelination. The bottom figures show the types of neurons that innervate the cortical layers at different ages.

Conel's work has been popular in developmental cognitive neuroscience because of the specificity of the information about the neurophysiological processes being studied and its large age range. For example, Johnson (1990, 1995; Johnson et al., 1991, 1998) posits that development in the layers of the the primary visual cortex (e.g., Figure 1.3, bottom figures) acts as a limiting factor for visual behavior and visual attention controlled by brain systems. Such developmental changes in the layers of the primary cortex from birth to about 6 months act as a gateway for the onset of these eye movements in young infants.

There are limitations of these postmortem studies for developmental cognitive neuroscience. An implicit assumption is that the individuals measured at different ages are representative of that age and provide knowledge about the brain status of specific individuals of that age. It is likely true that the changes across age are large enough that groups of infants at one age will have neuroanatomic and cytoarchectural similarities differentially from groups at different ages. However the developmental status of the brain of an individual are likely to show idiosyncratic individual differences in brain development between individuals at the same age. Second, these studies typically are limited to small samples (single individual at each age) and restricted to infants who died. If the reasons for the death are related to the characteristics being studied, the results will not be applicable to a wide range of participants. Without some independent verification of the generality of the findings, these surely cannot be applied to determine the status of individual participants. These studies typically have used extremely limited samples for young infants and children.

One technique that may be used to examine the brains of individual infants is MRI. MRI has been described in several publications (e.g., Huettel, Song, & McCarthy, 2004; Thomas & Tseng, 2008) and I will provide a brief overview emphasizing its use for studying the brain. MRI applies a very large magnetic field to the head. The head's media (skull, cerebrospinal fluid [CSF], brain) have magnetic properties such that the magnetic field aligns spinning protons in the same direction as the field. Radiofrequency (RF) energy pulses cause disruption of the magnetic fields and disrupt the alignment of the protons. MRI measures the disruption in alignment due to the RF pulse and return of the alignment to the strong magnetic field. Different body tissue types have differing times to return to alignment, and these differing times (or different resonance frequencies and/or differing on/off durations of the RF pulses) may be used to identify where different types of media are located in the head. This allows the identification and visualization of skull, skin, CSF, white and gray matter, myelin, vascularization, and other components in the head. MRI measurement has been used to measure developmental changes in myelination (Sampaio & Truwit, 2001), distribution of white and gray matter in the cortex (O'Hare & Sowell, 2008), and biochemical characteristics of the developing brain (Sajja & Narayana, 2008). An interesting use of the MRI is the application of "diffusion tensor imaging," which details the connectivity of axons between different areas in the brain (Wozniak, Mueller, & Lim, 2008).

The use of structural MRI for determining brain developmental status is relatively new but well underway. The most comprehensive study of brain structural development with MRI is currently ongoing. The "NIH MRI Study of Normal Brain Development" (Almli, Rivkin, & McKinstry, 2007; Evans, 2006; NIH, 1998) is a multicenter research project sponsored by the National Institutes of Health to perform anatomical scans of about 800 children ranging in age from birth to 18 years. This study uses 1.5T scanners to get T1- and T2-weighted images, proton density excitation, DTI, and other scans. An interesting aspect of this study is the collection of a large battery of neuropsychological and developmental tests. This will allow the correlation of psychological processes, neuropsychological status, and developmental level with the brain status of individual participants. The study will provide individual MRIs to researchers interested in these aspects, and likely will provide standardized or stereotaxic scans in the "MNI" framework (Montreal Neurological Institute brain atlas, Mazziotta, Toga, Evans, Fox, & Lancaster, 1995; Evans, Collins, & Milner, 1992; Evans et al., 1993) or Talairach space (Talairach &Tournoux, 1988; also see Talairach Atlas Database Daemon, Fox & Uecker, 2005; Lancaster, Summerlin, Rainey, Freitas, & Fox, 1997; Lancaster et al., 2000). Currently (late 2007) MRIs are available for children ranging in ages from 4 to 18 years. Most of the MRIs for the infant participants have been collected but are undergoing quality control.

A second approach I am using in my current work is to acquire structural MRIs on infant participants who also participate in studies of attention, and relate the information found about specific individual's brain developmental status to performance in attention tasks. Parents of infants are contacted in the normal course of our contact system for psychological experiments. The parents who agree to participate in the MRI have several visits. First, the parent(s) and infant come to the MRI center located at a local community/teaching hospital. The parent is shown the equipment and the process is described. Second, the parents return to the MRI center for the scan. The procedures for the MRI recording use infants during sleep (Almli, Rivkin, & McKinstry, 2007; Evans, 2006; NIH, 1998). The infant and parent come to the MRI center in the evening at the infant's normal bedtime. The infant and parent go into the darkened room with the MRI and the infant is put to sleep. Then the infant is placed on the MRI table, earplugs and headphones put on, and then the recording is done. Figure 1.4 shows an infant lying on the MRI bed—the headphones and cloths surrounding the infant can be seen. When the infant is in the MRI tube, a research assistant reaches in and has a hand on the infant to see if the baby moves or wakens. Getting the baby to sleep usually takes about 45 to 60 min, and the MRI recording itself has scan sequences lasting in total about 20 min. Previous studies from several laboratories have described procedures for performing MRI recording of nonsedated infants with success rates that range from 66% to 90% (Almli et al., 2007; Dehaene-Lambertz, Dehaene, & Hertz-Pannier, 2002; Evans, 2006; Gilmore et al., 2004; Paterson, Badridze, Flax, Liu, & Benasich, 2004; Sury, Harker, Begent, & Chong, 2005). We have had 100% success *after* the infant is sleeping; several infants have not been able to get to sleep. The parent is in the scanner room during the scan, along with a pediatric nurse. Finally, the infant and parent then come to a psychophysiological laboratory for studies of attention (see the section "Brain and Infant Attention: Spatial Orienting").

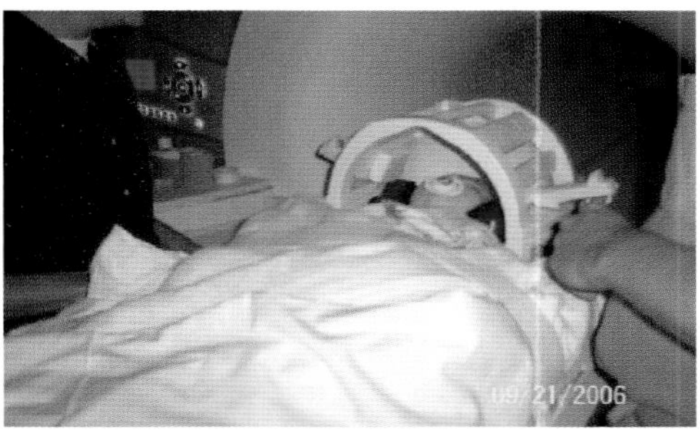

Figure 1.4 An infant lying on the MRI bed going into the MRI tunnel. The infant is covered with a sheet and has a restraining strap lightly placed across its body. The headphones and cloths surrounding the infant can be seen in this picture. A research assistant (left side of picture) and the parent (right side of picture) are close to the baby during the scan.

Several procedures are followed to insure the infant's safety, obtain a good recording, and minimize the amount of time in the scanner. Potential risks of MRI recording include scanner noise, the magnetic fields, and magnetic gradients. We use earplugs and earphones to minimize scanner noise. The scans in our 3T magnet are optimized for the lowest sound levels and fastest recording. The infants are placed on the bed on "memory foam," covered snugly with sheets, and have rolled washcloths around the head for restricting head movement comfortably. The U.S. FDA considers MRI recording in infants to be a "nonsignificant" risk when used within FDA-specified parameters (USFDA, 2003, 2006). This assessment is based on over 20 years of MRI recording in neonate and infants (e.g., Barkovich, Kjos, Jackson, & Norman, 1988; Rivkin, 1998) with no reports of deleterious long-term effects. Outcome studies of such effects show that the magnetic field or the magnetic gradients do not threaten the concurrent physiological stability of the infant during scanning (Battin, Maalouf, Counsell, Herlihy, & Hall, 1998; Taber, Hayman, Northrup, & Maturi, 1998; Stokowski, 2005) and there are several studies showing no short-term or long-term effects from this type of recording (Baker, Johnson, Harvey, Gowland, & Mansfield, 1994; Clements, Duncan, Fielding, Gowland, Johnson, & Baker, 2000; Kangarlu, Burgess, & Zu, 1999; Kok, de Vries, Heerschap, & van den Berg, 2004; Myers, Duncan, Gowland, Johnson, & Baker, 1998; Schenck, 2000). These risks are discussed in detail in several sources (Barkovich,

2005; Dehaene-Lambertz, 2001; Evans, 2006; Stokowski, 2005).

Three scans are done on each infant. First, we do a localizer sequence (45 s) to orient the subsequent high-resolution slices. This orients the longitudinal fissure parallel with the saggital plane, perpendicular to the coronal and axial planes, and the line between the anterior commisure (AC) and posterior commisure (PC) is on the center MRI slice. This will orient the scan so that the MRI may be oriented relative to the origin for the stereotaxic space defined by Talairach (Talairach & Tournoux, 1988). Second, the localizer scan is followed by a 3D MPRAGE T1-weighted scan. The T1-weighted (T1W) scan results in an MRI volume that shows maximal distinction between gray matter and white matter. The MPRAGE employs a TI of 960 ms, a delay of 3000 ms between shots and an 8° flip angle, with a very short TE (4.9 ms). Using this sequence, we can collect a 1 mm isotropic (150 × 256 × 256 mm FOV) in about 9 min. The gray matter, white matter, and CSF can be segmented from the T1W scan, but a subsequent T2-weighted (T2W) scan helps to discriminate white matter and CSF with automatic segmenting routines. The T2W scan emphasizes liquid in the brain, so CSF is very bright (high voxel values) relative to other brain matter. This is acquired as a dual contrast proton density and T2-weighted sequence with a dual echo fast spin echo sequence. The dual echo acquisition takes 4 min to acquire (256 × 256 matrix with rectangular FOV, 1 × 1mm pixel size, 2 mm slice thickness, no slice gap, 50 saggital slices in two interleaved packages, echo train length of 10, first TE=13 ms, second TE=101 ms, TR=4640 ms, parallel imaging factor = 2). Any of the sequences may be repeated if degraded by motion artifacts; however, all infants we have tested have been sleeping and still during the entire scanning protocol. If only the T1W scan is available, some automatic classification/segmentation routines are substituted with manual segmentation routines of the T1W scan.

What are the MRI scans used for? Briefly, the purpose of the attention studies is to identify areas of the brain involved in sustained attention and how they affect specific cortical/cognitive processes. Neural activity produces electrical currents that pass through the media of the head and can be recorded on the surface of the scalp. This electrical activity is the electroencephalogram (EEG). We use the EEG for cortical source analysis. One aspect of this analysis is the necessity to have a realistic head model for the quantification. We obtain this from the MRI. Figure 1.5 shows the MRI recorded from the infant pictured in Figure 1.4. The middle section shows the media identified inside this baby's head (i.e., gray matter, white matter, CSF, skull). The right section shows a tetrahedral wireframe model of the identified sections. This wireframe model is used in computer program such as BESA, EMSE, and my own computer program (Richards, 2006, submitted) to identify the current sources of the EEG on the head. I will describe the details of the EEG analysis in the next section (section on "How to Measure Brain Function") and some results from the study in a following section (section on "Brain and Infant Attention: Spatial Orienting"). Whereas our use of these MRIs is primarily as an adjunct to current source analysis of EEG signals, specific aspects of the MRI can be used such as amount of myelination in brain areas, structure of brain areas, and perhaps connectivity between brain areas.

Why is this approach important? The first and perhaps obvious answer is that "cognitive neuroscience" requires measurement of both the cognitive and the neural aspects of cognitive neuroscience. A developmental cognitive neuroscience study without measures of brain development will be extremely limited. Second, the structural MRI of individual infants is necessary to relate the findings for particular participants to the functional data of particular infants. This is especially important given the wide range of topographical changes over this age, and the possibility that large individual differences might occur in infant brains. An example of this problem is shown in Figure 1.6. This shows MRIs at a common stereotaxic position (axial level of anterior commisure) across a wide range of ages. The wide range of head sizes across this age, and some variability within

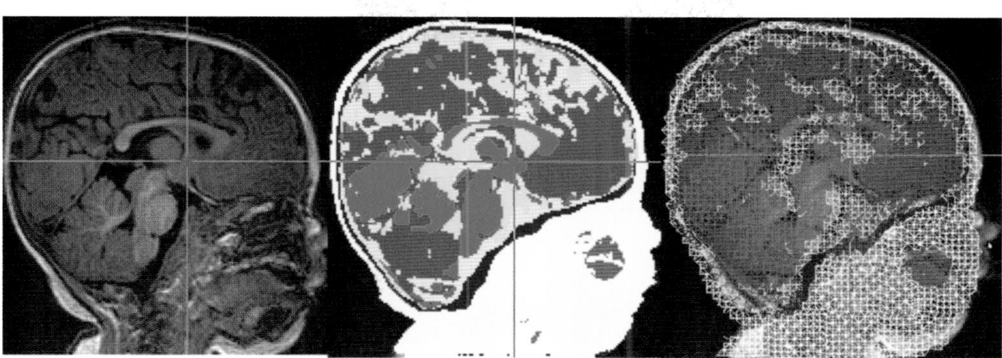

Figure 1.5 The MRI from the infant shown in Figure 1.4. The left scan is a saggital view of the T1-weighted scan, with the cross-hairs indicating the position of the anterior commisure. The middle figure is the brain segmented into skin and muscle (white), gray matter (red), white matter (green), CSF (cerebralspinal fluid, yellow), dura (pink), skull (blue), and nasal cavity (purple). The right figure is a representation of the tetrahedral wireframe used in EEG source analysis programs.

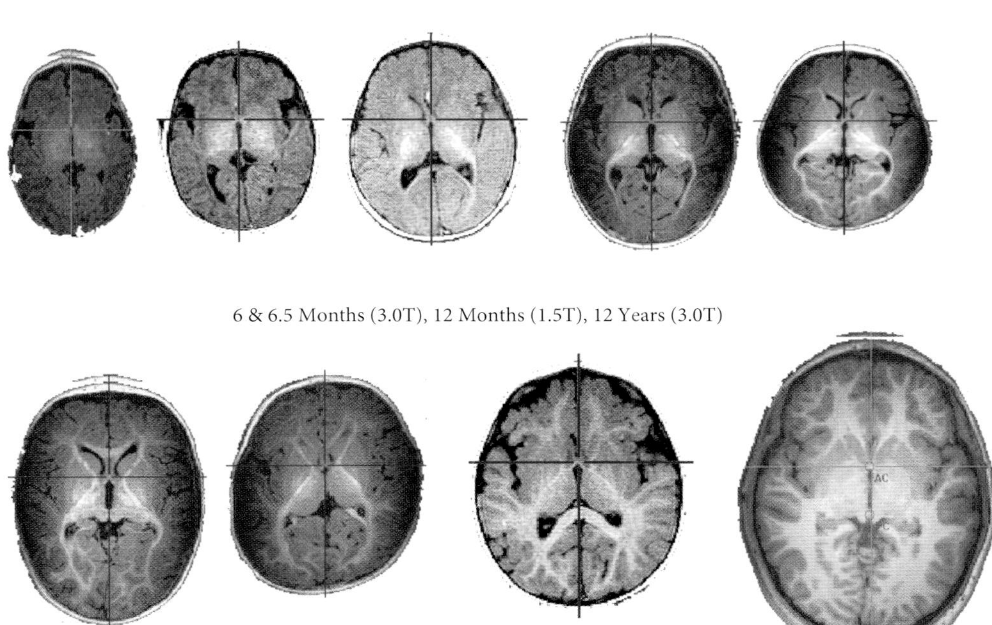

Figure 1.6 Axial T1-weighted MRI scans for participants ranging from birth to 12 years. Each scan is presented at the axial level of the anterior commisure (blue cross-hairs). Note the large change in shape and size, differences in the type of brain underlying similar skull locations, and the changes in myelination across these ages.

ages, is clear in these examples. Additionally, the exact type of brain media under the same skull location differs across the infants. It is important for the study of brain development to have structural information on particular infants.

A third reason why this approach is important is that this allows specific comparisons across age in related structures. Figure 1.7 shows brains of infants at 3 and 6 months, and a 10-year-old child. The MNI brain is also shown (Montreal Neurological Institute brain atlas, Mazziotta et al., 1995; Evans et al., 1992, 1993). The MNI brain consists of the average of 152 college-age participants. Several brain areas have been identified for the MNI brain. For example, Figure 1.7 (bottom right panel) shows various anatomical structures that have been identified on the MNI brain. The MNI brain and associated brain areas may be used as a stereotaxic atlas to identify structures in children at younger ages. The bottom part of the figure shows the structure identified on the MNI brain (bottom right panel), which is then transformed to the head size and shape of the participants at the other ages (three bottom panels on left). This may allow the direct comparison of the development of specific brain areas across a wide range of participants.

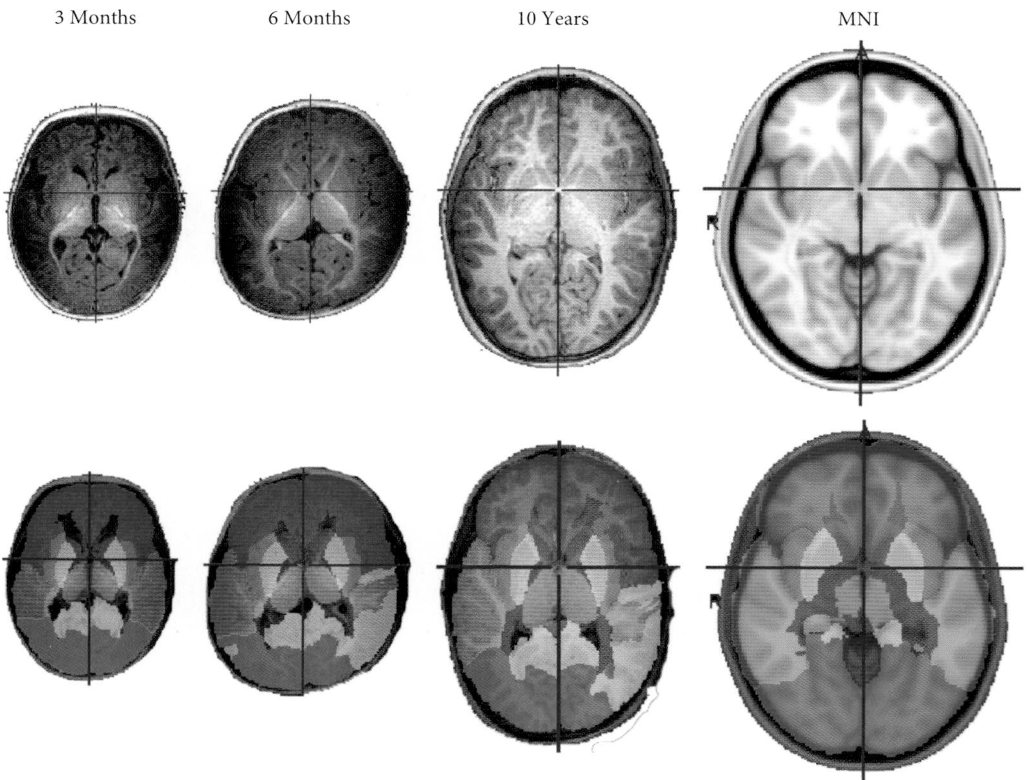

Figure 1.7 Axial T1-weighted MRI scans for participants at 3 and 6 months, 10 years, and the "MNI" brain, located on the axial level of the anterior commisure (cross-hairs). The bottom right MRI has the anatomical locations overlaid in color derived from the MNI brain, and structures such as the prefrontal cortex (blue), temporal (red) and occipital (green) cortex, and several subcortical structures may be seen. The three figures on the bottom left are the single participant brains with the stereotaxic anatomical areas translated from the MNI brain to the individual participant.

How to measure brain activity in infants

There are multiple aspects of brain development that might be important in the development of cognitive processes. The previous section gave some illustrative examples of the development of brain anatomy (brain structure). The field of cognitive neuroscience is interested in the functioning the relationship between the brain, and cognitive and psychological processes. The development of brain functioning is as important for developmental cognitive neuroscience as is the development of brain structure.

The measurement of brain activity during psychological tasks in infant participants has been as difficult as the measure of brain structure. Most of the neurodevelopmental models of infant attention mentioned in section 1 were based on the brain function of nonhuman animals, so-called "marker tasks," or speculative relations between overt behavioral measures and putative brain markers. I will briefly review the older measurement techniques and then comment on three new techniques.

Most neurodevelopmental models have relied either on measurement of brain function in animal models, or the measurement of overt behavior putatively linked to brain activity. Johnson (1997) calls the latter measures "marker tasks." Marker tasks are behavioral activities that can be measured overtly but which are thought to be controlled by specific brain areas. Johnson proposes that such tasks may be used in infants with the understanding that development in these tasks implies brain development in the associated areas. I have discussed this proposal previously (Richards, 2002, 2008; Richards & Hunter, 2002). Similarly, there are a wide range of studies using physiological indices in the infant in psychological tasks (Richards, 2004c; Reynolds and Richards, 2007). These psychophysiological measures (e.g., heart rate, EEG) have known physiological processes that cause their activity and thus may show changes in these processes linked to experimental manipulations or cognitive processing. Like the marker tasks, psychophysiological measures are indirect measures of brain function and do not tell us about the developmental status of the brain for an individual participant. With proper caution, marker tasks and psychophysiological measures allow inferences to be made about brain development and help to inform a developmental cognitive neuroscience approach to attention.

I have been using the EEG and scalp-recorded event-related potentials (ERP) as measures of brain activity. The EEG is electrical activity located on the scalp that is generated by neural activity occurring in cell bodies or extracellular neural tissue. ERP are EEG activity that is time-locked either to experimental events or to cognitive events. Recently I have been advocating the use of these measures with "cortical source analysis" (Reynolds & Richards, 2007, 2009; Richards, 2003b, 2005, 2006, 2007a, 2007b, submitted). Cortical source analysis uses high-density EEG recording (Johnson et al., 2001; Reynolds & Richards, 2009; Tucker, 1993; Tucker, Liotti, Potts, Russell, & Posner, 1994) to hypothesize cortical sources of the electrical activity and identifies the location of the brain areas generating the EEG or ERP (Huizenga & Molenaar, 1994; Michel et al., 2004; Nunez, 1990; Scherg, 1990, 1992; Scherg & Picton, 1991; Swick, Kutas, & Neville, 1994). The activity of these cortical sources may be directly linked to ongoing behavioral manipulations or psychological processes. This results in a description of the functional significance of the brain activity, i.e., functional cognitive neuroscience. Greg Reynolds and I have been using this technique to study infant recognition memory in the paired-comparison visual-preference procedure (Reynolds, Courage, & Richards, 2006; Reynolds & Richards, 2005) and have recently reviewed our use of this technique (Reynolds & Richards, 2009). I will present a brief introduction to this work but we have reviewed it elsewhere (Reynolds & Richards, 2007, 2009).

The basic outlines of this technique are as follows. Recording of electrical activity on the head (EEG, ERP) is made. The cortical source analysis hypothesizes electrical dipoles generating current inside the head as the sources of the EEG (ERP) changes measured on the scalp. The source analysis estimates the location and amplitude of the dipole. Figure 1.8 (top left MRI slices) shows the dipoles for an ERP component known as the "Nc" that occurs in young infants in response to brief familiar and novel stimuli (from Reynolds & Richards, 2005; also see Reynolds et al., 2006, and Richards, 2003a). The spatial resolution of EEG for localizing brain activity is typically believed to be about 5 cm (Huettel et al., 2004), whereas source analysis with realistic models has spatial resolutions closer to 1 cm (Richards, 2006).

The activity of the dipoles can be estimated over time and in relation to psychological events. Figure 1.8 (bottom figures) shows the activity of these dipoles for stimuli that were novel or familiar, and which elicited attention or did not. The activity of the dipoles distinguishes the type of stimuli (experimental manipulation), the attention state of the infant (psychological process), and the temporal unfolding of the brain activity. Since neural activity is generating the EEG, the temporal resolution of this procedure is on the same time course of neural activity (1 ms). Our conclusion from this analysis is that we have identified the brain areas that generate the scalp-recorded

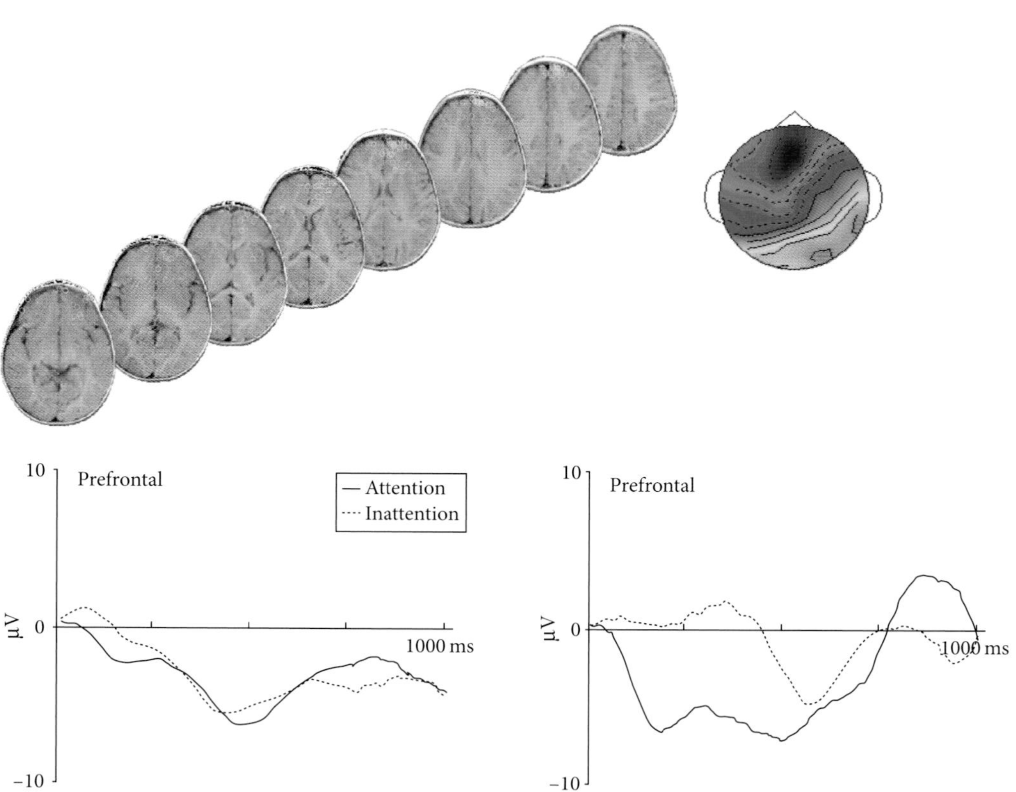

Figure 1.8 **The sequence of MRI slides shows the dipole locations (yellow circles) for an ERP component known as the Nc (topographical scalp potential maps on upper right figures). The activity of the dipoles is shown in the bottom figures as a function of experiment condition (familiar stimuli on left, novel on right), psychological process (attentive dark line, inattentive solid line), and temporal pattern (0 to 1000 ms following stimulus onset).**

Nc ERP component. The effects of attention on this brain activity are to enhance the amplitude of the brain activity and make it occur more quickly to novel stimuli. This technique offers a noninvasive tool for the measurement of brain activity, with spatial resolution sufficient to locate anatomical areas in the brain and temporal resolution occurring on the same time frame as activity in neurons (Reynolds & Richards, 2009; Richards, 2006).

I will mention two other techniques that might be useful to measure brain activity in young infants. Both measure the change in blood flow that occurs following neural activity. Neural activity occurring in a localized area of the brain results in changes in brain tissue resulting from the neural activity (e.g., neurotransmitter release, ionic exchange between neuron and surrounding media). These local changes affect arterial capillaries and arteries to effect the transport of oxygen and nutrients to the area. Some of these changes occur over wide areas of the brain whereas some are limited to the area in which the neural activity occurred.

Two techniques have been used in adult participants in cognitive neuroscience to measure these blood flow changes. The most familiar is "functional MRI" (fMRI; Huettel et al., 2004; Thomas & Tseng, 2008). Oxygenated and deoxygenated blood have differing magnetic properties that may be distinguished in MRI recording. When the blood flow (and resulting oxygenation) change occurs immediately after neural activity, the MRI may be used to localize these areas and show their time course. This signal may then be related to the experimental manipulations or cognitive processes, i.e., functional neuroimaging. This procedure has been used extensively in young children and adolescents (Thomas & Tseng, 2008), but has been applied only rarely in infant participants. The less-familiar technique for measuring activity-dependent blood flow is near-infrared optical spectroscopy (NIRS) or optical topography (OT). An infrared emitter placed on the skull can send an infrared signal that penetrates several millimeters (2 to 3 cm) into the skull. Infrared light of differing wavelengths is differentially absorbed/reflected by oxygenated and deoxygenated hemoglobin. The reflected light can be measured with a detector placed near the emitter, and the time course of the oxygenated and deoxygenated blood flow can be measured. This procedure is being applied to infant participants routinely (Mehler, Gervain, Endress, & Shukla, 2008).

Both techniques have been applied to infant participants. The recording of fMRI was done in young infants of 2–3 months of age to study speech perception (Dehaene-Lambertz et al., 2002). Infants were presented with speech and backward speech in 20 s blocks, alternating with 20 s periods of silence. MRI sequences were recorded about every 2 s (usually done in 3 mm slices). The fMRI technique examines the blood flow in the brain during the presentation of the sounds, subtracting the blood flow measurements during the periods of silence. Figure 1.9 shows where in the brain these changes occurred. The MRI slices on the top left are from three different levels. Brain activity during speech was larger than during the silent periods in the colored areas on the MRI slices. This occurred over a wide range of areas in the left temporal cortex. The time course of this activity is shown in Figure 1.9 (top left figure). There was a gradual increase in blood flow to these areas that peaked about 6 to 7 s after sound onset, continued during the presentation of the sound, and lasted for nearly 10 s into the silent period.

The NIRS procedure has been used to study functional brain activity in newborns and young infants (Mehler et al., 2008). For example, one study investigated language perception in newborns (Peña et al., 2003). Figure 1.9 (bottom left figure) shows the location on the scalp on which the emitters and detectors were placed. The numbers indicate the area on the scalp under which the blood flow is reflected. The middle figure shows the same locations overlaid on the brain. This study presented newborn infants with forward and backward speech, with 15 s stimulus periods and 25 to 35 s silent periods. The bottom left figure shows the changes in the total blood flow as a function of time for the 12 recording locations. The blood flow changes for

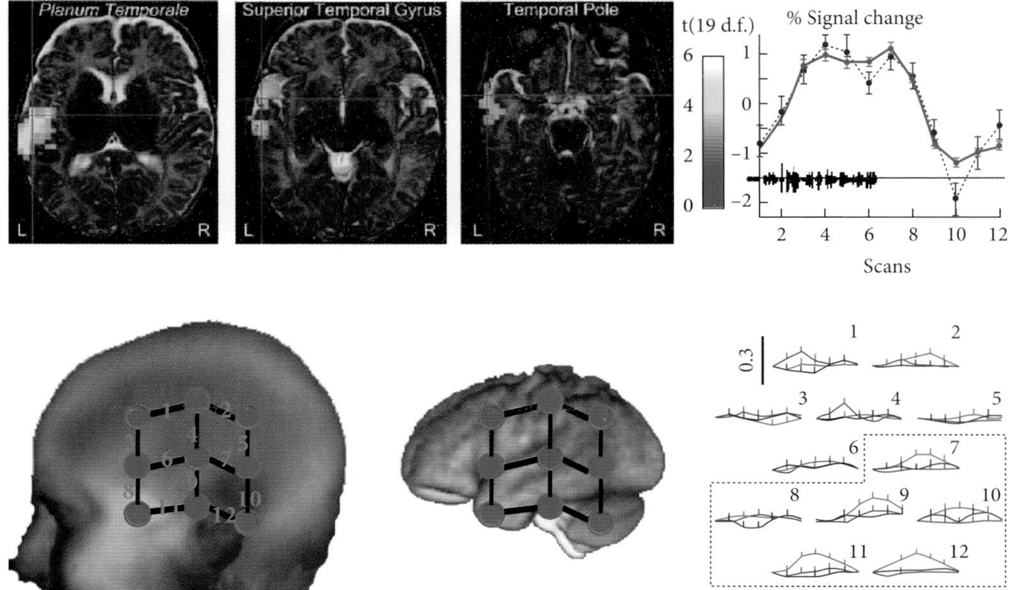

Figure 1.9 Blood-flow-based neuroimaging techniques in infant participants. The upper figures show the fMRI activations for activity at three levels of the temporal cortex, and the time course of this activity is seen in the upper right figure (about 6 scans per 10 s). The bottom left figure shows the positioning of the NIRS detector (blue) and emitter (red) probes, and the lines and numbers between the probes are the location of the scalp under which blood flow is measured. The middle figure shows the putative brain locations being measured, and the right figure shows the time course of total hemoglobin activity for forward speech (red), backward speech (green) and silent periods (blue).

the forward speech (red lines) were different in the recordings over the left temporal cortex than those for backward speech (green) or silent periods (blue). Comparable regions on the right temporal cortex (not shown) were not different for forward, backward, and silent periods. The onset of the maximal peak was 10 to 15 s following stimulus onset and the blood flow changes lasted 10–15 s after sound offset. These results show that infants are sensitive to the properties of speech at birth. Areas of the brain similar to those in older infants (i.e., Figure 1.9. top MRI figures) respond differentially to forward and backward speech.

I will comment briefly on the relative advantages of these three techniques (EEG source localization, fMRI, NIRS) for the measurement of brain function in infant participants. First, the fMRI technique provides the most direct measure of brain structure and function since the procedure is directly measuring blood flow in the location of the cortical activity. The EEG source analysis procedure uses quantitative inferential techniques to estimate such locations. The NIRS is limited to the analysis of the scalp-recorded optical changes. This restricts its value for localizing brain activity. The exact type of brain material under the same skull location differs across infants at the same age and across ages (Figure 1.6). Second, the NIRS and fMRI have a slower temporal resolution than EEG/source analysis. The underlying measurement phenomenon in the former are changes in blood flow, which occur over seconds (6–7 s for fMRI, 10–15 s for NIRS, Figure 1.9) and continues to respond for several seconds after stimulation. Alternatively, the EEG changes are caused by neural electrical activity occurring around the time of the synaptic potential changes of the neuron and are responsive to short-latency changes in this neural activity (e.g., 100–200 ms in Figure 1.8). Third, the spatial resolutions of the three techniques vary. MRI recording has <1 mm resolution for structural scans, and fMRI uses 3 mm slices and needs to perform averaging over a wide area. Motion artifacts may also degrade the spatial resolution of fMRI, especially for infant participants. The EEG techniques typically have resolution in the 5 cm range, though EEG source analysis with realistic head models probably lowers this to about 1 cm (10 mm). The NIRS technique has the poorest spatial resolution, since its measurement technique demands that emitter/detector distance be about 2–3 cm. It also may have its resolution blurred by larger arterial vascular changes occurring on the surface of the cortex carrying blood to intracortical capillaries. Fourth, the three techniques vary in "ease of use." The NIRS and EEG recordings are noninvasive and can be done easily on infant participants behaving in relatively unrestrained situations. The fMRI recording is extremely sensitive to motion artifacts and is best done in sleeping infants. This restricts its use for the study of a wide range of psychological processes in infant participants. The NIRS has the fewest quantitative requirements; EEG source analysis and fMRI requires extensive and sophisticated modeling with computer programs. The most used measure of the three for infant cognitive neuroscience is EEG, and NIRS is beginning to be used. The fMRI technique has rarely been used. Whereas I prefer the EEG source analysis technique as a temporally relevant and spatially appropriate method for infant cognitive neuroscience, the three techniques offer complementary information about infants' developmental cognitive neuroscience. They provide measurement of brain activity (and structure) in individual participants, rather than relying on brain measurement in other participants (i.e., nonhuman animals, postmortem or autopsy studies) or on techniques, which at best only indirectly measure brain activity (marker tasks, indirect psychophysiological recording).

Brain and Infant Attention: Spatial Orienting

The previous sections have outlined the proposal that brain development and attention development were closely related (section "Hypothesis: Infant Attention Development is Controlled by Infant Brain Development), and elaborated on methods used to measure brain structure (section "What's Inside a Baby's Head?") and function ("How to Measure Brain Function in Infants"). The current section details a type of attention, "covert attention" or "covert orienting" that has been studied behaviorally, psychophysiologically, and with the functional brain measurement described in the previous two sections.

Studies with adult participants have shown that attention may be moved around our environment flexibly. This is shown by the voluntary movement of the eyes from one location to another, which requires disengaging fixation (and attention) at one location, moving fixation (attention) to another location, and engaging attention in the new location. The flexibility of spatial attention is shown most dramatically in "covert attention" or "covert orienting." Michael Posner first studied this type of flexibility with the spatial cueing procedure (Posner, 1980; Posner & Cohen, 1984). In this procedure, a participant is directed to pay attention to a location in space where a target will occur. The target identifies some action needed to be done by the participant. The target occurs in the periphery and target identification is done without moving the eyes to the location, either during the target or in the time preceding target onset. The participant's response to the target is affected by several factors, which show that attention may be moved about in space covertly. The cueing procedure can use a cue in the same location as the target, in which case the psychological process is called "covert orienting." Alternatively, when a cue in a different location than the target, or cues are based on simple directions to "pay attention to the right side," the resulting psychological processes are called "covert attention."

Behavioral studies of this type of spatial orienting have been done in infant participants.

The spatial cueing procedure developed by Posner was first adapted by Hood (1995) to study covert orienting in infant participants. Hood presented 3- to 6-month-old infants with an interesting (color and movement) pattern on the center of a video monitor. When the infant began to fixate on this pattern, a stimulus was presented on the right or left side of the center; the center pattern remained on. Infants at this age will not shift fixation from a center pattern that is engaging fixation to the peripheral pattern. Thus, any differential response to the side on which the cue was presented, or the cue on the side, would indicate that the infant was able to covertly orient toward the peripheral pattern in the absence of overt eye movements. Note that this procedure differs from the typical Posner-type spatial cueing procedure in which verbal instructions are given to the participant to keep fixation oriented toward the center of the display.

There are a number of behavioral findings for infants in this spatial cueing procedure. A common variant is to present the peripheral pattern when the central stimulus is present, then turn both stimuli off, then present a pattern, functioning as a target, to which an eye movement will be made. The target can be presented on the same side as the cue ("valid trials"), on the opposite side ("invalid trials"), not presented ("no-target control"), or can be presented on a trial without the cue being presented ("neutral"). A number of studies show that in 2- and 3-month-old infants, the time to move the eyes from the center location to the target is faster when the cue and target are on the same side (valid trials) than when no cue was presented or the cue and target were on opposite sides (Hood, 1993, 1995; Hood & Atkinson, 1992; Johnson & Tucker, 1996; Richards, 2000a, 2000b, 2001, 2004a, 2004b, 2006, 2007). Figure 1.10 shows this finding for 14-, 20-, and 26-week-old infants (Richards, 2000a). The left-hand figures show the time to move the eyes from the center location to the target when the stimulus-onset asynchrony (SOA) was 350 ms. This time was

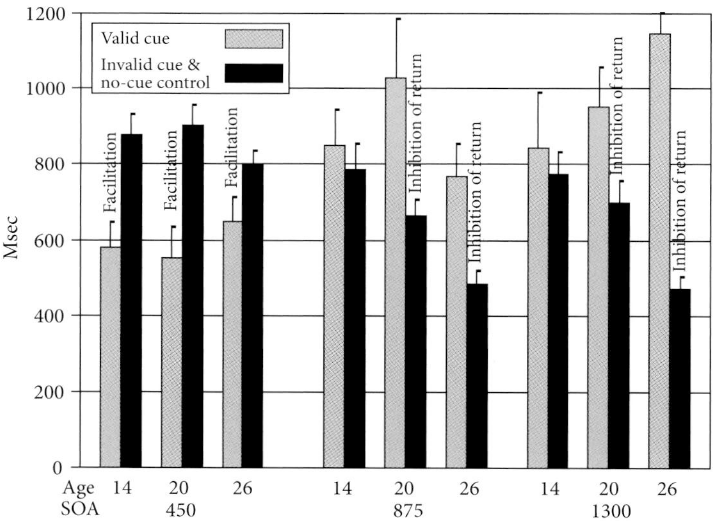

Figure 1.10 **Reaction time in the spatial cueing procedure for infants at 14, 20, and 26 weeks of age, as a function of stimulus onset asynchrony (SOA) and cueing type. The short SOA shows faster response times for the valid cued trials than the invalid and neutral trials for the three testing ages, whereas the medium and long SOA show inhibition of return only for the 20 and 26 week old infants. From Richards (2000a).**

shorter on the valid trials for the three testing ages. This facilitation shows that the presence of the cue registered in the infant's cognitive system even though fixation continued on the central stimulus; i.e., covert orienting.

An additional finding comes from the 20- and 26-week-old (4.5 and 6 months) infants. On trials when the time between the cue and target was relatively brief (e.g., 350 ms in Richards, 2000a), infants showed the facilitation of the response to valid targets. Alternatively, if the SOA was large enough (e.g., 700 to 1000 ms), the opposite occurred. The movement of the eye from the center position to the target was longer on the valid trials than on either the invalid trials or neutral trials with no cue stimulus. This longer response time may be seen in Figure 1.10 for the middle and right sets of bars. The 20- and 26-week-old infants showed lengthened reaction times for the valid trials at the 750 and 1300 ms SOA in this figure. Posner labeled this slowing of the response at intermediate SOA levels "inhibition of return." Interestingly, the inhibition of return occurs at late ages only for "covert orienting." If the cue is shown and fixation is moved to the cue, and then back to the center pattern, "overt orienting," young infants and newborns take longer and are less likely to move fixation back to the cued location (Butcher, Kalverboer, & Gueze, 1999; Clohessy, Posner, Rothbart, & Vecera, 1991; Simion, Valenza, Umilta, & Barba, 1995; Valenza, Simion, & Umilta, 1994).

The effects showing covert shifts of attention (covert orienting, covert attention) in adult participants have been studied with methods to determine the brain bases of these responses. Study methods have included fMRI, ERP, study of pathological populations, and invasive studies in animal preparations. The response facilitation that occurs at short SOAs is hypothesized to be due to the enhancement of sensory processing of information occurring in the attended portion of visual space (Hillyard, Luck, & Mangun, 1994; Hillyard, Mangun, Woldroff, & Luck, 1995). This has been shown with ERP studies that find enhanced amplitude of the early components of the ERP elicited by the target (Hillyard et al., 1994, 1995), and by studies linking these ERP changes with fMRI recording (Martinez et al., 1999). For example, in response to a target occurring in one part of the visual space, there is an enhanced ERP component labeled "N1" that occurs on the posterior scalp on the contralateral side, i.e., where the occipital brain areas for the opposite visual field are. This enhanced N1 seems to be caused by areas in the extrastriate occipital cortex and the fusiform gyrus (Martinez et al., 1999). The inhibition of return effect is thought to be mediated by the superior colliculus (Posner, Rafal, Choate, & Vaughan, 1985; Rafal, 1998; Rafal, Calabresi, Brennan, & Sciolto, 1989). It is thought that the activation of pathways in the superior colliculus responsible for fixation shifts, and the inhibition of those pathways during the spatial cueing procedure, results in inhibition of return.

Researchers studying infants in the spatial cueing procedure have adopted this neurophysiological perspective (Hood, 1993, 1995; Johnson & Tucker, 1996; Richards, 2000a, 2000b, 2001, 2004b, 2005, 2007b; Richards & Hunter, 2002). The spatial cueing effects have three putative developmental phases for infants. First, the superior colliculus is relatively mature at birth and should support inhibition of return. One can find in newborns, using the procedure in which there are overt shifts of fixations, examples of inhibition of return (Simion et al., 1995; Valenza et al., 1994). Second, the facilitation of response times at short SOAs must occur in cortical areas supporting visual processing. Only by 3 or 4.5 months is this area mature enough to support such response facilitation; thus the emergence of shortened response times to valid targets occurs by about 3 months of age (Richards, 2000a, 2000b, 2001, 2005, 2007b). Finally, the emergence of inhibition of return following covert attention shifts by 4.5 or 6 months of age must be due to the increasing influence of cortical systems on fixation in this task. Perhaps these cortical systems inhibit fixation to the peripheral stimulus during the presentation of the cue, leading to an inhibition of return of the attention system to the cued area. The changes in covert attention shifts found between 3 and 6 months of age must therefore be due to cortical changes in areas such as the parietal cortex and frontal eye fields involving saccadic planning and attention shifting. This interpretation is consistent with the general view that that there is an increase in the first 6 months of life of cortical control over eye movements that occur during attention and increasing cortical control over general processes involved in attention shifting (e.g., Hood, 1995; Richards, 2008; Richards & Hunter, 1998, 2002).

I have studied the areas of the brain involved in covert orienting effects in infants using ERPs and cortical source analysis. I briefly presented the use of scalp-recorded EEG for the measure of brain activity (section "How to Measure Brain Activity in Infants"). An EEG recording is made of the electrical activity occurring on the scalp. The EEG is generated by neural activity occurring in neural tissue inside the head. The infant is placed in the experimental situation with the spatial cueing procedure and changes in EEG are measured that are linked in time to the experimental presentations, i.e., ERP. The ERP thus is a measure of brain activity, recorded on the scalp, which is synchronized with the experimental manipulations or the psychological processes occurring in the spatial cueing procedure. The link between the scalp-recorded activity and the experimental manipulations is therefore a functional neuroscience method.

The studies I have done have tested infants at 14, 20, and 26 weeks of age (e.g., Richards, 2000a, 2000b, 2001, 2005, 2007b). The spatial cueing procedure adapted for infants was used and the ERP was measured at the beginning of target onset or immediately before saccade onset. Figure 1.11 shows the ERP changes occurring at target onset for the occipital electrode that was contralateral to the target (Richards, 2000a). This contralateral occipital electrode is interesting because visual information from the eye first reaches the cortex in the contralateral occipital cortex, which is just underneath the scalp near this electrode. A large positive deflection in the ERP occurred about 135 ms following target onset. This potential was the same size for the 14-week-old infants for the valid and other conditions, slightly larger for the valid condition for the 20-week-old infants, and largest for the valid condition for the 26-week-old infants. This ERP component occurred about the same time and has similar morphology to the "P1" ERP component often found in adults. This enhanced P1 is often found in response to a valid target in adult participants, and has been labeled the "P1 validity effect" (Hillyard et al., 1994, 1995). The study suggests that areas of the brain that control this response are developing over this age range. Presumably this brain development is related to the behavioral changes occurring in response facilitation or inhibition of return.

The cortical locations that generate the P1 validity effect was further examined with

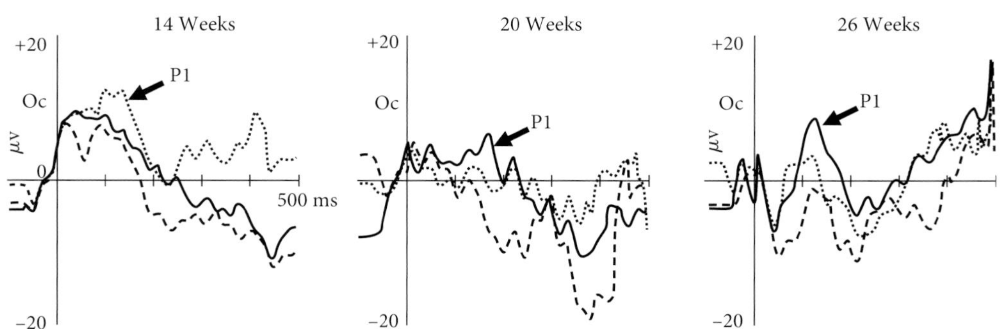

Figure 1.11 The ERP changes occurring at target onset in the occipital electrode contralateral to the target side. The valid (solid), invalid (dotted), and neutral (dashed) targets produced the same ERP response in the 14-week-old infants. The P1 ERP component was larger for the valid trials in the 20- and 26-week-old infants. From Richards (2000a).

cortical source analysis (Richards, 2005, 2007b). The section "How to Measure Brain Activity in Infants" introduced cortical source analysis. In this analysis, electrical dipoles that can generate the current resulting in the ERP component may be identified. The dipoles represent the location of the source of the cortical activity that is related to the experimental manipulations or psychological processes, i.e., functionally localized brain sources. Activity in these dipoles changes over time so that cortical activity that generates the temporal characteristics of the ERP can be shown.

I first will discuss the change over time occurring in several locations. Cortical sources for ERP recording were found in several areas of the cortex, including the posterior occipital cortex, extrastriate occipital cortex (including fusiform gyrus), and temporal cortex. Figure 1.12 shows the activity of these areas over time. A significant difference between the valid and the invalid/neutral trials is highlighted with the hatched bars. The posterior occipital cortex and the temporal cortex showed a large negative activity (brain activity resulting in negative scalp recordings), whereas the extrastriate occipital cortical areas

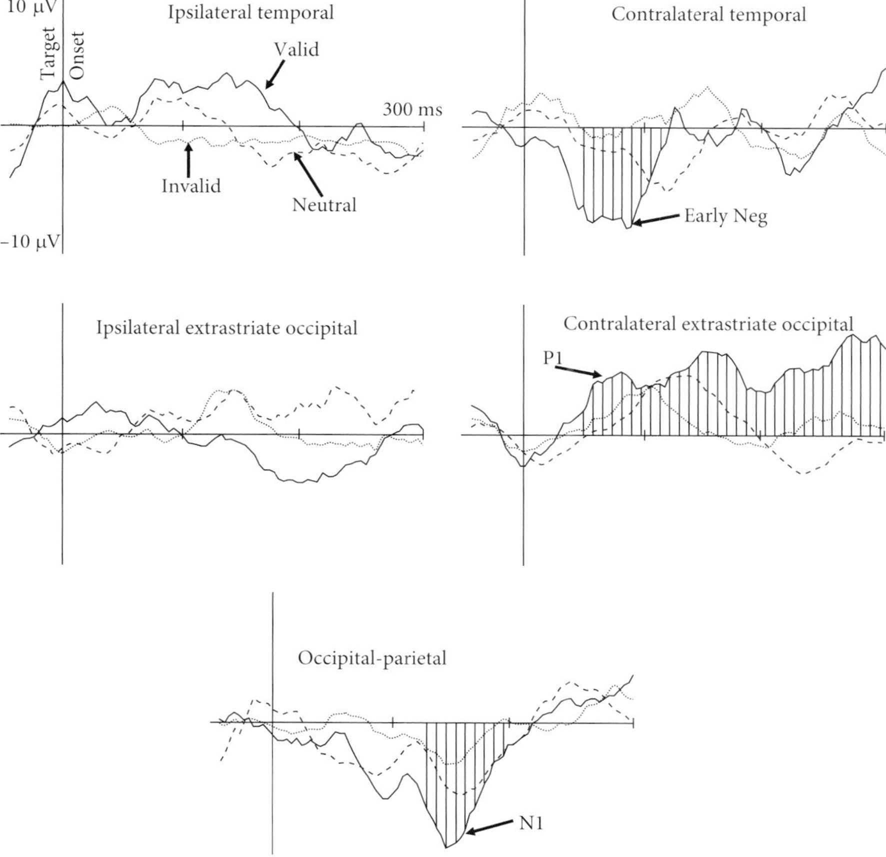

Figure 1.12 The time course of activity for the dipoles located with cortical source analysis. The valid trials (solid line) produced a significantly larger response in the posterior occipital cortex, extrastriate occipital (including lateral occipital, lateral-medial occipital, fusiform gyrus), and temporal regions (hatched areas). The cortical source analysis identifies only "activity" of the sources, and the direction of the source is determined from the direction of the ERP occurring in these locations.

showed the positive activity. This latter activity was similar in time course and electrical current direction to the P1 ERP component.

The activity for the contralateral extrastriate occipital areas will be examined further. Figure 1.13 (top left figures) shows a topographical scalp potential map for the ERP activity occurring in this area. The cortical sources for this brain area may be seen in the figure on the top right. These sources occurred in middle and superior occipital areas (Brodmann areas 18, 19) and in the fusiform gyrus. These areas are pathways that lead from the primary visual area to the object identification areas in the temporal cortex ("ventral processing stream"). Figure 1.13 also shows these activations in a bar graph separately for 14- and 20-week-old infants, and separately for the valid, invalid, and neutral conditions. The largest response was for the 20-week-old infants. This parallels the earlier finding of the gradual increase in the P1 validity effect over this age (Figure 1.11; Richards, 2000a). This implies that changes occurring in this area of the cortex underlie the P1 validity effect changes and perhaps some of the behavioral changes occurring in this task.

An interesting comparison can be made between the findings that areas of the contralateral extrastriate occipital cortex are the brain sources for the P1 validity effect in infants and a combined ERP/fMRI study in adults (Martinez et al., 1999). The Martinez study used a spatial cueing procedure in which participants were instructed to direct fixation to either the right or left side, and then targets were presented in either the attended or the unattended side. This procedure was done separately in a psychophysiological session using ERP and in a functional MRI session. They found the typical P1 validity effects in the ERP and localized the cortical sources to extrastriate occipital areas. These areas showed enhanced blood oxygen level–dependent (BOLD) activity in the fMRI experiment when attention was directed to the contralateral visual field. Alternatively, areas of the primary visual cortex did not show the ERP validity effect.

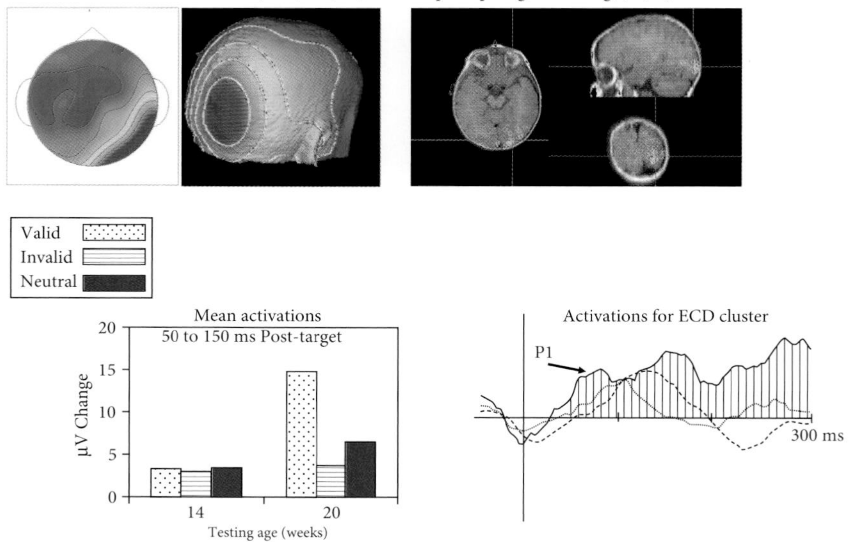

Figure 1.13 Topographical scalp potential maps for the contralateral extrastriate occipital areas (top left) and the cortical sources located in the brain (top right). The activity in this area was largest for the 20-week-olds in the valid cueing condition (bottom left figure).

Figure 1.14 compares the findings from the Martinez et al. (1999) study to the Richards (2005) results. Figure 1.14 shows the fMRI areas in the Martinez et al. study (upper left corner) and the cortical sources plotted on MRI slices from the Richards (2005) study. The green and red arrows point from the fMRI areas where an attention effect was observed to the comparable areas in the cortical sources of Richards, representing the contralateral extrastriate occipital areas that was the basis for the infant P1 validity effect. These areas are very similar in both studies. The yellow arrows point to the areas in the primary visual cortex in the studies of Martinez et al. (1999) and Richards (2005) where no validity effects occurred.

The Martinez et al. (1999) and the Richards (2005) results are compared further in Figure 1.15. The average MRI from several infants in the range from 3 to 6 months is shown as the MRI in Figure 1.15. Superimposed upon the MRI in the cross-hatched area are the middle and superior occipital cortex (top figures) or lateral-occipital cortex/occipital-fusiform gyrus (bottom figures). These areas were identified from the relevant anatomical areas derived from the MNI brain (Figure 1.7). The small yellow circles represent individual source dipoles from the cortical sources found in Richards (2005), both areas which show a P1 validity effect in their activation. The larger filled circles are the average Talairach locations for the superior occipital

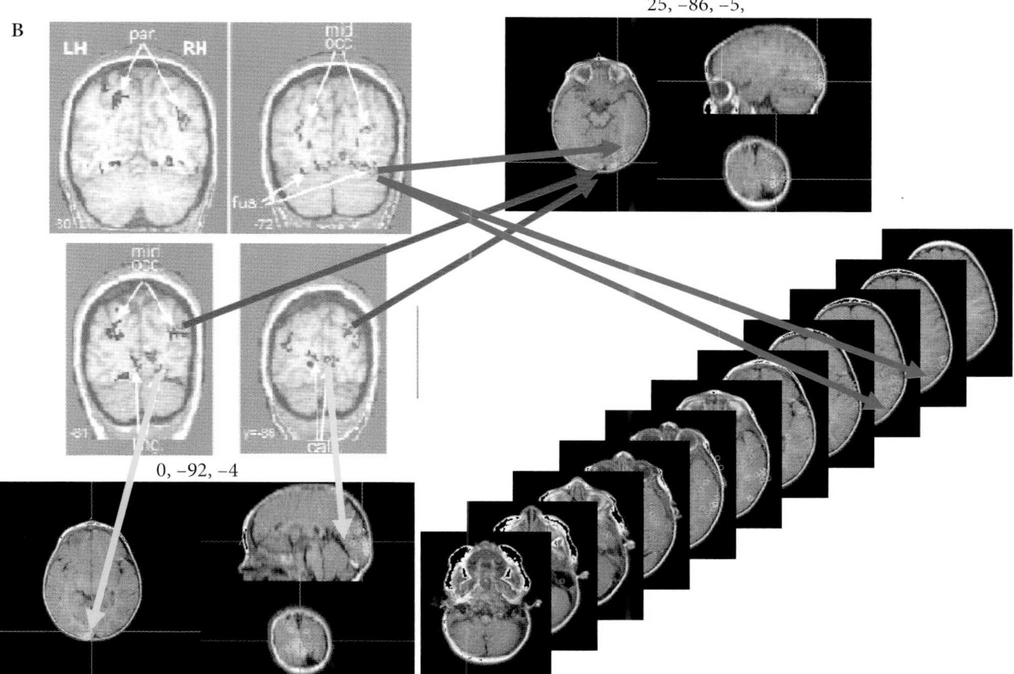

Figure 1.14 Comparison of results from a study of adults with fMRI (Martinez et al., 1999) and infants with source analysis of ERP (Richards, 2005). The upper left panels show the sources that were active in the fMRI study. The green lines are areas in the lateral occipital cortex and fusiform gyrus that were more active when attention was shifted to the contralateral side (fMRI) and the lateral occipital and fusiform gyrus locations that showed a P1 validity effect (infant ERP). The red arrows point to middle and superior occipital areas showing attention effects in both studies. The yellow areas are occipital cortex areas representing the primary visual cortex, showing attention effects in the adult fMRI but not in the infant ERP.

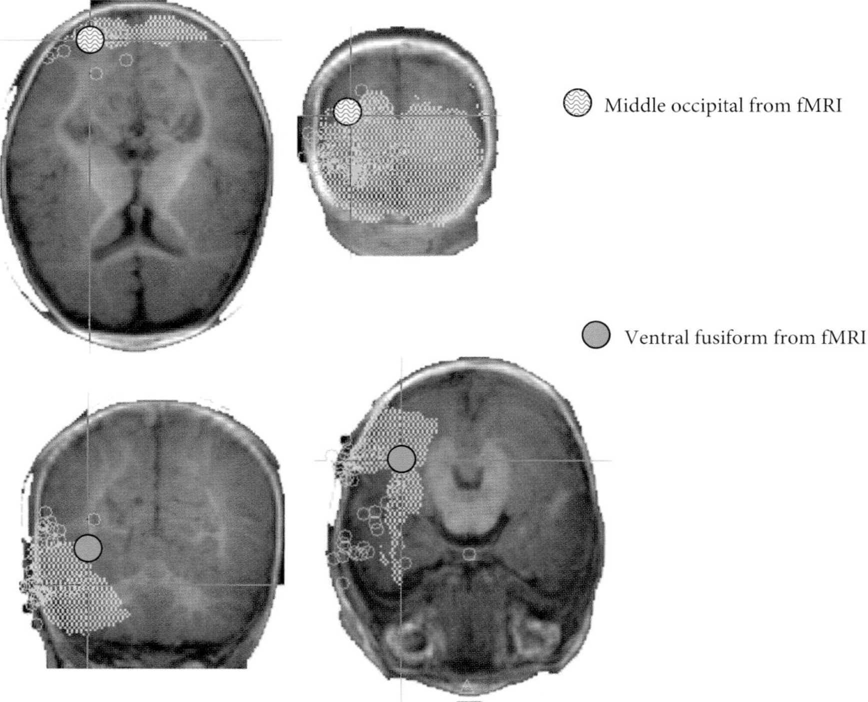

Figure 1.15 The distribution of cortical sources in Richards (2005) which were the cortical sources for the P1 validity effect in the ERP (yellow circles), compared with the cortical source locations found with adult ERP for this effect (large circles). The light purple hatched areas represent the anatomical locations of these areas translated from the MNI stereotaxic atlas (Figure 1.7) to an average of infant MRIs from 3 to 6 months of age.

and fusiform gyrus locations identified in the Martinez et al. study as showing the P1 validity effect in the ERP. Figure 1.15 shows how similar are the locations of the cortical source analysis found in these two studies.

There are two implications of the work showing the ERP components accompanying covert orienting in young infants and their cortical bases. The first implication is that the brain areas involved in the control of sensory processing and the effects of attention on these brain areas may form the basis for the changes in attention to peripheral stimuli in young infants. These techniques may be useful in showing how brain changes in these areas parallel developmental changes in the behavioral components of these tasks. The use of scalp-recorded ERP and the source analysis allow a "functional cognitive neuroscience" for infant participants. Second, the brain changes found in the P1 validity effect (Figures 1.11 and 1.13) parallel those findings of the inhibition of return rather than those of the response facilitation (Figure 1.10). This suggests that the development of the inhibition of return may be linked to the enhanced processing of stimuli occurring initially in the sensory systems. I have argued that cortical areas involved with saccade planning (presaccadic ERP; frontal eye fields; see Richards, 2000a, 2001, 2005, 2007b) may be more closely related to the inhibition of return effect. This may occur as attention-based saccade planning and fixation control comes to inhibit the movement of the eyes from the center to the cued location. These areas are likely in prefrontal cortex rather than posterior regions.

Brain and Infant Attention: Future Directions

This chapter reviewed the hypothesis that changes in brain areas controlling attention strongly influence the development of attention in infant participants. A considerable portion of the chapter examined the methodological advances in imaging showing what is inside the infant's head and how to measure brain activity in infant participants. I have focused on my work using cortical source analysis of ERP in the spatial cueing procedure as an example of how this might be done. The goal of research in this area is to link measures of infant brain development and measures of attention development.

There are aspects of this work that require further advances. Greg Reynolds and I (Reynolds & Richards, 2009) describe in more detail the application of cortical source analysis to infant participants. One limitation we note is that the cortical source analysis has been based on parameters for use with adult participants. The forward solution used impedance values for the matter inside the head (gray matter, white matter, CSF, skull) that are derived from adult participants. We know these are incorrect—adult skin has higher impedance than infant skin because of the accumulation of dead skin cells in adults, and infant skulls are less dense and thinner than adult skulls so that adult skulls have higher impedance than infants. This is being addressed by taking individual participant MRIs (section "What's Inside a Baby's Head?") from infants and using source analysis based on that infants head topography and infant-based values of the impedance of head materials (Reynolds & Richards, 2009; Richards, 2006, 2007a, submitted).

A second aspect of this work that requires advancement is the association of specific cortical changes with specific behavior changes in individual infant participants. The work discussed in the previous section (section "Brain and Infant Attention: Spatial Orienting") relied on average change in the group on the measures of behavior (Figure 1.10), ERP validity effect (Figure 1.11), and source activation and brain change (Figures 1.12 to 1.15). An individual approach would be to first identify aspects of brain development in individual participants and relate those aspects to that infant's behavioral performance. For example, perhaps extent of myelination (Figure 1.1) of the occipital areas (Figures 1.13 to 1.15) in an infant would be related to the existence of response facilitation but not inhibition of return for that infant, and the inhibition of return would be closely related to the size of the P1 validity effect. Alternatively, myelination in frontal areas occurring in this age range may be closely related to ERP changes indicating attention-directed saccade planning and the presence of inhibition of return. Such analyses would show directly the relation between brain development and attention development. An example of this kind of work is that of Klingberg (2008) showing in children and adolescents a close relation between myelination characteristics and cognitive and linguistic status.

Finally, I am working on several improvements to the spatial cueing procedure to make it more amenable to EEG and ERP analysis. One advance I have made is to create a testing protocol that results in a large number of presentations. In prior studies (Richards, 2000a, 2000b, 2001, 2005), the infants were presented with a single presentation of center stimulus, cue, target, and reaction time, interspersed with intertrial intervals with no stimulus present. This took from 5 to 15 s and resulted in 20 to 40 trials per participant. This allowed us to obtain numbers of trials sufficient for ERP analysis, but not optimal for relating individual performance with brain areas active in the task. Currently, I am using a procedure that presents a variegated background with continuous presentation of a stimulus that is foveated, cue, target, response, and then continued presentations. Between 75 and 200 trials can be obtained with this procedure and the infants are very cooperative. This allows for more manipulations in a single participant, larger numbers of trials for ERP averages, and examination of the relation between ERP characteristics, brain source activation, and different behavior patterns on a trial-by-trial basis. I have presented some results from this procedure (Richards, 2007b) and am continuing with other studies using this procedure. We also are using this procedure to test individual participants who have had anatomical MRIs. This allows the correlation between the structural characteristics of the individual infant's brain and its performance in the task.

Acknowledgment

This research was supported by grants from the National Institute of Child Health and Human Development, R01-HD18942.

References

Almli, C. R., Rivkin, M. J., & McKinstry, R. C. (2007). The NIH MRI study of normal brain development (Objective-2): Newborns, infants, toddlers, and preschoolers. *Neuromage, 35,* 308–325.

Bachevalier, J. (2008). Non-human models of primate memory development. In C.A. Nelson & M. Luciana (Eds.), *Developmental cognitive neuroscience* (pp. 499–508). Cambridge, MA: MIT Press.

Baker, P. N., Johnson, I. R., Harvey, p. R., Gowland, P. A., & Mansfield, P. (1994). A three-year follow-up of children imaged in utero with echo-planar magnetic resonance. *American Journal of Obstetrics and Gynecology, 170,* 32–33.

Barkovich, A. J. (2005). *Pediatric neuroimaging.* Philadelphia, PA: Lippincott Williams & Wilkins.

Barkovich, A.J., Kjos, B.O., Jackson, D.E., & Norman, D. (1988) Normal maturation of the neonatal and infant brain: MR imaging at 1.5 T. *Radiology, 166,* 173 Philadelphia, PA 180.

Battin, M., Maalouf, E.F., Counsell, S., Herlihy, A., & Hall A. (1998). Physiologic stability of preterm infants during magnetic resonance imaging. *Early Human Development, 52,* 101–110.

Bourgeois, J. P. (1997). Synaptogenesis, heterochrony and epigenesis in the mammalian neocortex. *Acta Paediatrica Supplement, 422,* 27–33.

Bronson, G. W. (1974). The postnatal growth of visual capacity. *Child Development, 45,* 873–890.

Bronson, G. W. (1997). The growth of visual capacity: Evidence from infant scanning patterns. In C. Rovee-Collier & L.P. Lipsitt, *Advances in infancy research* (Vol. 11, pp. 109–141). Greenwich, CT: Ablex.

Butcher, P. R., Kalverboer, A. F., & Gueze, R. H. (1999). Inhibition of return in very young infants: A longitudinal study. *Infant Behavior and Development, 22,* 303–319.

Clements, H., Duncan, K. R., Fielding, K., Gowland, P.A., Johnson, I. R., & Baker, P. N. (2000). Infants exposed to MRI in utero have a normal paediatric assessment at 9 months of age. *British Journal of Radiology, 73,* 190–194.

Clohessy, A. B., Posner, M. I., Rothbart, M. K., & Vecera, S. P. (1991). The development of inhibition of return in early infancy. *Journal of Cognitive Neuroscience, 3,* 345–350.

Conel, J. L. (1939). *Postnatal development of the human cerebral cortex: The cortex of the newborn* (Vol. 1). Cambridge, MA: Harvard University Press.

Conel, J. L. (1941). *Postnatal development of the human cerebral cortex: The cortex of the one-month infant* (Vol. 2). Cambridge, MA: Harvard University Press.

Conel, J. L. (1947). *Postnatal development of the human cerebral cortex: The cortex of the three-month infant* (Vol. 3). Cambridge, MA: Harvard University Press.

Conel, J. L. (1951). *Postnatal development of the human cerebral cortex: The cortex of the six-month infant* (Vol. 4). Cambridge, MA: Harvard University Press.

Conel, J. L. (1955). *Postnatal development of the human cerebral cortex: The cortex of the fifteen-month infant* (Vol. 5). Cambridge, MA: Harvard University Press.

Conel, J. L. (1959). *Postnatal development of the human cerebral cortex: The cortex of the twenty-four-month infant* (Vol. 6). Cambridge, MA: Harvard University Press.

Conel, J. L. (1963). *Postnatal development of the human cerebral cortex: The cortex of the forty-eight-month infant* (Vol. 7). Cambridge, MA: Harvard University Press.

Conel, J. L. (1967). *Postnatal development of the human cerebral cortex: The cortex of the seventy-two-month infant* (Vol. 8). Cambridge, MA: Harvard University Press.

Dehaene-Lambertz, G. (2001). Practical and ethical aspects of neuroimaging research in infants http://www.unicog.org/main/pages.php?page=InfantEthics. Accessed 2009.

Dehaene-Lambertz, G., Dahaene, S., & Hertz-Pannier, L. (2002). Functional neuroimaging of speech perception in infants. *Science, 298,* 2013–2015.

Evans, A. C. (2006). The NIH MRI study of normal brain development. *NeuroImage, 30*, 184–202.

Evans, A. C., Collins, D. L., & Milner, B. (1992). An MRI-based stereotactic atlas from 250 young normal subjects. *Journal of the Society for Neuroscience Abstracts, 18*, 408.

Evans, A. C., Collins, D. L., Mills, S. L., Brown, E. D., Kelly, R. L., & Peters, T. M. (1993). 3D statistical neuroanatomical models from 305 MRI volumes. *Proceedings of the IEEE-Nuclear Science Symposium and Medical Imaging Conference*, 1813–1817.

Fox, M. & Uecker, A. (2005). Talairach daemon client. University of Texas Health Sciences Center, San Antonio, TX http://ric.uthscsa.edu/projects/talairachdaemon.html. Accessed 2005.

Gilmore, J. H., Zhai, G., Wilber, K., Smith, J. K., Lin, W., & Gerig, G. (2004) 3 Tesla magnetic resonance imaging of the brain in newborns. *Neuroimaging, 132*, 81–85.

Hillyard, S. A., Luck, S. J., & Mangun, G. R. (1994). The cueing of attention to visual field locations: Analysis with ERP recordings. In H. J. Heinze, T. F. Munte, & G. R. Mangun (Eds.), *Cognitive electrophysiology* (pp. 1–25). Botson: Birkhauser.

Hillyard, S. A., Mangun, G. R., Woldroff, M. G., & Luck, S. J. (1995). Neural systems mediating selective attention. In M. S. Gazzaniga (Ed.), *Cognitive neurosciences* (pp. 665–682). Cambridge, MA: MIT Press.

Hood, B. M. (1993). Inhibition of return produced by covert shifts of visual attention in 6-month-old infants. *Infant Behavior and Development, 16*, 245–254.

Hood, B. M. (1995). Shifts of visual attention in the human infant: A neuroscientific approach. *Advances in Infancy Research, 10*, 163–216.

Hood, B. M., & Atkinson, J. (1991). Shifting covert attention in infants. Paper presented at the meeting of the Society for Research in Child Development, Seattle, WA, April, 1990.

Hood, B. M., Atkinson, J., & Braddick, O. J. (1998). Selection-for-action and the development of orienting and visual attention. In J. E. Richards (Ed.), *Cognitive neuroscience of attention: A developmental perspective* (pp. 219–250). Hillsdale, NJ: Lawrence Erlbaum Press.

Huettel, S.A., Song, A.W., & McCarthy, G. (2004). *Functional magnetic resonance imaging.* Sunderland, MA: Sinauer Press.

Huizenga, H. M., & Molenaar, P. C. M. (1994). Estimating and testing the sources of evoked potentials in the brain. *Multivariate Behavioral Research, 29*, 237–262.

Hunter, S. K., & Richards, J. E. (2003). Peripheral stimulus localization by 5- to 14-week-old infants during phases of attention. *Infancy, 4*, 1–25.

Hunter, S. K., & Richards, J. E. Characteristics of eye movements to a "Sesame Street" movie from 8 to 26 weeks of age, Manuscript submitted for publication.

Huttenlocher, P. R. (1990). Morphometric study of human cerebral cortex development. *Neuropsychologia, 28*, 517–527.

Huttenlocher, P. R. (1994). Synaptogenesis, synapse elimination, and neural plasticity in human cerebral cortex. In C.A. Nelson (Ed.), *Threats to optimal development, the Minnesota Symposia on Child Psychology* (Vol. 27, pp. 35–54). Hillsdale, NJ: Lawrence Erlbaum.

Iliescu, B. F., & Dannemiller, J. L. (2008). Brain–behavior relationships in early visual development. In C. A. Nelson & M. Luciana (Eds.), *Developmental cognitive neuroscience* (pp. 127–146) Cambridge, MA: MIT Press.

Johnson, M. H. (1990). Cortical maturation and the development of visual attention in early infancy. *Journal of Cognitive Neuroscience, 2*, 81–95.

Johnson, M. H. (1995). The development of visual attention: A cognitive neuroscience perspective. In M. S. Gazzaniga (Eds.), *The cognitive neurosciences* (pp. 735–747). Cambridge, MA: MIT Press.

Johnson, M. H. (1997). *Developmental cognitive neuroscience*. London: Blackwell.

Johnson, M. H., de Haan, M., Oliver, A., Smith, W., Hatzakis, H., Tucker, L. A., et al. (2001). Recording and analyzing high-density event-related potentials with infants using the Geodesic Sensor Net. *Developmental Neuropsychology, 19*, 295–323.

Johnson, M. H., Gilmore, R. O., & Csibra, G. (1998). Toward a computational model of the development of saccade planning. In J.E. Richards (Ed.), *Cognitive neuroscience of attention: A developmental perspective* (pp. 103–130). Hillsdale, NJ: Lawrence Erlbaum Press.

Johnson, M. H., Posner, M. I., & Rothbart, M. K. (1991). Components of visual orienting in early infancy: Contingency learning, anticipatory looking and disengaging. *Journal of Cognitive Neuroscience, 3*, 335–344.

Johnson, M. H., Posner, M. I., & Rothbart, M. K. (1994). Facilitation of saccades toward a covertly attended location in early infancy. *Psychological Science*, 90–93.

Johnson, M. H., & Tucker, L. A. (1996). The development and temporal dynamics of spatial orienting in infants. *Journal of Experimental Child Psychology, 63*, 171–188.

Kangarlu, A., Burgess, R. E., & Zu, H. (1998). Cognitive, cardiac and physiological studies in ultra high field magnetic resonance imaging. *Magnetic Resonance Imaging, 17*, 1407–1416.

Kinney, H., Brody, B., Kloman, A., & Gilles, F. (1988). Sequence of central nervous myelination in human infancy: Pattern of myelination in autopsied infants. *Journal of Neuropathology and Experimental Neurology, 47*, 217–234.

Kinney, H., Karthigasan, J., Borenshteyn, N., Flax, J., & Kirschner, D. (1994). Myelination in the developing human brain: Biochemical correlates. *Neurochemistry Research, 19*, 983–996.

Klingberg, T. (2008). Development of white matter as a basis for cognitive development during childhood. In C.A. Nelson & M. Luciana (Eds.), *Developmental cognitive neuroscience* (pp. 237–244). Cambridge, MA: MIT Press.

Kok, R. D., de Vries, M. M., Heerschap, A., & van den Berg, P. P. (2004). Absence of harmful effects of magnetic resonance exposure at 1.5 T in utero during the third trimester of pregnancy: A follow-up study. *Magnetic Resonance Imaging, 22*, 851–854.

Lancaster, J. L., Summerlin, J. L., Rainey, L., Freitas, C. S., & Fox, P. T. (1997), The Talairach Daemon, a database server for Talairach Atlas Labels. *Neuroimage, 5*, S633.

Lancaster, J. L., Woldorff, M. G., Parsons, L. M., Liotti, M., Freitas, C. S., Rainey, L., et al. (2000). Automated Talairach Atlas labels for functional brain mapping. *Human Brain Mapping 10*, 120–131.

Martinez, A., Anllo-Vento, L., Sereno, M. I., Frank, L. R., Buxton, R. B., Dubowitz, D. J., et al. (1999). Involvement of striate and extrastriate visual cortical areas in spatial attention. *Nature Neuroscience, 2*, 364–369.

Maurer, D. & Lewis, T. L. (1979). A physiological explanation of infants' early visual development. *Canadian Journal of Psychology, 33*, 232–252.

Maurer, D., & Lewis, T. L. (1991). The development of peripheral vision and its physiological underpinnings. In M. J. S. Weiss & P. R. Zelazo (Eds.), *Newborn attention: Biological constraints and the influence of experience* (pp. 218–255). Norwood, NJ: Ablex.

Maurer, D., & Lewis, T. L. (1998). Overt orienting toward peripheral stimuli: Normal development and underlying mechanisms. In J. E. Richards (Ed.), *Cognitive neuroscience of attention: A developmental perspective* (pp. 51–102). Hillsdale, NJ: Lawrence Erlbaum.

Mazziotta, J. C., Toga, A. W., Evans, A., Fox, P., & Lancaster, J. (1995). A probablistic atlas of the human brain: Theory and rationale for its development. *NeuroImage, 2*, 89–101.

Mehler, J., Gervain, J., Endress, A., & Shukla, M. (2008). Mechanisms of language acquisition: imaging and behavioral evidence. In C. A. Nelson & M. Luciana (Eds.), *Developmental cognitive neuroscience* (pp. 325–336). Cambridge, MA: MIT Press.

Michel, C. M., Murray, M. M., Lantz, G., Gonzalez, S., Spinelli, L., & Grave de Peraltz, R. (2004). EEG source imaging. *Clinical Neurophysiology, 115*, 2195–2222.

Myers, C., Duncan, K. R., Gowland, P. A., Johnson, I. R., & Baker, P. N. (1998). Failure to detect intrauterine growth restriction following in utero exposure to MRI. *British Journal of Radiology, 71*, 549–551.

Nelson, C.A., & Luciana, M. (2008). *Developmental cognitive neuroscience*. Cambridge, MA: MIT Press.

NIH (1998). Pediatric study centers (PSC) for a MRI study of normal brain development. NIH RFP NIHNINDS-98-13, sponsored by National Institute of Neurological Disorders and Stroke, National Institute of Mental Health, National Institute of Child Health and Human Development.

Nunez, P. L. (1990). Localization of brain activity with electroencephalography. *Advances in Neurology, 54*, 39–65.

O'Hare, E. D. & Sowell, E. R. (2008). Imaging developmental changes in grey and white matter in the human brain. In C. A. Nelson & M. Luciana (Eds.), *Developmental cognitive neuroscience* (pp. 23–38). Cambridge, MA: MIT Press.

Paterson, S. J., Badridze, N., Flax, J. F., Liu, W.-C., & Benasich, A. A. (2004). *A method for structural MRI scanning of non-sedated infants*. Chicago: International Conference for Infancy Studies.

Peña, M., Maki, A., Kovacic, D., Dehaene-Lambertz, G., Koizumi, H., Bouquet, F., et al. (2003). Sounds and silence: An optical topography study of language recognition at birth.

Proceedings of the National Academy Sciences, 100, 11702–11705.

Posner, M. I. (1980). Orienting of attention. *Quarterly Journal of Experimental Psychology, 32,* 3–25.

Posner, M. I., & Cohen, Y. (1984). Components of visual orienting. In H. Bouma & D. G. Bouwhis (Eds.), *Attention and performance X* (pp. 531–556). Hillsdale, NJ: Erlbaum.

Posner, M. I., Rafal, R. D., Choate, L. S., & Vaughan, J. (1985). Inhibition of return: Neural basis and function. *Cognitive Neuropsychology, 2,* 211–228.

Rafal, R. D. (1998). The neurology of visual orienting: A pathological disintegration of development. In J. E. Richards (Ed.), *Cognitive neuroscience of attention: A developmental perspective* (pp. 181–218). Hillsdale, NJ: Lawrence Erlbaum.

Rafal, R. D., Calabresi, P. A., Brennan, C. W., & Sciolto, T. K. (1989). Saccade preparation inhibits reorienting to recently attended locations. *Journal of Experimental Psychology Human Perception and Performance, 15,* 673–685.

Reynolds, G. D., Courage, M., & Richards, J. E. (2006). Infant visual preferences within the modified-oddball ERP paradigm. Poster presented at the International Conference on Infant Studies, Kyoto, Japan.

Reynolds, G. D., & Richards, J. E. (2005). Familiarization, attention, and recognition memory in infancy: An ERP and cortical source localization study. *Developmental Psychology, 41,* 598–615.

Reynolds, G. D., & Richards, J. E. (2007). Infant heart rate: A developmental psychophysiological perspective. In L. A. Schmidt & S. J. Segalowitz (Eds.), *Developmental psychophysiology* (pp. 106–117). Cambridge: Cambridge University Press.

Reynolds, G. D., & Richards, J. E. (2009). Cortical source analysis of infant cognition, *Developmental Neuropsychology,34,*312–329.

Richards, J. E. (2000a). Localizing the development of covert attention in infants using scalp event-related-potentials. *Developmental Psychology, 36,* 91–108.

Richards, J. E. (2000b). The development of covert attention to peripheral targets and its relation to attention to central visual stimuli. Paper presented at the International Conference for Infancy Studies, Brighton, England, July 2000.

Richards, J. E. (2001). Cortical indices of saccade planning following covert orienting in 20-week-old infants. *Infancy, 2,* 135–157.

Richards, J. E. (2002). Development of attentional systems. In M. De Haan & M. H. Johnson (Eds.), *The cognitive neuroscience of development.* East Sussex, UK: Psychology Press.

Richards, J. E. (2003a). Attention affects the recognition of briefly presented visual stimuli in infants: An ERP study. *Developmental Science, 6,* 312–328.

Richards, J.E. (2003b). Cortical sources of event-related-potentials in the prosaccade and antisaccade task. *Psychophysiology. 40,* 878–894.

Richards, J.E. (2004a). Recovering cortical dipole sources from scalp-recorded event-related-potentials using component analysis: Principal component analysis and independent component analysis. *International Journal of Psychophysiology, 54,* 201–220.

Richards, J. E. (2004b). Development of covert orienting in young infants. In L. Itti, G. Rees, & J. Tsotsos (Eds.), *Neurobiology of attention* (Chap. 14, pp. 82–88). London: Academic Press/Elsevier.

Richards, J. E. (2004c). The development of sustained attention in infants. In M. I. Posner (Ed.), *Cognitive neuroscience of attention* (Chap. 25, pp. 342–356). Guilford Press.

Richards, J. E. (2005). Localizing cortical sources of event-related potentials in infants' covert orienting. *Developmental Science, 8,* 255–278.

Richards, J. E. (2006). Realistic cortical source models of ERP. Unpublished manuscript. http://jerlab.psych.sc.edu./PDF%20Files/RealisticSourceModels.pdf. Accessed 2009.

Richards, J. E. (2007a). Realistic head models for cortical source analysis in infant participants. Society for Research in Child Development, Boston.

Richards, J. E. (2007b). Infant sustained attention affects brain areas controlling covert orienting. Society for Research in Child Development, Boston.

Richards, J. E. (2008). Attention in young infants: A developmental psychophysiological perspective. In C. A. Nelson & M. Luciana (Eds.), *Developmental cognitive neuroscience* (pp. 479–497) Cambridge, MA: MIT Press.

Richards, J. E.(2009) Cortical sources of ERP in the prosaccade and antisaccade task using realistic source models based on individual MRIs. Manuscript submitted for publication.

Richards, J. E., & Casey, B. J. (1992). Development of sustained visual attention in the human infant. In B. A. Campbell, H. Hayne, R. Richardson (Eds.), *Attention and information processing in infants and adults: Perspectives from human and animal research* (pp. 30–60). Hillsdale: Lawrence Erlbaum Associates.

Richards, J. E., & Holley, F. B. (1999) Infant attention and the development of smooth pursuit tracking. *Developmental Psychology, 35*, 856–867.

Richards, J. E., & Hunter, S. K. (1997). Peripheral stimulus localization by infants with eye and head movements during visual attention. *Vision Research, 37*, 3021–3035.

Richards, J. E. & Hunter, S. K. (1998). Attention and eye movement in young infants: Neural control and development. In J. E. Richards (Ed.), *Cognitive neuroscience of attention: A developmental perspective* (pp. 131–162). Mahway, NJ: Erlbaum.

Richards, J. E., & Hunter, S. K. (2002). Testing neural models of the development of infant visual attention. *Developmental Psychobiology, 40*, 226–236.

Rivkin, M. J. (1998). Developmental neuroimaging of children using magnetic resonance techniques. *Mental Retardation and Developmental Disabilities Research Reviews, 6*, 68–80.

Sajja, B. R., & Narayana, P. A. (2008). Magnetic resonance spectroscopy of developing brain. In C.A. Nelson & M. Luciana (Eds.), *Developmental cognitive neuroscience* (pp. 337–350). Cambridge, MA: MIT Press.

Sampaio, R. C., & Truwit, C. L. (2001). Myelination in the developing human brain. In C. A. Nelson & M. Luciana (Eds.), *Developmental cognitive neuroscience* (pp. 35–44) Cambridge, MA: MIT Press.

Schenck, J. F. (2000). Safety of strong, static magnetic fields. *Journal of Magnetic Resonance Imaging, 12*, 2–19.

Scherg, M. (1990). Fundamentals of dipole source potential analysis. In F. Grandori, M. Hoke, & G. L. Romani (Eds.), *Auditory evoked magnetic fields and potentials* (pp. 40–69). Basel: Karger.

Scherg, M. (1992). Functional imaging and localization of electromagnetic brain activity. *Brain Topography, 5*, 103–111.

Scherg, M., & Picton, T. W. (1991). Separation and identification of event-related potential components by brain electrical source analysis. In Brunia, C. H. M., Mulder, G., & Verbaten, M. N. (Eds.), *Event-related brain research* (pp. 24–37). Amsterdam: Elsevier Science.

Shankle, W. R., Romney, A. K., Landing, B. H., & Hara, J. (1998). Developmental patterns in the cytoarchitecture of the human cerebral cortex from birth to 6 years examined by correspondence analysis. *Proceedings of the National Academy of Sciences, 95*, 4023–4028.

Simion, F., Valenza, E., Umilta, C., & Barba, B. D. (1995). Inhibition of return in newborns is temporo-nasal asymmetrical. *Infant Behavior and Development, 18*, 189–194.

Stokowski, L. A. (2005). Ensuring safety for infants undergoing magnetic resonance imaging. *Advances in Neonatal Care, 5*, 14–27.

Sury, J., Harker, H., Begent, J., & Chong, W. K. (2005) The management of infants and children for painless imaging. *Clinical Radiology, 60*, 731–741.

Swick, D., Kutas, M., & Neville, H. J. (1994). Localizing the neural generators of event-related brain potentials. In A. Kertesz (Ed.), *Localization and neuroimaging in neuropsychology. Foundations of neuropsychology* (pp. 73–121). San Diego: Academic Press.

Taber, K. H., Hayman, L. A., Northrup, S. R., & Maturi, L. (1998). Vital sign changes during infant magnetic resonance examinations. *Journal of Magnetic Resonance Imaging, 8*, 1252–1256.

Talairach, J., & Tournoux, P. (1988). *Co-planar stereotaxic atals of the human brain.* New York: Thieme Medical Publishers.

Thomas, K. M., & Tseng, A. (2008). Functional MRI methods in developmental cognitive neuroscience. In C.A. Nelson & M. Luciana (Eds.), *Developmental cognitive neuroscience* (pp. 311–324). Cambridge, MA: MIT Press.

Tucker, D. M. (1993). Spatial sampling of head electrical fields: the geodesic sensor net. *Electroencephalography and Clinical Neurophysiology, 87*, 154–163.

Tucker, D. M., Liotti, M., Potts, G. F., Russell, G. S., & Posner, M. I. (1994). Spatiotemporal analysis of brain electrical fields. *Human Brain Mapping, 1*, 134–152.

U. S. Food and Drug Administration (2003). Criteria for significant risk investigations of magnetic resonance diagnostic devices. http://www.fda.gov/cdrh/ode/guidance/793.pdf. Accessed 2009.

U.S. Food and Drug Administration (2006). Information Sheet Guidance For IRBs, Clinical

Investigators, and Sponsors Significant Risk and Nonsignificant Risk Medical Device Studies. http://www.fda.gov/oc/ohrt/irbs/devrisk.pdf. Accessed 2009.

Valenza, E., Simion, F., & Umilta, C. (1994). Inhibition of return in newborn infants. *Infant Behavior and Development, 17*, 293–302.

Wozniak, J.R., Mueller, B.A., & Lim, K.O. (2009). Diffusion tensor imaging. In C.A. Nelson & M. Luciana (Eds.), *Developmental cognitive neuroscience* (pp. 301–310). Cambridge, MA: MIT Press.

Yakolev, P. I., & Lecours, A. R. (1967). The myelogenetic cycles of regional maturation of the brain. In A. Mankowski (Ed.), *Regional development of the brain in early life* (pp. 3–69). Philadelphia: Davis.

CHAPTER 2
All Together Now: Learning through Multiple Sources

Natasha Kirkham

The exciting promise of developmental psychology is that it can produce coherent explanations of development instead of merely describing behavior. It is, therefore, our business as developmental psychologists to find mechanistic explanations, which can be traced back to their origins, as opposed to delineating behavior at only one time slice. We must account for how infants and children build complex representations and acquire sophisticated knowledge, and then how they go on to use that knowledge to define and modulate their behavior. And we must show how all this occurs in real time. This is a daunting task, which requires analyzing the cognitive system from the bottom up, as learning occurs over time.

Such a study of learning is, in part, a study of perception, since the building blocks of complex knowledge must presumably be extracted from the world. Fortunately for the infant, the world is rich with perceptual redundancies that help guide attention (e.g., Bahrick & Lickliter, 2000; Lewkowicz, 2000). The same information, such as the location of an event or the number of an event's occurrences, can be conveyed simultaneously in visual, auditory, and tactile cues: We hear the voice of our partner coming from the direction of our front door, we see his face come through the doorway, and we reach out to greet him. The ability to integrate perceptual information across different modalities (as well as within them) is a key element in learning about events and objects.

In this chapter, I shall discuss the importance and the usefulness of such cross-modal integration in learning about basic structure, suggesting that it provides the foundations for more complex knowledge, and outline a theory of multiple cue integration. Data from a variety of paradigms will show the effect that richer, more numerous, and cross-modal cues have on infants' ability to learn visual sequences and events. As the infant develops, her tolerance for coherence between these cues changes, as she is able to acquire more sophisticated representations for a narrower set of cues. It may be that rich scenery, with the many cues available that highlight environmental structure, is processed more efficiently by infants than a scene containing sparser features. If this is so, then emergent sensitivities to probabilistic spatiotemporal information might require more contextual support in order to glean structure from the environment.

In order for humans to effectively use probabilistic information (i.e., to draw conclusions about the likelihood of potential events), they must be sensitive to the relative frequencies of various events. Indeed, there is much evidence to suggest that humans are very sensitive to frequencies of occurrence (and co-occurrence; Jonides & Jones, 1992; Jonides & Naveh-Benjamin, 1987). Some examples include the ability to accurately judge the relative frequencies of encounters with other people (e.g., Saegert, Swap, & Zajonc, 1972), the ability to judge the frequency of lethal events (e.g., Lichenstein, Slovic, Fischoff, Layman, & Combs, 1978), and in the language domain, judgments of the frequency of words (e.g., Shapiro, 1969), syllables (e.g., Rubin, 1974), letters (e.g., Attneave, 1953), and position of letters (e.g., Sedmeier, Hertwig, & Gigerenzer, 1998). Zajonc (1968) showed that this sensitivity to frequency can implicitly bias judgments of liking, the "mere exposure" effect that has been used widely by experimental psychologists across numerous fields.

Infants are sensitive not just to frequency of events, but also their probabilistic structure. As I shall discuss below, it has become evident that infants and young children have access to a powerful domain-general learning device. In laboratory experiments they can quickly learn statistically defined (or probabilistic) patterns in both auditory and visual domains (Fiser & Aslin, 2003; Kirkham, Slemmer, & Johnson, 2002; Saffran, Aslin, & Newport, 1996). Young children, as well, are quickly capable of understanding probabilistic information implicitly (Meulemans, Van der Linden, & Perruchet, 1998) or with explicit feedback (Kirkham & Shohamy, 2007). I posit that this learning device, coupled with a rich and accessible environment, provides the building blocks for mature knowledge.

Multiple cues

What happens when there are multiple probabilistic information sources available? From basic vision to language acquisition, multiple perceptual cues have been cited as providing important information to the system. How these cues are weighted, and what parameters determine differential weighting, has been of great interest in the perception literature. Weighted sum models of perception have been proffered as explanations for how adults perform many different tasks, including detecting an auditory signal with two frequency components that activate different auditory channels (e.g., Green, 1958), combining redundant stimulus properties in complex figures (e.g., Kinchla, 1977), combining multiple depth cues (e.g., Landy, Maloney, Johnston, & Young, 1995), and combining information across different senses (e.g., Ernst, Banks, & Bülthoff, 2000). Research on depth perception has shown the benefit of differential visual cues such as binocular disparity (e.g., Mayhew & Frisby, 1980), texture gradients (e.g., Todd & Akerstrom, 1987), and motion (e.g., Sperling, Landy, Dosher, & Perkins, 1989). Object motion, binocular disparity, occlusion and texture gradients, to name a few, are integrated to produce coherent visual percepts of objects, surface layout, and scenes (e.g., Bruno & Cutting, 1988; Mayhew & Frisby, 1980; Sperling et al., 1989; Todd & Akerstrom, 1987). In the adult vision literature, theories of multiple cue integration, or weighted sum models, have been offered as explanations for how observers combine stimulus property cues (e.g., Kinchla, 1977; Landy et al., 1995; Massaro, 1999).

In the cognitive domain too, multiple cues are often integrated in complex decision making, such as medical diagnosis (Brehmer & Qvarnstrom, 1976). A doctor uses all the pieces of information available to her, not just one. The information will be weighted differentially depending on the context and the nature of the information, but each bit will be used. This instance is an example of a complex cognitive problem, but multiple cue use is evident in the simplest, most mundane situations. When you decide to go to a restaurant for dinner, for example, there are a great many bits of information that will help produce a decision of the specific restaurant: What kind of food do you want to eat? Who else is going, and what food do they want to eat? Who is paying? Are either time spent at or distance from the restaurant issues for anyone attending the dinner? No one bit will be the conclusive bit, but a combination of all of them will get you to the correct decision. And these cue weightings are done in a matter of minutes, or even seconds.

So, given that multiple sources of information are available to solve problems in both perception and cognition, and that these sources tend to be probabilistic in nature, reliance on multiple cues should therefore produce greater success than reliance on any one individual cue. Furthermore, since many problem domains are characterized by probabilistic solutions, sensitivity to variables such as frequency and correlation should be a domain-general ability, and perhaps a fundamental characteristic of the developing mind. In order for infants to make use of this information available in the environment, she must be sensitive to probabilistic patterns. This sensitivity then creates the foundation upon which higher-order knowledge is based.

Infant sensitivity to multimodal regularities

Infants show great sensitivity to multimodal regularities. Similar to adults, infants use multiple cues to organize their visual perception: For example, when making decisions about an occluded object, infants may exploit such cues as edge alignment, synchronous motion, and depth to support perception of unity (Johnson, 1997; Smith, Johnson, & Spelke, 2003). In addition, investigations of language acquisition have led Christiansen and colleagues (Christiansen, Allen, & Seidenberg, 1998; Christiansen & Dale, 2001; Christiansen & Monaghan, 2006; see also the chapter in this volume by Christiansen, Dale, & Reali) to put forward a multiple cue hypothesis. They propose that the mechanism underlying language acquisition has the capacity to extract and store various statistical properties of language, and integrate different sources of information. They go on to suggest that it might be the conjunctions of these cues that provide evidence about aspects of linguistic structure that is not available from any single source of information.

A great deal of our perceptual understanding (as well as a great many of our responses to the environment) requires correctly correlating events across modalities. Gibson (1969) suggested that the responsiveness to invariant intersensory relations is a necessary part of the development of perception and learning. Indeed, during the first 6 months of life, infants develop many intersensory capacities, which allow them to perceive correlations across modalities (Lewkowicz, 2000; see also Richardson & Kirkham, 2004). Newborns bind a visual stimulus with an auditory stimulus to the extent that they expect the sound to move with the associated object (Morrongiello, Fenwick, & Chance, 1998). Lewkowicz and Turkewitz (1980) showed that very young infants (3 weeks of age) bind sound and vision together by attending to the intensity of the stimuli. By 4 months of age, infants can not only perceive the bimodal nature of objects (Spelke, 1979, 1981), but they can also perceive speech bimodally (Kuhl and Meltzoff, 1982; Rosenblum, Schmuckler, & Johnson, 1997). Infants of 5 months, when habituated to a bimodal presentation of rhythm (e.g., an audiovisual movie of a hammer tapping out a rhythm), dishabituated to a unimodal presentation of a novel rhythm (e.g., just the visual of a hammer tapping, without the sound; Bahrick & Lickliter, 2000). By 5–7 months, infants can match faces with voices based on the age, gender, and affective expression of the speaker (Bahrick, Netto, & Hernandez-Reif, 1998).

Multiple cue integration theory

It seems clear from the evidence presented in the earlier section that infant learning in the natural environment would exploit multiple cues across different modalities. Certainly, infants' sensitivity to cross-modal information stands in contrast to the sparse, unimodal presentations of many laboratory experiments. If laboratory studies do not fully exploit the cross-modal sensitivity of infants, then perhaps they risk underestimating the full capacity of their learning abilities. For example, Bahrick and Lickliter and colleagues have presented beautiful evidence that "intersensory redundancy," the overlap of information provided by amodal stimuli, drives selective attention (e.g., Bahrick & Lickliter, 2000; Bahrick, Lickliter, & Flom, 2004). Thus, it seems to follow nicely that intersensory redundancy should also drive basic perceptual learning. Broadly speaking, this theory predicts that there are three factors that will affect an infant's ability to learn a particular sequence or set of events: (1) the availability of multiple cues, (2) the coherence of the cues presented, and (3) the age of the infant. Thus, learning of basic visuospatial patterns or events should be facilitated if the same information is present in multiple cues within or across modalities. For example, infants will be better able to learn the statistical structure of a sequence of events when that pattern is conveyed by the shape, color, position, and sound of the events, rather than one of those cues alone. Cues can interfere with learning when they do not coherently co-occur. So if particular sounds are associated with particular locations, but the visual features that appear in that location are random or constant, learning will suffer. At younger ages, infants will require a higher number of cues and a higher degree of coherence between them. At later ages, infants will be able to learn statistical structure from a smaller set of cues and be able to tolerate a degree of incoherence between multiple cues.

Sequence learning

Both adults and infants are sensitive to the statistical structure of perceptual events. Adults are extremely competent at exploiting complex spatiotemporal sequences in order to guide behavior (Chun & Jiang, 1998; Howard, Mutter, & Howard, 1993). In serial reaction time studies, for example, adult observers view a single repetitive stimulus presented sequentially at different locations and respond to each position by pressing a corresponding key (e.g., Nissen & Bullemer, 1987). Stimulus locations follow a particular spatial and temporal pattern that a participant may be unable to describe explicitly, yet reaction times typically decrease reliably across trials (Cohen, Ivry, & Keele, 1990; Curran & Keele, 1993; Nissen & Bullemer, 1987). There is evidence that such learning is independent of the specific motor response: Observation of a sequential pattern can also lead to knowledge of serial order (Howard et al., 1993), and there appears to be no special benefit to learning imparted by manual responses, relative to oculomotor responses (Heyes & Foster, 2002). Perception of scenes can be guided by statistical information (Chun, 2000). Fiser and Aslin (2001, 2002) presented adults with probabilistically structured sequences of single shapes and shape arrays and found that observers were sensitive to the statistical correlations among multipart objects presented simultaneously, as well as to the joint and conditional probabilities of successive shape pairs.

Are infants also sensitive to the statistical structure of events? Research concerned with the development of sequence learning has revealed a capacity to pick up temporal patterns under many conditions. Saffran, Aslin, and colleagues found that 8-month-old infants parse a stream of auditory stimuli based solely on the transitional probabilities within and between the syllables (Aslin, Saffran, & Newport, 1998; Saffran et al., 1996; see also Gomez's and Saffran's chapters in this book for more discussion of infant auditory sequence learning). Gomez and Gerken (1999) exposed 12-month-olds to a subset of strings produced by one of two artificial grammars and then tested the infants on their ability to discriminate new strings from both the familiar and the unfamiliar grammar. Infants preferred to listen to new strings from their training set relative to strings from the novel grammar. These grammars differed only in terms of the ordering of word pairs: Individual words in the two sets, and the starting and ending words, were always the same. The only cues to provide recognition, therefore, were contained in word order, implying that the infants encoded the temporal patterns of word co-occurrences. Infants' ability to extract regularities in sequential input does not seem to be a language-specific mechanism, but exists broadly across audition. Infants parse auditory streams based on statistical probabilities even when the stimuli are tones (Saffran, Johnson, Aslin, & Newport, 1999), and at least one species of nonhuman primates, cotton-top tamarins (which never develop humanlike language skills), learns statistically structured sounds (Hauser, Newport, & Aslin, 2001).

There is evidence from other paradigms, however, that infants show some sensitivity to visual spatial relations among repetitive events under certain conditions. For example, young infants learn simple (two-location), predictable spatial sequences in the visual expectation paradigm, which uses oculomotor anticipation as the index of learning (Haith, 1993). Infants also show sensitivity to spatial contingency in temporal sequences: Wentworth, Haith, and Hood

(2002) presented 3-month-old infants with a spatiotemporal sequence in which a stimulus appeared on the left, in the center, or on the right of a computer monitor. Infants viewed either a fixed or a random pattern of locations, and in some cases, there was a contingent relation between the identity of the central stimulus and the location of the next peripheral picture. The fixed sequence of three locations resulted in more eye movement anticipations, and there were more anticipatory saccades to the correct location when there was a contingent relation between central and peripheral events. In displays of greater complexity than the simple two- and three-location events described previously, infants are still responsive to statistical structure. Upon exposure to a sequence of static multielement scenes, for example, 9-month-olds appeared to acquire the underlying statistical structure of the scene layout, attending longer following habituation to isolated element pairs that had co-occurred with a higher frequency within the familiar scenes (Fiser & Aslin, 2003).

Visual statistical learning: color and shape

There is clear and compelling evidence that infants are sensitive to patterns of events. Much of the work discussed has focused on the types of abstract statistical structure that infants are capable (and not capable) of learning at specific ages. This leaves open the question of the effect of the range and type of stimuli that infants are exposed to in such learning paradigms. For example, in earlier work, my colleagues and I tested the hypothesis that infants' ability to learn the statistical structure of event sequences was not limited to the auditory domain.

We examined visual statistical learning in infants using a habituation/dishabituation technique (Kirkham et al., 2002). Two-, 5-, and 8-month-olds were familiarized with a series of six discrete colored shapes that loomed from the center of a display monitor. Presentation order was defined in part by statistical regularities: The shapes were organized into pairs, and the pairs were ordered randomly (see Figure 2.1). That is,

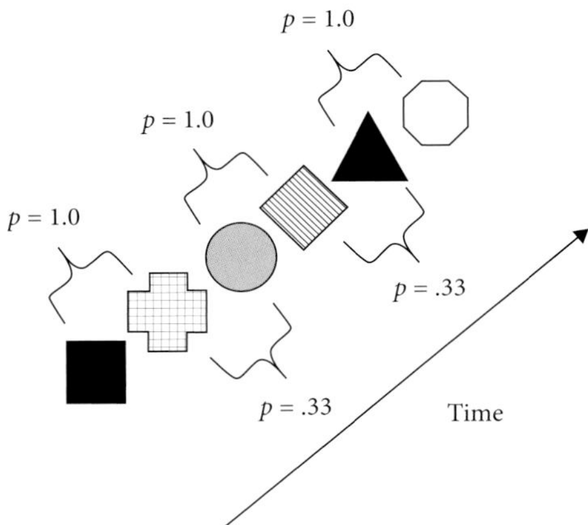

Figure 2.1. Schematic of Kirkham et al. (2002): An example of the visual sequence shown to the infants (NB. In the actual experiment, the shapes were different colors and not black-and-white).

the first shape in a pair reliably predicted the second, but the next shape to appear could be any of the first members of a pair. Following habituation, infants viewed six test displays alternating between familiar sequences, composed of the same three pairs of shapes, and novel sequences, produced by randomly ordering the same shapes. The only difference between familiar and novel sequences was the transitional probabilities between the shapes. We hypothesized that visual statistical learning would be evinced by a consistent preference for the random post-habituation sequence (i.e., a novelty preference). Our prediction was supported: Infants in all three age-groups exhibited a reliable preference for the random (novel) sequence. Indeed, there were no statistically significant age differences in the strength of novelty preferences, indicating that statistical learning under these conditions is available even to very young infants.

In the Kirkham et al. (2002) study, sequence information was contained in two cues, shape and color. Although the information conveyed by the cues was completely redundant, a multiple cue integration theory would suggest that such a redundancy supports learning. In the first test of a multiple cue integration theory, this prediction was supported by several experiments in which infants of ages 5 and 8 months failed to learn the same sequences when they consisted of either monochrome looming shapes or different colors of the same shape (Kirkham & Wagner, in preparation).

Spatiotemporal Statistical Learning: Color, Shape, and Location

The world will only seem coherent if one can process an object's spatial location and understand what its present location might predict about future events. Acquisition of this type of knowledge is essential for motion perception and for the production of action sequences, because one has to learn not only which actions are appropriate, but also where and when they should be performed. In recognition of the importance of location information, Kirkham, Slemmer, Richardson, and Johnson (2007) adapted the Kirkham et al. (2002) visual statistical learning paradigm to examine spatiotemporal statistical learning. Multiple cue integration theory was tested by isolating location from visual feature cues and examining learning with the support of different cue combinations across the first year of life. Could infants extract purely spatiotemporal correlations, and if so, at what age and under what conditions?

Infants were familiarized to stimuli appearing in one of six different locations on a grid and then were shown the familiar spatial pattern alternating with a novel spatial sequence. These spatial patterns mirrored the structure of the randomized shape pairs used by Kirkham et al. (2002). In Experiment 1, a red circle appeared in a statistically defined spatial pattern, and 11-month-olds, but not 8-month-olds, exhibited significantly greater interest in the novel spatial sequence (Figure 2.2A). In Experiment 2, six different color/shape stimuli were presented (Figure 2.2B). There was a statistical structure to both the features and the locations of the stimuli, but crucially, only the spatial sequence was violated during the test phase. Eight-month-olds, but not 5-month-olds, showed a novelty preference for an altered spatial sequence. Although they provided only redundant information, these multiple visual cues allowed 8-month-olds to learn the spatiotemporal sequence as

A

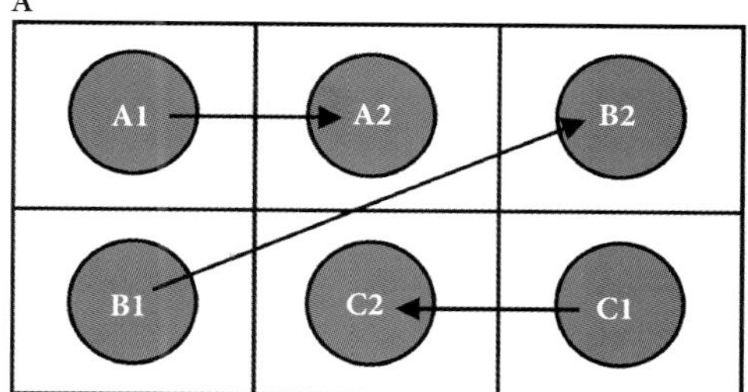

B

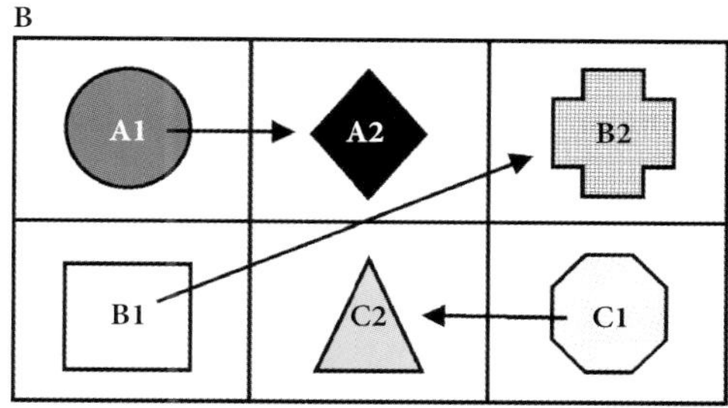

Figure 2.2 **(A) Experiment 1 in Kirkham et al. (2007): An example of the location statistics. (B) Experiment 2 in Kirkham et al. (2007): An example of the location statistics**

the 11-month-olds had. Experiment 3 suggested that perhaps 5-month-olds were simply not able to encode spatiotemporal information sufficiently, since they showed renewed interest in the novel sequence when the sequence of locations but not the sequence of color/shape pairings was held constant in the test trials.

There is an alternative explanation for 8-month-olds' performance in Experiment 2. It is possible that the infants were not sensitive to a probabilistic pattern of location changes: They merely picked up on individual shape–location pairings and showed a novelty preference when those pairings were violated. To rule out this explanation, Experiment 4 used an "on-line learning" paradigm, in which 8-month-olds' eye movements were recorded as they watched the habituation sequence employed in Experiment 2. Saccadic latencies to the newly appearing shapes were recorded as a measure of sequence learning. After exposure to the sequence, latencies to the first shape in a pair were longer on average than latencies to the second shape in a pair. This is because the second shape in a pair could be predicted once the first had appeared. If, as the alternative explanation holds, the 8-month-olds in Experiment 2 only learnt associations between a particular shape and a particular location, they would have no information about how one location can predict the next and should not show any saccade latency decrease in this experiment. In contrast, the decrease in anticipatory saccades that was found revealed the role multiple cue integration can play in generating expectations about the world.

These four experiments present evidence concerning a fundamental cognitive skill in infancy—the ability to learn probabilistic event sequences across space and time. Evidence was also obtained of an important developmental limitation in learning: Only the oldest infants observed (11-month-olds) responded solely on the basis of location statistics, showing a post-habituation novelty preference to a display in which the positions of stimulus elements were randomly placed. The youngest infants (5-month-olds), in contrast, appeared largely insensitive to location statistics, although they were able to detect probabilistic sequences based on a combination of color and shape. Infants at an intermediate age (8 months) provided evidence of learning location statistics only when color and shape contributed additional (redundant) cues for the spatiotemporal sequence. This suggests that temporal order statistics that involve spatial relations may become available to infants over the course of the first year after birth and that integrating multiple cues can bolster such learning.

SPATIAL INDEXING: COLOR, SHAPE, LOCATION, AND SOUND

At a certain stage of their development, infants can learn spatiotemporal sequences by exploiting redundant information of multiple cues. The cues used in Kirkham et al. (2007), however, were all visual. Infants do not live in a silent world, as a trip to any toy store will show. Do the sounds of particular objects act as redundant, cross-modal cues that can help infants to learn?

Dynamic spatial indexing is defined as the ability to encode the locations of multimodal events, track the locations as they move, and later, look back to the correct location when a particular event is relevant (Richardson & Kirkham, 2004). This behavior has been shown in adult subjects. For example, in Experiment 1 of Richardson and Kirkham (2004), adult participants looked at a spinning cross that appeared in two squares ports on a computer screen. While the cross span, adults heard a piece of factual information. After two facts, the ports moved around the screen. Participants then answered a question relating to one of the facts. While answering, they looked at the empty port that had previously been associated with the fact (see also, Richardson & Spivey, 2000). We hypothesized that a propensity for dynamic spatial indexing is not just a feature of the mature adult visual system, but emerges by 6 months along with some of the first uses of adult-like spatial reference frames. At that age, infants are still learning to orientate their attention properly (Colombo, 2001) and are only beginning to represent spatial locations egocentrically (Gilmore & Johnson, 1997).

Consistent Visual Cues

In Experiment 2 (Richardson & Kirkham, 2004), infants saw movies of two brightly colored toys that moved in time to two different sounds (see Figure 2.3). The toys appeared in square ports on a computer screen. Test phases consisted of the two empty ports and the auditory element of one of the movies. We found that infants looked longer at the empty port that had previously been associated with the toy, even when the ports had moved round the screen in between the presentation and test phases (Experiment 3). We argued that the ability to spatially index under these challenging circumstances was supported by the rich, multimodal nature of the events. So, how does the relative coherence of these three types of cues (visual features, location, and sound) affect dynamic spatial indexing?

Uninformative Visual Cues

The multiple cue integration theory predicts that even though the visual features

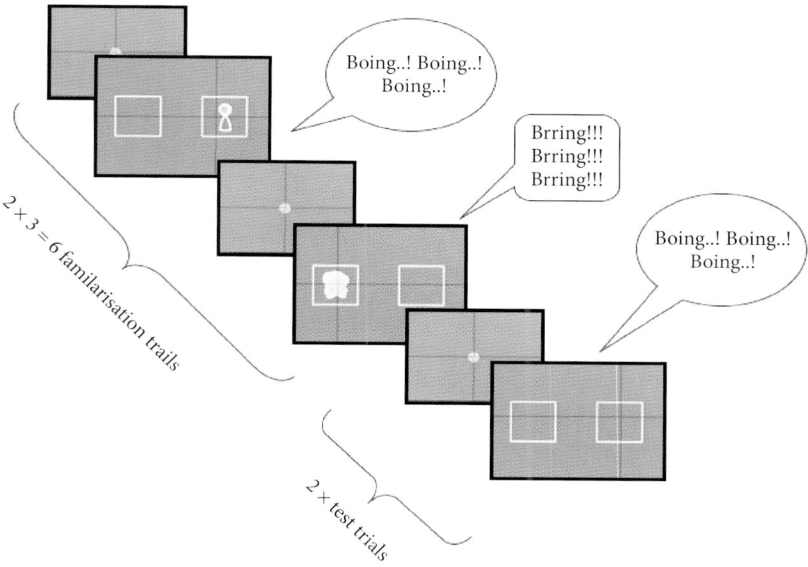

Figure 2.3. An example of what was presented to infants in Experiment 2 of Richardson and Kirkham (2004) with crosshair showing fixation. *Note*: In Experiment 3, the location of the ports during the familiarization phase was at the top and bottom of the screen; during test the empty ports translated to the horizontal positions.

provide information that is redundant for spatial indexing, their presence will support the infants' behavior. In contrast, it has been argued that infants below 9 months of age have an "object concept" governed by spatial–temporal continuity and that changes in visual features can go unnoticed (e.g., Xu & Carey, 1996). This account predicts that visual features would be irrelevant to dynamic spatial indexing.

Kirkham, Richardson, Johnson, and Wu (in preparation) tested these predictions in a series of experiments that modified Richardson and Kirkham's (2004) paradigm (see Figure 2.3). In the inconstant visual cues condition, the infants saw a different object on each presentation trial. In the constant visual cues condition, infants saw the same object on every presentation trial. In other words, the same auditory stimulus and the same synchronized motion were always associated with a certain location, but the visual features either changed on every trial (inconstant cues) or stayed the same (constant cues). To replicate the original finding, an informative cue condition was included where two objects seemed to be reliably associated with two locations. In every case, on test trials, only the auditory element was presented, and infants' looking times to empty frames were measured.

Infants of 6 and 10 months were run in the three conditions. Three-month-olds were run only in the original condition. The original dynamic spatial indexing finding (informative cue) was replicated in all three age groups; even the 3-month-olds performed well. Infants looked longer at the empty port previously associated with the toy after the ports had moved around the screen. The behavior is different, however, in the inconstant and constant visual cues conditions. Six-month-old infants failed to look significantly longer at either port in both the inconstant and constant visual cues conditions. Changing the visual features of the multimodal events on each presentation, or keeping them the same, reduced the infants' ability to discriminate locations during the test trial. When we presented 10-month-old infants with the same stimuli, however, they successfully looked at the critical location in both conditions. As predicted by a multiple cue integration theory, without the support of reliable and informative (though still redundant) multiple cues, younger infants find it harder to learn about their world. Older infants, however, are capable of learning these associations from a narrower set of reliable cues.

Object trajectory: objects, motion, and sound

So far in this chapter, I have discussed the usefulness of multiple cues on various forms of pattern detection. I would like to introduce the idea that multiple cues are useful in supporting more complex representations. This can be shown in investigations of young infants' understanding of objects as enduring across space and time, regardless of temporary occlusion. In most experimental settings, this experiment is unimodal: Infants watch a ball move across a screen, disappearing briefly behind a rectangular occluder. Accompanying sound tends to be stationary, coming at the infant from both sides of the screen that is used to keep the infants focused. Successful understanding of the object's trajectory is determined by number of anticipatory saccades directed toward the emerging ball. The typical results are that 4-month-olds appear to construe partly occluded trajectory events in terms of disconnected trajectories on either side of the occluder (suggesting that they are not expecting its reemergence), whereas by 6 months of age, infants are beginning to perceive the continuity of the trajectory behind the occluder (Johnson et al., 2003). This skill is not on a fixed path, however: Johnson, Amso, and Slemmer (2003) showed that 4-month-old infants, who are right at the beginning of a transition toward success at perceptual completion in the ball-and-box display, benefit greatly from "training." When exposed to an unoccluded trajectory prior to viewing an occluded trajectory, 4-month-olds showed a reliable increase in anticipatory saccades (relative to a control group of untrained 4-month-olds). This visual experience with the object's complete trajectory facilitated a representation of the persistent motion of the object even when interrupted by occlusion. Given that outside of the laboratory infants have more than just visual experience of moving objects, perhaps

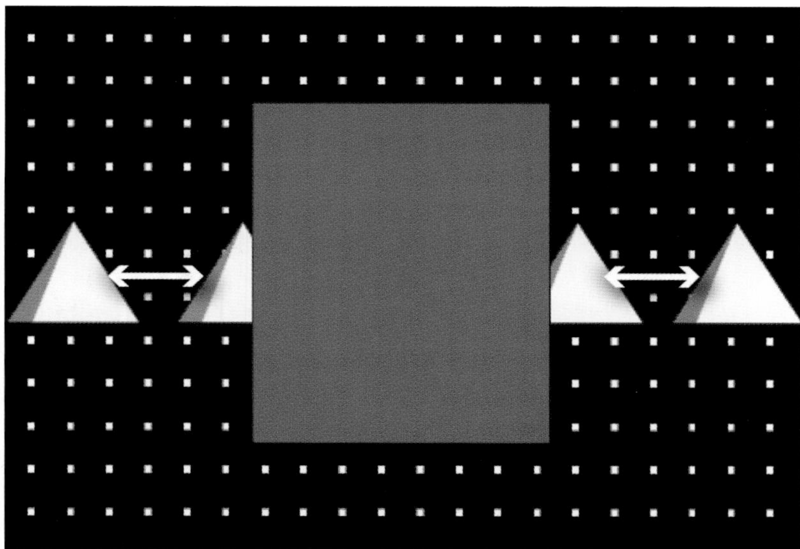

Figure 2.4. An example of one of the trajectories presented to the babies in Kirkham, Johnson, and Wagner (in preparation).

the addition of another source of information would help. Kirkham, Johnson, and Wagner (in preparation) incorporated a continuous moving sound into the ball-and-box paradigm, such that the sound traveled with the object from one side of the occluder to the other side (see Figure 2.4). Results from this study showed that 4-month-olds integrate multiple auditory and visual cues to infer a continuous trajectory. Control conditions examining whether static lateralized sounds would help or whether a sound moving in the opposite direction of the object would produce anticipations in the opposite direction support the initial finding. Four-month-olds show more anticipations only when the sound travels with the object. Indeed, when given these multiple, cross-modal cues, 4-month-old infants appear to be anticipating trajectories as well as 6-month-olds in the unimodal condition.

Conclusion

In this chapter, I have tried to describe a theory of multiple cue integration, supporting the acquisition of complex knowledge. As we now know, the "great blooming, buzzing confusion" (James, 1890, p. 462) of the perceptual world actually holds a wealth of information for an infant in the form of statistical structure and cross-modal regularities. It also contains many distractions, in terms of noise and extraneous information. When learning about the world, how do infants pay attention to the right set of multiple cues at the right time? This theory posits a developmental trajectory out of this problem: At early ages, infants rely on multiple, cross-modal cues in learning about sequences and locations; later on, they are better able to ignore unhelpful information and learn from a narrower set of cues.

In conclusion, I would like to suggest that the impact of multiple cue integration on infant learning in a probabilistic environment remains largely unexplored. How does multiple cue integration interact with statistical learning? What kinds of expectations about objects can be supported by this type of learning? The theory outlined in this chapter is an attempt to unify research from statistical learning and cross-modal perception perspectives and ascertain the capabilities of infants' hypothesized statistical learning mechanism.

Acknowledgments

The research discussed in this chapter was supported, in part, by Grant RO3 HD050613-01 from the National Institute of Health. I would like to thank all the parents and children who came to our laboratory and participated in our research. I would also like to thank Daniel Richardson for helpful comments on this chapter.

References

Aslin, R. N., Saffran, J. R., & Newport, E. L. (1998). Computation of conditional probability statistics by 8-month-old infants. *Psychological Science, 9,* 321–324.

Attneave, F. (1953). Psychological probability as a function of experienced frequency. *Journal of Experimental Psychology, 46,* 81–86.

Bahrick, L. E., & Lickliter, R. (2000). Intersensory redundancy guides attentional selectivity and perceptual learning in infancy. *Developmental Psychology, 36,* 190–201.

Bahrick, L. E., Lickliter, R., & Flom, R. (2004). Intersensory redundancy guides the development of selective attention, perception, and cognition in infancy. *Current Directions in Psychological Science, 13,* 99–102.

Bahrick, L. E., Netto, D., & Hernandez-Reif, M. (1998). Intermodal perception of adult and child faces and voices by infants. *Child Development, 69,* 1263–1275.

Brehmer, B., & Qvarnstrom, G. (1976). Information integration and subjective weights in multiple-cue judgments. *Organizational Behavior & Human Performance, 17,* 118–126.

Bruno, N., & Cutting, J. E. (1988). Minimodularity and the perception of layout. *Journal of Experimental Psychology: General, 117,* 161–170.

Christiansen, M. H., Allen, J., & Seidenberg, M. S. (1998). Learning to segment speech using multiple cues: A connectionist model. *Language and Cognitive Processes, 13,* 221–268.

Christiansen, M. H., & Dale, R. A. C. (2001). Integrating distributional, prosodic and phonological information in a connectionist model of language acquisition. *Proceedings of the 23rd Annual Conference of the Cognitive Science*

Society (pp. 220–225). Mahwah, NJ: Lawrence Erlbaum.

Christiansen, M. H., & Monaghan, P. (2006). Discovering verbs through multiple-cue integration. In K. Hirsh-Pasek & R.M. Golinkoff (Eds.), *Action meets words: How children learn verbs* (pp. 88–107). New York: Oxford University Press.

Chun, M. M. (2000). Contextual cueing of visual attention. *Trends in Cognitive Sciences, 4,* 170–178.

Chun, M. M., & Jiang, Y. (1998). Contextual cueing: Implicit learning and memory of visual context guides spatial attention. *Cognitive Psychology, 36,* 28–71.

Cohen, A., Ivry, R. I., & Keele, S. W. (1990). Attention and structure in sequence learning. *Journal of Experimental Psychology: Learning, Memory, and Cognition, 16,* 17–30.

Colombo, J. (2001). The development of visual attention in infancy. *Annual Review of Psychology, 52,* 337–367.

Curran, T., & Keele, S. W. (1993). Attentional and nonattentional forms of sequence learning. *Journal of Experimental Psychology: Learning, Memory, and Cognition, 19,* 189–202.

Ernst, M. O., Banks, M. S., & Bülthoff, H. H. (2000). Touch can change visual slant perception. *Nature Neuroscience 3,* 69–73.

Fiser, J., & Aslin, R. N. (2001). Unsupervised statistical learning of higher-order spatial structures from visual scenes. *Psychological Science, 12,* 499– 504.

Fiser, J. & Aslin, R. N. (2002). Statistical learning of higher-order temporal structure from visual shape sequences. *Journal of Experimental Psychology: Learning, Memory, and Cognition, 28,* 458–467.

Fiser, J., & Aslin, R. N. (2003). Statistical learning of new visual feature combinations by infants. *Proceedings of the National Academy of Sciences of The United States of America, 99,* 15822–15826.

Gibson, E. J. (1969). *Principles of perceptual learning and development.* New York: Appleton Century Crofts.

Gilmore, R. O., & Johnson, M. H. (1997). Egocentric action in early infancy: Spatial frames of reference for saccades. *Psychological Science, 8,* 224–230.

Gomez, R. L., & Gerken, L. (1999). Artificial grammar learning by 1-year-olds leads to specific and abstract knowledge. *Cognition, 70,* 109–135.

Green, D. M. (1958). Detection of multiple component signals in noise. *Journal of the Acoustical Society of America, 30,* 904–911.

Haith, M. M. (1993). Future-oriented processes in infancy: The case of visual expectations. In. C. Granrud (Ed.), *Visual perception and cognition in infancy* (pp. 235–264). Hillsdale, NJ: Erlbaum.

Hauser, M. D., Newport, E. L., & Aslin, R. N. (2001). Segmentation of the speech stream in a non-human primate: Statistical learning in cotton-top tamarins. *Cognition, 78,* B53–B64.

Heyes, C. M., & Foster, C. L. (2002). Motor learning by observation: Evidence from a serial reaction time task. *The Quarterly Journal of Experimental Psychology, 55A,* 593–607.

Howard, J. H., Mutter, S. A., & Howard, D. V. (1993). Serial pattern learning by event observation. *Journal of Experimental Psychology: Learning, Memory, and Cognition, 18,* 1029–1039.

James, W. (1890/1981). *The principles of psychology.* Cambridge, MA: Harvard University Press.

Johnson, S. P. (1997). Young infants' perception of object unity: Implications for development of attentional and cognitive skills. *Current Directions in Psychological Science, 6,* 5–11.

Johnson, S. P., Amso, D., & Slemmer, J. A. (2003). Development of object concepts in infancy: Evidence for early learning in an eye tracking paradigm. *Proceedings of the National Academy of Sciences USA, 100,* 10568–10573.

Johnson, S. P., Bremner, J. G., Slater, A., Mason, U., Foster, K., & Cheshire, A. (2003). Infants' perception of object trajectories. *Child Development, 74,* 94–108.

Jonides, J., & Jones, C. M. (1992). Direct coding of frequency of occurrence. *Journal of Experimental Psychology: Learning, Memory, and Cognition, 18,* 368–378.

Jonides, J. M., & Naveh-Benjamin, M. (1987). Estimating frequency of occurrence. *Journal of Experimental Psychology: Learning, Memory, and Cognition, 13,* 230–240.

Kinchla, R. A. (1977). The role of structural redundancy in the perception of visual targets. *Perception and Psychophysics, 22,* 19–30.

Kirkham, N. Z., Johnson, S. P., & Wagner, J. *Moving sounds: The role of inter-modal perception in solving the problem of occlusion.* Manuscript in preparation.

Kirkham, N.Z., & Shohamy, D (2007). *Feedback modulation of probabilistic learning: A developmental perspective.* Poster presented at the

Annual Meeting of the Cognitive Neurosciences Society, May 2007.

Kirkham, N. Z., Richardson, D. C., & Johnson, S. P., & Wu, R. *The importance of 'what' The usefulness of multiple redundant cues across the first year of life.* Manuscript in preparation.

Kirkham, N. Z., Slemmer, J. A., & Johnson, S. P. (2002). Visual statistical learning in infancy. *Cognition, 83,* B35–B42.

Kirkham, N. Z., Slemmer, J. A., Richardson, D. C., & Johnson, S. P. (2007). Location, location, location: Development of spatiotemporal sequence learning in infancy. *Child Development, 78,* 1559–1571.

Kuhl, P. K., & Meltzoff, A. N. (1982). The bimodal perception of speech in infancy. *Science, 218,* 1138–1140.

Landy, M. S., Maloney, L. T., Johnston, E. B., & Young, M. (1995). Measurement and modelling of depth cue combination: In defense of weak fusion. *Vision Research, 35,* 389–412.

Lewkowicz, D. J. (2000). The development of intersensory temporal perception: An epigenetic systems/limitations view. *Psychological Bulletin, 126,* 281–308.

Lewkowicz, D. J., & Turkewitz, G. (1980). Cross-modal equivalence in early infancy: Auditory–visual intensity of matching. *Developmental Psychology, 16,* 597–607.

Lichenstein, S. P., Slovic, P., Fischoff, B., Layman, M., & Combs, B. (1978). Judged frequency of lethal events. *Journal of Experimental Psychology: Human Learning and Memory, 4,* 551–578.

Massaro, D. W. (1999). Speechreading: Illusion or window into pattern recognition. *Trends in Cognitive Science, 3,* 310–317.

Mayhew, J. E., & Frisby, J. P. (1980). The computation of binocular edges. *Perception, 1,* 69–86.

Meulemans, T., Van der Linden, M., & Perrouchet, P. (1998). Implicit learning in children. *Journal of Experimental Child Psychology, 69,* 199–221.

Morrongiello, B. A., Fenwick, K. D., & Chance, G. (1998). Cross modal learning in newborn infants: Inferences about properties of auditory–visual events. *Infant Behavior and Development, 21,* 543–554.

Nissen, M. J., & Bullemer, P. (1987). Attentional requirements of learning: Evidence from performance measures. *Cognitive Psychology, 19,* 1–32.

Richardson, D. C., & Kirkham, N. Z. (2004). Multi-modal events and moving locations: Eye movements of adults and 6-month-olds reveal dynamic spatial indexing. *Journal of Experimental Psychology: General, 133,* 46–62.

Richardson, D. C., & Spivey, M. J. (2000). Representation, space, and Hollywood Squares: Looking at things that aren't there anymore. *Cognition, 76,* 269–295.

Rosenblum, L. D., Schmuckler, M. A., & Johnson, J. A. (1997). The McGurk effect in infants. *Perception & Psychophysics, 59,* 347–357.

Rubin, D. C. (1974). The subjective estimation of syllable frequency. *Perception and Psychophysics, 16,* 193–196.

Saegert, S., Swap, W., & Zajonc, R. B. (1973). Exposure, context, and interpersonal attraction. *Journal of Personality and Social Psychology, 25,* 234–242.

Saffran, J. R., Aslin, R. N., & Newport, E. L. (1996). Statistical learning by 8-month-old infants. *Science, 274,* 1926–1928.

Saffran, J. R., Johnson, E. K., Aslin, R. N., & Newport, E. L. (1999). Statistical learning of tone sequences by human infants and adults. *Cognition, 70,* 27–52.

Sedmeier, P., Hertwig, R., & Gigerenzer, G. (1998). Are judgments of the positional frequencies of letters systematically biased due to availability? *Journal of Experimental Psychology: Learning, Memory, and Cognition, 24,* 754–770.

Shapiro, B., J. (1969). The subjective estimation of relative word frequency. *Journal of Verbal Learning and Verbal Behavior, 8,* 248–251.

Smith, W. C., Johnson, S. P., & Spelke, E. S. (2003). Motion and edge sensitivity in perception of object unity. *Cognitive Psychology, 46,* 31–64.

Spelke, E. S. (1979). Perceiving bimodally specified events in infancy. *Developmental Psychology, 15,* 626–636.

Spelke, E. S. (1981). The infant's acquisition of knowledge of bimodally specified events. *Journal of Experimental Child Psychology, 31,* 279–299.

Sperling, G., Landy, M. S., Dosher, B. A., & Perkins, M. E. (1989). Kinetic depth effect and identification of shape. *Journal of Experimental Psychology: Human Perception and Performance, 15,* 826–840.

Todd, J. T., & Akerstrom, R. A. (1987). Perception of three-dimensional form from patterns of optical texture. *Journal of Experimental Psychology:*

Human Perception and Performance, 13, 242–255.

Wentworth, N. Haith, M. M., & Hood, R. (2002). Spatiotemporal regularity and interevent contingencies as information for infants' visual expectations. *Infancy, 3,* 303–321.

Xu, F. & Carey, S. (1996). Infants' metaphysics: the case of numerical identity. *Cognitive Psychology, 30,* 111–153.

Zajonc, R. B. (1968). Attitudinal effects of mere exposure. *Journal of Personality and Social Psychology Monograph Supplement, 9,* 1–28.

CHAPTER 3
Perceptual Completion in Infancy

Scott P. Johnson

Sensory systems provide information about the environment so that we might prepare and enact actions appropriate for the context. Visual perception, in particular, is useful in acquiring information about near and distant objects in our surroundings. Consider, for example, the scene in Figure 3.1, adjacent to the beach in Venice, California. This scene is typical of what we might encounter when we move about in the world: the ground extends into the distance and consists of different materials (concrete, grass, sand) that might dictate our route, and there are many objects that might either be avoided or approached as we move about, depending on our goals.

In everyday contexts, we hold certain commonsense expectations about the objects we see. We expect most objects, for example, to be solid and three-dimensional, persistent across space and time, and we plan our actions around these expectations. How are these commonsense expectations about objects achieved? Object perception and action planning typically seem so effortless and rapid that we may fail to appreciate their complexity. But there are many steps involved in perceiving objects:

- Segmentation of a scene into its component surfaces based on differences in color, luminance, motion, shape, orientation, distance, and so forth.
- Assembly of the surfaces into units (units, or collections of units, constitute objects).
- Perception of units as complete across space and time despite gaps in perception due to occlusion and movement of objects.
- Deduction of 3D shape from limited views due to objects' self-occlusion.
- Recognition of objects encountered before.
- Tracking the identity of previously encountered objects over time.
- Categorization of similar objects.
- Detecting affordances for action.

This way of decomposing object perception underscores its complexity, and also provides hints as to how investigations into its mechanisms and development might proceed. In this chapter, I will describe a program of research whose goal is to elucidate the developmental origins of object perception, with particular focus on *perceptual completion*, which constitutes a subset of the steps just described: assembly of visible surfaces into units despite gaps in perception due to occlusion by other objects, and perception of 3D shape despite self-occlusion. I will describe three kinds of perceptual completion and consider the developmental mechanisms involved in each: *spatial completion*, perceiving the unity of partly occluded surfaces; *spatiotemporal completion*, perceiving the unity of partly occluded trajectories; and *3D object completion*, perceiving the 3D shape of objects seen from a limited vantage point.

In principle, perceptual completion might be accomplished innately—in the absence of visual

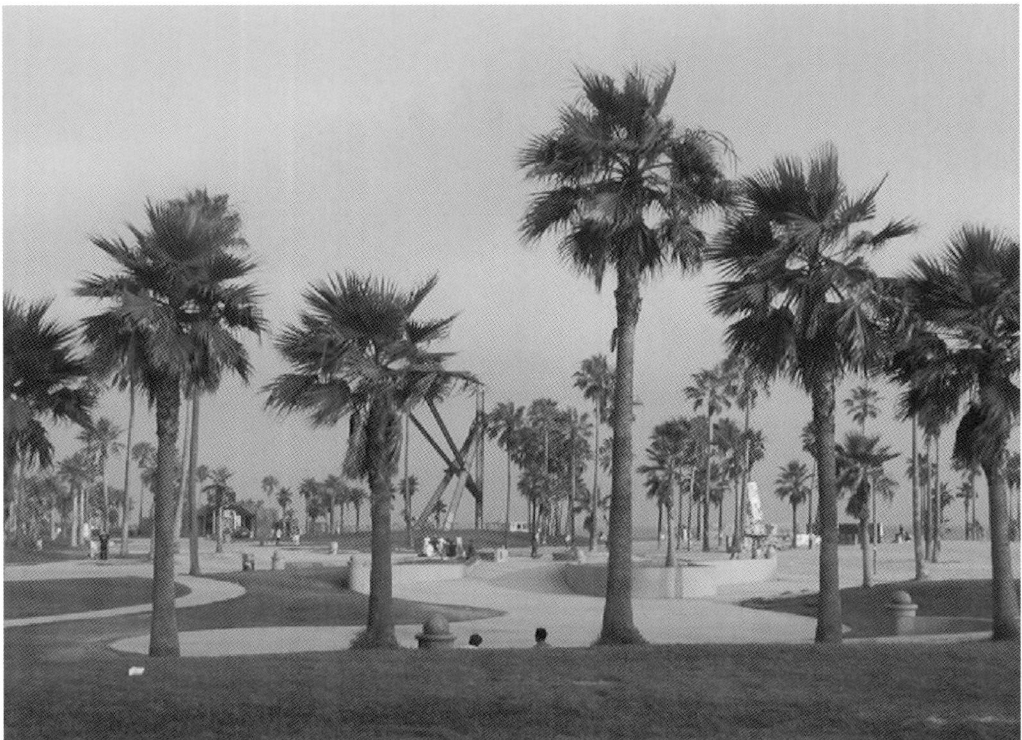

Figure 3.1 **A scene in Venice, California.**

experience—if the developmental processes that build those parts of the visual system that support it were complete at birth. In the mature primate visual system, for example, spatial completion is accomplished in part by interactions among neurons in relatively low levels of the visual system (V1 and V2), which, when firing in response to a visible edge, connect with other neurons that are tuned to similar edge orientations (Peterhans & von der Heydt, 1991). In this way, activation "spreads" among neurons coding for a specific edge orientation when that orientation is detected—so-called "local" circuits—and activation can propagate across a spatial gap. As it happens, connections among low-level local circuits in the human visual system are likely first formed at about 2 postnatal months (Burkhalter, 1993; Burkhalter, Bernardo, & Charles, 1993), and consistent with this timing, infants begin to provide evidence of perceptual completion at about 2 months after birth (Johnson, 2004). It is unknown if there is a one-to-one correspondence between these developmental events, as might be predicted on a strictly maturational account (e.g., if growth of neural connections causes spatial completion), but maturation is likely an important part of the overall developmental story. The evidence is clearer, however, for a direct and important role for learning as a principal means of development of perceptual completion. I will describe this evidence subsequently.

The remainder of this chapter is organized as follows. In the next section, I will describe two theoretical views of object perception in infancy, one of Jean Piaget and the other of theorists espousing a nativist view. In the following sections, I will describe in more detail the three kinds of perceptual completion mentioned previously (spatial, spatiotemporal, and 3D object completion), and some of the developmental mechanisms involved. The chapter will conclude by considering implications of our research for constructivist theory, which of course is the theme of this book.

THEORETICAL CONSIDERATIONS

Piaget (1954) described the first systematic investigations of how infants, beginning at birth and extending across the next several years, respond to objects and their spatial relations. According to Piagetian theory, the development of object knowledge consists of construction of two related concepts: first, that objects persist across time and space, and second, that objects exist external to the self in a particular spatial arrangement. Piaget devised a series of clever activities involving objects, often occluded objects, which he presented to infants and children, and he recorded the children's responses. These observations revealed a developmental sequence of behaviors thought to reflect underlying knowledge of objects and their spatial relations. Initially, infants provided no responses to indicate knowledge of object permanence, though there was recognition of familiar objects. Between 3 and 6 months, infants begin to show evidence of a sense of objects as having boundaries that extend beyond the visible, such as searching for (whole) objects that are only partly visible, and directing gaze toward the expected point of emergence of a moving object that became hidden. Later, at around 8 months of age, infants search for fully hidden objects; still later (around 18–24 months), infants solve more complex hiding tasks involving more than one location, at which point Piaget ascribed them full object permanence.

At birth, therefore, the infant experiences not objects per se but rather surfaces that appear and disappear erratically—fleeting images that are arbitrary and subjective, rather than substantial, predictable, and permanent. Piaget suggested, furthermore, that the principal mechanisms of development were rooted in the infant's own behavior: engaging with objects, following their motions, and taking note of the consequences of self-directed actions.

Many of Piaget's observations have been replicated repeatedly, but his interpretation of infants' behavior has been disputed on the basis of more recent experiments employing methods claimed to be more sophisticated and sensitive than reaching in tapping infants' cognitive constructs. Some of these methods capitalize on infants' tendency to show clear visual preferences for particular stimuli over others; one such method, known as the "violation of expectation" method, is claimed to demonstrate infants' knowledge of event sequences that are physically impossible. For example, in an experiment described by Baillargeon, Spelke, and Wasserman (1985), 5-month-old infants viewed a box and a screen arranged such that the screen rotated and appeared to move through the space occupied by the box, a so-called "impossible" event, accomplished with one-way mirrors. Infants were reported to look longer at this event than at a "possible" version in which the screen stopped at an appropriate place in its rotation, before moving through the box, therefore providing evidence for object permanence earlier than acknowledged by Piagetian theory.

A second example comes from an experiment described by Bower (1967) in which 1-month-old infants viewed a triangle made of wire, its center occluded by a rectangular object. Bower did not record looking times toward the object; instead, he recorded rates of sucking on a pacifier during viewing and reasoned that a change in sucking rates upon presentation of a novel stimulus would indicate perceptual discrimination of the new stimulus from the original. Following the occluded object, infants viewed four new stimuli presented individually: a whole triangle, a triangle with crossed lines in the center, and two different kinds of incomplete triangles, each with a gap in the center. All four test stimuli were consistent with the visible portions of the triangle seen during training. The infants maintained sucking rates in response to the complete object, and reduced sucking rates most when viewing the two incomplete forms. This implies generalization of the complete form to the partly occluded object, and response to the incomplete forms as novel.

Noting the inconsistencies between the Bower study and Piaget's observations, Kellman and Spelke (1983) undertook a more thorough examination of young infants' perception of partly occluded objects. In one such experiment, infants were first presented with a moving, partly occluded rod until habituation of looking occurred; that is, looking times declined according to a predetermined criterion. The infants were then tested with incomplete (or broken) and complete versions of this display without the occluder (see Figure 3.2). The test stimulus that attracted the most attention was assumed to be perceived as most novel relative to the initial stimulus. Four-month-old infants showed reliable preferences for a broken rod test display when the partly occluded rod (the habituation stimulus) was seen to move laterally relative to the background and occluder (as depicted in Figure 3.2). (In this study, and the others described in this chapter that use habituation methods, a separate age-matched control group was observed for evidence of spontaneous preference for one of the test stimuli; in all cases, none were found.) There was no evidence of unity perception, however, in displays in which the rod remained stationary, in contradiction to the results reported by Bower. The discrepancies between the findings of the Kellman and Spelke study concerning unity perception and the Bower experiment are difficult to reconcile, but it is noteworthy that the Kellman and Spelke finding has been replicated on multiple occasions.

These studies and others have been suggested to provide support for a nativist theory of cognitive development stressing an innate knowledge component (i.e., independent of experience) that guides infant responses to objects. This theory is founded principally on the assumption that object knowledge is innate because responses to occlusion are observed at an early age, and there is inadequate opportunity for infant learning of foundational concepts, such as persistence and permanence (Baillargeon, 1995). On a nativist account, Piaget may have underestimated infants' object knowledge and the age at which competence at object permanence can be elicited because of the insensitivity of his methods. Piaget's methods are thought to rely too heavily on overt manual responses, such as coordinated reaching. Difficulties with reaching may mask latent cognitive capacities that can be revealed with methods that rely on relatively simpler action sequences, such as looking and sucking.

Yet the nativist account has three fundamental flaws with respect to infants' responses to partly and fully occluded objects. First, findings from experiments using measures that do not require manual search skills, such as looking times, in reality are broadly consistent with Piaget's observations: Infants provide evidence of representing partly occluded objects a few months after birth, and fully occluded objects by about the middle of the first year. Some have claimed that infants have a sense of object permanence on the basis of evidence from looking time studies (e.g., Baillargeon et al., 1985), but

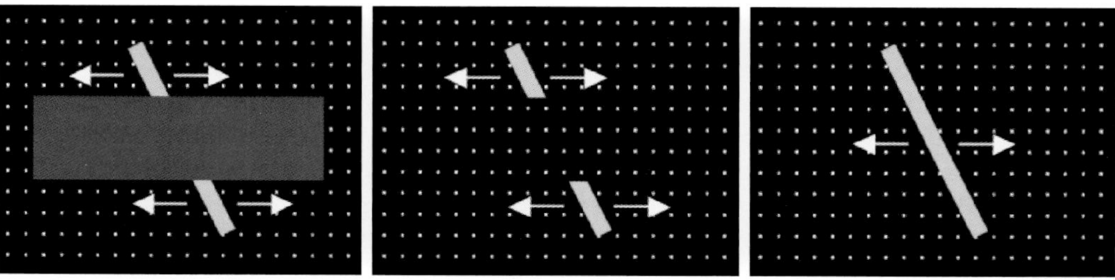

Figure 3.2 Schematic depictions of displays used to assess infants' perception of object unity, or spatial completion. Left: The display shown during habituation consists of two aligned rod parts moving in tandem above and below an occluder. Center: Broken test display. Right: Complete rod test display. Note: Real, 3D objects were used in the original Kellman and Spelke (1983) experiments; displays depicted here are adapted from 2D versions (Johnson & Náñez, 1995).

in fact the best that can be said about infant performance in most such paradigms is that there is a short-term representation of an object that is maintained for a matter of seconds (cf. Haith, 1998; Kagan, 2008). This is a far cry from Piaget's criteria for full object permanence, which requires accurate search in multiple locations for a desired hidden object, accessing knowledge of both persistence and the spatial relations between the object, the hiding locations, and the infant.

Second, nativist theories contribute little if any substantive knowledge about developmental mechanisms underlying object perception. Even on a strictly maturational account stipulating developments that are exclusive of visual experience, there are means by which the infant comes to perceive and represent objects, and these means may be amenable to empirical investigation.

Third, there is substantial evidence that newborn infants do not perceive moving, partly occluded objects as having hidden parts. Instead, neonates appear to construe such stimuli solely in terms of their visible parts, failing to achieve spatial completion (Slater, Johnson, Brown, & Badenoch, 1996; Slater et al., 1990; but see Valenza, Leo, Gava, & Simion, 2006, for evidence against this possibility). This and other findings show clear evidence for a developmental progression in perceptual completion and call for an explanation of underlying mechanisms of change. This is the goal of the experiments described in the following sections of this chapter.

Spatial Completion

Adults and 4-month-old infants construe the occlusion display depicted in Figure 3.2 as consisting of two parts, a single rod or bar moving back and forth behind an occluding rectangle (Kellman & Spelke, 1983). Neonates, by contrast, perceive this display as consisting of three separate parts: two disjoint rod parts and an occluder (Slater et al., 1990, 1996). These conclusions arise from looking time experiments described previously in which posthabituation looking patterns are thought to reflect a novelty preference; the 4-month-olds and neonates show opposite patterns of preference. This has led to the more general conclusion that neonates are unable to perceive occlusion, and that occlusion perception emerges over the first several postnatal months (Johnson, 2004). That is, "piecemeal" or fragmented perception of the visual environment extends from birth through the first several months afterward, implying a fundamental shift in the infant's perceptual experience: "During the first few months of existence the child's universe is really lacking permanent objects... this means that perceived figures simply appear and disappear like moving tableaux and exhibit a series of changing shapes in between" (Piaget & Inhelder, 1956, p. 9).

Because neonates and 4-month-olds appear to regard rod-and-box displays differently—as separate surfaces and as occluded objects, respectively—an important step in understanding development of spatial completion is investigations of performance in infants between these ages. In the first such investigation, 2-month-olds were found to show an "intermediate" pattern of performance—no reliable posthabituation preference—implying that spatial completion is developing at this point but not yet complete (Johnson & Náñez, 1995). A follow-up study examined the possibility that 2-month-olds will perceive unity if given additional perceptual support. The amount of visible rod surface revealed behind the occluder was enhanced by reducing box height and by adding gaps in it, and under these conditions 2-month-olds provided evidence of unity perception (Johnson & Aslin, 1995). With newborns, however, this manipulation failed to reveal similar evidence: Even in enhanced displays, newborns seemed to perceive disjoint rather than unified rod parts (Slater et al., 1996; Slater, Johnson, Kellman, & Spelke, 1994). These experiments served to pinpoint more precisely the time of emergence of spatial completion in infancy: the first several weeks or months after birth under typical circumstances.

Additional experiments explored the kinds of visual information infants use to perceive spatial completion. Our starting point was the Gestalt cues of good continuation and common

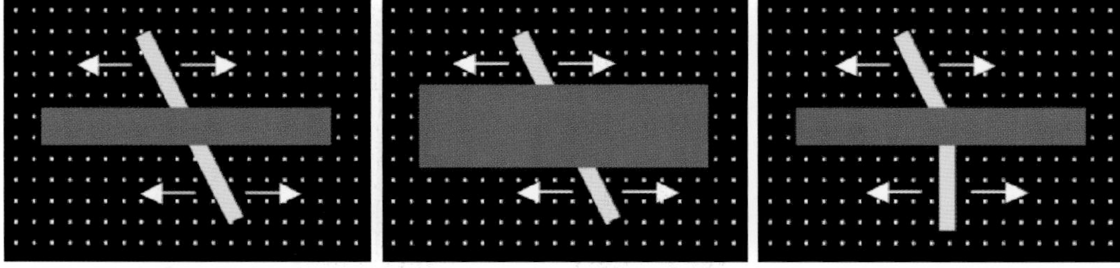

Figure 3.3 Schematic depictions of displays used to assess 2-month-olds' spatial completion. Infants perceived completion only when rod parts were aligned and the occluder was relatively narrow (left). Infants provided evidence of perceiving disjoint surfaces in the other displays. Adapted from Johnson (2004).

motion, also known as common fate. The Kellman and Spelke (1983) experiments provided evidence that 4-month-olds perceived object unity only when the rod parts moved in tandem behind a stationary occluder. We replicated and extended this finding, showing in addition that 4-month-olds provided evidence of completion only when the rod parts were aligned (Johnson & Aslin, 1996). Later experiments revealed similar patterns of performance in 2-month-olds when tested using displays with different occluder sizes and edge arrangements, as seen in Figure 3.3 (Johnson, 2004). Perceptual completion obtained only when rod parts were aligned across a narrow occluder; in the other displays, infants provided evidence of disjoint surface perception.

One possible interpretation of these findings is that alignment, motion, and occluder width (i.e., the spatial gap) are interdependent contributions to spatial completion, such that common motion is detected most effectively when rod parts are aligned (Kellman & Arterberry, 1998). I evaluated this possibility in experiments probing 2-month-olds' discrimination of different patterns of rod motion with varying orientations of rod parts and occluder widths. Under all tested conditions, infants discriminated the motion patterns, implying that motion discrimination was neither impaired nor facilitated by misalignment or occluder width. The precise contributions of motion to spatial completion in infants remain unknown; one possibility is that motion serves multiple functions, first serving to segment the scene into its constituent surfaces, and then serving to bind moving surfaces into a single object (Johnson, Davidow, Hall-Haro, & Frank, 2008).

In summary, experiments that examine development of spatial completion provide support for the possibility that young infants analyze the motions and arrangements of visible surfaces and initially (at birth) perceive them as separate from one another and the background. Only later do infants integrate these surfaces into percepts of coherent, partly occluded objects. According to this view, therefore, development of object knowledge begins with perception of visible object components, and proceeds with increasing proficiency at representation of those object parts that cannot be discerned directly.

Learning to Perceive Spatial Completion

In this section, I will describe experiments designed to elucidate developmental mechanisms of spatial completion. An important part of the developmental explanation revealed by these experiments is the strong relation between oculomotor scanning patterns—eye movements—and unity perception. Amso and Johnson (2006) and Johnson, Slemmer, and Amso (2004) observed 3-month-old infants in a spatial completion task using the habituation paradigm described previously. Infants' eye movements were recorded with a corneal reflection eye tracker during the habituation phase of the experiment. We found systematic differences in scanning patterns between infants

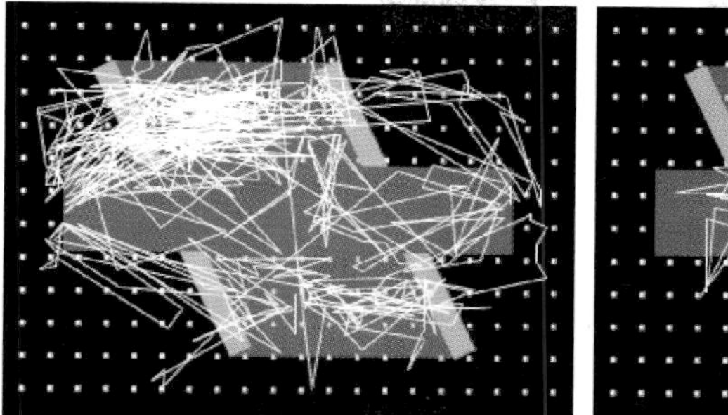
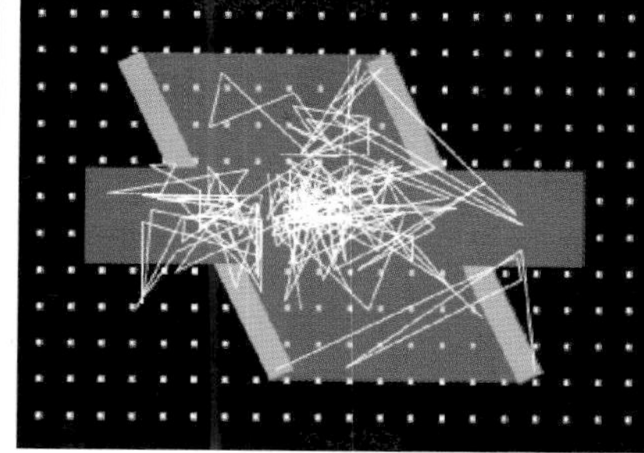

Figure 3.4 Scan patterns of a "perceiver" (left) and a "nonperceiver" (right), both 3-month-olds, from Amso and Johnson (2006). The leftmost and rightmost positions of the rod during its motion are shown. Scan paths are depicted as lines between points, which represent fixations.

whose posthabituation test display preferences indicated unity perception and infants who provided evidence of perception of disjoint surfaces: "Perceivers" tended to scan more in the vicinity of the two visible rod segments, and to scan back and forth between them (Figure 3.4). In a somewhat younger sample (58 to 97 days), Johnson et al. (2008) found a reliable correlation between posthabituation preference—our index of spatial completion—and targeted visual exploration, the proportion of eye movements directed toward the moving rod parts, which we reasoned was the most relevant aspect of the stimulus for perception of completion. Spatial completion was not predicted by other measures of oculomotor performance, including mean number of eye movements per second, mean distance between fixations, and the "dispersion" of visual attention, an assessment of "global" versus "local" scanning activity. Spatial completion was best predicted by saccades directed toward the vicinity of the moving rod parts. This can be a challenge for a developing oculomotor system, attested by the fact that targeted scans almost always followed the rod as it moved, rarely anticipating its position.

How targeted visual exploration emerges in infancy to maximize effective uptake of visual information is not yet known. Very young infants' ability to perceive occlusion may be challenged by difficulties in accessing visual information for unity such as alignment and common motion of edges across a spatial gap. Alternatively, insufficient information acquisition may lead to a "default" response to the visible surfaces only, characteristic of neonates, yielding a novelty preference for the complete rod at test. Either of the possibilities is consistent with the idea that efficient visual exploration is an important mechanism of development in object perception.

How do these findings provide evidence for learning as a mechanism of spatial completion? A nativist view stressing innate mechanisms that are independent of experience might posit that spatial completion stems exclusively from maturation of neural structures responsible for object perception, such as connections in V1 and V2 mentioned previously. Then, as infants begin to perceive occlusion, their eye movement patterns support or confirm this percept. Unequivocal evidence for a direct role for targeted visual exploration in development of spatial completion would come from experiments in which individual differences in oculomotor patterns were observed in both spatial completion and some other visual task, and this was recently reported by Amso and Johnson (2006). We found that both spatial completion and scanning patterns were strongly related to performance in an independent visual search task in which targets were selected amongst distracters. This finding is inconsistent with the possibility that scanning patterns were tailored specifically to perceptual completion, and instead suggests that a general facility with targeted visual behavior leads to improvements across multiple tasks.

How might developing object perception systems benefit from targeted scans? Eye movements may serve as a vital binding mechanism due to the relatively restricted visual field and poor acuity characteristic of young infants' vision. Visual information in the periphery is more difficult to access with a single glance, increasing the need to scan between features to ascertain their relations to one another. Infants who are more likely to do this will increase their processing of relevant features and their correspondences, as irrelevant features are ignored.

In summary, the individual differences in targeted visual exploration that we have observed suggest that scanning patterns make a vital contribution to the emergence of veridical object perception. Evidence suggests that as scanning patterns develop, they enable learning of relevant visual features of the environment, and support binding of these features into coherent percepts of unified objects.

Spatiotemporal completion

A number of studies using different methods (e.g., looking times, reaching in the dark) have shown that young infants can maintain representations for hidden objects across brief delays (e.g., Aguiar & Baillargeon, 1999; Clifton, Rochat, Litovsky, & Perris, 1991; Spelke, Breinlinger, Macomber, & Jacobson, 1992). Yet, as mentioned previously, newborns provide little evidence of perceiving partly occluded objects—that is, spatial completion—findings that raise the question of how perception of complete occlusion emerges during the first few months after birth. Apart from Piaget's theory, this question has received relatively little serious attention until recently, in favor of accounts that stress innate object concepts (e.g., Baillargeon, 2008; Spelke, 1990).

To address this gap in our knowledge, my colleagues and I have conducted experiments with computer-generated displays in which objects moved on a trajectory, disappeared behind an occluder, reappeared on the far side, and reversed direction, repeating the cycle. We reasoned that manipulation of spatial and temporal characteristics of the stimuli, and the use of different age groups, might provide insights into development of spatiotemporal completion, as they did in the case of spatial completion.

These investigations revealed a fragmented-to-holistic developmental pattern, and revealed spatial and temporal processing constraints as well. Both sets of results are in parallel with the investigations of spatial completion described in the previous section. Spatiotemporal completion was tested using similar methods: habituation to an occlusion display (Figure 3.5), followed by broken and complete test displays, and different versions of the partly hidden trajectory seen during habituation. At 4 months, infants treat the ball-and-box display depicted in Figure 3.5 as consisting of two disconnected trajectories, rather than a single, partly hidden

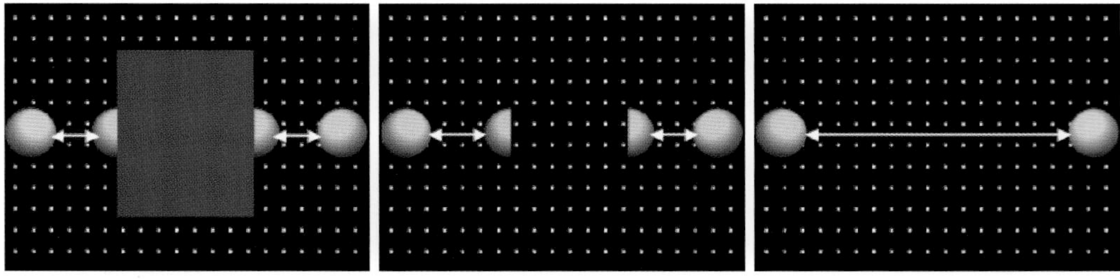

Figure 3.5 Schematic depictions of displays used to assess infants' perception of occluded trajectories, or spatiotemporal completion. Left: The display shown during habituation consists of two segments of object trajectory. Center: Discontinuous trajectory test display. Right: Continuous trajectory rod test display. Adapted from Johnson, Bremner et al. (2003).

path (Johnson et al., 2003); evidence comes from a reliable preference for the continuous version of the test trajectory. By 6 months, infants perceived this trajectory as unitary, as revealed by a reliable preference for the discontinuous trajectory test stimulus. When occluder size was narrowed, however, reducing the spatiotemporal gap across which the trajectory had to be interpolated, 4-month-olds' posthabituation preferences (and thus, by inference, their percepts of spatiotemporal completion) were shifted toward the discontinuous, partway by an intermediate width, and fully by a narrow width, so narrow as to be only slightly larger than the ball itself. In 2-month-olds, this manipulation appeared to have no effect.

Reducing the spatiotemporal gap, therefore, facilitates spatiotemporal completion. Reducing the temporal gap during which an object is hidden, independently from the spatial gap, also supports spatiotemporal completion. Increasing the ball size (Figure 3.6) can minimize the time out of sight as it passes behind the occluder, and this led 4-month-olds to perceive its trajectory as complete. Accelerating the speed of a smaller ball as it passed behind the occluder (and appeared more quickly) had a similar effect (Bremner et al., 2005). On the other hand, altering the orientation of the trajectory-impaired path completion (Figure 3.6), unless the edges of the occluder were orthogonal to the path; these findings are similar to outcomes of experiments on edge misalignment described in the previous section (Bremner et al., 2007).

This work leads to two conclusions. First, there may be a lower age limit for trajectory completion (between 2 and 4 months), just as there appears to be for spatial completion (between birth and 2 months). Second, young infants' spatiotemporal completion is based on relatively simple parameters. Either a short time or short distance out of sight leads to perception of continuity, and this may occur because the processing load is reduced by these manipulations. The fragile nature of emerging spatiotemporal completion is underscored as well by results showing its breakdown when either occluder or path orientation is nonorthogonal.

Learning to Perceive Spatiotemporal Completion

Piaget (1954) described a series of infants' behaviors providing evidence for an emerging ability to track objects that became occluded. Before the development of skilled manual search at about 4 to 6 months, search for hidden objects was exclusively visual. For example, Piaget's son Laurent, at 2 months, was reported to maintain gaze at a point where Piaget had been seen previously, a passive expectation of his father's reappearance. More active visual search behavior emerged after 4 months, such as visual "accommodation," as when an infant would respond to a dropped object by looking down toward the floor, a behavior observed in Laurent at 6.5 months. On Piaget's theory, visual accommodation or anticipation becomes more consistent as the infant learns from self-directed manipulation of objects, providing

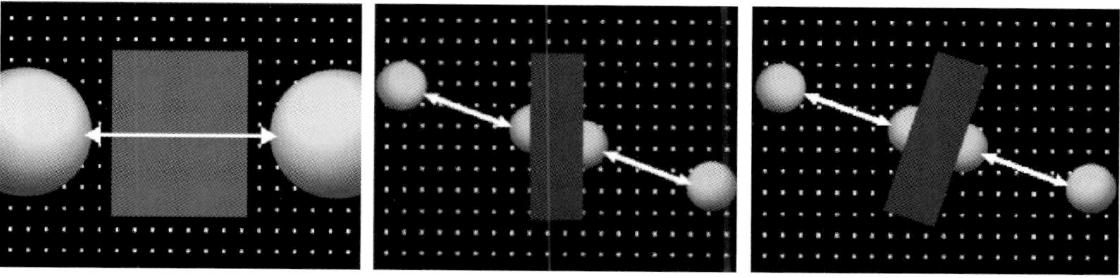

Figure 3.6 Schematic depictions of displays used to examine conditions under which infants show evidence of spatiotemporal completion. Adapted from Bremner et al. (2005, 2007).

direct experience with dropping and retrieval, and develops alongside reconstruction of partly occluded objects from visible fragments, which I have referred to in this chapter as spatial completion. Piaget suggested that increasing visual, tactile, and manual experience is a vital developmental mechanism in developing more complex concepts of objects.

More recent research has shown that by 6 months, infants' representations of hidden objects are sufficiently robust to guide reaching prospectively to intercept objects on occluded trajectories (Clifton et al., 1991; von Hofsten, Vishton, Spelke, Feng, & Rosander, 1998). Researchers have built on these ideas by recording infants' eye movements as they view repetitive events in which objects move behind an occluder and subsequently reemerge, such as that shown in Figure 3.5. The question is the extent to which infants produce anticipatory eye movements toward the place of reemergence while the object is out of view, implying a functional representation of the object that guides oculomotor behavior.

At 4 months, prospective behavior—anticipations from eye and head movements to the place of reappearance of an object seen to move behind an occluder—is adapted to variations in occluder width and object speed, implying that under some conditions, infants may track with their "mind's eye" (von Hofsten, Kochukhova, & Rosander, 2007). At 6 months, infants begin to respond to nonlinear trajectories, showing spatially accurate predictive eye movements when a target moves on a partly occluded circular path (Gredebäck & von Hofsten, 2004; Gredebäck, von Hofsten, & Boudreau, 2002). Yet the evidence from habituation experiments described previously indicates 4-month-olds process partly occluded trajectories in terms of visible components only, not complete paths, when tested under conditions that challenge spatiotemporal completion (Johnson, Bremner, et al., 2003), and, notably, the lower bound for predictive tracking is about 12 weeks (Rosander & von Hofsten, 2004). These results indicate that representations of occluded objects in 4-month-olds may be rather fragile and not completely established, and, more broadly, that representations of occluded objects are weak if not nonexistent in very young infants, and gradually strengthen across the first year after birth (Munakata, 2001; Piaget, 1954).

To examine the possibility that learning plays an important role in development of spatiotemporal completion, my colleagues and I presented ball-and-box displays to 4- and 6-month-olds as we recorded their eye movements (Johnson, Amso, & Slemmer, 2003). The stimulus was identical to the displays used by Johnson, Bremner et al. (2003) (Figure 3.5). Because 6-month-olds provided evidence of spatiotemporal completion in these displays when tested with a habituation paradigm, we predicted that oculomotor anticipations would be more frequent in the older age group. This prediction was supported. A higher proportion of 6-month-olds' eye movements was classified as anticipatory (i.e., initiated prior to the ball's emergence from behind the occluder) relative to 4-month-olds, corroborating the likelihood that spatiotemporal completion strengthens between 4 and 6 months.

As noted previously, 4 months is a time of transition toward spatiotemporal completion, raising questions about the role of experience in oculomotor anticipation performance at this age. There is mixed evidence for short-term gains in predictive performance, gains that hypothetically might arise from repeated exposure to a target object that moves in a perfectly predictable manner (to adults). In other words, we might expect infants to show more reliable anticipation as they view multiple instances of an object emerging from behind an occluder. Rosander and von Hofsten (2004) found that predictive performance of the oldest infants they observed (21-week-olds) improved with repeated exposure to four complete cycles of motion, in terms of decreasing eye movement latencies as a function of trial. By contrast, Gredebäck et al. (2002) and Johnson, Amso, and Slemmer (2003) found that oculomotor anticipations declined across trials in infants ranging from 4 to 9 months. In these studies, infants were exposed to several dozen opportunities to learn about the repetitive event during the sequence of trials, yet performance declined consistently. In general, therefore, infants do not seem to capitalize on the predictable nature of occlusion stimuli in producing predictive eye movements, implying that infants do not acquire spatiotemporal completion solely by means of this kind of experience.

But of course the visual environment in the real world is not limited to dynamic occlusion events. There are many instances of objects that move in full view, and infants will track moving objects from the first opportunities to do so, at birth (Slater, 1995). What do infants learn by watching such events? We addressed this question with a "training" paradigm: presenting infants with unoccluded object trajectory displays for 2 min immediately preceding the occlusion stimulus seen in Figure 3.5 (Johnson, Amso, & Slemmer, 2003). Following training, the 4-month-olds' performance was statistically indistinguishable from that of the 6-month-olds, providing evidence for rapid learning of spatiotemporal completion. Data from a second training condition indicates that we were not simply facilitating horizontal eye movements that carried over from training to test. This second training condition used a vertical unoccluded trajectory for training, followed as before by the (horizontal) occlusion display. Again, performance was statistically indistinguishable from that of the older infants.

Brief training, therefore, brought 4-month-olds to a level of predictive performance similar to that of older infants. How might this work in infants' everyday environment? In the real world, infants are exposed to many different objects moving in different ways, presenting multiple opportunities for learning. It may be that repeated exposure to moving objects, and repeated viewing of objects as they move in and out of view due to occlusion, leads to an associative link between the two scenarios. These associations accrue gradually in everyday learning, attested by the relatively long span between improvements in performance (between 4 and 6 months), but the learning mechanisms themselves are remarkably efficient, attested by the very brief training interval (2 min) necessary to bridge this gap in performance in the laboratory.

For associative learning about occlusion to be a viable means of dealing with real-world events, associations between visible and partly occluded paths must be committed to memory. How long do such rapidly acquired associations last? To address this question, we replicated the Johnson, Slemmer, and Amso (2003) methods and observed a nearly identical pattern of anticipatory behaviors by 4-month-olds in baseline and training conditions (Johnson & Shuwairi, 2009). A third group received a half-hour break between training and test, and performance reverted to baseline, implying that memory for the association was lost during the delay. But a fourth group, provided with a single "reminder" trial after an identical delay, showed a recovery of oculomotor anticipations equivalent to the no-delay training condition. (A fifth group, provided only a single training trial, showed no benefit in the form of anticipatory looking.) These findings suggest that accumulated exposure to occlusion events may be an important means by which spatiotemporal completion arises in infancy.

In summary, research that examines infants' oculomotor anticipations as they view repetitive dynamic occlusion events is broadly consistent with Piaget's original descriptions of infant performance: There is little evidence of systematic predictive behavior prior to 4 months, after which time anticipations become robust and flexible, and performance continues to improve with age. It seems unlikely, however, that direct manual experience with objects is a principal developmental mechanism driving the emergence of this predictive behavior, because oculomotor anticipations begin to become established prior to the onset of functional goal-directed reaching and manual object manipulation in developmental time. Experiments described in the next section, however, provide evidence for a vital role for manual experience in development of perception of objects as coherent in 3D space.

3D OBJECT COMPLETION

Spatial and spatiotemporal completion consist of filling in the gaps in object surfaces that have been occluded by nearer ones. Solid objects also occlude parts of themselves such that we cannot see their hidden surfaces from our present vantage point, yet our experience of most objects is that of filled volumes rather than hollow shells. Perceiving objects as solid in 3D space despite limited views constitutes 3D object completion. In contrast to spatial and spatiotemporal completion, little is known about development of 3D object completion. We recently addressed this question with a looking time paradigm similar to those described previously (Soska & Johnson, 2008a). Four- and 6-month-olds were habituated to a wedge rotating through 15° around the vertical axis such that the far sides were never revealed (Figure 3.7). Following habituation, infants viewed two test displays in alternation, one an incomplete, hollow version of the wedge, and the other a complete, whole version, both undergoing a full 360° rotation revealing the entirety of the object shape. Four-month-olds showed no consistent posthabituation preference, but 6-month-olds looked longer at the hollow stimulus, indicating perception of the wedge during habituation as a solid, volumetric object in 3D space.

In a follow-up study (Soska & Johnson, 2008b), we used these same methods with a more complex stimulus: a solid "L"-shaped object with eight faces and vertices, as opposed to the five faces and six vertices in the wedge-shaped object described previously. We tested 4-, 6-, and 9.5-month-olds. As in the Soska and Johnson (2008a) study with the wedge stimulus, we found a developmental progression in 3D object completion: 4-month-olds' posthabituation looking times revealed no evidence for completion, whereas 9.5-month-olds consistently looked longer at the hollow test display, implying perception of the habituation object as volumetric in 3D space. At 6 months, interestingly, only the male infants showed this preference; females looked about equally at the two test displays. (At 9.5 months, the male advantage had disappeared: both males and females looked longer at the hollow shape.)

Data from the Soska and Johnson (2008a, 2008b) studies provide evidence for a developmental progression in infants' 3D object completion abilities, and for a sex difference in these abilities that is revealed at a transitional period in this skill—6 months—but only when infants'

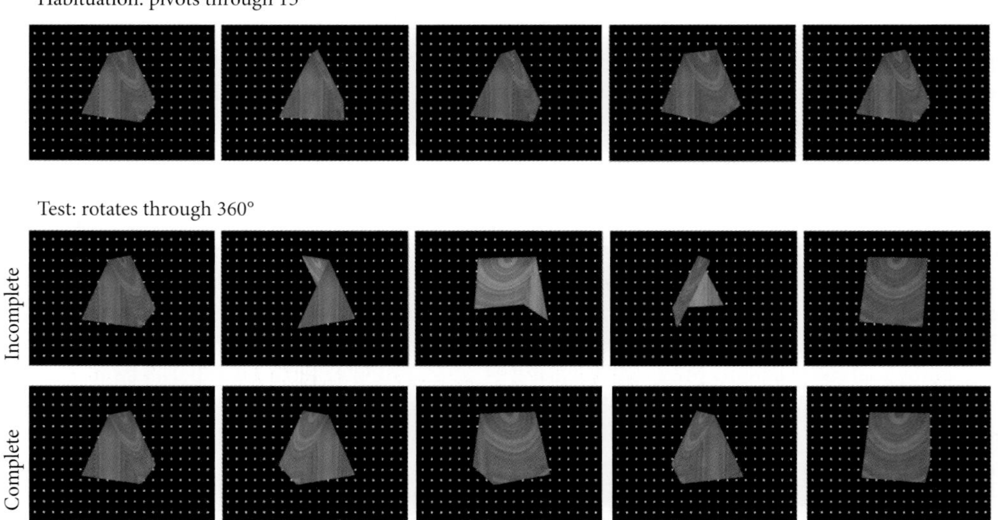

Figure 3.7 Schematic depictions of displays used to investigate 3D object completion in infants. Adapted from Soska and Johnson (2008a).

views were tested with relatively complex stimuli. It may be that the infants who were successful at 3D object completion engaged in mental rotation in this task: manipulation of a mental image of the object and imagining it from a different perspective. Mental rotation is a cognitive skill for which men have an advantage relative to women (Shepard & Metzler, 1971; Zacks, 2008), and two recent reports have provided evidence of a male advantage in young infants as well (Moore & Johnson, 2009; Quinn & Liben, 2009). It remains to be determined definitely whether mental rotation is involved in 3D object completion; at present, it is clear that it develops early in postnatal life, alongside spatial and spatiotemporal completion.

Learning to Perceive 3D Object Completion

How does 3D object completion arise? One possibility is that emerging motor skills support perception of objects as coherent volumes. Two types of motor skills, both of which undergo dramatic improvements between 4 and 6 months, may be particularly important: self-sitting ability and coordinated visual–manual object exploration. Independent sitting frees the hands for play and promotes gaze stabilization during manual actions (Rochat & Goubet, 1995). Thus, self-sitting might spur coordination of object manipulation (e.g., rotating and transferring objects hand-to-hand) with visual inspection, providing infants with multiple views of objects. Stroking, poking, turning, and transferring objects hand to hand may promote learning about object form by supplying tactile information and would provide multiple views at the same time.

To examine these possibilities, we tested infants between 4.5 and 7.5 months in a replication of the Soska and Johnson (2008a) habituation experiment with the rotating wedge stimuli (Soska, Adolph, & Johnson, in press). In addition, we assessed infants' manual exploration skills by observing their spontaneous object manipulation in a controlled setting and obtained parental reports of the duration of infants' sitting experience. We reasoned that infants who showed a greater tendency to explore objects from multiple viewpoints would also have had more opportunities to learn about objects' 3D forms outside the laboratory. Thus, within this age range, individual differences in coordinated visual–manual exploration (rotations, fingerings, and transfers with looking at toys) and self-sitting experience should predict individual differences in infants' looking preferences to the complete and incomplete object displays, our index of 3D object completion.

These predictions were supported. We found strong and significant relations between both self-sitting and visual–manual coordination (from the motor skills assessment) and our measure of 3D object completion (from the habituation paradigm). (Other motor skills we recorded, such as holding skill and manual exploration without visual attention to the objects, did not predict 3D object completion.) Self-sitting experience and coordinated visual–manual exploration were the strongest predictors of performance on the visual habituation task, but it seems that the role of self-sitting was indirect, influencing 3D completion chiefly because of its support of infants' visual–manual exploration. Self-sitting infants performed more manual exploration while looking at objects than did nonsitters, and visual–manual object exploration is precisely the skill that provides active experience viewing objects from multiple viewpoints, thereby facilitating perceptual completion of 3D form. These results provide evidence for a cascade of developmental events following from the advent of visual–motor coordination, including learning from self-produced experiences.

In principle, 3D object completion might develop from more passive perceptual experiences, but the findings yielded by the Soska et al. (in press) experiment indicate that passive experience may be insufficient to learn about 3D object form. Active exploration provides information to the infant about her own control of an event while simultaneously generating multimodal information to inform developing object perception skills. Coordinating visual inspection with manual exploration seems to be critical: Only the visual–manual skills involved in generating changes in object viewpoint—rotating, fingering, and transferring while looking—were related to 3D object completion.

SUMMARY AND CONCLUSIONS

I have described a set of object perception skills that develop early in infancy, focusing on three ways in which observers fill in the gaps in perception imposed by occlusion: spatial completion, spatiotemporal completion, and 3D object completion. And I have described experiments designed to examine developmental mechanisms of perceptual completion in infants. The best evidence to date suggests that newborn infants do not fill in the gaps in perception, and therefore, do not perceive objects as do adults. Instead, the visual world of neonates seems to consist solely of surface fragments that have no substance, volume, or continuity. Infants initially appear to process complex stimuli as simple isolated units, and subsequently integrate them into higher-order patterns.

This developmental progression is consistent with a constructivist view of cognitive development, and consistent with developmental patterns in other domains, as described in the remainder of the chapters in this book. A constructivist view attempts to understand development in terms of information processing principles (Cohen & Cashon, 2006). According to this approach, infants process information at the highest level of complexity possible, but this level depends on the infant's individual capacity and on task demands. Processing capacity expands with development, which helps to explain why older infants and children are better able to see configurations and relations among parts, and it is constrained by task complexity, which helps to explain why perception of intricate, multielement stimuli may break down when perceptual systems become "overloaded" (see the chapter by Cohen in this volume).

Each of the three kinds of filling-in I have described appears to proceed on a separate developmental timetable with a unique set of developmental mechanisms, yet they have in common a prominent role for learning: *learning by doing*, evinced by the importance of oculomotor and manual action systems in spatial and 3D object completion, respectively, and *learning by observation*, evinced by the importance of associating views of fully visible and partly occluded trajectories in spatiotemporal completion. The potential role of learning fundamental object concepts and their developmental antecedents is becoming increasingly clear from the experiments I have described in this chapter, in their suggestion that infants use developing perceptual, cognitive, and action systems to learn about the visual environment, and to assemble its constituent parts into coherent wholes.

ACKNOWLEDGMENT

Preparation of this article was supported by NIH grants R01-HD40432 and R01-HD48733.

REFERENCES

Aguiar, A., & Baillargeon, R. (1999). 2.5-month-old infants' reasoning about when objects should and should not be occluded. *Cognitive Psychology, 39*, 116–157.

Amso, D., & Johnson, S. P. (2006). Learning by selection: Visual search and object perception in young infants. *Developmental Psychology, 6*, 1236–1245.

Baillargeon, R. (1995). A model of physical reasoning in infancy. In C. Rovee-Collier & L. P. Lipsitt (Eds.), *Advances in infancy research* (Vol. 9, pp. 305–371). Norwood, NJ: Ablex.

Baillargeon, R. (2008). Innate ideas revisited: For a principle of persistence in infants' physical reasoning. *Perspectives on Psychological Science, 3*, 2–13.

Baillargeon, R., Spelke, E. S., & Wasserman, S. (1985). Object permanence in five-month-old infants. *Developmental Psychology, 20*, 191–208.

Bower, T. G. R. (1967). Phenomenal identity and form perception in an infant. *Perception & Psychophysics, 2*, 74–76.

Bremner, J. G., Johnson, S. P., Slater, A., Mason, U., Cheshire, A., & Spring, J. (2007). Conditions for young infants' failure to perceive trajectory continuity. *Developmental Science, 10*, 613–624.

Bremner, J. G., Johnson, S. P., Slater, A. M., Mason, U., Foster, K., Cheshire, A., et al. (2005). Conditions for young infants' perception of object trajectories. *Child Development, 74*, 1029–1043.

Burkhalter, A. (1993). Development of forward and feedback connections between areas V1 and V2 of human visual cortex. *Cerebral Cortex, 3*, 476–487.

Burkhalter, A., Bernardo, K. L., & Charles, V. (1993). Development of local circuits in human visual cortex. *The Journal of Neuroscience, 13*, 1916–1931.

Clifton, R. K., Rochat, P., Litovsky, R. Y., & Perris, E. E. (1991). Object representation guides infants' reaching in the dark. *Journal of Experimental Psychology: Human Perception and Performance, 17*, 323–329.

Cohen, L. B., & Cashon, C. H. (2006). Infant cognition. In D. Kuhn & R. S. Siegler (Eds.), *Handbook of child psychology: Vol. 2. Cognition, perception, and language* (6th ed., pp. 214–251). New York: Wiley.

Gredebäck, G., & von Hofsten, C. (2004). Infants' evolving representations of object motion during occlusion: A longitudinal study of 6- to 12-month-old infants. *Infancy, 6*, 165–184.

Gredebäck, G., von Hofsten, C., & Boudreau, J. P. (2002). Infants' visual tracking of continuous circular motion under conditions of occlusion and non-occlusion. *Infant Behavior & Development, 25*, 161–182.

Haith, M. M. (1998). Who put the cog in infant cognition? Is rich interpretation too costly? *Infant Behavior & Development, 21*, 167–179.

Johnson, S. P. (2004). Development of perceptual completion in infancy. *Psychological Science, 15*, 769–775.

Johnson, S. P., Amso, D., & Slemmer, J. A. (2003). Development of object concepts in infancy: Evidence for early learning in an eye tracking paradigm. *Proceedings of the National Academy of Sciences, USA, 100*, 10568–10573.

Johnson, S. P., & Aslin, R. N. (1995). Perception of object unity in 2-month-old infants. *Developmental Psychology, 31*, 739–745.

Johnson, S. P., & Aslin, R. N. (1996). Perception of object unity in young infants: The roles of motion, depth, and orientation. *Cognitive Development, 11*, 161–180.

Johnson, S. P., Bremner, J. G., Slater, A., Mason, U., Foster, K., & Cheshire, A. (2003). Infants' perception of object trajectories. *Child Development, 74*, 94–108.

Johnson, S. P., Davidow, J., Hall-Haro, C., & Frank, M. C. (2008). Development of perceptual completion originates in information acquisition. *Developmental Psychology, 44*, 1214–1224.

Johnson, S. P., & Náñez, J. E. (1995). Young infants' perception of object unity in two-dimensional displays. *Infant Behavior & Development, 18*, 133–143.

Johnson, S. P., Slemmer, J. A., & Amso, D. (2004). Where infants look determines how they see: Eye movements and object perception performance in 3-month-olds. *Infancy, 6*, 185–201.

Kagan, J. (2008). In defense of qualitative changes in development. *Child Development, 79*, 1606–1624.

Kellman, P. J., & Arterberry, M. E. (1998). *The cradle of knowledge: The development of perception in infancy*. Cambridge, MA: MIT Press.

Kellman, P. J., & Spelke, E. S. (1983). Perception of partly occluded objects in infancy. *Cognitive Psychology, 15*, 483–524.

Moore, D. S., & Johnson, S. P. (2008). Mental rotation in human infants: A sex difference. *Psychological Science, 19*, 1063–1066.

Munakata, Y. (2001). Graded representations in behavioral dissociations. *Trends in Cognitive Sciences, 5*, 309–315.

Peterhans, E., & von der Heydt, R. (1991). Subjective contours—bridging the gap between psychophysics and physiology. *Trends in Neurosciences, 3*, 112–119.

Piaget, J. (1954). *The construction of reality in the child* (M. Cook, Trans.). New York: Basic Books. (Original work published 1937).

Piaget, J., & Inhelder, B. (1956). *The child's conception of space*. New York: Routledge. (Original work published 1948).

Quinn, P. C., & Liben, L. S. (2008). A sex difference in mental rotation in young infants. *Psychological Science, 19*, 1067–1070.

Rochat, P., & Goubet, N. (1995). Development of sitting and reaching in 5- to 6-month-old infants. *Infant Behavior & Development, 18*, 53–68.

Rosander, K., & von Hofsten, C. (2004). Infants' emerging ability to represent occluded object motion. *Cognition, 91*, 1–22.

Shepard, R. N., & Metzler, J. (1971). Mental rotation of three-dimensional objects. *Science, 171*, 701–703.

Slater, A. (1995). Visual perception and memory at birth. In C. Rovee-Collier & L. P. Lipsitt (Eds.), *Advances in infancy research* (Vol. 9, pp. 107–162). Norwood, NJ: Ablex.

Slater, A., Johnson, S. P., Brown, E., & Badenoch, M. (1996). Newborn infants' perception of partly occluded objects. *Infant Behavior & Development, 19*, 145–148.

Slater, A., Johnson, S. P., Kellman, P. J., & Spelke, E. S. (1994). The role of three-dimensional depth cues in infants' perception of partly occluded objects. *Early Development and Parenting, 3*, 187–191.

Slater, A., Morison, V., Somers, M., Mattock, A., Brown, E., & Taylor, D. (1990). Newborn and older infants' perception of partly occluded objects. *Infant Behavior & Development, 13*, 33–49.

Soska, K. C., Adolph, K. A., & Johnson, S. P. (in press). Systems in development: Motor skill acquisition facilitates 3D object completion. *Developmental Psychology.*

Soska, K. C., & Johnson, S. P. (2008a). Development of 3D object completion in infancy. *Child Development, 79*, 1230–1236.

Soska, K. C., & Johnson, S. P. (2008b). *Infants' 3D object completion in complex displays.* Manuscript in preparation.

Spelke, E. S. (1990). Principles of object perception. *Cognitive Science, 14*, 29–56.

Spelke, E. S., Breinlinger, K., Macomber, J., & Jacobson, K. (1992). Origins of knowledge. *Psychological Review, 99*, 605–632.

Valenza, E., Leo, I., Gava, L., & Simion, F. (2006). Perceptual completion in newborn human infants. *Child Development, 77*, 1810–1821.

von Hofsten, C., Kochukhova, O., & Rosander, K. (2007). Predictive tracking over occlusions in 4-month-old infants. *Developmental Science, 10*, 625–640.

von Hofsten, C., Vishton, P., Spelke, E. S., Feng, Q., & Rosander, K. (1998). Predictive action in infancy: Tracking and reaching for moving objects. *Cognition, 67*, 255–285.

Zacks, J. M. (2008). Neuroimaging studies of mental rotation: A meta-analysis and review. *Journal of Cognitive Neuroscience, 20*, 1–19.

CHAPTER 4
Numerical Identity and the Development of Object Permanence

M. Keith Moore and Andrew N. Meltzoff

INTRODUCTION

Numerical identity refers to an object being the selfsame individual over time. Our principal way of knowing an object's numerical identity is by tracing its spatial history. This is how we find "our" Coke can on a table full of Coke cans that all look alike. Numerical identity allows us to construe the changes in an object's appearance, location, motion, orientation, and visibility, as different manifestations of a single object rather than as many objects. It enables us to differentiate an encounter with a new object from a reencounter with the same one again. In this chapter, we propose that infants' developing understanding of numerical identity underlies their discovery of object permanence. We also suggest a mechanism for developmental change that derives from this view.

Object permanence refers to the fact that material objects are preserved over breaks in perceptual contact. When an occluder moves in front of an object, adults understand that the occluder blocks visual access to it. They know that the object still exists in a specific location in the world for every moment it is occluded. This understanding is what we mean when we say that objects are permanent over occlusion events. Thus conceived, object permanence provides a powerful tool for extracting structural regularity from experience.

Psychologists have been fascinated by infant object permanence ever since Piaget (1954) described the curious fact that young infants would not search for a highly desired object when it was hidden. For Piaget, a central task for infants was to extract an independent, enduring concept of objects from the infants' sensorimotor experience with them. Piaget's first key theoretical assumption was the primacy of the role of action. In early infancy, to "know" an object was to act upon it. Development derived from relating actions to one another and to consequences in the perceptual world (sensory–motor connections). The second key assumption was that a lack of sensory contact, especially invisibility, was an insurmountable problem for young infants. When sensory contact with objects was lost, objects ceased to exist for the infant ("out of sight is out of mind"). The development of representation around 18 months of age was postulated as the way infants transcended a purely sensorimotor world to realize that objects were permanent over all occlusion events. An object was not deemed to be fully independent of perception and action, and thus permanent, until infants could represent the invisible movements of an object that was stationary when it was occluded, an invisible displacement in Piaget's terms, at 18–24 months of age. His age-ordered search tasks were seen as measures of progress toward that end (see Table 4.1).

Many studies have replicated Piaget's stages of search for hidden objects. Yet, modern empirical research has largely undermined his key theoretical assumptions. We are left then with

Table 4.1 Summary of Piaget's Stages of Object Permanence Development

Stage	Age (months)	Sensorimotor Level	Object Permanence	Manual Search Behavior
1	0–1	Reflex repetition	None	None
2	1–4	Reflexes are coordinated by action on a common O	Search is only an extension of current action; visual tracking	None
3	4–8	Action is differentiated from its result; acts to prolong the result	Manual acts on part to conserve visible whole O	Finds partially hidden O, but not one totally hidden
4	8–12	Actions can be coordinated to achieve results; means–ends acts	O's existence is dependent on the last action on O	Finds totally hidden O in one location, but returns there if O is hidden in a new location (the A-not-B error)
5	12–18	Explores all variations of a new means act discovered by chance	O's existence depends on prior perception, but not prior action	Finds O where last displaced visibly, but not if moved invisibly
6	18–24	Representation allows invention of new means; hidden causes	O is independent of action and perception because represented	Finds O after invisible displacement from its last visible location

Note. O indicates object.

the puzzle of his ordered sequence in infants' manual search for hidden objects. A comprehensive theory of object permanence should explain the development of manual search for occluded objects and the invariant ordering of these steps.

Here we offer a solution to this puzzle that does not rely on Piagetian theory. In our view, the fundamental issue of object permanence is how infants use the visible transformations of their perceptual world, such as an object's occlusion and disocclusion, to develop an understanding of an invisible world that links these visible events. The infant's primary data are their encounters with objects disappearing and reappearing, which immediately poses a question about numerical identity. Thus, we propose that the origins and development of object permanence are preceded by development in infants' understanding of how to determine and trace numerical identity. We call this view the identity development (ID) account of object permanence (Moore & Meltzoff, 1999).

Identity Development Account's Relation to Other Theoretical Positions

Several strands of contemporary research, including ours, have been influenced by Bower's (1967, 1971) assertion that infants' notion of object identity influences their behavior. Studies building on this insight have explored how infants individuate different objects to determine how many are involved in a visual event (e.g., two objects seen simultaneously in different locations are different objects; Wilcox & Baillargeon, 1998; Xu & Carey, 1996). Leslie and colleagues (e.g., Leslie, Xu, Tremoulet, & Scholl, 1998) demonstrated that object identification (i.e., distinguishing which objects are involved in an event) is a related but more difficult task than individuation (for a review, see Krøjgaard, 2004). Still another strand of research on object identity has focused on how infants determine that the object before them is the same unique individual that they encountered previously—that it is the same one again (e.g., Moore, Borton, & Darby, 1978; Moore & Meltzoff, 1978). In this strand, infants' notions of numerical identity are said to develop and change as they experience objects in the world.

Structure of the Argument

As required of all developmental theories, the ID account has the burden of specifying (a) the foundational primitives underlying the earliest notions of object identity, (b) the principles that determine the course of successive developments, and (c) a mechanism of change accounting for how the transition from having no concept of permanence to having permanence occurs. This is a substantial challenge, and few developmental theories have met it.

We turn first to the theoretical assumptions and hypotheses of the ID account, and then take up the empirical methods needed to test it using manual search, and new evidence obtained with such methods. We then propose a detailed mechanism of change for the transition from treating occluded objects as impermanent to treating them as permanent. We conclude by evaluating four theories of object permanence: Piagetian, dynamical systems, nativist, and the ID account.

THEORETICAL UNDERPINNINGS OF THE IDENTITY DEVELOPMENT ACCOUNT

The ID account utilizes three theoretical terms that are often conflated—representation, identity, and permanence. We wish to differentiate them and show the resulting implications for describing infants' understanding of object permanence.

Identity and Permanence

The first fundamental assumption of the ID account, and one that cannot be overstressed, is that the infant's notion of the relation between permanence and numerical identity is radically different from that of adults. For adults, permanence entails identity, and identity entails permanence. Adults do not interpret an object as being permanent over a disappearance–reappearance unless they got the same object back. The permanence judgment depends on identity. Conversely, an adult does not interpret such an event as two encounters with the same object unless it continued to exist between encounters. The identity judgment depends on permanence. We hypothesize that as infants begin to understand permanence, it is only understood for certain kinds of disappearances and not others. We capture this by saying that permanence is constrained to the kinds of disappearance events that the infant can construe as preserving the numerical identity of the object. Thus, permanence depends on identity, but not the other way round.

In our view, the infants' prepermanence world is stranger still. They can determine object identity but do not treat objects as permanent. To illustrate this by analogy, infants' unusual cognitive representation of their prepermanence world would be like projecting an adult's 3-D perceptual world onto a 2-D TV screen. All of the interactions of objects would be visible because there are no invisible dimensions. Objects disappear at edges by deletion and reappear by accretion; there is no image overlap, so nothing is hidden. In this 2-D world, an individual image can be reidentified after absences on the basis of its place or trajectory of motion, without requiring that it be somewhere between appearances. It is spatiotemporally the same image, but it does not exist constantly, because there is nowhere for it to exist out of sight.

Identity and Representation

A second assumption of the ID account is that the infant representational system can relate a currently perceived object to a stored representation of that object. Identity criteria provide a means of linking the currently perceived object to its previously formed representation (i.e., the criteria describing the object representation match the criteria of the perceived object). We have argued that infants have such a representational system from birth, and that it is sufficient to maintain the numerical identity of visible objects participating in events with visible outcomes in a steady-state world—for example, reidentifying objects after looking away from them—and enabling infants to learn to predict object appearances after disappearances (for details, see Meltzoff & Moore, 1998).

Representation and Permanence

Another tenet of the ID account is that a further change in the representational system is needed to account for permanence. Object permanence, as we define it, is not simply maintaining a representation in mind, no matter how long it lasts. Nor, is it reidentifying the object as the same one again after it disappears and then reappears. Object permanence is the understanding that an individual object, while it is still invisible, continues to exist in a hidden location in the external world. To encompass permanence, the representational system has to link the representation of the object and the representation of its location, while neither object nor location is currently visible. When this is achieved, the infant can be said to know where the object is while it is out of sight. Such understanding is necessary to support intentional, permanence-directed search for an occluded object.

Identity Development Account

In this section, we elucidate a series of 10 interlocking hypotheses that comprise the ID account. The series describes the development and interrelationship of infants' notions of identity and permanence over the first 2 years of life. Because they are hypotheses, we cite relevant evidence where available. Finally, we propose a theoretically appropriate way to describe occlusion events.

Identity and Permanence Development: 10 Hypotheses

1. *The fundamental criteria for numerical identity are spatiotemporal parameters.* This idea draws on "quantitative" or "numerical" identity as described by philosophers (e.g., Strawson, 1959). The primary way of knowing that an object at one point in time is numerically identical to an object perceived at another point in time is by tracing the object's spatiotemporal history between these points of contact: If it is in the right place in space at the right time whenever it is seen, it is numerically the same object. The psychological reality of this analysis has been demonstrated by the use of spatiotemporal coordinates to address "object files" in studies of adult attention (Kahneman, Treisman, & Gibbs, 1992; Treisman, 1992) and object identity and indexing in infants (Bower, 1982; Carey & Xu, 2001; Leslie et al., 1998).

2. *Infants are innately prepared for a Newtonian world operating according to the first law of kinematics: Objects at rest remain at rest; objects in motion continue in motion.* Infants are evolutionarily prepared for interacting with objects in a Newtonian steady-state world, and the first spatiotemporal distinction is whether the object is at rest or in motion. The spatiotemporal parameters that capture this distinction are its *place* in space for a stationary object or its *trajectory* of motion for a moving object. Neuroscientists have shown that the location of objects in space and their trajectories of motion can be established by perceptual processing (Haxby et al., 1991; Köhler, Kapur, Moscovitch, Winocur, & Houle, 1995; Watamaniuk & McKee, 1995; Watamaniuk, McKee, & Grzywacz, 1995).

To be "evolutionarily prepared" does not mean that infants are born with an adult-like notion of trajectory, for example, but rather that they are predisposed to detect a trajectory of visual motion—the constant movement of a visual feature in a particular direction—from a background of random-direction noise. These "trajectory detectors" are thought to be higher-level units in the visual system extracting coherent signals in space and time from lower-level motion detectors (Grzywacz, Watamaniuk, & McKee, 1995). Such evolutionary preparedness underlies the development of smooth pursuit visual tracking, the perception of object trajectories, and their representation (Aslin, 1981;

Bremner et al., 2005; Johnson, Bremner et al., 2003).[1]

3. *The spatiotemporal parameters of an object's place and/or trajectory act as identity criteria, allowing the object to be identified as the same one again after breaks in perceptual contact.* The earliest identity logic used by infants is that a stationary object encountered in the same place as one seen previously in that place is the same object again. Similarly, a moving object encountered on the same trajectory of motion as one seen previously on that trajectory is the same object again. Spatiotemporal parameters initially override featural appearance in judgments of numerical identity. Young infants do not treat a pre- to postdisappearance change of object features as specifying a different object as long as the altered object reappears in the place or on the trajectory established by their first encounter with it (Bower, Broughton, & Moore, 1971; Krøjgaard, 2007; Newcombe, Huttenlocher, & Learmonth, 1999; Van de Walle, Carey, & Prevor, 2000; Wilcox & Baillargeon, 1998; Xu & Carey, 1996).

4. *Experience from repeated encounters with visible objects allows infants to learn which object properties are preserved over events (so long as the object can be construed as the same one—i.e., in the same place or on the same trajectory).* Initially, an object's properties play no role in judgments of numerical identity (#3 above). Thus, the utility of object properties to confirm or disconfirm numerical identity is learned (although there is some disagreement over the age at which this learning occurs, see: Krøjgaard, 2007; Van de Walle et al., 2000).

5. *Young infants use the spatiotemporal parameters to reidentify an object as the numerically same individual over a disappearance-reappearance event, without implying that the object was located anywhere in the external world during the period of occlusion.* Initially, infants are using the spatiotemporal parameters to identify individual objects over changes in the visible world, and even to anticipate where the same one is likely to be seen again (e.g., extrapolating an object's visible trajectory across an occluder to anticipate its next appearance in the visible world). These spatiotemporal identity criteria provide an overarching structure, allowing young infants to extract predictable regularities from visible events. However, unlike adults, the criteria do not specify the object's location while it is invisible, which is consistent with young infants' failure to search for occluded objects (Meltzoff & Moore, 1998). There is broad consensus for such failure before 8 or 9 months of age, despite infants' ability to anticipate reappearances.

6. *Object permanence is the understanding that a particular object continues to exist in an invisible location or on an invisible trajectory in the external world during the period of occlusion or break in perceptual contact—while it is still invisible.* Permanence refers to a state of affairs that is beyond the infant's perception. It is the basis for infants' prediction of an object's occluded location after disappearance and during the time when it is still invisible. Such predictions about the object's location while it cannot be seen provide the goals for infants' intentional search acts and are the hallmarks of permanence-governed search.

7. *Object permanence develops from numerical identity. An infant must be able to construe*

[1] A trajectory of motion can be described as a vector specifying direction and speed. As an example of the predisposition to detect trajectories, 4-month-old infants visually extrapolated the left to right order in the sequential illumination of a linear array of lights into the space beyond the array. This occurred even though there was no "object" in motion and the pattern of illumination did not continue in that direction (Haith, Kessen, & Collins, 1969). A broad range of infant behavior is consonant with the idea that a notion of trajectory underlies it: The prospective control of head tracking and reaching for visibly moving objects (von Hofsten, Vishton, Spelke, Feng, & Rosander, 1998); learning to extrapolate the trajectory of a moving object across an occluder to predict its reappearance (Johnson, Amso, & Slemmer, 2003; Rosander & von Hofsten, 2004); the facilitation of predictive tracking over occlusions by unoccluded trajectory experience, and subsequent generalization to a new trajectory direction (Johnson, Amso, et al., 2003); and adjusting the time of an object's expected appearance over varying occluder widths by the trajectory's velocity (von Hofsten, Kochukhova, & Rossander, 2007). Conversely, when a constant velocity is not maintained, reappearances are not predicted (e.g., if the object is decelerating as it disappears; Rosander & von Hofsten, 2004) and overtrial learning to do so does not occur (e.g., if the object moves constantly while behind an occluder on some trials and delays behind it on others; Bertenthal, Longo, & Kenny, 2007).

the disappearance and reappearance of an object as involving a single individual, a numerical identity, before the answer to where the object was located during the period of occlusion can be obtained. Unless numerical identity can be established, objects appearing after an occlusion are new and different ones, rather than reappearances of the same one again. And, if new and different objects are popping into view after occlusions, the question of what happens to a single object between appearances, while it is invisible, never arises and could not be learned "from experience." Numerical identity renders this problem solvable.

Disappearance events can be described in spatiotemporal terms relevant to numerical identity as the places and trajectories of objects and their occluders over the time course of an occlusion. Rather than describe disappearances in terms of the recovery actions needed for search (as Piagetian theory did), the ID account describes them in terms of the places and trajectories of all the objects involved. For example, "a stationary object's occlusion in place by the movement of an occluder" specifies one type of disappearance transform and implies that the object can be reidentified as the same one again by its place of disappearance—reappearance (Moore & Meltzoff, 1999).

Since the spatiotemporal parameters serve as criteria for reidentifying the reappearing object as the same one again (see #5 above), the nature and development of these spatiotemporal parameters for numerical identity provide the skeleton underlying permanence development. In other words, the age ordering of disappearance transforms over which infants treat objects as permanent depends on the order of disappearance transforms for which the numerical identity of an object can be maintained. When infants can understand a disappearance transform as one in which "the same object has come back," they can then use subsequent experience to learn that the object is permanent over this disappearance transform. Thus, we say infants' understanding of permanence is dependent on the type of disappearance transform involved, or "permanence is transformationally dependent knowledge."

8. *Initially, object permanence understanding is an interpretation infants make of observed physical events that satisfy two conditions: the object participating in an occlusion event is identified as a single individual, and both the object and its occluded location can be independently represented.* Permanence understanding unites the object and its hidden location by an interpretation of the occlusion event—a deduction based on the occlusion—that links the now-hidden but represented object with the now-hidden but represented location. This is the representational basis for infants' knowing where that particular object is after it disappears. We hypothesize that development proceeds by infants at first reinterpreting the event after the reappearance of the object—"the same object was there before it reappeared"—and only with further experience is the interpretation prompted by the occlusion event itself.

9. *Once objects as wholes are interpreted as permanent over a particular class of disappearance events (a disappearance transform), further experience with that same transformation allows infants to learn which object properties are also preserved over that disappearance transform.* This learning process is parallel to the one in hypothesis #4 above except that now it is based on the object's permanence over the disappearance transform, and the preserved properties are taken to be permanent properties of the object in its occluded state.

Infant cognition is conservative. Infants do not assume that all properties of a predisappearance object are preserved in that same object postdisappearance. Conservation of the whole has priority, and initially infants accept a reappearing object satisfying the spatiotemporal identity criteria regardless of its visual features or function. They then learn that some properties, such as orientation and perspective, often are not preserved over occlusions; and that others, such as shape and functional properties like sound, usually are (referred to here as the object's "distinctive features and functions").

10. *Once some object features and functions are also known to be permanent over a particular disappearance transform, they can play an independent role in determining an object's* *numerical identity for that transformation.* Object features and functions that are permanent over a particular transform allow infants to use three identity criteria—spatiotemporal, featural, and functional—to determine numerical identity. Now infants do not have to accept a featurally or functionally different object as the same one again just because its reappearance satisfies the spatiotemporal identity criteria. For example, an object reappearing in the expected place with the wrong (unexpected) features or functions given the disappearance transform could lead to further search for the original object. Similarly, if an object was moved to a new location when infants were not watching, they can weigh whether the identity of the one they see is the same as the one that disappeared (because it looks the same but is in the wrong place). The answer is not completely determined by its location, all three of the identity criteria can be taken into account in decision-making.

Describing an Occlusion Event

An occlusion event can be characterized by three components, all of which bear on permanence understanding: (a) the psychophysics of the transition to invisibility, (b) the degree of object occlusion, and (c) the type of disappearance transform. All three components are incorporated in the ID account.

(a) *Psychophysics of transition: Michottean disappearance events.* Different types of visual events are specified psychophysically by the nature of the transition to invisibility (Michotte, 1962) and have been shown to differentially affect looking, sucking, predictive tracking, and electroencephalogram (EEG) responses in young infants (e.g., Bertenthal, Longo, & Kenny, 2007; Bower, 1967; Kaufman, Csibra, & Johnson, 2005). For example, a progressive deletion of the visible portion of an object at an edge is a necessary, though not always sufficient, condition to perceptually specify that the object slipped behind/under the edge during the transition, and has not been destroyed by the disappearance (Bremner et al., 2007; Gibson, Kaplan, Reynolds, & Wheeler, 1969). In the ID account, this innate, Michottean perceptual mechanism serves as a filter, separating out disappearance transitions that destroy the object (e.g., implosions, dissolutions, instantaneous disappearances, etc.) from ones that do not. Only events that survive this filtering engage the next two components and feed into infants' determination of identity and permanence.

(b) *Degree of object occlusion.* The degree of object occlusion refers to the extent of occlusion—that is, how much of the whole object is occluded (totally, partially, or not obscured at all; Moore & Meltzoff, 2008).

(c) *The disappearance transform.* Both descriptions of the Michottean transition and the degree of occlusion apply to disappearance transforms, but a transform is not reducible to them. As we define the term, the "disappearance transform" describes the spatiotemporal arrangement of object(s) and occluder(s) over the entire course of the occlusion event (e.g., the occlusion of a stationary object in place by the movement of an occluder). A disappearance transform refers to a class of equivalent events; they are spatiotemporally equivalent. Thus, any total occlusion of a stationary object in place by the movement of an occluder is the same disappearance transform—the objects, locations, and occluders can all vary. This means that many events, which are different on the surface, can be grouped as the same abstract disappearance transform. In the ID view, it should not matter to infants whether a cloth covers a stationary object or a vertical barrier is placed in front of it—both are occlusions of a stationary object in place.

Requirements for Testing a Strong Form of Object Permanence

Testing the ID account of infants' object permanence development presents two major empirical challenges. Object permanence refers to infants' understanding of a postocclusion state of affairs. The first challenge is how to assure that infants' search acts are actually launched on the basis of the object in its occluded state, rather than on some other basis. We call this the "occluded object standard." The second challenge is how to assess whether infants represent the object in a specific, invisible location. We call this the "invisible location standard." The point of this section is to provide the logic of an empirical method that can meet both standards and why it is necessary to adopt these safeguards in order to be sure one is tapping infants' object permanence understanding rather than some lower-order action.

Occluded Object Standard

In order to force infants to act off of their representation of the occluded object while it is invisible, we hide the object while it is out of reach. Infants are thus prevented from initiating search until after the occlusion is complete and they are brought back within reach. This procedure protects against one kind of artifact—continuations of search action already in progress before the disappearance is complete. From that point on, any action taken toward the hidden object would have to be governed by their representation of the object in its occluded state.

There are other potential artifacts that must also be prevented: (a) acts based on prior practice with occluder removal in the test situation (e.g., extensive warm-up trials in a study); (b) acts based on clues from the experimenter such as drawing attention to an occluder by "touching it last" (Diamond, Cruttenden, & Neiderman, 1994; Smith, Thelen, Titzer, & McLin, 1999); or (c) acts based on contingencies set up by the experimenter accidentally or by training (e.g. continued testing after chance success has uncovered the object in a particular place). Search based on any of these do not meet the occluded object standard because it need not be based on the object's disappearance (Moore & Meltzoff, 2008).

Invisible Location Standard

Under the conditions above, correct manual search coupled with spatially directed visual anticipation of the object's reappearance locus is evidence about where infants think the object is located while it is out of sight. Such behavior implies that the location of the object is represented while both the object and its location are occluded.

In short, if infants' search acts are initiated after the object is fully occluded, and if infants are looking to where the object should reappear as a consequence of their acts, before the object is visible, then such acts are valid evidence of object permanence. Permanence measured this way is called the strong form of object permanence for clarity, because it meets both standards. These more rigorous requirements lead to slightly more conservative age estimates than studies that use "occluder removal" alone as a direct measure of permanence. We believe that these precautions allow a more valid measure of infants' object permanence understanding, and will use them in assessing the ID account.

Empirical Evidence

Of the 10 ID account hypotheses, those numbered 1–4 have substantial empirical support. There is less evidence bearing on hypotheses 5–10, because few studies have assessed the strong form of object permanence until recently. We turn now to consider such evidence.

Is a Strong Form of Object Permanence Needed to Account for Search Behavior in Infancy?

Studies of object permanence, whether using visual habituation or manual search methods, are typically conducted within one spatial setting and the infant situated in one position within it. Thus, an object's permanence may be put in doubt by an occlusion, but permanence of the spatial setting is preserved through unbroken perceptual contact. Many other circumstances in infants' lives lead to an object's disappearance where the setting is changed before they ever see it reappear or get an opportunity to act. Infants are removed from the setting, they go to sleep, they travel, and objects are moved to new settings unobserved by them. Obviously, the adult notion of permanent objects is rich enough to encompass these situations. For the adult, absent objects continue to exist in hidden locations after all forms of perceptual contact with the original setting have been severed. And, if another agent has moved the objects, the adult believes they continue to exist in some new location. Do infants view the world in this way? Most studies of object permanence, regardless of method, are silent on this fundamental point.

In a recent study, 14-month-old infants watched an object being hidden, left the test environment, and returned 24 h later. The results showed that when they were brought back to the same room the next day, they searched successfully (Moore & Meltzoff, 2004). This test satisfies both standards for strong object permanence. Successful search under these conditions shows that in addition to representing the object, a representation of the hiding place was also set up at the disappearance event (concordant with hypothesis # 8). For at least one basic disappearance transform, "the occlusion of an object in place," 14-month-olds' search after a 24-h break suggests that the object's existence in the world is not dependent on maintaining any kind of perceptual contact with the disappearance locale.

Does Numerical Identity Play a Role in This Strong Form of Infant Object Permanence?

The ID account holds that the aim of infants' permanence-governed search is to recover exactly the same object that disappeared. Leaving the locale of an object's disappearance and returning after 24 h poses a question of numerical identity. If one returns to the same locale, the object hidden on day 1 could be found here; but, if this is a different locale, then the expectation should be that the original object could not be found here. To test this idea, we instituted a "room change" condition. The findings were that the 14-month-old infants in the room-change group did not search while the same-room infants searched successfully (Moore & Meltzoff, 2004). This result comports with the idea that infants were seeking the original object and supports hypothesis # 7 that numerical identity underlies permanence-governed search.

A new behavior was also discovered that points up the importance of numerical identity to object permanence. In these experiments, no object was in the hiding place on day 2, so no infants found it there. When the original object was later shown in the middle of the room to infants who had seen it hidden on day 1, they engaged in "verifying search." They went across the room to the hiding place and looked inside, even though the object was in full view (Moore & Meltzoff, 2004). Despite the fact that the features and functions of the visible object matched the one they saw hidden, they checked in the hiding place before playing with it. Our interpretation of this behavior is that the 14-month-olds were searching the disappearance place to verify that the original object was not there. This would help them determine if the visible object was the numerically correct individual or merely one that looked and acted like it. This behavior supports hypothesis # 10 on the interplay of the three identity criteria, because the object's features and functions were sufficient to tentatively identify it (as the same one), and the spatiotemporal information (the place of its expected reappearance) was used to confirm or disconfirm that provisional identity.

Taken together, the room-change results and the verifying search behavior suggest that these infants were seeking, in the same hiding place, within the same disappearance locale, the selfsame object that they saw hidden on day 1. Violating the global spatiotemporal criterion for the identity of a stationary object (the room) led to no search at all if it was the wrong locale. Violating the local spatiotemporal criterion (the place in the room) led to verifying search if the object was in the wrong place within the correct global locale. The role of numerical identity in object permanence understanding provides an explanatory concept for both behavior patterns.

Is a Strong Form of Object Permanence Present from Birth?

If the strong form of object permanence is present at some time during infancy, is it present at all times? The classic argument has been that attempts to answer this question using manual search tend to underestimate competence because of "performance constraints" (e.g., Baillargeon, Graber, DeVos, & Black, 1990).

A recent study investigated whether four commonly cited performance constraints presumed to limit infant search actually caused failures: motor skills, means–ends coordination, spatial understanding, and memory span (Moore & Meltzoff, 2008).

A new partial occlusion task was used to assess whether 8.75-month-old infants had the means–ends coordination and motor skills needed to remove an occluder (see also Johnson, this volume, for more on partial occlusions). In the standard Piagetian task, the visible part extends toward the infants, and they typically pull on the visible part because it is close and easy to reach. In the new task, the object's visible part projected laterally from the occluder, so both part and occluder were equally available. The first question was whether the infants would recover the object by removing the occluder. If infants do this, their lifting or displacing of the occluder demonstrates the same motor and means–ends skills needed to remove it on total occlusions. The next question was whether the infants who removed the occluder on partial occlusions also removed it on total occlusions, as would be expected if they understood permanence. The findings showed they did not: Fully half of the 32 8.75-month-old infants tested had the requisite skills, but only two used them to remove the occluder from a totally hidden object (Moore & Meltzoff, 2008, Experiment 1).

If motor skills and means–ends coordination were not the limiting factors, what was the impediment? Bower (1982) has argued that a source of difficulty is the spatial relationship between an occluder and the object it occludes. He predicted that when some distance separates a stationary object and a totally occluding vertical screen, the object is perceived as behind the occluder. However, if there is no spatial separation between object and occluder (e.g., under cloths or inside cups), the search task is more difficult, because the occluder appears to be taking the place of the object rather than hiding it during the disappearance event. Therefore, he argued that using cloth occluders would underestimate infants' understanding of object permanence. When we tested this idea with 8.75- and 10-month-old infants, there were no differences in search success whether the object was behind an occluder or under an occluder: The younger infants failed even when the object was behind an upright occluder (Moore & Meltzoff, 2008).

Another commonly cited performance constraint for young infants concerns memory. If the memory span required by a total occlusion were too great, infants might forget the object before they could search (Diamond, 1985; Harris, 1987). This limitation was addressed by hiding an object that emitted a continuous sound to prevent forgetting. Even with this memory aid, 8.75-month-olds did not succeed. Older infants were also tested. The introduction of the sounding object more than doubled the success rate for the 10-month-olds, but it did not help the younger infants (Moore & Meltzoff, 2008, Experiment 2).

In sum, these findings show that infants at 8.75 months of age possess the requisite skills to search for the hidden object. But they did not search. Taken together, with the fact that 14-month-olds demonstrate the strong form of object permanence for this same disappearance transform, we infer that a notion of permanence begins to develop between 8.75 and 10 months of age and is quite robust by 14 months.

If Object Permanence Develops, Is the Change Once and for All or a Series of Steps?

In the work discussed thus far, only the degree of the object's occlusion has been manipulated—partial hidings are easier to solve than total hidings. On the ID account, however, changes in the type of disappearance transform should also affect search success even when the degree of occlusion is exactly the same. A study testing this idea compared two types of total occlusions in which the same object was hidden in the same place behind the same screen (Moore & Meltzoff, 1999). If infants solved one task but not the other, this task differentiation could not be attributed to the types of performance constraints previously mentioned, because the same search response to the same totally

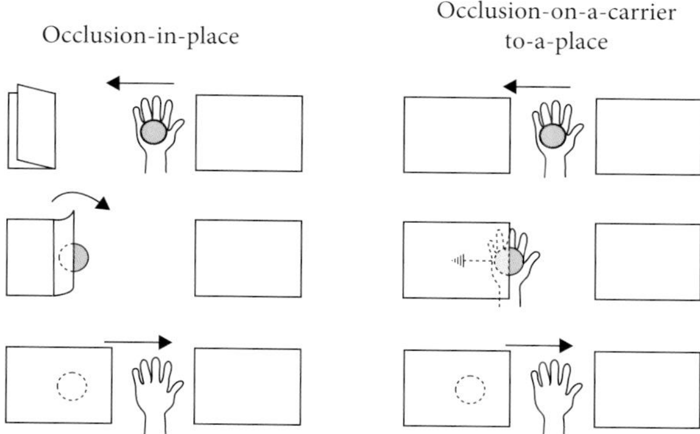

Figure 4.1 Two types of disappearance transforms. The left column depicts occlusion-in-place and the right column depicts occlusion-on-a-carrier-to-a-place. Occlusion-in-place begins with the experimenter carrying the object to a place on the table next to the folded cloth and depositing it there. The occlusion occurs by unfolding the cloth over the object. The experimenter's hand then returns to the starting point in the center of the table. Occlusion-on-a-carrier-to-a-place begins with the experimenter carrying the object toward the cloth. The occlusion occurs as the object goes under the cloth; it is then deposited on the table. The experimenter's hand returns to the starting point in the center of the table. Adapted from Moore & Meltzoff (1999).

occluded object, in the same spatial location was needed in both (Figure 4.1). In one occlusion, a stationary object in place on the table was totally hidden by the movement of a screen. In the other, the object was carried under the stationary screen by hand, occluding it on the carrier/hand, and deposited on the table; then the carrier emerged empty.

Three age groups were tested and the occlusion-in-place was significantly easier than the occlusion-on-a-carrier-to-a-place at 10 and 12 months of age; only the 14-month-old group was equally successful on both tasks. Even though a majority of the younger infants succeeded on the total occlusion-in-place, only a small minority succeeded on the total occlusion-on-a-carrier-to-place. Importantly, therefore, the permanence understanding that enables success on one total occlusion is insufficient to solve the other. In fact, about 4 months elapse before a majority of infants can solve both tasks. These findings suggest that object permanence is not a once-and-for-all attainment: The nature of the disappearance transform matters.

Identity Development Interpretation of the Empirical Data

On the ID account, the occlusion-in-place is a total disappearance of an object at rest on the table by the movement of a cloth occluder. In an occlusion-on-a-carrier-to-place, an object at rest on the carrier is moved under the cloth. At this point in the occlusion-on-a-carrier, both tasks occlude an object that is at rest relative to the surface it is on (table or carrier). For both, the object would be identified by the spatiotemporal criterion of place of disappearance and expected to reappear there. For infants who understand permanence for the occlusion-in-place transform, the object in its invisible state continues to exist in that place (table or carrier) for both tasks. However, in the occlusion-on-a-carrier, the object is deposited on the table under the cloth and the carrier is withdrawn empty. No object is present on the carrier where that same one would be expected. If infants use their permanence understanding to uncover the place of disappearance in order to find the hidden object, on the occlusion-in-place task they succeed because they uncover the place on the table; but on the occlusion-on-a-carrier task they fail, because the disappearance place (the carrier) is empty. Thus, the identity criterion or rule that underlies infants' comprehension of one task leads to noncomprehension of the other.[2]

In terms of numerical identity for the 10- and 12-month-old infants, the original object has to reappear on the carrier to be the same object—there is no other place in the external world where that object could be identified as the same one. If numerical identity guides search, it also follows that there is nowhere else to search for that same object. The 10-month-olds who failed this task provide support for this interpretation because the overwhelming majority of them did not search at all (even when they searched correctly on the other occlusion task).

In terms of permanence, if there is no place in the world for that same object to be after disappearance except on the carrier, then, when the carrier is empty, it is evidence for the infant that the object is not permanent. In this sense, one transform preserves the object over an occlusion (permanent for occlusion-in-place) and the other transform does not (impermanent for occlusion-on-a-carrier-to-place). This provides support for a key claim of the ID account: An infant can understand objects as permanent for one type of disappearance transform, but still think that objects are not permanent and are nowhere to be found under a different transform. This is what we mean when we say object permanence understanding is transformation-dependent; it is not an all-or-none attainment. The pattern of these findings and their interpretation suggests that permanence development proceeds in a transformationally dependent manner and also that the steps can be described by the spatiotemporal parameters for numerical identity.

[2] For ease of exposition, we often characterize these spatiotemporal criteria as "rules" because the spatiotemporal parameters yield a rule-governed pattern of operation (e.g., a place rule for permanence, a trajectory rule for identity, a place-to-place rule, etc). They are functional descriptions; we are not speculating on the underlying neurophysiology.

Violations of Strong Object Permanence Cause Negative Emotion in Infants

Adults can be driven to distraction when something important is inexplicably lost. If object permanence were an equally fundamental understanding of the world for infants, then violations of permanence should generate strong negative affect—conflict, upset, and avoidance. The 10-month-olds' response to the occlusion-on-a-carrier-to-place in the Moore and Meltzoff (1999) study provides a test of this idea. As argued above, the empty carrier emerging from under the occluder violates the place rule for where the hidden object should be. By contrast, the place rule is not violated when the object disappears by an occlusion-in-place, because a majority of infants at this age understand that the object still resides in the now invisible place that it disappeared. Therefore, there should be a difference in their emotional reactions to the two tasks.

Infants' active avoidance was the measure of affect used. The results were that avoidance was strongly associated with the occlusion-on-a-carrier-to-place. The avoidance of the occlusion-on-a-carrier did not simply reflect infants' frustration at not finding the object. This was examined using infants who failed both tasks. Significantly more of these infants avoided occlusion-on-a-carrier but did not avoid occlusion-in-place than infants who did the converse (Moore & Meltzoff, 1999). Thus, infants' avoidance of occlusion-on-a-carrier-to-place appears to be a reaction to the disappearance transform, rather than to search consequences.

This differential avoidance pattern suggests that infants were treating the "empty hand" as a violation of their understanding of permanence, which is apparently important enough to produce conflict when violated, and as argued above, for which their identity rules provide no alternative understanding. These findings suggest that the strong form of object permanence reflects a fundamental understanding of the infants' world as early as 10-months of age. When this understanding is violated, there is a strong emotional response (not just increases in looking time, but avoidance and even upset).

A Mechanism of Change for Developing Object Permanence

We have argued that the strong form of object permanence is not innately specified, but develops. We sketched the ID account that permanence develops from infants understanding of numerical identity and reviewed the new empirical evidence bearing on this claim. The results suggest that permanence is the understanding that allows infants to make sense of what happens between encounters with objects that can be reidentified as the same one again. Object permanence fills the spatiotemporal gap between an object's disappearance and its reappearance.

The theoretical problem is now sharply posed. If permanence is a discovery that arises from a precondition in which objects are not permanent, how does the concept develop? This raises the classic nativist challenge to all developmental theories and all claims for conceptual change (Fodor, 1981). In particular, how can a concept of object permanence evolve from precursors that do not already entail a notion of permanence?

Genesis of Object Permanence for the Occlusion of an Object in Place

The crux of the developmental problem is the transition from impermanence to permanence. Here, we will describe a mechanism of permanence development for a particular case of occlusion. In the next section, we extend these ideas to provide a generative mechanism of permanence discovery and development. Two key findings for theory construction emerged from the Moore and Meltzoff (2008) study. First, the infants' pattern of success established an invariant ordering: Many infants solved partial occlusions by removing the occluder and failed total occlusions, but none of the infants failed partial occlusions and solved total occlusions. This suggests that understanding the easier, partial occlusion serves as a foundation for understanding the more difficult, total occlusion. Second, as noted above, 8.75-month-olds were no more successful searching for a sounding object than a silent one. However, the sounding object markedly improved the success rate of the 10-month-olds. This change in the use of sound suggests that a developmental transition occurs between these ages.

Our specific mechanism of permanence development has two interwoven parts. First, infants' understanding of partial occlusions is a necessary precursor to locating stationary objects that are totally occluded and to establishing their identity when they are out of sight. Second, infants' discovery of permanence for a total occlusion is a process of reinterpreting the occlusion event based on their existing understanding of the precursor, the partial occlusion.

Transition From Impermanence to Permanence: The Crucial Role of Partial Occlusions

When an object is hidden on a table, the total occlusion of the object is only a partial occlusion of the table surface on which it sits. The occluded place on the partially occluded table continues to exist after occlusion (for infants who understand partial occlusions) and provides an invisible location for the totally occluded object to reside while it is out of sight. Thus, infants could understand that there is somewhere in the external world for the totally occluded object to be. Moreover, if that invisible place continues to exist, then it could satisfy the place criterion that identifies the object in that place, when it is out of sight, as the same one that disappeared there. We suggest that this development in spatial cognition lays the groundwork for discovering permanence over total occlusions in place. Infants can use the permanence of the partially hidden portion of the table supporting the object to provide an invisible, but still existing, location for the object to reside after it is totally occluded, and also to provide a place criterion identifying it as the same one while it is invisible and when it is disoccluded.

Sounding Objects as a Window on the Process of Discovery

There are at least three ways that sound from an occluded object could help infants search. First, sound from the object could aid in remembering and localizing the object. If this were true, then sound should help both age groups, but the younger group more than the older. Second, infants might not be able to interpret sound as coming from a hidden object unless they knew that the object still existed in the hidden location (i.e., the object is already permanent). If this were true, then only infants who could solve occlusions with silent objects would solve them with sounding ones. Third, sound could function as a catalyst, triggering a new way to understand the occlusion that was not accessible when the object was silent. The data showed that a sounding object was of no help to the younger infants, but significantly more of the older infants succeeded with the sounding object than with the silent one (Moore & Meltzoff, 2008). This pattern suggests that sound acted as a catalyst. How might that work?

The fact that partial occlusions appear to be a precursor to solving total occlusions suggests that infants who understand partial occlusions are developmentally poised to discover how to understand total occlusions from experience. Once infants have this framework, a characteristic sound from the object could provide additional spatial and identity information about how to interpret an object's disappearance. Sound from the hidden object, localized as coming from the partially occluded surface, could help catalyze a reinterpretation: the same object that disappeared is the source of this sound and remains unseen on that partially occluded surface. Based on this view, permanence is an interpretation infants make of the occlusion event. The logic is concordant with hypothesis #8, the object is interpreted as permanent over a transform if it is identified as a single individual, and both the object and the occluded location are independently represented.

We are not arguing that the role of sound is a general explanation for how infants acquire object permanence for total occlusions in place. Nor are we arguing that the 10-month-olds who did not succeed on total occlusions with silent objects, but did with sounding objects, acquired object permanence from that experience alone. Rather, we think that the results with the sounding object give us a window on the process of how permanence is acquired for total occlusions: It is a deductive inference that restructures what the infants already know about partial occlusions to yield the new understanding.

How did sound from the object help? We think it provided an interpretive aid. Hypothesis # 8 suggests that the normal developmental course would be for infants to first reinterpret the disappearance as conserving the object in place after reappearance (because they can confirm the reappearing object's identity after disocclusion); subsequently, they begin to make that interpretation after the object's disappearance but before it reappears. On this view, the characteristic sound from the object provides a shortcut enabling the interpretation to be made at disappearance, because it allowed infants to confirm the object's identity by its sound from the represented place before it reappeared. Thus, the auditory provision of identity and localization information before disocclusion fostered interpretation by infants who were already able to represent the hidden place.

In sum, search for the sounding object is a special case, but illustrates a process of interpretation that could be applied more generally. According to the specific mechanism of change described here, permanence arises only when an existing means for determining numerical identity and a developing understanding of partial hidings have prepared the ground. On this foundation, an occlusion event that was previously interpreted as not preserving the object can be interpreted in a new way, and confirmed by subsequent experience, as actually preserving the object in a precise hidden location—it is now permanent over this disappearance transform, a total occlusion in place.

Generalizing the Mechanism of Change: From Transform T to Transform T+1

We have suggested that the process of developmental change is one in which an understanding of permanence and the experience gained with a simpler disappearance transform make a harder transform amenable to reinterpretation so long as the numerical identity of the object can be maintained. In the case of total occlusions, the advance occurred because infants could use the permanence of the partially hidden portion of the table supporting the object to provide (a) an invisible, but still existing, location for the object to reside after it was totally occluded, and (b) a continuously existing "place" criterion identifying it as the same individual from disappearance to reappearance. In this context, a reinterpretation of total occlusions became possible. In what follows, we utilize this analysis and our new findings to extend the developmental process toward a more general mechanism of change and development.

There are two major problems confronting a general mechanism. One is how to explain the step-like progression of occlusion tasks that infants can solve as they develop. We have reviewed data on two ordered steps here: the partial to total occlusion transition, and the occlusion-in-place to occlusion-on-a-carrier-to-place transition. Other steps have been suggested by previous longitudinal studies (Kramer, Hill, & Cohen, 1975; Piaget, 1954). A second problem arises when infants find that applying their current permanence rule to a disappearance transform does not preserve the object. This obstacle was illustrated in the Moore and Meltzoff (1999) study. Infants, who had a place rule to solve an occlusion-in-place, found that applying it to an occlusion-on-a-carrier resulted in an empty reappearance place, and an apparently upsetting violation of permanence.

The general process of developmental change focuses on what else develops once a transform is understood as conserving an occluded object as a whole. The major claim is that infants learn which features and functions of an object are themselves permanent over that transform and can bear independently on identity determination (hypotheses # 9 & 10). Thus, an object's permanent features and functions could also serve as identity criteria for distinguishing that object when spatiotemporal parameters are absent, neutral, or even in disagreement. We term these criteria the object's "distinctive" features and functions. This discovery offers new developmental leverage because the spatiotemporal parameters, the object's properties, and its permanence can all interact in interpreting occlusion events.

The phenomenon of "verifying search" provides relevant evidence (Moore & Meltzoff, 2004). Infants treated the properties of an object seen hidden on day 1 as bearing on numerical identity because, when the object was presented in a new location on day 2, infants searched in the original hiding place before playing with it. Even though it was in the wrong place, the featural and functional identity criteria conflicted with the spatiotemporal criterion and raised the question of its identity. For this disappearance transform then, the distinctive features and functions of the object implied its numerical identity at 14 months of age.

This suggests a general mechanism of change that could account for the ordering of search tasks found in the longitudinal studies and how infants might use apparent violations of permanence. We will state the hypothesis in its most abstract form and illustrate it with a simple transform that violates the place rule for permanence and identity. The general problem is how "rule R" for the identity and permanence of an object and its features over transform T changes to rule "R+1" for a new disappearance transform. The proposed mechanism is shown schematically in Figure 4.2. Here it is applied to a task in which the object is moved after disappearance in place *X* to a second place *Y* by means of the screen (e.g., a cup covers an object and is then pushed to a new location with the object still underneath). According to rule R, the infant searches place *X* on the table and finds it empty, which violates the spatiotemporal logic of rule R. Meanwhile, the object reappears at place *Y*, which confirms the featural logic of rule R—it can be interpreted provisionally as the same one again. This produces conflict because rule R is both confirmed and violated. The infant has to weigh the apparent violation of permanence for the object at *X* and the appearance of a featurally identical object at *Y* against the validity of rule R. This conflict is resolved by reinterpreting the spatiotemporal logic of rule R to encompass the change of location ($X \rightarrow Y$). This reorganization provides the new spatiotemporal logic of rule R+1, maintaining an object's identity and permanence over a new transform T+1.

In the terms we have been using, the example above captures the process of reinterpreting a place rule for identity and permanence to yield

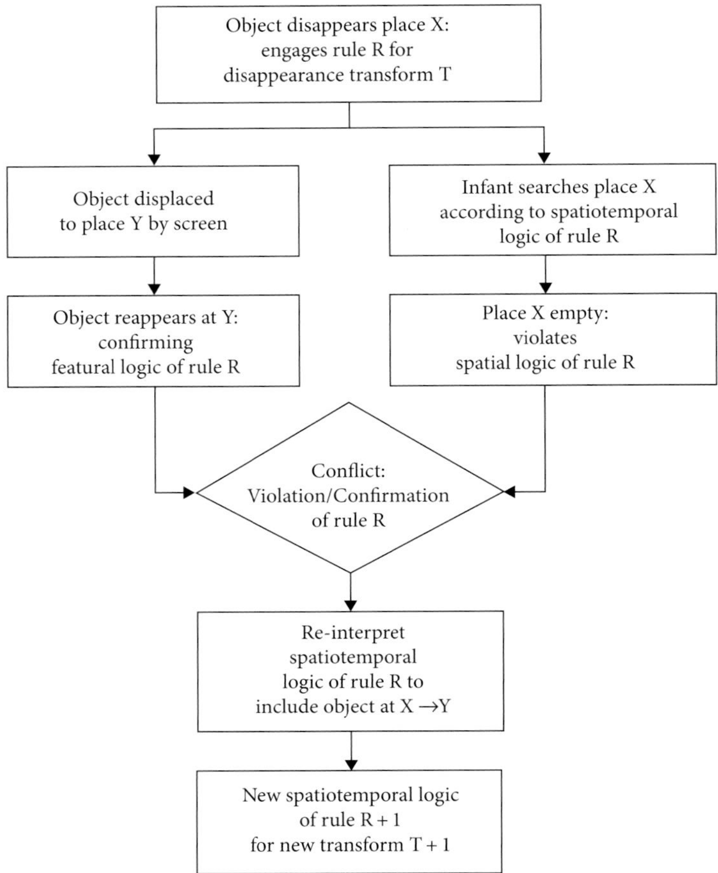

Figure 4.2 A mechanism of change for developing object permanence. An object disappears at place *X* and reappears at place *Y*. The infant expects the object to reappear at *X* according to permanence rule R. The flowchart illustrates the hypothesized process for changing the spatiotemporal component of rule R to rule R+1. Conflict occurs between confirmation of the featural component of rule R, which is satisfied by the object appearing at *Y*, and disconfirmation of the spatiotemporal component, which is violated by the object's failure to appear at *X*. Changing the spatiotemporal component of rule R to rule R+1 resolves the conflict. See text for details. Adapted from Moore (1975).

a new place-to-place rule. An object disappearing in place *X* can be the same one again when it reappears in place *Y*. The identity and permanence of the whole object are preserved over the new transform and the process of learning which properties of an object are also preserved can begin again for the R+1 transform. Note that rule R+1 does not overwrite rule R. Rather, rule R is engaged by observing transform T (i.e., after occlusion the occluder remains at the place of disappearance) and rule R+1 is engaged by transform T+1 (i.e., after occlusion, the occluder moves from the place disappearance to a new place). The particular rules are engaged by the spatiotemporal structure of the various disappearance transforms. We think that this kind of mechanism of development would account for the stepwise progression of infant success on search tasks because the steps are generated by the order of the underlying spatiotemporal criteria for identity and the resulting understandings of object permanence.

More broadly, when an object is occluded, the goal of search is quite specific: Infants are seeking the same object that disappeared—no other object will do. Successful search reconnects the infant with the same predisappearance object and maintains order in the infant's cognitive world; failed search confronts infants with disorder, which can have affective consequences. Infants' striving to preserve order and coherence in their world is the motivation for permanence development, and tracing an object's identity over transformational events is a means to achieve it.

Implications for Existing Theories of Object Permanence in Infancy

Infant object permanence has been the focus of attention for seven decades. Four basic approaches have been articulated. We consider them in light of the evidence and arguments presented here and make suggestions for future research.

Piagetian Approaches

According to Piaget (1952, 1954), infants develop a concept of objects as permanent by increasingly separating the object itself from the matrix of actions upon it, culminating in an object's representation independent of both perception and action (Table 4.1). A number of theorists have broadened his theoretical terms to include a "gradual strengthening of representation" or "movement of the observer either by actions of the infant or by being carried through space" as the sources of development while narrowing their focus to explaining how infants first solve a total occlusion or overcome the A-not-B search error (Bremner, 1989; Campos et al., 2000; Mareschal, Plunkett, & Harris, 1999; Munakata, McClelland, Johnson & Siegler, 1997; Newcombe & Huttenlocher, 2000). Piaget's manual search tasks are differentiated in terms of three major factors: (a) the actions required for recovery, (b) the degree of occlusion, and (c) the number of hiding locations. The research reviewed here showing that infants can solve one type of total occlusion (an occlusion-in-place) 4 months before solving a different type of total occlusion (an occlusion-on-a-carrier-to-a-place) demonstrates that Piaget's developmental sequence is incomplete. The same search action at the same location was required to find the object in both tasks. For Piaget (1954), there is no easy explanation for how total hidings in one place, solved by the same recovery act, can be developmentally different.

Moreover, there is further evidence that does not comport with Piagetian theory. Piaget is correct in claiming that success on partial occlusions precedes success on total occlusions. But, his theory provides no explanation for the new data showing that infants fail to remove the occluder of a totally hidden object when they have the means–ends coordination to do so. Such coordination characterizes Piaget's stage 4, and infants who uncovered the partially occluded object should have uncovered the totally occluded object, but they did not.

Taken together, the new studies suggest that Piaget's diagnosis of infants' problems in developing object permanence was off target, and his action-based theory of development does not fit the evidence. The infant's conceptual problem is not separating objects from the matrix of action, representing them in mind, or positioning them in visible space—the early perceptual and representational systems do all three.

Dynamic Systems Theory

Dynamic systems theorists believe that infants' initial appreciation of objects is embedded in the dynamics of their acts of attending, reaching, and remembering (Thelen & Smith, 1994). They think that objects are so inextricably bound up in attention and action that a concept of permanence is not developed in infancy (Thelen, Schoner, Scheier, & Smith, 2001), and in that sense, postulate an even less cognitive, more action-bound infant than Piaget. The study of 14-month-olds' search after a 24-h delay tests this assertion (Moore & Meltzoff, 2004). Infants observed an object's disappearance with no familiarization play with the hiding places and immediately left the laboratory. Upon return 24 h later, no attention was drawn to the hiding place, yet infants successfully found the object.

From the dynamic systems perspective, there were no practiced acts to repeat, no directing of infants' attention to the hiding place. Infants searched based on a stored representation of the absent object and its location in space. This suggests that some conception of permanence is needed to guide search on the second day contrary to the dynamic systems' model of infancy.

Nativist Theory

Object permanence nativists claim that it is logically impossible for infants to learn that objects are permanent from the chaos of sensory experience (Spelke, 1994). In this approach, object is an innate conception resulting from perceptual processing that entails permanence (Baillargeon, 2008; Spelke, 1990). Permanence does not develop; it is present from the beginning and part of what it means to perceive an object.

Nativists claim that search necessarily underestimates infants' competence. Instead, increased looking time to events in which occluded objects do not reappear when/where they are expected to reappear is the appropriate measure. This method leads to the paradox that infant's putative knowledge of permanence at birth as inferred from looking time measures does not guide action: Infants fail to search manually for hidden stationary objects (for review: Marcovitch & Zelazo, 1999), and they fail to "catch" moving objects that briefly disappear and reappear (Berthier et al., 2001; Jonsson & von Hofsten, 2003; Spelke & von Hofsten, 2001) until about 9 months of age. This age discrepancy is usually explained as a result of performance constraints on the innate knowledge.

However, the new finding of a developmental difference in search for occluded objects, when performance factors are controlled and search skills are available, casts doubt on this explanation for the failure to search. Infants who succeeded on partial hidings by removing the occluder should also succeed in removing the occluder on total hidings if they understood permanence. But they did not succeed. We interpret this to mean that the 8.75-month-olds do not understand permanence for a total occlusion. The results showed that by 10 months of age, infants could understand permanence for a total occlusion-in-place. Importantly, that was not the end of development. Recall that 10-month-olds, who solved this form of total occlusion, did not succeed on a total occlusion-on-a-carrier to-a-place until 14 months of age. These data suggest there are at least two steps in permanence development, unexplained by performance constraints, which challenge nativist theory. Permanence neither seems to be innate nor a once-and-for-all acquisition.

Identity Development Theory

On the ID account, object permanence develops from a prior understanding of numerical identity—the spatiotemporal criteria infants use to reidentify an object as the same one again after a break in perceptual contact. When infants can parse a particular disappearance transform as maintaining the identity of the object, they are in a position to discover what happens to it between appearances. Then, experience with object reappearances can be understood in a new way, allowing infants to reinterpret the occlusion as preserving the object in a hidden place.

Once infants understand the total occlusion of an object in place as preserving it invisibly in that place, they still do not understand all total occlusions (as argued above). The ID claim is that the interplay of an object's spatiotemporal parameters and its permanent features and functions afford a mechanism of developmental change, which enables the discovery of other disappearance transforms over which the object's identity and its permanence are preserved. Hence, permanence understanding is constrained to specific types of disappearance transforms, and develops one transform at a time. The ID account holds that object permanence develops in ordered steps, and that search tasks, properly conducted, can assess this development.

On the surface, the ID account resembles Piaget's in arguing for a step-like development in object permanence and for the validity of manual search as a measure of it. However, this resemblance is more apparent than real. There are profound differences. Empirically, the ID account encompasses additional steps in permanence development and in visual search not included in Piaget's account. Theoretically, the ID account bases infant development on an initial capacity for representation and numerical identity rather than seeing representation as the culmination of development at 18 months of age. Moreover, the ID engine of development is cognitive, and stems from infants' striving to understand which objects in the external world are the same ones encountered previously, rather than from Piaget's hierarchical coordination of sensorimotor action schemes. This striving for a coherent understanding of the appearance and disappearance of the same object, which leads to the discovery of permanence and orders the course of development, is more objective and independent of action than envisaged by Piaget.

Future Directions in Object Permanence Research

At present, the field has two methods that yield diametrically opposed results, yet both claim to measure the same concept—object permanence. This dichotomy poses deep difficulties. According to the nativists, permanence is an innately perceived property of objects, and increased looking time to events incompatible with permanence demonstrates this implicit knowledge of permanence. According to ID theory, permanence is a function of the disappearance transforms that infants understand, and the order of the manual search tasks solved by infants demonstrates the development of this understanding. A paradox arises because the innate knowledge shown by looking time measures does not lead to search before 9 months of age. This paradox still engenders considerable debate (e.g., Cohen & Cashon, 2006; Kagan, 2008; Meltzoff & Moore, 1998; Newcombe, & Huttenlocher, 2006; Quinn, 2008).

In this chapter, we have tried to narrow the gap to some extent. On the one hand, we have clarified the definition of object permanence—it refers to a prereappearance understanding that an occluded object continues to exist in a particular hidden location in the external world. Permanence is knowledge of an invisible state of affairs. This contrasts with the nativists' equating object permanence with continuity in space and time (Spelke, Breinlinger, Macomber, & Jacobson, 1992), but being unable, using preferential looking or habituation methods, to assess infants' reactions to continuity/discontinuity *while the object is still invisible*. Essentially, what is measured by looking time is postreappearance knowledge. That is, what is directly measured is whether the visible, preocclusion state of affairs is consistent with or discrepant from the visible, postocclusion state. Looking time measures are retrospective and based on the visible structure of the entire disappearance–reappearance cycle. By contrast, the search measures described here (i.e., incorporating spatially directed visual anticipation of the object's reappearance locus) are predictive. Search success under these conditions shows that infants are seeking the object where it is located while it is still in its occluded state. In light of this distinction, one resolution of the dilemma is that we are not in fact assessing the same concept at all.

On the other hand, we have identified some markers of the strong form of object permanence that nativists could use to demonstrate that the two approaches are measuring the same concept. It would be interesting if the looking time methods could be adapted to allow young infants to leave the locale where the object disappeared and return later for assessment. Or, could the violation-of-expectation method be adapted to show strong emotion for a violation of permanence (rather than simply increased looking time), as shown by search tests with 10-month-olds? One corollary of the nativists' view seems less persuasive in light of our new data: It is difficult to maintain that infants fail to search due to known performance constraints. We found no evidence for this in two independent studies and three different ages.

Conversely, one might wonder then whether the ID account has any explanation for the looking-time phenomena demonstrated by the nativist approach. We have taken up this challenge for some of the phenomena (Meltzoff & Moore, 1998). Essentially, our argument is that many of the looking time effects result from the early representational system operating to maintain an object's numerical identity even in the absence of object permanence (hypothesis # 5). The ID account contends that this representational system allows infants to learn and retain the spatiotemporal structure of disappearance and reappearance events in the visible world, and to form expectations about the visible outcomes of such events (Johnson, Amso, et al., 2003; Kochukhova & Gredebäck, 2007). When discrepancies from expected outcomes occur, they will recruit increased attention. Thus, on the ID account, such discrepancies could explain increased looking times to the events that have been studied, without implying actual infant knowledge of permanence (for details, see Meltzoff & Moore, 1998).

In the end, a full developmental theory has to be compatible with the facts: Infants learn, develop, and change seemingly based on input; they solve problems; they care about consequences and show emotion; and they act. They do not just sit and perceive, receive, and parse events in the world. They go out and change it. We have begun to provide an account of object permanence development compatible with these facts.

Summary

We have proposed an ID account of object permanence that locates the origins and development of permanence in infants' notions of how to determine and trace numerical identity. The arguments and evidence generated from this approach suggest a number of conclusions: (a) object permanence understanding is not an all-or-none attainment; (b) permanence is understood for some disappearance transforms but not others; (c) the development of infants' spatiotemporal criteria for numerical identity provide the form and ordering of the disappearance transforms over which they understand permanence; (d) apparent violations of permanence can cause negative emotion; and (e) taking seriously the conceptual distinctions between representation, identity, and permanence offers considerable theoretical power. Finally, we proposed a mechanism of change to account for the transition from having no concept of permanence to having permanence.

Acknowledgments

This work was supported by NIH (HD-22514), NSF (SBE-0354453), and the Tamaki Foundation. Any opinions, findings, and conclusions expressed in the paper are those of the authors and do not necessarily reflect the views of these agencies. We thank Calle Fisher and Craig Harris for their assistance and S.J. for very helpful comments on an earlier version of this chapter.

References

Aslin, R. (1981). Development of smooth pursuit in human infants. In D. F. Fischer, R. A. Monty, & E. J. Senders (Eds.), *Eye movements: cognition and visual perception* (pp. 31–51). Hillsdale, NJ: Erlbaum.

Baillargeon, R. (2008). Innate ideas revisited: For a principle of persistence in infants' physical reasoning. *Perspectives on Psychological Science, 3*, 2–13.

Baillargeon, R., Graber, M., DeVos, J., & Black, J. (1990). Why do young infants fail to search for hidden objects? *Cognition, 36*, 255–284.

Bertenthal, B. I., Longo, M. R., & Kenny, S. (2007). Phenomenal permanence and the development of predictive tracking in infancy. *Child Development, 78*, 350–363.

Berthier, N. E., Bertenthal, B. I., Seaks, J. D., Sylvia, M. R., Johnson, R. L., & Clifton, R. K. (2001). Using object knowledge in visual tracking and reaching. *Infancy, 2*, 257–284.

Bower, T. G. R. (1967). The development of object-permanence: Some studies of existence constancy. *Perception & Psychophysics, 2*, 411–418.

Bower, T. G. R. (1971). The object in the world of the infant. *Scientific American, 225*, 30–38.

Bower, T. G. R. (1982). *Development in infancy* (2nd ed.). San Francisco: Freeman.

Bower, T. G. R., Broughton, J. M., & Moore, M. K. (1971). Development of the object concept as manifested in changes in the tracking behavior of infants between 7 and 20 weeks of age. *Journal of Experimental Child Psychology, 11*, 182–193.

Bremner, G. (1989). Development of spatial awareness in infancy. In A. Slater & G. Bremner (Eds.), *Infant Development* (pp. 123–141). Hillsdale, NJ: Erlbaum.

Bremner, J. G., Johnson, S. P., Slater, A., Mason, U., Cheshire, A., & Spring, J. (2007). Conditions for young infants, failure to perceive trajectory continuity. *Developmental Science, 10*, 613–624.

Bremner, J. G., Johnson, S. P., Slater, A., Mason, U., Foster, K., Cheshire, A., et al. (2005). Conditions for young infants, perception of object trajectories. *Child Development, 76*, 1029–1043.

Campos, J. J., Anderson, D. I., Barbu-Roth, M. A., Hubbard, E. M., Hertenstein, M. J., & Witherington, D. (2000). Travel broadens the mind. *Infancy, 1*, 149–219.

Carey, S., & Xu, F. (2001). Infants' knowledge of objects: Beyond object files and object tracking. *Cognition, 80*, 179–213.

Cohen, L. B, & Cashon, C. H. (2006). Infant cognition. In D. Kuhn, R. S. Siegler, W. Damon, & R. M. Lerner, (Eds.). *Handbook of child psychology*, (Vol. 2, pp. 214–251). Hoboken, NJ: Wiley.

Diamond, A. (1985). Development of the ability to use recall to guide action, as indicated by infants' performance on A$\bar{B}$. *Child Development, 56*, 868–883.

Diamond, A., Cruttenden, L., & Neiderman, D. (1994). A$\bar{B}$ with multiple wells: 1. Why are multiple wells sometimes easier than two wells? 2. Memory or memory + inhibition? *Developmental Psychology, 30*, 192–205.

Fodor, J. A. (1981). *Representations: Philosophical essays on the foundations of cognitive science.* Cambridge, MA: MIT Press.

Gibson, J. J., Kaplan, G. A., Reynolds, H. N., & Wheeler, K. (1969). The change from visible to invisible: A study of optical transitions. *Perception & Psychophysics, 5*, 113–116.

Grzywacz, N. M., Watamaniuk, S. N. J., & McKee, S. P. (1995). Temporal coherence theory for the detection and measurement of visual motion. *Vision Research, 35*, 3183–3203.

Haith, M. M., Kessen, W., & Collins, D. (1969). Response of the human infant to level of complexity of intermittent visual movement. *Journal of Experimental Child Psychology, 7*, 52–69.

Harris, P. L. (1987). The development of search. In P. Salapatek & L. Cohen (Eds.), *Handbook of infant perception* (Vol. 2, pp. 155–207). New York: Academic Press.

Haxby, J. V., Grady, C. L., Horwitz, B., Ungerleider, L. G., Mishkin, M., Carson, R. E., et al. (1991). Dissociation of object and spatial visual processing pathways in human extrastriate cortex. *Proceedings of the National Academy of Sciences, USA, 88*, 1621–1625.

Johnson, S. P., Amso, D., & Slemmer, J. A. (2003). Development of object concepts in infancy: Evidence for early learning in an eye-tracking paradigm. *Proceedings of the National Academy of Sciences, USA, 100*, 10568–10573.

Johnson, S. P., Bremner, J. G., Slater, A., Mason, U., Foster, K., & Cheshire, A. (2003). Infants' perception of object trajectories. *Child Development, 74*, 94–108.

Jonsson, B., & von Hofsten, C. (2003). Infants' ability to track and reach for temporarily occluded objects. *Developmental Science, 6*, 86–99.

Kagan, J. (2008). In defense of qualitative changes in development. *Child Development, 79*, 1606–1624.

Kahneman, D., Treisman, A., & Gibbs, B. J. (1992). The reviewing of object files: Object-specific integration of information. *Cognitive Psychology, 24*, 175–219.

Kaufman, J., Csibra, G., & Johnson, M. H. (2005). Oscillatory activity in the infant brain reflects object maintenance. *Proceedings of the National Academy of Sciences, USA, 102*, 15271–15274.

Kochukhova, O., & Gredebäck, G. (2007). Learning about occlusion: Initial assumptions and rapid adjustments. *Cognition, 105*, 26–46.

Köhler, S., Kapur, S., Moscovitch, M., Winocur, G., & Houle, S. (1995). Dissociation of pathways for object and spatial vision: A PET study in humans. *Neuroreport, 6*, 1865–1868.

Kramer, J. A., Hill, K. T., & Cohen, L. B. (1975). Infants' development of object permanence: A refined methodology and new evidence for Piaget's hypothesized ordinality. *Child Development, 46*, 149–155.

Krøjgaard, P. (2004). A review of object individuation in infancy. *British Journal of Developmental Psychology, 22*, 159–183.

Krøjgaard, P. (2007). Comparing infants' use of featural and spatiotemporal information in an object individuation task using a new event-monitoring design. *Developmental Science, 10*, 892–909.

Leslie, A. M., Xu, F., Tremoulet, P. D., & Scholl, B. J. (1998). Indexing and the object concept: Developing 'what' and 'where' systems. *Trends in Cognitive Sciences, 2*, 10–18.

Marcovitch, S., & Zelazo, P. D. (1999). The A-not-B error: Results from a logistic meta-analysis. *Child Development, 70*, 1297–1313.

Mareschal, D., Plunkett, K., & Harris, P. (1999). A computational and neuropsychological account of object-oriented behaviors in infancy. *Developmental Science, 2*, 306–317.

Meltzoff, A. N., & Moore, M. K. (1998). Object representation, identity, and the paradox of early permanence: Steps toward a new framework. *Infant Behavior & Development, 21*, 201–235.

Michotte, A. (1962). *Causalité, permanence, et réalité phénoménales: Études de psychologie expérimentale.* Louvain: Publications Universitaires.

Moore, M. K. (1975, April). Object permanence and object identity: A stage-developmental model. In M. K. Moore (Chair), *Object identity: The missing link between Piaget's stages of object permanence.* Symposium conducted at the meeting of the Society for Research in Child Development, Denver, CO.

Moore, M. K., Borton, R., & Darby, B. L. (1978). Visual tracking in young infants: Evidence for object identity or object permanence? *Journal of Experimental Child Psychology, 25*, 183–198.

Moore, M. K., & Meltzoff, A. N. (1978). Object permanence, imitation, and language development in infancy: Toward a neo-Piagetian perspective on communicative and cognitive development. In F. D. Minifie & L. L. Lloyd (Eds.), *Communicative and cognitive abilities—Early behavioral assessment* (pp. 151–184). Baltimore: University Park Press.

Moore, M. K., & Meltzoff, A. N. (1999). New findings on object permanence: A developmental difference between two types of occlusion. *British Journal of Developmental Psychology, 17*, 623–644.

Moore, M. K., & Meltzoff, A. N. (2004). Object permanence after a 24-hr delay and leaving the locale of disappearance: The role of memory, space, and identity. *Developmental Psychology, 40*, 606–620.

Moore, M. K., & Meltzoff, A. N. (2008). Factors affecting infants' manual search for occluded objects and the genesis of object permanence. *Infant Behavior & Development, 31*, 168–180.

Munakata, Y., McClelland, J. L., Johnson, M. H., & Siegler, R. S. (1997). Rethinking infant knowledge: Toward an adaptive process account of successes and failures in object permanence tasks. *Psychological Review, 104*, 686–713.

Newcombe, N. S., & Huttenlocher, J. (2006). Development of spatial cognition. In D. Kuhn, R. S. Siegler, W. Damon, & R. M. Lerner, (Eds.). *Handbook of child psychology* (Vol. 2, pp. 734–776). Hoboken, NJ: Wiley.

Newcombe, N. S., & Huttenlocher, J. (2000). *Making space: The development of spatial representation and reasoning.* Cambridge, MA: MIT Press.

Newcombe, N., Huttenlocher, J., & Learmonth, A. (1999). Infants' coding of location in continuous space. *Infant Behavior & Development, 22*, 483–510.

Piaget, J. (1952). *The origins of intelligence in children* (M. Cook, Trans.). New York: International Universities Press.

Piaget, J. (1954). *The construction of reality in the child* (M. Cook, Trans.). New York: Basic Books.

Quinn, P. C. (2008). In defense of core competencies, quantitative change, and continuity. *Child Development, 79*, 1633–1638.

Rosander, K., & von Hofsten, C. (2004). Infants' emerging ability to represent occluded object motion. *Cognition, 91*, 1–22.

Smith, L. B., Thelen, E., Titzer, R., & McLin, D. (1999). Knowing in the context of acting: The task dynamics of the A-not-B error. *Psychological Review, 106*, 235–260.

Spelke, E. S. (1990). Principles of object perception. *Cognitive Science, 14*, 29–56.

Spelke, E. S. (1994). Initial knowledge: Six suggestions. *Cognition, 50*, 431–445.

Spelke, E. S., Breinlinger, K., Macomber, J., & Jacobson, K. (1992). Origins of knowledge. *Psychological Review, 99*, 605–632.

Spelke, E. S., & von Hofsten, C. (2001). Predictive reaching for occluded objects by 6-month-old infants. *Journal of Cognition and Development, 2*, 261–281.

Strawson, P. F. (1959). *Individuals: An essay in descriptive metaphysics.* London: Methuen.

Thelen, E., Schöner, G., Scheier, C., & Smith, L. B. (2001). The dynamics of embodiment: A field theory of infant perseverative reaching. *Behavioral and Brain Sciences, 24*, 1–86.

Thelen, E., & Smith, L. B. (1994). *A dynamic systems approach to the development of cognition and action.* Cambridge, MA: MIT Press.

Treisman, A. (1992). Perceiving and re-perceiving objects. *American Psychologist, 47*, 862–875.

Van de Walle, G. A., Carey, S., & Prevor, M. (2000). Bases for object individuation in infancy: Evidence from manual search. *Journal of Cognition and Development, 1*, 249–280.

von Hofsten, C., Kochukhova, O., & Rosander, K. (2007). Predictive tracking over occlusions by 4-month-olds. *Developmental Science, 10*, 625–640.

von Hofsten, C., Vishton, P., Spelke, E. S., Feng, Q., & Rosander, K. (1998). Predictive action in infancy: Tracking and reaching for moving objects. *Cognition, 67,* 255–285.

Watamaniuk, S. N. J., & McKee, S. P. (1995). Seeing motion behind occluders. *Nature, 377,* 729–730.

Watamaniuk, S. N. J., McKee, S. P., & Grzywacz, N. M. (1995). Detecting a trajectory embedded in random-direction motion noise. *Vision Research, 35,* 65–77.

Wilcox, T., & Baillargeon, R. (1998). Object individuation in infancy: The use of featural information in reasoning about occlusion events. *Cognitive Psychology, 37,* 97–155.

Xu, F., & Carey, S. (1996). Infants' metaphysics: The case of numerical identity. *Cognitive Psychology, 30,* 111–153.

PART II

Words, Language, and Music

CHAPTER 5
Connectionist Explorations of Multiple-Cue Integration in Syntax Acquisition

Morten H. Christiansen, Rick Dale, and Florencia Reali

Among the many feats of learning that children showcase in their development, syntactic abilities appear long before many other skills, such as riding bikes, tying shoes, or playing a musical instrument. This is achieved with little or no direct instruction, making it both impressive and even puzzling, because mastering natural language syntax is one of the most difficult learning tasks that humans face. One reason for this difficulty is a "chicken-and-egg" problem involved in acquiring syntax. Syntactic knowledge can be characterized by constraints governing the relationship between grammatical categories of words (such as noun and verb) in a sentence. At the same time, the syntactic constraints presuppose the grammatical categories in terms of which they are defined; and the validity of grammatical categories depends on how they support those same syntactic constraints. A similar "bootstrapping" problem faces a student learning an academic subject such as physics: understanding momentum or force presupposes some understanding of the physical laws in which they figure; yet these laws presuppose these very concepts. The bootstrapping problem solved by very young children seems much more daunting, both because the constraints governing natural language are so intricate, and because these children do not have the intellectual capacity or explicit instruction present in conventional academic settings. Determining how children accomplish the astonishing feat of language acquisition remains a key question in cognitive science.

By 12 months, infants are attuned to the phonological and prosodic regularities of their native language (Jusczyk, 1997; Kuhl, 1999). This perceptual attunement may provide an essential scaffolding for later learning by biasing children toward aspects of language input that are particularly informative for acquiring grammatical knowledge. In this chapter, we hypothesize that integrating multiple probabilistic cues (phonological, prosodic, and distributional) by perceptually attuned general-purpose learning mechanisms may hold promise for explaining how children solve the bootstrapping problem. Multiple cues can provide reliable evidence about linguistic structure that is unavailable from any single source of information.

In the remainder of this chapter, we first review empirical evidence suggesting that infants may use a combination of phonological, prosodic, and distributional cues to bootstrap into syntax. We then report a series of simulations demonstrating the computational efficacy of multiple-cue integration within a connectionist framework (for modeling of other aspects of cognitive development, see the chapter by Mareschal & Westermann, this volume). Simulation 1 shows how multiple-cue integration results in better, faster, and more uniform learning. Simulation 2 uses this initial model to mimic the effect of grammatical and prosodic manipulations in a sentence comprehension study with 2-year-olds (Shady & Gerken, 1999). Simulation 3 uses an idealized representation of prenatal exposure to gross-level phonological and prosodic cues, leading to facilitation of postnatal learning of syntax by the model. Simulation 4 demonstrates that adding additional distracting cues, irrelevant to the syntactic acquisition task, does not hinder learning. Finally, Simulation 5 scales up these initial simulations, showing that connectionist models can acquire aspects of syntactic structure from cues present in actual child-directed speech.

The Need for Multiple Language-Internal Cues

In this section, we identify three kinds of constraints that may serve to help the language learner solve the syntactic bootstrapping problem. First, innate constraints in the form of linguistic universals may be available to discover to which grammatical category a word belongs, and how they function in syntactic rules. Second, language-external information, concerning observed semantic relationships between language and the world, could help map individual words onto their grammatical function. Finally, language-internal information, such as aspects of phonological, prosodic, and distributional patterns, may indicate the relation of various parts of language to each other, thus bootstrapping the child into the realm of syntactic relations. We discuss each of these potential constraints below, and conclude that some form of language-internal information is needed to break the circularity.

Although innate constraints likely play a role in language acquisition, they cannot solve the bootstrapping problem. Even with genetically prescribed abstract knowledge of grammatical categories and syntactic rules (e.g., Pinker, 1984), the problem remains: Innate knowledge requires building in universal mappings across languages, but the relationships between words and grammatical categories clearly differ cross-linguistically (e.g., the sound /su/ is a noun in French (*sou*) but a verb in English (*sue*)). Even with rich innate knowledge, children still must assign sound sequences to appropriate grammatical categories while determining the syntactic relations between these categories in their native language. Recently, a wealth of compelling experimental evidence has accumulated, suggesting that children do not initially use abstract linguistic categories. Instead, they seem to employ words at first as concrete individuals (rather than instances of abstract kinds), thereby challenging the usefulness of hypothesized innate grammatical categories (Tomasello, 2000). Whether we grant the presence of extensive innate knowledge or not, it seems clear that other sources of information are necessary to solve the bootstrapping problem.

Language-external information, such as correlations between the environment and semantic categories, may contribute to language acquisition by supplying a "semantic bootstrapping" solution (Pinker, 1984). However, because children learn linguistic distinctions that have no semantic basis (e.g., gender in French: Karmiloff-Smith, 1979), semantics cannot be the only source of information involved in solving the bootstrapping problem. Other sources of language-external constraints include cultural learning, indicated by a child's imitation of linguistic forms in socially conventional contexts (Tomasello, Kruger & Ratner, 1993). For example, a child may perceive that the idiom "*John let the cat out of the bag*," used in the appropriate context, means that John has revealed some sort of secret, and not that he released a feline from captivity. Despite both of these important language-external sources, to break down the linguistic forms into relevant units, it appears that correlation and cultural learning must be coupled with language-internal information.

We do not challenge the important role that the two foregoing sources of information play in language acquisition. We would argue, however, that language-internal information is fundamental to bootstrapping the child into syntax. Because language-internal input is rich in potential cues to linguistic structure, we offer a requisite feature of this information for syntax acquisition: Cues may only be partially reliable individually, and a learner must integrate an array of these cues to solve the bootstrapping problem. For example, a learner could use the tendency for English nouns to be longer than verbs to conjecture that *bonobo* is a noun, but the same strategy would fail for *ingratiate*. Likewise, although speakers tend to pause at syntactic phrase boundaries in a sentence, pauses also occur elsewhere during normal language production. And although it is a good distributional bet that the definite article *the* will precede a noun, so might adjectives, such as *silly*. The child therefore needs to integrate a great diversity of probabilistic cues to language structure. Fortunately, as we review in the next section, there is now extensive evidence that multiple probabilistic cues are available in language-internal input, that children are sensitive to them, and that they facilitate learning through integration.

Bootstrapping through Multiple Language-Internal Cues

We explore three sources of language-internal cues: phonological, prosodic, and distributional. Phonological information includes stress, vowel quality, and duration, and may help distinguish grammatical function words (e.g., determiners, prepositions, and conjunctions) from content words (nouns, verbs, adjectives, and adverbs) in English (e.g., Cutler, 1993; Gleitman & Wanner, 1982; Monaghan, Chater & Christiansen, 2005; Monaghan, Christiansen & Chater, 2007; Morgan, Shi, & Allopenna, 1996; Shi, Morgan, & Allopenna, 1998). Phonological information may also help separate nouns and verbs (Monaghan et al., 2005, 2007; Onnis & Christiansen, 2008). For example, English disyllabic nouns tend to receive initial-syllable (trochaic) stress whereas disyllabic verbs tend to receive final-syllable (iambic) stress, and adults are sensitive to this distinction (Kelly, 1988). Acoustic analyses have also shown that disyllabic words that are noun–verb ambiguous and have the same stress placement can still be differentiated by syllable duration and amplitude cue differences (Sereno & Jongman, 1995). Even 3-year-old children are sensitive to this stress cue, despite the fact that few multisyllabic verbs occur in child-directed speech (Cassidy & Kelly, 1991, 2001). Additional noun/verb cues in English likely include differences in word duration, consonant voicing, and vowel types, and many of these cues may be cross-linguistically relevant (see Kelly, 1992; Monaghan & Christiansen, 2008, for reviews).

Prosodic cues help word and phrasal/clausal segmentation and may reveal syntactic structure (e.g., Gerken, Jusczyk & Mandel, 1994; Gleitman & Wanner, 1982; Kemler-Nelson, Hirsh-Pasek, Jusczyk, & Wright Cassidy, 1989; Morgan, 1996). Acoustic analyses find that pause length, vowel duration, and pitch all mark phrasal boundaries in English and Japanese child-directed speech (Fisher & Tokura, 1996). Perhaps from utero (Mehler et al., 1988) and beyond, infants seem highly sensitive to such language-specific prosodic patterns (Gerken et al., 1994; Kemler-Nelson et al., 1989; for reviews, see Gerken, 1996; Jusczyk & Kemler-Nelson, 1996; Morgan, 1996). Prosodic information also improves sentence comprehension in 2-year-olds (Shady & Gerken, 1999). In experiments using adult participants, artificial language learning is facilitated in the presence of prosodic marking of syntactic phrase boundaries (Morgan, Meier & Newport, 1987; Valian & Levitt, 1996). Neurophysiological evidence in the form of event-related brainwave potentials (ERP) in adults shows that prosodic information has an immediate effect on syntactic processing (Steinhauer, Alter, & Friederici, 1999), suggesting a rapid, on-line role for this important cue. While prosody is influenced to some extent by a number of nonsyntactic factors, such as breathing patterns, resulting in an imperfect mapping between prosody and syntax (Fernald & McRoberts, 1996), infants' sensitivity to prosody argues for its likely contribution to syntax acquisition (Fisher & Tokura, 1996; Gerken 1996; Morgan, 1996).

Distributional characteristics of linguistic fragments at or below the word level may also provide cues to grammatical category. Morphological patterns across words may be informative—e.g., English words that are observed to have both *-ed* and *-s* endings are likely to be verbs (Maratsos & Chalkley, 1980). In artificial language learning experiments, adults acquire grammatical categories more effectively when they are cued by such word-internal patterns (Brooks, Braine, Catalano & Brody, 1993; Frigo & McDonald, 1998). Corpus analyses reveal that word co-occurrence also gives useful cues to grammatical categories in child-directed speech (e.g., Mintz, 2003; Monaghan et al., 2005, 2007; Redington, Chater, & Finch, 1998). Given that function words primarily occur at phrase boundaries (e.g., initially in English and French and finally in Japanese), they can also help the learner by signaling syntactic structure. This idea has received support from corpus analyses (Mintz, Newport & Bever, 2002) and artificial language learning studies (Green, 1979; Morgan et al., 1987; Valian & Coulson, 1988). Finally, artificial language learning experiments indicate that duplication of morphological patterns across related items in a phrase (e.g., Spanish: Los *Estad*os *Unid*os) <COMP: Keep underline for clarity.> facilitates learning (Meier & Bower, 1986; Morgan et al., 1987).

It is important to note that there is ample evidence that children are sensitive to these multiple sources of information. After just 1 year of language exposure, the perceptual attunement of children likely allows them to make use of language-internal probabilistic cues (for reviews, see Jusczyk, 1997, 1999; Kuhl, 1999; Pallier, Christophe & Mehler, 1997; Werker & Tees, 1999). Through early learning experiences, infants already appear sensitive to the acoustic differences between function and content words (Shi, Werker & Morgan, 1999) and the relationship between function words and prosody in speech (Shafer, D. W. Shucard, J. L. Shucard & Gerken, 1998). Young infants are able to detect differences in syllable number among isolated words (Bijeljac, Bertoncini & Mehler, 1993). In addition, infants exhibit rapid distributional learning (e.g., Gómez & Gerken, 1999; Saffran, Aslin, & Newport, 1996; see Gómez & Gerken, 2000; Saffran, 2003 for reviews), and importantly, they are capable of multiple-cue integration (Mattys, Jusczyk, Luce, & Morgan, 1999; Morgan & Saffran, 1995). When facing the bootstrapping problem, children probably also benefit from characteristics of child-directed speech, such as the predominance of short sentences (Newport, Gleitman & Gleitman, 1977) and exaggerated prosody (Kuhl et al., 1997).

In summary, phonological information helps to distinguish function words from content words and nouns from verbs. Prosodic information helps word and phrasal/clausal segmentation, thus serving to uncover syntactic structure. Distributional characteristics aid in labeling and segmentation, and may provide further cueing of syntactic relations. Despite the value of each source, none of these cues in isolation suffices to solve the bootstrapping problem. The learner must integrate these multiple cues to overcome the limited reliability of each individually. This review has indicated that a range of language-internal cues is available for language acquisition, that these cues affect learning and processing, and that mechanisms exist for multiple-cue integration. What is yet unknown is how far these cues can be combined to solve the bootstrapping problem (Fernald & McRoberts, 1996). Here we present connectionist simulations to demonstrate that efficient and robust computational mechanisms exist for multiple-cue integration (see also the chapters in this volume by Hannon, Kirkham, and Saffran, for evidence from human infant learning).

SIMULATION 1: MULTIPLE-CUE INTEGRATION

Although the multiple-cue approach is gaining support in developmental psycholinguistics, its computational efficacy still remains to be established. The simulations reported in this chapter are therefore intended as a first step toward a computational approach to multiple-cue integration, seeking to test its potential value in syntax acquisition. Based on our previous experience with modeling multiple-cue integration in speech segmentation (Christiansen, Allen, & Seidenberg, 1998), we used a simple recurrent network (SRN; Elman, 1990) to model the integration of multiple cues. The SRN is feed-forward neural network equipped with an additional copy-back loop that permits the learning and processing of temporal regularities in the stimuli presented to it (see Figure 5.1). This makes it particularly suitable for exploring the acquisition of syntax, an inherently temporal phenomenon.

The networks were trained on corpora of artificial child-directed speech generated by a grammar that includes three probabilistic cues to grammatical structure: word length, lexical stress, and pitch. The grammar (described further below) was motivated by considering frequent constructions in child-directed speech in

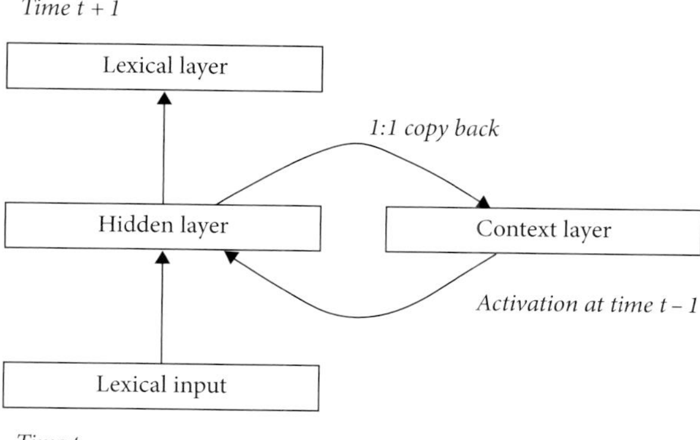

Figure 5.1 The general architecture of the simple-recurrent network (SRN) employed across simulations. An input layer representing information relevant for individual words along with an utterance boundary marker feeds into a hidden layer, and then to an output that predicts information relevant to the following word in a corpus. The hidden layer copies itself to a context layer, which supplies a limited memory for past words.

the CHILDES database (MacWhinney, 2000). Simulation 1 demonstrates how the integration of these three cues benefits the acquisition of syntactic structure by comparing performance across the eight possible cue combinations ranging from the absence of cues to the presence of all three.

Method

Networks

Ten networks were trained per condition, with an initial randomization of network connections in the interval [–0.1, 0.1]. Learning rate was set to 0.1, and momentum to 0. Each input to the networks contained a localist representation of a word (one unit = one word) and a set of cue units depending on cue condition. Words were presented one by one, and networks were required to predict the next word in a sentence along with the corresponding cues for that word. With a total of 44 words (see below) and a pause marking boundaries between utterances, the networks had 45 input units. Networks in the condition with all available cues had an additional five input units. The number of input and output units thus varied between 45 and 50 across conditions. Each network had 80 hidden units and 80 context units.

Materials

We constructed an idealized but relatively complex grammar based on independent analyses of child-directed speech corpora (Bernstein-Ratner, 1984; Korman, 1984) and a study of child-directed speech by mother–daughter pairs (Fisher & Tokura, 1996). As illustrated in Table 5.1, the grammar included three primary sentence types: declarative, imperative, and interrogative sentences. Each type consisted of a variety of common utterances reflecting the child's exposure. For example, declarative sentences most frequently appeared as transitive or intransitive verb constructions (*the boy chases the cat*, *the boy swims*), but also included predication using *be* (*the horse is pretty*) and second person pronominal constructions commonly found in child-directed corpora (*you are a boy*). Interrogative sentences were composed of wh-questions (*where are the boys?*, *where do the boys swim?*), and questions formed by using auxiliary verbs (*do the boys walk?*, *are the cats pretty?*). Imperatives were the simplest class of sentences, appearing as intransitive or transitive verb phrases (*kiss the bunny*, *sleep*). Subject–verb agreement was upheld in the grammar, along with appropriate determiners accompanying nouns (*the cars* vs. **a cars*).

Table 5.1 The Stochastic Phrase-Structure Grammar Used to Generate Training Corpora for Simulations 1–4

S → Imperative [0.1] | Interrogative [0.3] | Declarative [0.6]
Declarative → NP VP [0.7] | NP-ADJ [0.1] | That-NP [0.075] | You-P [0.125]
NP-ADJ → NP *is/are* adjective That-NP → *that/those is/are* NP You-P → *you are* NP
Imperative → VP
Interrogative → Wh-Question [0.65] | Aux-Question [0.35] Wh-Question → *where/who/what is/are* NP [0.5] | *Where/who/what do/does* NP VP [0.5] Aux-Question → *do/does* NP VP [0.33] | *Do/does* NP *wanna* VP [0.33] | *is/are* NP adjective [0.34]
NP → *a/the* N-sing/N-plur
VP → V-int | V-trans NP

Each word was assigned a unit for input into the model, and we added a number of units to represent cues. Two basic cues were available to all networks. The fundamental distributional information inherent in the grammar could be exploited by all networks in this simulation. As a second basic cue, utterance-boundary pauses signaled grammatically distinct utterances with 92% reliability (Broen, 1972). This was encoded as a single unit that was activated at the end of all but 8% of the sentences. Other semireliable prosodic and phonological cues accompanied the phrase-structure grammar: word length, stress, and pitch. Network groups were constructed using different combinations of these three cues. Cassidy and Kelly (1991) demonstrated that syllable count is a cue available to English speakers to distinguish nouns and verbs. They found that the probability of a single syllable word to be a noun rather than a verb is 38%. This probability rises to 76% at two syllables, and 92% at three. We selected verb and noun tokens that exhibited this distinction, whereas the length of the remaining words was typical for their class (i.e., function words tended to be monosyllabic). Word length was represented in terms of three units using thermometer encoding—that is, one unit would be on for monosyllabic words, two for bisyllabic words, and three for trisyllabic words. Pitch change is a cue associated with syllables that precede pauses. Fisher and Tokura (1996) found that these pauses signaled grammatically distinct utterances with 96% accuracy in child-directed speech, allowing pitch to serve as a cue to grammatical structure. In the networks, this cue was a single unit that would be activated at the final word in an utterance. Finally, we used a single unit to encode lexical stress as a possible cue to distinguish stressed content words from the reduced, unstressed form of function words. This unit would be on for all content words.

Procedure

Eight groups of networks, one for each combination of cues (all cues, 2 cues, 1 cue, or none), were trained on corpora consisting of 10,000 sentences generated from the grammar. Each network within a group was trained on a different randomized training corpus. Training consisted of 200,000 input/output presentations (words), or approximately 5 passes through the training corpus. Each group of networks had cues added to its training corpus depending on cue condition. Networks were expected to predict the next word in a sentence, along with the appropriate cue values. A corpus consisting of 1,000 novel sentences was generated for testing. Performance was measured by assessing the networks' ability to predict the next set of grammatical items given prior context. Importantly, this measure did not include predictions of cue information, and all network conditions were thus evaluated by exactly the same performance criterion.

To provide a statistical benchmark with which to compare network performance, we trained bigram and trigram models on the same corpora as the networks. These finite-state models, borrowed from computational linguistics, provide a simple prediction method based on strings of two (bigrams) or three (trigrams) consecutive words. Comparisons with these simple models provide an indication of whether the networks are learning more than simple two- or three-word associations.

Results

After training, SRNs trained with localist output representations will produce a distributional pattern of activation closely corresponding to a probability distribution of possible next items. In order to assess the overall performance of the SRNs, we made comparisons between network output probabilities and the full conditional probabilities given the prior context. For example, the full conditional probabilities given the context of "*The boy chases...*" can be represented as a vector containing the probabilities of being the next item in this sentence for each of the 44 words in the vocabulary and the pause. To ensure that our performance measure can deal with novel test sentences not seen during training, we estimate the prior conditional probabilities based on lexical categories rather than individual words (Christiansen & Chater, 1999). Suppose, in the example above, that every continuation of this sentence fragment in the training corpus always involved the indefinite determiner "*a*" (as in "*The boy chases a cat*"). If we did not base our full conditional probability estimates on lexical categories, we would not be able to assess SRN performance on novel sentences in which the definite determiner "*the*" followed the example fragment (as in "*The boy chases the cat*"). Formally, we thus have the following Equation 1 with c_i denoting the category of the ith word in the sentence:

$$P(c_p \mid c_1, c_2, \ldots, c_{p-1}) \cong \frac{\text{Freq}(c_1, c_2, \ldots, c_{p-1}, c_p)}{\text{Freq}(c_1, c_2, \ldots, c_{p-1})} \qquad (5.1)$$

where the probability of getting some member of a given lexical category as the pth item, c_p, in a sentence is conditional on the previous p–1 lexical categories. Note that for the purpose of performance assessment, singular and plural nouns are assigned to separate lexical categories throughout Simulations 1–4, as are singular and plural verbs. Given that the choice of lexical items for each category is independent, and that each word in a category is equally frequent, the probability of encountering a particular word w_n, which is a member of a category c_p, is simply inversely proportional to the number of items, C_p, in that category. So, overall, we have the following equation:

$$P(w_n \mid c_1, c_2, \ldots, c_{p-1}) \cong \frac{\text{Freq}(c_1, c_2, \ldots, c_{p-1}, c_p)}{\text{Freq}(c_1, c_2, \ldots, c_{p-1}) C_p} \qquad (5.2)$$

If the networks are performing optimally, then the vector of output unit activations should exactly match these probabilities. We evaluate the degree to which each network performs successfully by measuring the mean squared error between the vectors representing the network's output and the conditional probabilities (with 0 indicating optimal performance).

All networks achieved better performance than the standard bigram/trigram models (p-values < .0001), suggesting that the networks had acquired knowledge of syntactic structure beyond the information associated with simple pairs or triples of words. Figure 5.2A illustrates the best performance achieved by the trigram model as well as SRNs provided with no cues (the baseline network), a single cue (length, stress, or prosody), and three cues. The nets provided with one or more phonological/prosodic cues achieved significantly better performance than baseline networks (p-values < .02). Using trigram performance as criterion, all multiple-cue networks surpassed this level of performance faster than the baseline networks as shown in Figure 5.2B (p-values < .002). Moreover, the three-cue networks were significantly faster than the single-cue networks (p-values < .001). Finally, using Brown-Forsyth tests for variability in the final level of performance, we found that the three-cue networks also exhibited significantly more uniform learning than the baseline networks ($F(1,18) = 5.14$, $p < .04$), as depicted in Figure 5.2C.

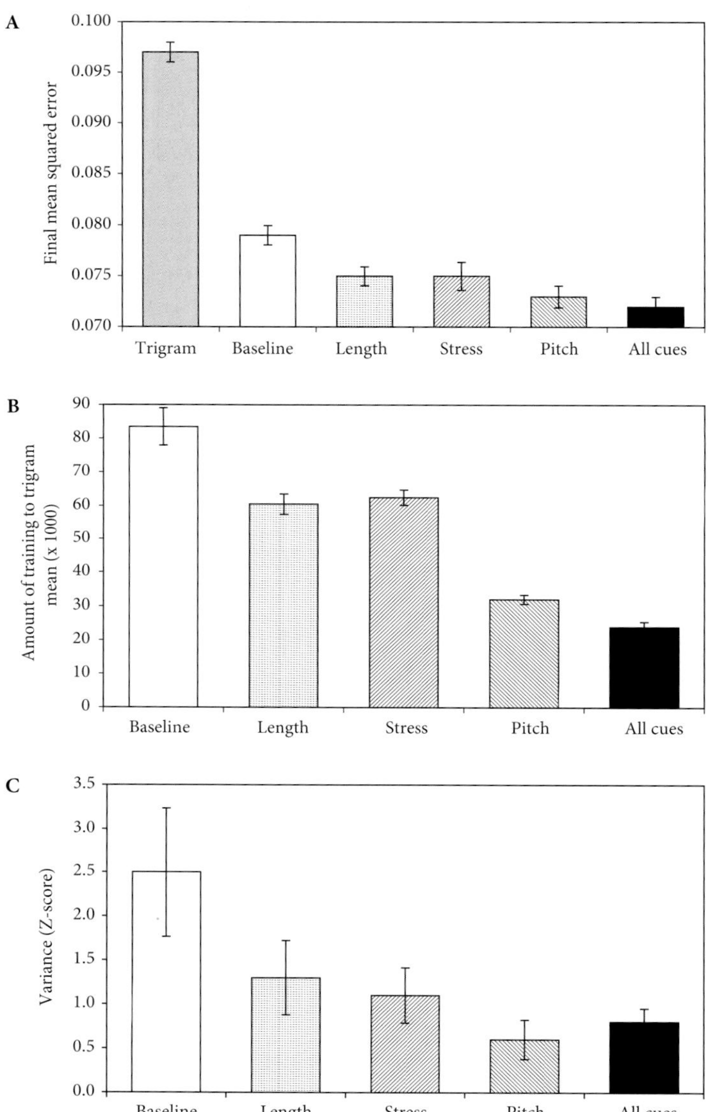

Figure 5.2 Comparison of learning performance for different cue combinations in Simulation 1, showing that multiple-cue integration leads to (A) better learning (as measured by the lowest error obtained on the test corpus), (B) faster learning (measured in terms of the amount of training needed to surpass the performance of the trigram model), and (C) more uniform learning (as indicated by less variance across the performance of the different instances of the network). (Error bars = S.E.M.)

SIMULATION 2: SENTENCE COMPREHENSION IN 2-YEAR-OLDS

Simulation 1 provides evidence for the general feasibility of multiple-cue integration for supporting syntax learning. To further demonstrate the relevance of the model to language development, closer contact with human data is needed (Christiansen & Chater, 2001). In the current simulation, we demonstrate that the three-cue networks from Simulation 1 are able to accommodate experimental data showing that 2-year-olds can integrate grammatical markers (function words) and prosodic cues in sentence comprehension (Shady & Gerken, 1999: Experiment 1). In this study, children heard sentences, such as (1) [see below], in one of three prosodic conditions depending on pause location: early natural [e], late natural [l], and unnatural [u]. Each sentence moreover involved one of three grammatical markers: grammatical (*the*), ungrammatical (*was*), and nonsense (*gub*).

1. Find [e] the/was/gub [u] dog [l] for me.

The child's task was to identify the correct picture corresponding to the target noun (*dog*). Children performed the task best when the pause location delimited a phrasal boundary (early/late), and with the grammatical marker *the*. Simulation 2 models these data by using comparable stimuli and assessing noun unit activations.

Method

Networks

Twelve three-cue networks of the same architecture and training used in Simulation 1 were used in each prosodic condition in the infant experiment. This number was chosen to match the number of infants in the Shady and Gerken (1999) experiment. An additional unit was added to the networks to encode the nonsense word (*gub*) in Shady and Gerken's experiment.

Materials

We constructed a sample set of sentences from our grammar that could be modified to match the stimuli in Shady and Gerken. Twelve sentences for each prosody condition (pause location) were constructed. Pauses were simulated by activating the utterance-boundary unit. Because these pauses probabilistically signal grammatically of distinct utterances, the utterance-boundary unit provides an approximation of what the children in the experiment would experience. Finally, the nonsense word was added to the stimuli for the within group condition (grammatical vs. ungrammatical vs. nonsense). Adjusting for vocabulary differences, the networks were tested on comparable sentences, such as (2):

2. Where does [e] the/is/gub [u] dog [l] eat?

Procedure

Each group of networks was exposed to the set of sentences corresponding to its assigned pause location (early vs. late vs. unnatural). No learning took place, since the fully trained networks were used. To approximate the picture selection task in the experiment, we measured the degree to which the networks would activate the groups of nouns following *the/is/gub*. The two conditions were expected to affect the activation of the nouns.

Results

The human results for the prosody condition in Shady and Gerken (1999) is depicted in Figure 5.3A. They reported a significant effect of prosody on the picture selection task. The same was true for our networks ($F(2,33) = 1{,}253.07$, $p < .0001$), and the pattern of noun activations closely resembles that of the toddlers' correct picture choice as evidenced by Figure 5.3B. The late natural condition elicited the highest noun activation, followed by the early natural condition, and with the unnatural condition yielding the least activation. The experiment also revealed an effect of grammaticality as can be seen from the human data shown in Figure 5.3C. We similarly obtained a significant grammaticality effect for our networks ($F(2,70) = 69.85$, $p < .0001$), which, as illustrated by Figure 5.3D, produced the highest noun activation

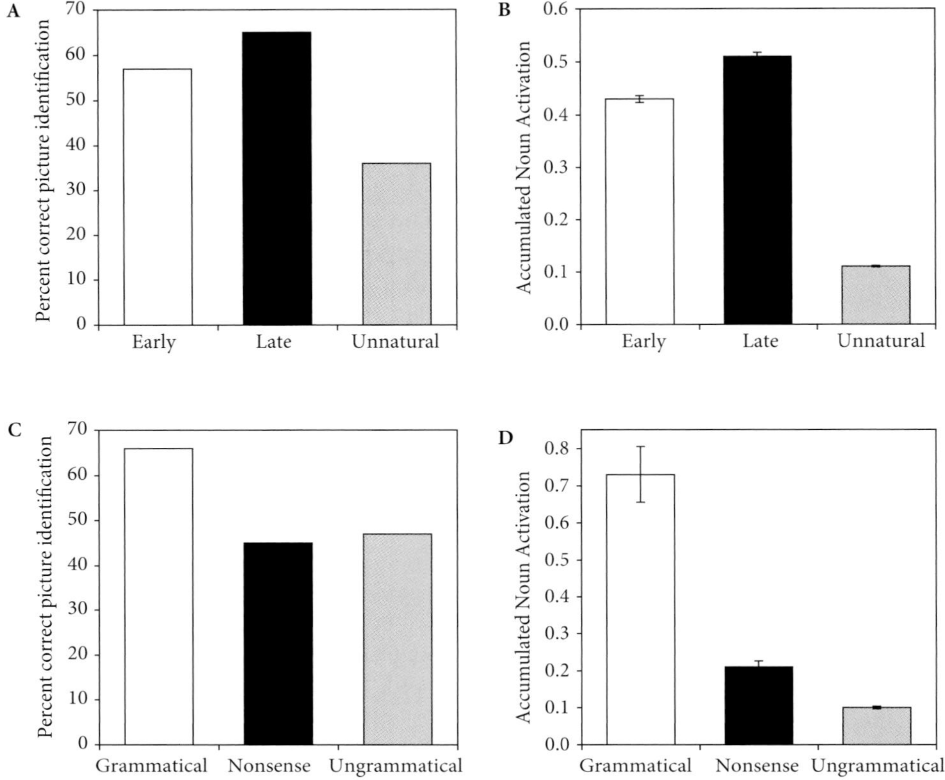

Figure 5.3 The effect of prosody and grammatical markers on human and SRN sentence processing. (A) Percent correct picture identification by 2-year-olds in the prosody condition of the Shady and Gerken (1999) experiment, with pauses inserted early, late, or in the unnatural position between the determiner and the noun. (B) Total activation of nouns by the SRN when exposed to the same prosodic manipulation as the human children. (C) Picture identification performance in the grammatical marker condition in Shady and Gerken (1999), involving a grammatical, nonsense, or ungrammatical word before the target noun. (D) Matching SRN activation of nouns for the same three types of grammatical markers. (Error bars = S.E.M.)

following the determiner, followed by the nonsense word, and lastly for the ungrammatical word. Again, the network results match the pattern observed for the toddlers. One slight discrepancy is that the networks are producing higher noun activation following the nonsense word compared to the ungrammatical marker. This result is however consistent with the results from a more sensitive picture selection task, showing that children were more likely to end up with a semantic representation of the target following nonsense syllables compared to incorrectly used morphemes (Carter & Gerken, 1996). Thus, the results suggest that the syntactic knowledge acquired by the networks mirrors the kind of sensitivity to syntactic relations and prosodic content observed in human children. Together with Simulation 1, the results also demonstrate that multiple-cue integration may both facilitate syntax acquisition, and underlie some patterns of linguistic skill observed early on in human performance. In the next simulation, we show that the multiple-cue perspective can simulate possible prosodic scaffolding that occurs much earlier in development: prenatal attunement to prosody.

Simulation 3: The Role of Prenatal Exposure

Studies of 4-day-old infants suggest that the attunement to prosodic information may begin prior to birth (Mehler et al., 1988). We suggest that this prenatal exposure to language may provide a scaffolding for later syntactic acquisition by initially focusing learning on certain aspects of prosody and gross-level properties of phonology (such as word length) that later will play an important role in postnatal multiple-cue integration. In the current simulation, we test this hypothesis using the connectionist model from Simulations 1 and 2. If this scaffolding hypothesis is correct, we would expect that prenatal exposure corresponding to what infants receive in the womb would result in improved acquisition of syntactic structure.

Method

Networks

Ten SRNs were used in both prenatal and non-prenatal groups, with the same initial conditions and training details as Simulation 1. Each network was supplied with the full range of cues used in Simulation 1.

Materials

A set of "filtered" prenatal stimuli was generated using the same grammar as previously (Table 5.1), with the exception that input/output patterns now ignored individual words and only involved the units encoding word length, stress, pitch change and utterance boundaries. The postnatal stimuli were the same as in Simulation 1.

Procedure

The networks in the prenatal group were first trained on 100,000 input/output filtered presentations drawn from a corpus of 10,000 new sentences. Following this prenatal exposure, the nets were then trained on the full input patterns exactly as in Simulation 1. The non-prenatal group only received training on the postnatal corpora. As previously, networks were required to predict the following word and corresponding cues. Performance was again measured by the prediction of following words, ignoring the cue units.

Results

Both network groups exhibited significantly higher performance than the bigram/trigram models ($F(1,18) = 25.32$, $p < .0001$ for prenatal, $F(1,18) = 12.03$, $p < .01$ for non-prenatal), again indicating that the networks are acquiring complex grammatical regularities that go beyond simple adjacency relations. We compared the performance of the two network groups across different degrees of training using a two-way analysis of variance with training condition (prenatal vs. non-prenatal) as the between-network factor and amount of training as within-network factor (five levels of training measured in 20,000 input/output presentation intervals). There was a main effect of training condition ($F(1,18) = 12.36$, $p < .01$), suggesting that prenatal exposure significantly improved learning. A main effect of degrees of training ($F(9,162) = 15.96$, $p < .001$) reveals that both network groups benefited significantly from training. An interaction between training conditions and degrees of training indicates that the prenatal networks learned significantly better than postnatal networks ($F(1,18) = 9.90$, $p < .01$). Finally, as illustrated by Figure 5.4, prenatal input also resulted in faster learning (measured in terms of the amount of training needed to surpass the trigram model; $F(1,18) = 9.90$, $p < .01$). The exposure to prenatal input—void of any information about individual words—promotes better performance on the prediction task as well as faster learning overall. This provides computational support for the prenatal scaffolding hypothesis, derived as a prediction from the multiple-cue perspective on syntax acquisition.

Simulation 4: Multiple-Cue Integration with Useful and Distracting Cues

So far, simulations have demonstrated the importance of cue integration in syntax acquisition, that integration can match data obtained in infant experiments, and that this perspective can provide novel predictions in language

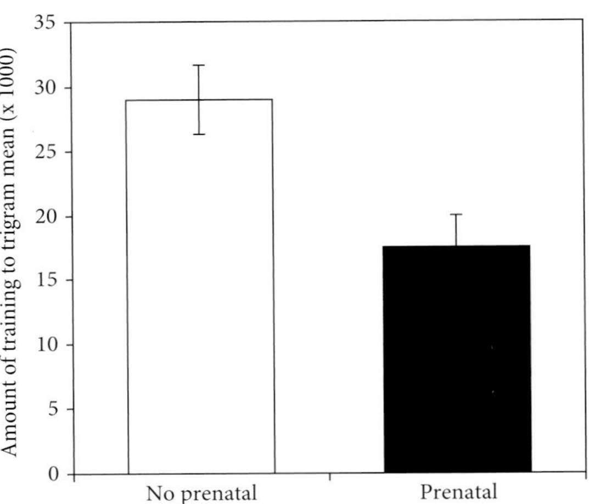

Figure 5.4 Speed of learning for networks trained with or without prenatal exposure to prosody and gross-level properties of phonology. (Error bars = S.E.M.)

development. A possible objection to these simulations is that our networks succeed at multiple-cue integration because they are only provided with cues that are at least partially relevant for syntax acquisition. Consequently, performance may potentially drop significantly if the networks themselves had to discover which cues were partially relevant and which are not. Simulation 4 therefore tests the robustness of our multiple-cue approach when faced with additional, uncorrelated distractor cues. Accordingly, we added three distractor cues to the previous three reliable cues. These new cues encoded the presence of word-initial vowels, word-final voicing, and relative (male/female) speaker pitch—all acoustically salient in speech, but which do not appear to cue syntactic structure.

Method

Networks

Networks, groups, and training details were the same as in Simulation 3, except for three additional input units encoding the distractor cues.

Materials

The three distractor cues were added to the stimuli used in Simulation 3. Two of the cues were phonetic and therefore available only in postnatal training. The word-initial vowel cue appears in all words across classes. The second distractor cue, word-final voicing, also does not provide useful distinguishing properties of word classes. Finally, as an additional prenatal and postnatal cue, overall pitch quality was added to the stimuli. This was intended to capture whether the speaker was female or male. In prenatal training, this probability was set to be extremely high (90%), and lower in postnatal training (60%). In the womb, the mother's voice naturally provides most of the input during the final trimester when the infant's auditory system has begun to function (Rubel, 1985). The probability used here was intended to capture the likelihood that some experience would derive from other speakers as well. In postnatal training, this probability drops, representing exposure to male members of the linguistic community, but still favoring mother–child interactions.

Procedure

Prenatal stimuli included the three previous semireliable cues, and only the additional prosodic, distractor cue encoding relative speaker pitch. In the postnatal stimuli, all three distractor cues were added. Training and testing details were the same as in Simulation 3.

Results

As in Simulations 1 and 3, both groups performed significantly better than the bigram/trigram models ($F(1,18) = 18.95$, $p < .0001$ for prenatal, and $F(1,18) = 14.27$, $p < .001$ for non-

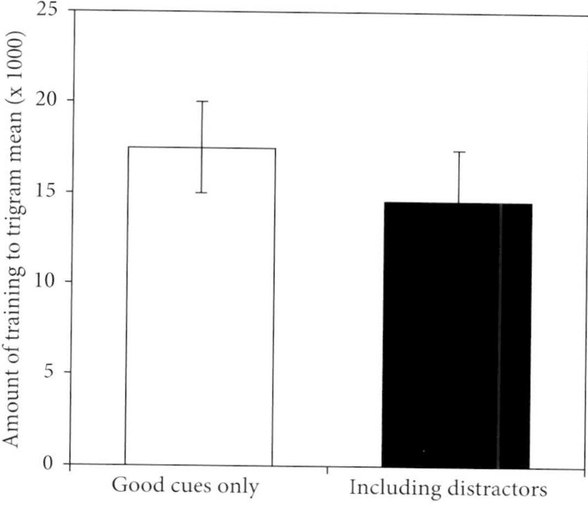

Figure 5.5 Speed of learning for networks trained with or without distractor cues. (Error bars = S.E.M.)

prenatal). We repeated the two-factor analysis of variance computed for Simulation 2, revealing a main effect for training condition ($F(1,18) = 4.76, p < .05$) and degrees of training ($F(9,162) = 13.88, p < .0001$). This indicates that the presence of the distractor cues did not hinder the improved performance following prenatal language exposure. As in Simulation 3, the prenatal networks learned comparatively faster than the non-prenatal networks ($F(1,18) = 5.31, p < .05$). To determine how the distractor cues affected performance, we compared the prenatal condition in Simulation 3 with that of the current simulation. There was no significant difference in performance across the two simulations ($F(1,18) = 0.13, p = .72$). Moreover, as shown in Figure 5.5, there was no difference in the speed of learning between the SRNs trained only with good cues and those whose input included distractor cues ($F(1,18) = .57, p = .46$). A further comparison between these non-prenatal networks and the bare networks in Simulation 1 showed that the networks trained with cues of mixed reliability significantly outperformed networks trained without any cues ($F(1,18) = 14.27, p < .001$). This indicates that the uncorrelated cues did not prevent the networks from integrating the partially reliable ones toward learning grammatical structure. Together with the first three simulations, Simulation 4 demonstrates that SRNs can integrate multiple cues efficiently when exposed to relatively complex artificial corpora. Next, we scale up the model to deal with naturalistic child-directed speech.

Simulation 5: Multiple-Cue Integration with Full-Blown Child-Directed Speech

In this final simulation, we take a further step toward describing the computational underpinnings of multiple-cue integration. The previous series of simulations have demonstrated that SRNs provide a suitable model for integrating multiple cues when exposed to input generated by a psychologically motivated artificial grammar. Here we further show that the SRN scales up to deal with real child-directed speech. In particular, we seek to determine the extent to which these networks are sensitive to the lexical category information present in the set of phonological cues. To accomplish this task, we set up two identical groups of networks, each provided with a different encoding of the corpus. The encoding of the first corpus was based on 16 phonological cues, previously shown by Monaghan et al. (2005) to provide information useful for syntax acquisition. The second set of input was encoded using the same cue vectors but randomized across lexical categories. Possible performance differences in networks trained with these different input sets would be due to lexical category information revealed by the multiple phonological cues.

Method

Networks

Ten SRNs were used for the phonetic-input condition and the random-input condition, with an initial weight randomization in the interval [−0.1, 0.1]. A different random seed was used for each simulation. Learning rate was set to 0.1 and momentum to 0.7. Each input to the network contained a thermometer encoding for each of the 16 phonological cues from Monaghan et al. (2005), listed in Table 5.2. This encoding required 43 units (each of them in a range from 0 to 1) and a pause marking boundaries between utterances, resulting in the networks having 44 input units. Each output was encoded using a localist representation consisting of 14 different lexical categories and a pause marking boundaries between utterances, resulting in networks with 15 output units. Each network furthermore was equipped with 88 hidden units and 88 context units.

Materials

We trained and tested the network on a corpus of child-directed speech (Bernstein-Ratner, 1984). This corpus contains speech recorded from nine mothers speaking to their children over a 4- to 5-month period when the children were between the ages of 1 year and 1 month to 1 year and 9 months. The corpus includes 1,371 word types and 33,035 tokens distributed over 10,082 utterances. The sentences incorporate a number of different types of grammatical structures, showing the varied nature of the linguistic input to children. Utterances range from declarative sentences (*Oh you need some space*) to wh-questions (*Where's my apple*) to one-word utterances ("*Uh*" or "*hello*"). Each word in the corpus corresponded to one of the 14 following lexical categories: nouns (19.5%), verbs (18.5%), adjectives (4%), numerals (<0.1%), adverbs (6.5%), articles (6.5%), pronouns (18.5%), prepositions (5%), conjunctions (4%), interjections (7%), complex contractions (8%), abbreviations (<0.1%), infinitive markers (1.2%), and proper names (1.2%). The training set consisted of 9,072 sentences (29,930 word tokens) from the original corpus. A separate test set consisted of 963 additional sentences (2,930 word tokens).

Each word was encoded in terms of the following 16 phonological cues from Table 5.2: number of phonemes (1–11), number of syllables (1–5), stress position (0 = no stress, 1 = 1st syllable stressed, etc.), proportion of reduced vowels (0–1), proportion of coronal consonants

Table 5.2 Phonological Cues that Distinguish between Lexical Categories

Nouns and Verbs
Nouns have more syllables than verbs (Kelly, 1992)
Bisyllabic nouns have 1st syllable stress, verbs tend to have 2nd syllable stress (Kelly & Bock, 1988)
Inflection -ed is pronounced /d/ for verbs, /@d/ or /Id/ for adjectives (Marchand, 1969)
Stressed syllables of nouns have more back vowels than front vowels. Verbs have more front vowels than back vowels (Sereno & Jongman, 1990)
Nouns have more low vowels, verbs have more high vowels (Sereno & Jongman, 1990)
Nouns are more likely to have nasal consonants (Kelly, 1992)
Nouns contain more phonemes per syllable than verbs (Kelly, 1996)
Function and Content Words
Function words have fewer syllables than content words (Morgan, Shi & Allopenna, 1996)
Function words have minimal or null onsets (Morgan, Shi & Allopenna, 1996)
Function word onsets are more likely to be coronal (Morgan, Shi & Allopenna, 1996)
/D/ occurs word-initially only for function words (Morgan, Shi & Allopenna, 1996)
Function words have reduced vowels in the first syllable (Cutler, 1993)
Function words are often unstressed (Gleitman & Wanner, 1982)

(0–1), number of consonants in onset (1–3), consonant complexity (0–1), initial /D/ (1 if begins /D/, 0 otherwise), reduced first vowel (1 if first vowel is reduced, 0 otherwise), any stress (0 if no stress, 1 otherwise), final inflection (0 if none, /@d/ or /Id/, 1 if present), stress vowel position (from front to back, 1–3), vowel position (mean position of vowels, from front to back, 1–3), final consonant voicing (0: vowel, 1: voiced, 2: unvoiced), proportion of nasal consonants (0–1) and mean height of vowels (0–3). The cues that assume only binary values were encoded using a single unit (e.g., "any stress", "initial /D/"). The cues that take on values between 0 and 1 (e.g., proportion of vowel consonants) were also encoded using a single unit with a decimal number, whereas the cues that assume values in a broader range (e.g., number of syllables) were represented using a thermometer encoding; for example, one unit would be on for monosyllabic words, two for bisyllabic words, and so on. Finally we used a single unit that would be activated at pauses between utterances.

The random-input networks were trained using input for which we randomly distributed the multiple-cue vectors among all the words in the corpus. Thus, the vector encoding for a given word would be randomly reassigned to a different word in the corpus regardless of its lexical category. Each phonological vector was assigned to only one word. Moreover, each token of a word was represented using the same random vector for all occurrences of that word in the test and training sets.

Procedure

Ten networks were trained on phonological cues and 10 control networks were trained on the random vectors. Training consisted of one pass through the training corpus. We used the same 10 random seeds for both simulation conditions. The networks were trained to predict the lexical category of the next word. The task of mapping phonological cues onto lexical categories may seem somewhat artificial because children are not provided directly with the lexical categories of the words to which they are exposed. However, children do learn early on to use pragmatic and other cues to discover the meaning of words. Given that the networks in our simulations only have access to linguistic information, we see lexical categories as a "stand-in" for more ecologically valid cues that we hope to be able to include in future work.

Results

We recorded the output vectors for the two groups of networks. Because the output consisted of localist representations for each lexical category (one unit = one lexical category) along with the utterance-final pause, we could use Equation 5.1 to estimate the full conditional probabilities, comparing network predictions to the full conditional probabilities for the next lexical category using the mean cosine of the angle between the two vectors (with 1 corresponding to optimal performance). We compared the predictions of the phonetic-input networks with those of the random-input networks. Figure 5.6A shows a comparison of test–set performance for the phonetic-input networks with that of the random-input networks. The phonetic-input networks were significantly better than the random-input networks at predicting the next combination of lexical categories (p-values < .00005). These results suggest that distributional information is generally a stronger cue than phonological information, even though the latter does lead to better learning overall. However, phonological information may provide the networks with a better basis for processing novel lexical items. Next, we probe the internal representations of the two sets of networks in order to gain further insight into their performance differences.

Probing the Internal Representations

Simulation 5 indicated that the phonetic-input networks did not benefit as much as one perhaps would have expected from the information provided by the phonological cues. However, the networks may nonetheless use this information to develop internal representations that better encode differences between lexical categories. This may allow them to go beyond the phonetic input and integrate it with the distributional

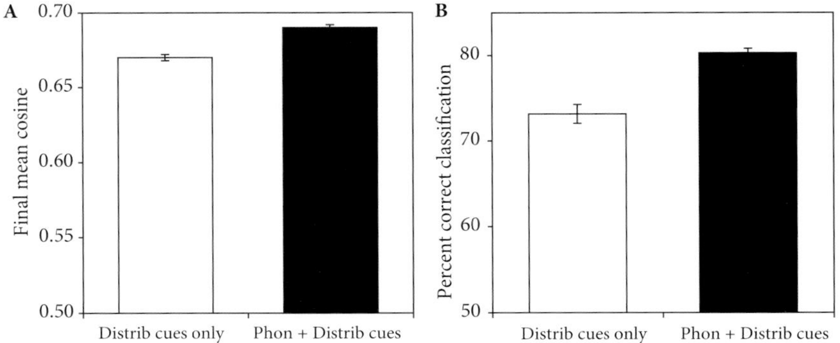

Figure 5.6 Performance of the network models trained on full-blown child-directed speech. (A) Test performance for networks provided only with distributional cues and networks provided with both phonological and distributional cues. (B) Results of the discriminant analyses, comparing the ability of the two types of networks to place themselves in a "noun state" and a "verb state" when processing novel nouns and verbs, respectively. (Error bars = S.E.M.)

information derived from the sequential order in which these vectors were presented. To investigate these possibilities, we carried out a series of discriminant analyses of network hidden unit activations as well as of the phonetic input vectors, focusing on the representations of nouns and verbs.

Method

Informally, a linear discriminant analysis allows us to determine the degree to which it is possible to separate a set of vectors into two (or more) groups based on the information contained in those vectors. In effect, we attempt to use a linear plane to split the hidden unit space into a group of noun vectors and a group of verb vectors. Using discriminant analyses, we can statistically estimate the degree to which this split can be accomplished given a set of vectors.

We recorded the hidden unit activations from the two sets of networks in Simulation 5. The hidden unit activations were recorded for 200 novel nouns and 200 novel verbs occurring in unique sentences taken from other CHILDES corpora (MacWhinney, 2000). The hidden unit activations were labeled such that each corresponded to the particular lexical category of the input presented to the network (though the networks did not receive this information as input). For example, a vector would be labeled a noun vector when the hidden unit activations were recorded for a noun (phonetic) input vector. We also included a condition in which the noun/verb labels were randomized with respect to the hidden unit vectors for both sets of networks, in order to establish a random control.

Results

We first compared the categorization performance of the two sets of networks, as illustrated in Figure 5.6B. The phonetic-input networks had developed hidden unit representations that allowed them to correctly separate 80.30% of the 400 nouns and verbs. This was significantly better than the random-input networks, which only achieved 73.15% correct separation ($t(8) = 5.89$, $p < .0001$). Both sets of networks surpassed their respective randomized controls (phonetic-input control: 69.05% – $t(8) = 11.51$, $p < .0001$; random-input control: 68.20% – $t(8) = 3.92$, $p < .004$). The controls for the two sets of networks were not significantly different from each other ($t(8) = 0.82$, $p > .43$). As indicated by our previous analyses of phonetic cue information in child-directed speech (Monaghan et al., 2005), the phonetic input vectors contained a considerable amount of information about lexical categories, allowing for 67.25% correct separation of nouns and verbs, but still significantly below the performance of the phonetic-input networks ($t(4) = 25.97, p < .0001$). The random-input networks also surpassed the level of separation afforded by their input vectors (59.00% – $t(4) = 12.80, p < .0001$).

The results of the hidden-unit discriminant analyses suggest that not only did the phonetic-input networks develop internal representations better suited for distinguishing between nouns and verbs, but they also went beyond the information afforded by the phonetic input and integrate it with distributional information. Crucially, the phonetic-input vectors were able to surpass the random-input networks, despite that the latter was also able to use distributional information to go beyond the input. Consistent phonological information thus appears to be important for network generalization to novel nouns and verbs.

General discussion

As described in an earlier part of this chapter, children who are learning syntax face a complex "chicken-and-egg" bootstrapping problem. A growing bulk of evidence from developmental cognitive science has suggested that a solution may come from a process of integrating multiple sources of probabilistic information, each of which is individually unreliable, but jointly advantageous (cf. Smith & Pereia chapter in this volume). What has so far been lacking is a demonstration of the computational feasibility of this approach and the series of simulations reported here takes a first step toward accomplishing this. We have demonstrated that providing SRNs with prosodic and phonological cues significantly improves their acquisition of syntactic structure (Simulation 1), and that the three-cue networks can mimic children's sensitivity to both prosodic and grammatical cues in sentence comprehension (Simulation 2). The model illustrates the potential value of prenatal exposure (Simulation 3) and provides evidence for the robustness of multiple-cue integration, since highly unreliable cues did not interfere with the integration process (Simulation 4). Finally, we expanded these results by showing that SRNs can also utilize highly probabilistic information found in 16 phonological cues in the service of syntactic acquisition when trained on a naturalistic corpus of child-directed speech (Simulation 5). Analysis of the networks' hidden unit activations provided further evidence that the integration of phonological and distributional cues during learning leads to more robust internal representations of lexical categories, at least when it comes to distinguishing between the two major categories of nouns and verbs.

Overall, the simulation results presented in this chapter provide support not only for the multiple-cue integration approach in general, but also for using neural network architectures to explore the integration of distributional, prosodic, and phonological information in language acquisition. Some researchers have challenged the value of multiple probabilistic cues (e.g., Fernald & McRoberts, 1996), but we have computationally demonstrated that their integration results in faster, better, and more uniform learning, even in the face of distracting information. Our simulations, along with artificial language learning experiments (Billman, 1989; Brooks et al., 1993; McDonald & Plauche, 1995; Morgan et al., 1987), underscore multiple-cue integration as a means of facilitating the complex task of syntax acquisition.

We have elsewhere explored the evolutionary emergence of phonological cues in agent-based simulations (Christiansen & Dale, 2004). In these evolutionary simulations, languages were mutated slightly across generations of randomized SRN learners. For any given generation, the languages best learned by the networks were allowed to be passed down to the next generation. Results showed that there emerges cross-linguistic variation in stable linguistic cues. Nevertheless, observed stable cue systems were consistent in that syntactic categories were marked by phonological cues, as found in English, French, Japanese, and other languages (as reviewed above). This stability was particularly strong when languages had larger lexicons, indicating that multiple-cue integration may have contributed to language evolution by aiding a learner's acquisition of growing set of lexical items and classes.

Because different natural languages employ different constellations of cues to signal syntactic distinctions, an important question for further research is exactly how a child's learning mechanisms discover which cues are relevant and for which aspects of syntax. This problem is compounded by the fact that the same cue may work in different directions across different languages. A case in point is that nouns tend to contain more vowels and fewer consonants than verbs in English, whereas nouns and verbs in French show the opposite pattern (Monaghan et al., 2007). So how can the child learn which cues are relevant and in which direction? One possibility may be to encode the correlations between cues in the linguistic environment. This view is supported by related mathematical analyses based on the Vapnik-Chervonenkis (VC) dimension (Abu-Mostafa, 1993), showing that the integration of multiple "hints" or cues of correlated information reduces the number of hypotheses a learning system has to entertain. The VC dimension specifies an upper bound for the amount of input needed by a learning process that starts with a set of hypotheses about a task solution. Cue information may lead to a reduction in the VC dimension by weeding out unhelpful hypotheses and thus lowering the number of examples needed to find a solution. In other words, the integration of multiple cues may reduce learning time by reducing the number of steps necessary to find an appropriate function approximation, as well as reduce the set of candidate functions considered, thus potentially ensuring better generalization.

More generally, the development of computational multiple-cue integration models is still in its infancy. There now exists a wealth of support for the usefulness of multiple probabilistic cues for language acquisition, and although theoretical models abound (e.g., Gleitman & Wanner, 1982; and contributions in Morgan & Demuth, 1996; Weissenborn & Höhle, 2001), only a few psychologically plausible computational models for multiple-cue integration are on offer (e.g., Cartwright & Brent, 1997). Extant models tend to capture the end-state of learning rather the developmental process itself. This approach cannot identify the time course of different cues as they become important for acquisition. For example, the ability to use visual context information to resolve a syntactically ambiguous sentence does not appear until about 8 years of age, considerably later than the knowledge of constraints on constructions that may follow specific verbs (Snedeker & Trueswell, 2004). To reveal cue integration and its development, models must capture the developmental trajectory of cue use across different phases of language acquisition. We anticipate that the availability of so-called "dense" corpora, which sample the child's input at a higher frequency (e.g., Behrens, 2006; Maslen, Theakston, Lieven, & Tomasello, 2004), will help the development of such constructivist-oriented models of language acquisition.

Future work should therefore provide more detailed analysis of the developmental trajectory of multiple-cue integration. Most work on cue availability in the child's environment makes the simplifying assumption that all information is available to the child simultaneously. This is an oversimplification: Children's productions indicate that the whole of language is not acquired in one step, but that overlapping phases of acquisition occur, where learning progress at any one time relies on progress that preceded it. Attempts to explain and exploit these learning phases in computational models has been successful in accounting for early processing constraints that facilitate later learning of complex syntactic structures (Elman, 1993), phrasal productions and errors in young children (Freudenthal, Pine, & Gobet, 2005), and the development of the lexicon (Steyvers & Tenenbaum, 2005). Such approaches could equally be applied to the computational simulation of multiple-cue integration reported in this chapter: The reliability of phonological, prosodic, or distributional cues could be based on the most frequent, or earliest-learned words, and constructed incrementally, and such a constructivist approach would enhance the cognitive plausibility of the availability and process of use of such cues by the developing child.

The wide array of phonological, prosodic, and distributional information sources in primary linguistic input may make the child's learning task substantially easier than it might seem when we consider only the complexities of syntax that they acquire. A domain-general learning mechanism, such as the SRN architecture used here, can capitalize on this rich information to acquire deep domain-specific knowledge that emerges through developmental time. Along with this language-internal information, surely innate and language-external constraints also contribute to the task, and future work should aim to integrate all three fundamental sources of constraints. We have nevertheless shown that even with relatively simple domain-general assumptions about the learner, multiple-cue integration can facilitate the complex task of syntax acquisition. Theories of the language learner therefore should not overburden innate and language-external constraints where language-internal multiple-cue integration can help.

Acknowledgments

This research was supported in part by a Human Frontiers Science Program Grant (RGP0177/2001-B) to M.H.C. Some of the material in this chapter was adapted from Christiansen, M. H., & Dale, R. (2001), Integrating distributional, prosodic and phonological information in a connectionist model of language acquisition, in *Proceedings of the 23rd Annual Conference of the Cognitive Science Society* (pp. 220–225), Mahwah, NJ: Lawrence Erlbaum, and Reali, F., Christiansen, M. H., & Monaghan, P. (2003), Phonological and distributional cues in syntax acquisition: Scaling up the connectionist approach to multiple-cue integration, in *Proceedings of the 25th Annual Conference of the Cognitive Science Society* (pp. 970–975), Mahwah, NJ: Lawrence Erlbaum.

References

Abu-Mostafa, Y. S. (1993) Hints and the VC dimension. *Neural Computation, 5*, 278–288.

Behrens, H. (2006). The input–output relationship in first language acquisition. *Language and Cognitive Processes, 21*, 2–24.

Bernstein-Ratner, N. (1984). Patterns of vowel modification in motherese. *Journal of Child Language, 11*, 557–578.

Bijeljac, R., Bertoncini, J., & Mehler, J. (1993). How do 4-day-old infants categorize multisyllabic utterances? *Developmental Psychology, 29*, 711–721.

Billman, D. (1989). Systems of correlations in rule and category learning: Use of structured input in learning syntactic categories. *Language and Cognitive Processes, 4*, 127–155.

Broen, P. (1972). *The verbal environment of the language-learning child.* ASHA Monographs, No. 17. Washington, DC: American Speech and Hearing Society.

Brooks, P. J., Braine, M. D., Catalano, L. & Brody, R. E. (1993). Acquisition of gender-like noun subclasses in an artificial language: The contribution of phonological markers to learning. *Journal of Memory and Language, 32*, 76–95.

Carter, A. & Gerken, L. A. (1996). Children's use of grammatical morphemes in on-line sentence comprehension. In E. Clark (Ed.), *Proceedings of the Twenty-Eighth Annual Child Language Research Forum* (Vol. 29). Palo Alto, CA: Stanford University Press.

Cartwright, T. A. & Brent, M. R. (1997). Syntactic categorization in early language acquisition: Formalizing the role of distributional analysis. *Cognition, 63*, 121–170.

Cassidy, K. W., & Kelly, M. H. (1991). Phonological information for grammatical category assignments. *Journal of Memory and Language, 30*, 348–369.

Cassidy, K. W., & Kelly, M. H. (2001). Children's use of phonology to infer grammatical class in vocabulary learning. *Psychonomic Bulletin and Review, 8*, 519–523.

Christiansen, M. H., Allen, J., & Seidenberg, M. S. (1998). Learning to segment speech using multiple cues: A connectionist model. *Language and Cognitive Processes, 13*, 221–268.

Christiansen, M. H., & Chater, N. (1999). Toward a connectionist model of recursion in human linguistic performance. *Cognitive Science, 23*, 157–205.

Christiansen, M. H., & Chater, N. (2001). Connectionist psycholinguistics: Capturing the empirical data. *Trends in Cognitive Sciences, 5*, 82–88.

Christiansen, M. H., & Dale, R. (2004). The role of learning and development in the evolution of language. A connectionist perspective. In D. Kimbrough Oller & U. Griebel (Eds.), *Evolution of communication systems: A comparative approach. The Vienna Series in Theoretical Biology* (pp. 90–109). Cambridge, MA: MIT Press.

Cutler, A. (1993). Phonological cues to open-and closed-class words in the processing of spoken sentences. *Journal of Psycholinguistic Research, 22*, 109–131.

Elman, J. L. (1990). Finding structure in time. *Cognitive Science, 14*, 179–211.

Elman, J. L. (1993). Learning and development in neural networks: The importance of starting small. *Cognition, 48*, 71–99.

Fernald, A., & McRoberts, G. (1996). Prosodic bootstrapping: A critical analysis of the argument and the evidence. In J. L. Morgan & K. Demuth (Eds.), *From Signal to syntax* (pp. 365–388). Mahwah, NJ: Lawrence Erlbaum Associates.

Fisher, C., & Tokura, H. (1996). Acoustic cues to grammatical structure in infant-directed speech: Cross-linguistic evidence. *Child Development, 67*, 3192–3218.

Freudenthal, D., Pine, J. M., & Gobet, F. (2006). Modelling the development of children's use of optional infinitives in English and Dutch using MOSAIC. *Cognitive Science, 30*, 277–310.

Frigo, L., & McDonald, J. L. (1998). Properties of phonological markers that affect the acquisition of gender-like subclasses. *Journal of Memory and Language, 39*, 218–245.

Gerken, L. A. (1996). Prosody's role in language acquisition and adult parsing. *Journal of Psycholinguistic Research, 25*, 345–356.

Gerken, L. A., Jusczyk, P. W., & Mandel, D. R. (1994). When prosody fails to cue syntactic structure: Nine-month-olds' sensitivity to phonological vs. syntactic phrases. *Cognition, 51*, 237–265.

Gleitman, L. & Wanner, E. (1982). Language acquisition: The state of the state of the art. In E. Wanner & L. Gleitman (Eds.), *Language acquisition: The state of the art* (pp. 3–48). Cambridge, UK: Cambridge University Press.

Gómez, R. L., & Gerken, L. A. (1999). Artificial grammar learning by 1-year-olds leads to specific and abstract knowledge. *Cognition, 70*, 109–135.

Gómez, R. L., & Gerken, L. A. (2000). Infant artificial language learning and language acquisition. *Trends in Cognitive Sciences, 4*, 178–186.

Green, T. R. G. (1979). The necessity of syntax markers: Two experiments with artificial languages. *Journal of Verbal Learning and Verbal Behavior, 18*, 481–496.

Jusczyk, P. W. (1997). *The discovery of spoken language*. Cambridge, MA: MIT Press.

Jusczyk, P. W. (1999). How infants begin to extract words from speech. *Trends in Cognitive Sciences, 3*, 323–328.

Jusczyk, P. W., & Kemler-Nelson, D. G. (1996). Syntactic units, prosody, and psychological reality during infancy. In J. L. Morgan & K. Demuth (Eds.), *Signal to syntax: Bootstrapping from speech to grammar in early acquisition* (pp. 389–408). Mahwah, NJ: Lawrence Erlbaum Associates.

Karmiloff-Smith, A. (1979). *A functional approach to child language: A study of determiners and reference*. Cambridge, UK: Cambridge University Press.

Kelly, M. H. (1988). Phonological biases in grammatical category shifts. *Journal of Memory and Language, 27*, 343–358.

Kelly, M. H. (1992). Using sound to solve syntactic problems: The role of phonology in grammatical category assignments. *Psychological Review, 99*, 349–364.

Kemler-Nelson, D. G., Hirsh-Pasek, K., Jusczyk, P. W., & Wright Cassidy, K. (1989). How the prosodic cues in motherese might assist language learning. *Journal of Child Language, 16*, 55–68.

Korman, M. (1984). Adaptive aspects of maternal vocalization in differing contexts at ten weeks. *First Language, 5*, 44–45.

Kuhl, P. K. (1999). Speech, language, and the brain: Innate preparation for learning. In M. Konishi & M. Hauser (Eds.), *Neural mechanisms of communication* (pp. 419–450). Cambridge, MA: MIT Press.

Kuhl, P. K., Andruski, J. E., Chistovich, I. A., Chistovich, L. A., Kozhevnikova, E. V., Ryskina, V. L., et al. (1997). Cross-language analysis of phonetic units in language addressed to infants. *Science, 277*, 684–686.

MacWhinney, B. (2000). *The CHILDES project: Tools for analyzing talk* (3rd ed.). Mahwah, NJ: Lawrence Erlbaum Associates.

Maratsos, M., & Chalkley, M. A. (1980). The internal language of children's syntax: The ontogenesis and representation of syntactic categories. In K. Nelson (Ed.), *Children's language* (Vol. 2, pp. 127–214). New York: Gardner Press.

Maslen, R., Theakston, A., Lieven, E., & Tomasello, M. (2004) A dense corpus study of past tense and plural overregularization in English. *Journal of Speech, Language and Hearing Research, 47*, 1319–1333.

Mattys, S. L., Jusczyk, P. W., Luce, P. A., & Morgan, J. L. (1999). Phonotactic and prosodic effects on word segmentation in infants. *Cognitive Psychology, 38*, 465–494.

McDonald, J. L., & Plauche, M. (1995). Single and correlated cues in an artificial language learning paradigm. *Language and Speech, 38*, 223–236.

Mehler, J., Jusczyk, P. W., Lambertz, G., Halsted, N., Bertoncini, J., & Amiel-Tison, C. (1988). A precursor of language acquisition in young infants. *Cognition, 29*, 143–178.

Meier, R. P., & Bower, G. H. (1986). Semantic reference and phrasal grouping in the acquisition of a miniature phrase structure language. *Journal of Memory and Language, 25*, 492–505.

Mintz, T.H. (2003). Frequent frames as a cue for grammatical categories in child directed speech. *Cognition, 90*, 91–117.

Mintz, T. H., Newport, E. L., & Bever, T. G. (2002). The distributional structure of grammatical categories in speech to young children. *Cognitive Science, 26*, 393–424.

Monaghan, P., Chater, N., & Christiansen, M. H. (2005). The differential contribution of phonological and distributional cues in grammatical categorisation. *Cognition, 96*, 143–182.

Monaghan, P., & Christiansen, M. H. (2008). Integration of multiple probabilistic cues in syntax acquisition. In H. Behrens (Ed.), *Trends in corpus research: Finding structure in data* (pp. 139–163) (TILAR Series). Amsterdam: John Benjamins.

Monaghan, P., Christiansen, M. H., & Chater, N. (2007). The phonological–distributional coherence hypothesis: Cross-linguistic evidence in language acquisition. *Cognitive Psychology, 55*, 259–305.

Morgan, J. L. (1996). Prosody and the roots of parsing. *Language and Cognitive Processes, 11*, 69–106.

Morgan, J. L., & Demuth, K. (1996). *Signal to syntax: Bootstrapping from speech to grammar in early acquisition.* Mahwah, NJ: Lawrence Erlbaum Associates.

Morgan, J. L., Meier, R. P., & Newport, E. L. (1987). Structural packaging in the input to language learning: Contributions of prosodic and morphological marking of phrases to the acquisition of language. *Cognitive Psychology, 19*, 498–550.

Morgan, J. L., & Saffran, J. R. (1995). Emerging integration of sequential and suprasegmental information in preverbal speech segmentation. *Child Development, 66*, 911–936.

Morgan, J. L., Shi., R., & Allopenna, P. (1996). Perceptual bases of grammatical categories. In J. L. Morgan & K. Demuth (Eds.), *Signal to syntax: Bootstrapping from speech to grammar in early acquisition.* (pp. 263–283). Mahwah, NJ: Lawrence Erlbaum Associates.

Newport, E. L., Gleitman, H., & Gleitman, L. R. (1977). Mother, I'd rather do it myself: Some effects and non-effects of maternal speech style. In C. E. Snow & C. A. Ferguson (Eds.), *Talking to children: Language input and acquisition* (pp. 109–149). Cambridge, UK: Cambridge University Press.

Onnis, L., & Christiansen, M. H. (2008). Lexical categories at the edge of the word. *Cognitive Science, 32*, 184–221.

Pallier, C., Christophe, A., & Mehler, J. (1997). Language-specific listening. *Trends in Cognitive Sciences, 1*, 129–132.

Pinker, S. (1984). *Language learnability and language development.* Cambridge, MA: Harvard University Press.

Redington, M., Chater, N., & Finch, S. (1998). Distributional information: A powerful cue for acquiring syntactic categories. *Cognitive Science, 22*, 425–469.

Rubel, E. W. (1985). Auditory system development. In G. Gottlieb & N. A. Krasnegor (Eds.), *Measurement of audition and vision in the first year of postnatal life* (pp. 53–89). Norwood, NJ: Ablex.

Saffran, J. R. (2003). Statistical language learning: Mechanisms and constraints. *Current Directions in Psychological Science, 12*, 110–114.

Saffran, J. R., Aslin, R. N., & Newport, E. L. (1996). Statistical learning by 8-month-old infants. *Science, 274*, 1926–1928.

Sereno, J. A., & Jongman, A. (1995). Acoustic correlates of grammatical class. *Language and Speech, 38*, 57–76.

Shady, M., & Gerken, L. A. (1999). Grammatical and caregiver cues in early sentence comprehension. *Journal of Child Language, 26*, 163–175.

Shafer, V. L., Shucard, D. W., Shucard, J. L., & Gerken, L. A. (1998). An electrophysiological study of infants' sensitivity to the sound patterns of English speech. *Journal of Speech, Language, and Hearing Research, 41*, 874–886.

Shi, R., Morgan, J., & Allopenna, P. (1998). Phonological and acoustic bases for earliest grammatical category assignment: A cross-linguistic perspective. *Journal of Child Language, 25*, 169–201.

Shi, R., Werker, J. F., & Morgan, J. L. (1999). Newborn infants' sensitivity to perceptual cues to lexical and grammatical words. *Cognition, 72,* B11–B21.

Snedeker, J., & Trueswell, J. (2004). The developing constraints on parsing decisions: The role of lexical-biases and referential scenes in child and adult sentence processing. *Cognitive Psychology, 49(3),* 238–299.

Steinhauer, K., Alter, K., & Friederici, A. D. (1999). Brain potentials indicate immediate use of prosodic cues in natural speech processing. *Nature Neuroscience, 2,* 191–196.

Steyvers, M., & Tenenbaum, J. (2005). The large scale structure of semantic networks: Statistical analyses and a model of semantic growth. *Cognitive Science, 29,* 41–78.

Tomasello, M. (2000). The item-based nature of children's early syntactic development. *Trends in Cognitive Sciences, 4,* 156–163.

Tomasello, M., Kruger, A. C., & Ratner, H. H. (1993). Cultural learning. *Behavioral and Brain Sciences, 16,* 495–552.

Valian, V., & Coulson, S. (1988). Anchor points in language learning: The role of marker frequency. *Journal of Memory and Language, 27,* 71–86.

Valian, V., & Levitt, A. (1996). Prosody and adults' learning of syntactic structure. *Journal of Memory and Language, 35,* 497–516.

Weissenborn, J., & Höhle, B. (Eds.) (2001). *Approaches to bootstrapping: Phonological, lexical, syntactic and neurophysiological aspects of early language acquisition.* Philadelphia, PA: John Benjamins.

Werker, J. F., & Tees, R. C. (1999). Influences on infant speech processing: Toward a new synthesis. *Annual Review of Psychology, 50,* 509–535.

CHAPTER 6
Shape, Action, Symbolic Play, and Words: Overlapping Loops of Cause and Consequence in Developmental Process

Linda B. Smith and Alfredo F. Pereira

Human beings are remarkably inventive, possessing the ability to solve problems and to create novel things. This chapter is about one early form of inventiveness that has long intrigued developmentalists—what is some times called symbolic play, but more narrowly, is also known as "object substitution in play." The specific phenomenon consists of young children using some object not for what it is but as a "stand in" for something else in play—a banana as a phone, a box as a doll bed, a shoe as a toy car. Piaget (1962) considered object-substitution in play—the using of a banana as phone, for example—as "symbolic" because the substituted object could be interpreted as "standing for" the real thing. This view that object-substitution is a form of symbolizing (whatever precisely that means) has been disputed (Namy, 2002; Perner, 1991). Regardless of different opinions on this issue, object substitution in play remains a signal of developmental achievement, emerging at the same time (18 to 24 months) as children's spoken vocabulary also expands. Perhaps most critically, object substitution in play is strongly linked to individual children's language development (see McCune, 1995; McCune-Nicolich, 1981; Shore, O'Connell, & Bates, 1984; Veneziano, 1981), with the lack of this behavior being a strong predictor of significant subsequent language delay (e.g., McCune-Nicolich, 1981; Weismer, 2007). This chapter is about how and why these object substitutions may be linked to language learning through developmental changes in visual object recognition.

At a broader level, this chapter is about the fundamentally constructive nature of developmental process itself: how development creates new forms of behaviors and abilities from interaction of multiple processes, engaged in different assemblies in overlapping tasks; how every developmental cause is itself a consequence of developmental process; how development is made of weird loops of causes and consequences with far-reaching and unexpected developmental dependencies.

A summary of the developmental story we will narrate is provided by Figure 6.1: Learning object names increases children's attention to shape, which in turn speeds up object name learning. Learning object names also changes how children perceive object shape, which facilitates learning and generalizing object names and of actions. Acting on objects, in turn, refines and tunes—making even more abstract—the representation of object shape. Along the way, we will suggest and provide evidence for the idea that the abstract representation of object shape is the critical link between object name learning and object substitutions in play.

Loop 1: Learning to Attend to Object Shape

Common object categories, categories such as chair, cup, spoon, house, and dog are (by adult

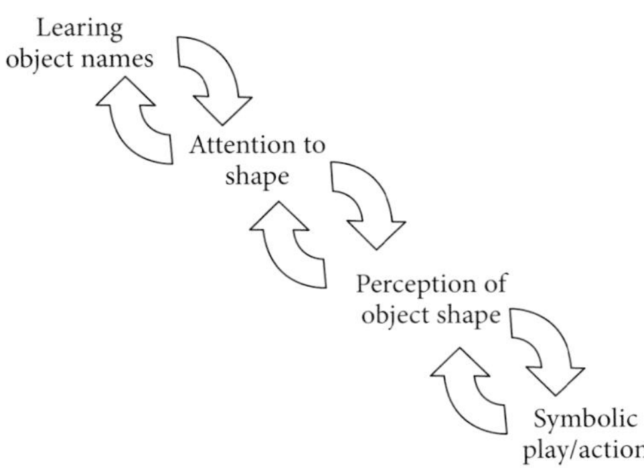

Figure 6.1 Loops of causes and consequences in the development of visual object recognition.

judgment) well organized by shape (Biederman, 1987; Rosch, Mervis, Gray, Johnson, & Boyes-Braem, 1976; Samuelson & Smith, 1999). More critically, in the vocabulary of typically developing 2-year-olds, over 70% of the nouns are for objects similar in shape (Samuelson & Smith, 1999). Accordingly, a large literature has been concerned with children's attention to three-dimensional object shape in the context of early word learning. Landau, Smith, and Jones (1988) reported one key result: They showed 2- and 3-year-old children a novel wooden object of a particular shape and named it with a novel count noun, "This is a dax." The children were then presented with test objects that matched the exemplar in shape, size, or texture and were asked about each of those objects "Is this a dax?" Children generalized the name to test objects that were the same in shape as the exemplar but not to test objects that were different in shape. The degree of children's selective attention to shape was considerable: for example, they extended the name "dax" to same-shaped test objects that were 100 times the size of the original. This "shape bias" in novel noun generalization tasks has been demonstrated in many different studies and by different experimenters using a variety of both specially constructed and real objects (e.g., Gathercole & Min, 1997; Imai, Gentner, & Uchida, 1994; Keil, 1994; Soja, 1992) and is evident in children learning a variety of languages (Colunga & Smith, 2005; Gathercole & Min, 1997; Yoshida & Smith, 2003). This substantial area of research has generated a large number of well-replicated results important to the first loop.

First, attention to shape increases as children learn object names. Children initially (12- to 18-month-olds, see Gershkoff-Stowe & Smith, 2004; Rakison & Butterworth, 1998a, 1998b) do not systematically attend to object shape in naming and categorization tasks, but increasingly do so in the period between 18 and 30 months. Moreover, longitudinal studies show that in individual children, the emergence of the shape bias is temporally linked to a measurable spurt in the growth of object name vocabulary (Gershkoff-Stowe & Smith, 2004). Attention to shape also predicts developmental delays. Late talkers—children delayed in their early noun acquisitions—show systematic deficits in attention to object shape in naming tasks (Jones, 2003; Jones & Smith, 2005).

Second, attention to shape is causally related to object name learning. Teaching children to attend to shape facilitates novel noun acquisitions and accelerates the rate of real-world vocabulary development (Smith, Jones, Landau, Gershkoff-Stowe & Samuelson, 2002; see also, Samuelson, 2002). This study was a 9-week longitudinal study. The children were 17 months of age at the start—too young to show a shape bias in novel noun generalization tasks and also on the early side of the increasing rate of new object names that begins around 18 to 22 months for most children. The children in the "Experimental" condition came to the laboratory once a week for 7 weeks. During that time, they played with 4 pairs of objects. The objects in each pair matched in shape but differed markedly in all other properties—color, texture, material, and size. The objects in each pair were named by the same novel name (e.g., "dax, riff, zup, toma") and during each weekly play session, the experimenter named each of these training objects by its designated name at least 20 times.

On week 8, children's ability to generalize these trained names was tested. If children learned that two particularly shaped objects were "daxes," would they judge a novel object—new size, new color, new material but the same shape—to also be "a dax?" The answer is yes; the children learned the category. On week 9, children were tested in a novel noun generalization task, with all new objects and all new names. If shown a new never-before-seen thing and told its name, would these children know how to generalize the name to new instances by shape? Again, the answer is yes. The children learned not just about particular categories and the importance of shape, but also that shape in general matters for naming objects. A variety of control conditions were run in these series of training studies, including grouping without naming, playing with objects with neither grouping or naming, or learning names for groups organized by texture or color. None of the children in these training groups generalized novel names for novel things on week 9 by shape.

The most dramatic result from these studies is the finding that training children to attend to shape in this laboratory task increased their rate of new object name acquisitions outside of the laboratory. Figure 6.2 shows the number of object names in children's productive vocabulary (as measured by the MCDI, Fenson et al., 1994) at the start and end of the experiment. There was a marked increase in new noun learning for children in the Experimental but not the Control conditions, and training influenced the rate with which children in the Experimental condition added new objects names to their vocabulary but not the rate with which they added other words. Learning names for things in shape-based categories teaches children to attend to shape when generalizing names for things, and doing so accelerates the learning of new object names, lexical categories that are in general well-organized by shape.

These training experiments may be microgenetic and targeted versions of what happens in the everyday development. In the real world, young children more slowly learn names for many different things at the same time. Although these categories are not as well organized by the shape as the training categories, many are categories of things that are mostly similar in shape. As children learn these categories, attention to shape in the context of naming things may increase, and, as a consequence, children may learn object names more rapidly, which should further tune attention to object

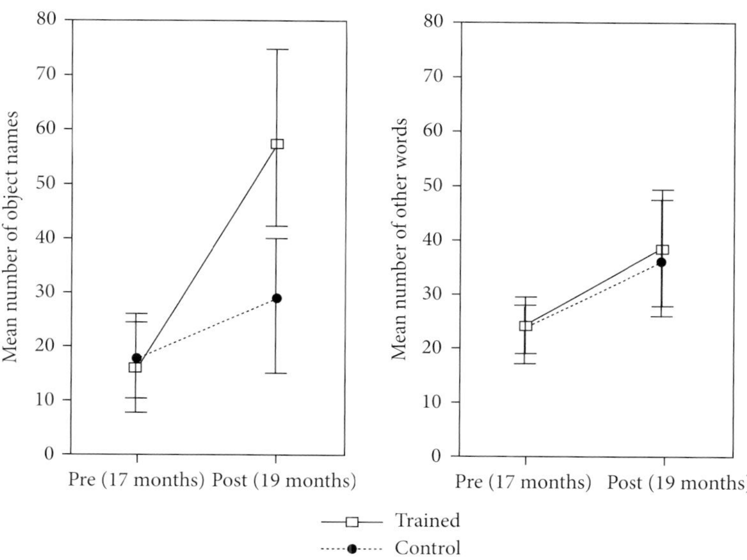

Figure 6.2 Object names and other words in children's productive vocabulary at the start and end of training in the Smith et al. (2002) study.

shape. Every word learned sets the stage for and constrains future learning. The shape bias in early noun learning is in this way both a cause and a consequence of learning object names.

Loop 2: building abstract representations of object shape

There is one critical unexplained aspect of Loop 1. In order for a shape bias to work to help children learn names for everyday object categories, children must be able to recognize sameness in shape across different instances of a category. This is trivial in artificial noun-learning tasks since all objects are relatively simple and "same-shaped" (objects are the *exact* same shape). But this is not trivial in the real world. In order for children to learn, for example, that chairs are "chair-shaped" and to use that knowledge to recognize a new chair, they must be able to abstract the common shape from a whole array of chairs that have been experienced, each with its own unique and detailed shape. Real world instances of common noun categories, though judged by adults to be the "same shape" (e.g., Samuelson & Smith, 1999) are not exactly the same shape, but only similar in shape at some appropriate level of abstraction. This then is the critical next question: What is the proper description of shape for common object categories? When and how do children discover that description? Before answering this question, we step back to consider what is known about adult shape representations and visual object recognition.

The first key fact about human visual object recognition is that it is impressive: it is fast, seemingly automatic, robust under degraded viewing conditions, and capable of recognizing novel instances of a very large number of common categories (Biederman & Gerhardstein, 1993; Cooper, Biederman, & Hummel, 1992; Fize, Fabre-Thorpe, Richard, Doyon, & Thorpe, 2005; Pegna, Khateb, Michel, & Landis, 2004). The second key fact is that object recognition is not a single skill but a consortium of abilities. For example, in their everyday lives, people routinely recognize the dog whose nose is sticking out from the blanket, the highly unique modernistic chair, and the cup on the table as a particular and favorite cup. Although competing theories of object recognition (Biederman, 1987; Edelman, 1999; Ullman, 2000) often pit different kinds of hypothesized processes and representations against each other, it is likely that human object recognition is dependent on a multitude of partially distinct and partially overlapping processes (Hayward, 2003; Hummel, 2000; Marr, 1982; Peissig & Tarr, 2007; Peterson, 1999). That is, no single mechanism is likely to explain the full range of contexts in which people recognize objects as individuals and as instances of categories.

Theories of object recognition that concentrate on how people rapidly recognize instances of novel categories (and approaches to machine vision that attempt to build devices that can recognize novel instances of categories) often propose processes of shape recognition that depend on abstract, sparse representations of the global shapes of things. There are two general classes of such theories. According to "view-based" theories, people store representations of specific views of experienced instances and use prototypes—a kind of average simplified shape that captures the global structure—to recognize new category instance (Edelman, 1995; Edelman & Duvdevani-Bar, 1997; Edelman & Intrator, 1997). In Edelman's (1995) account, category learning plays the critical role in creating prototypes of the holistic shape of category members. Novel instances are subsequently categorized by their overall similarity to these representations.

"Object-based" theories such as Biederman's (1987) recognition-by-components (RBC) account present another idea about what constitutes "sameness in shape." This theory proposes that objects are perceptually parsed, represented, and stored as configurations of geometric volumes ("geons"). Within this account, object shape is defined by 2 to 4 geometric volumes in the proper spatial arrangement, an idea supported by the fact that adults need only 2 to 4 major parts to recognize instances of common categories (Biederman, 1987; Hummel & Biederman, 1992) as illustrated at the bottom of Figure 6.3. This account thus posits sparse and impoverished representations that, through their high level of abstraction, can gather all

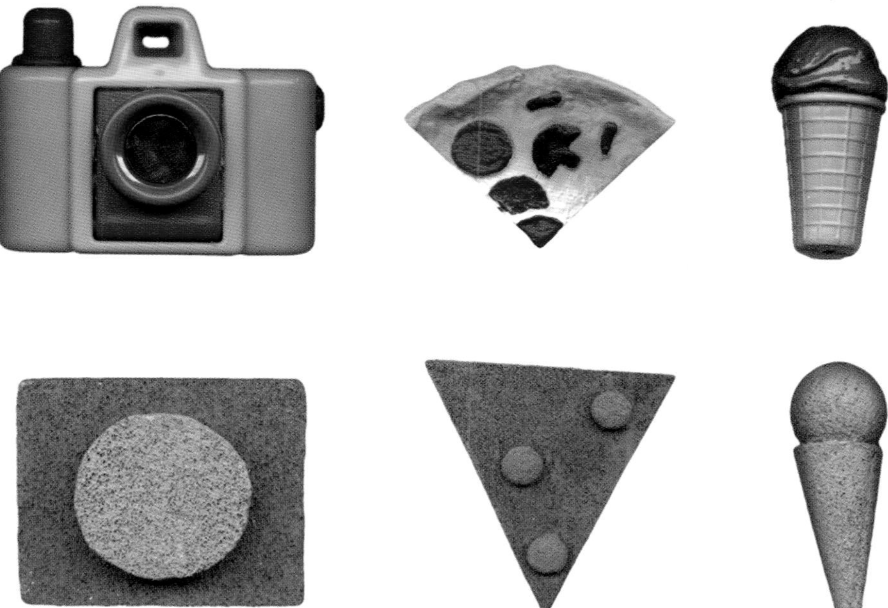

Figure 6.3 Pictures of some of the three-dimensional objects, richly detailed and shape caricatures, used in Smith (2003).

variety of highly different things into a "same shape" category. Both classes of theories fit aspects of the adult data, which include strong view dependencies in object recognition and also knowledge of part structure and relations. Accordingly, there is a growing consensus that both kinds of theories may capture important but different processes in mature object recognition (Hayward, 2003; Peissig & Tarr, 2007; Peterson, 1999; Stankiewicz, 2003; Tarr & Vuong, 2002). For this chapter, the important point is that both approaches posit that sparse and abstract representations of object shape support the recognition of instances of common object categories. The question we want to answer is when and how children develop these representations. Despite the importance of object recognition to many domains of cognitive development, there was, until recently, extraordinarily little developmental research in this area (see Kellman, 2001).

The first study (Smith, 2003) asked whether young children (18 to 24 months) could recognize instances of common object categories from sparse representations of the geometric structure as can adults (e.g., Biederman, 1987). The experiment specifically contrasted richly detailed typical examples with "shape caricatures" as shown in Figure 6.3. The task was name comprehension ("get the camera") and the 18- to 24-month participants were grouped into developmental level by the number of object names in their productive vocabulary. The main results were that children with smaller and larger vocabularies (below 100 object names versus more than 100 object names) recognized the richly detailed instances equally well. However, children with smaller noun vocabularies performed at chance levels when presented with the shape caricatures, whereas the children with high noun vocabularies recognized the shape caricatures as well as they did the richly detailed and typical instances.

These results have been replicated in two further studies (Son, Smith, & Goldstone, 2008; Pereira & Smith, 2009). Further, a study of older late talkers (children whose productive vocabulary is below the 20th percentile for their age) found a deficit in the recognition of shape caricatures but not richly detailed typical instances (Jones & Smith, 2005). Altogether, these results suggest a potentially significant change in how young children represent and compare object shape that is developmentally linked to the learning of objects names. In particular, sparse representations of object shape appear to emerge between 18 and 24 months.

One other line of research suggests that these developmental changes may also involve a shift in the kind of stimulus information used to categorize and recognize objects. In particular, a number of studies suggest that children younger than 20 months attend to the individual parts or local details of objects rather than overall shape (Rakison & Butterworth, 1998a). In a series of programmatic studies, Rakison and colleagues (Rakison & Butterworth, 1998b, Rakison & Cohen, 1999, Rakison and Cicchino, 2008) showed that 14- and 22-month old children based category decisions on highly salient parts (such as legs and wheels) and not on overall shape. For example, when children were presented with cows whose legs had been replaced by wheels, they classified the cows with vehicles rather than animals; likewise they categorized a vehicle as an animal when it had cow legs. Similarly, Colunga (2003) showed that 18-month-olds tended to only look at a small part of any pictured object, using clusters of local features such as the face when recognizing animals, or the grill and headlights when recognizing vehicles.

These results raise the possibility that very young children—perhaps before they develop more sparse representations of object structure—recognize objects via what Cerella (1986) called "particulate perception," concentrating on local components unintegrated into the whole. Such "part"-based object recognition is also suggestive of an approach to object recognition that has emerged in the machine vision literature: in particular, Ullman has developed a procedure through which objects are successfully recognized via stored representations of category specific fragments (Ullman & Bart, 2004; Ullman, Vidal-Naquet, & Sali, 2002). If adults possess multiple distinct processes of object recognition that are used in different contexts or for different kinds of tasks, perhaps these processes each have their own developmental trajectories with more "fragments" or "feature" processes developing earlier and sparse representations of global geometric structure emerging as a consequence of learning many shape-based object categories (see also the chapter in this volume by Johnson, for a similar developmental trajectory in young infants' perceptual completion).

Pereira and Smith (2009) provide support for this idea in a direct comparison of young children's ability to recognize objects given local featural details versus global geometric structure. The stimulus sets that they used resulted from a 2 × 2 design: the presence and absence of global information about geometric structure (which they labeled by *+Shape Caricature* and *–Shape Caricature*) and localized and fine detailed information predictive of the category (which they labeled by *+Local Details* and *–Local Details*). Examples of the four stimulus conditions are in Figure 6.4. The +Shape Caricatures, structured as in the Smith (2003) experiment were made from 1 to 4 geometric components in the proper spatial relations. The –Shape Caricatures were alterations of the +Shape caricatures: the shapes of at least two component volumes were altered and if possible the spatial arrangements of two volumes relative to each other were rearranged. The presence of detailed local information was achieved by painting surface details on these volumes that were predictive of the target category, for example, the face of a dog, wheels, and so forth.

Figure 6.5 shows the main result; the darker bars indicate performance when local details were present (+Local Details) and the solid bars indicate performance given the +Shape caricatures, that is, when the appropriate though sparse global shape structure was present. The children in the lowest vocabulary group show their highest level of performance (the darker bars) when the stimuli present local details, and for these stimuli, the presence or absence of appropriate shape structure does not matter. The children in the most advanced vocabulary group perform best given the appropriate sparse

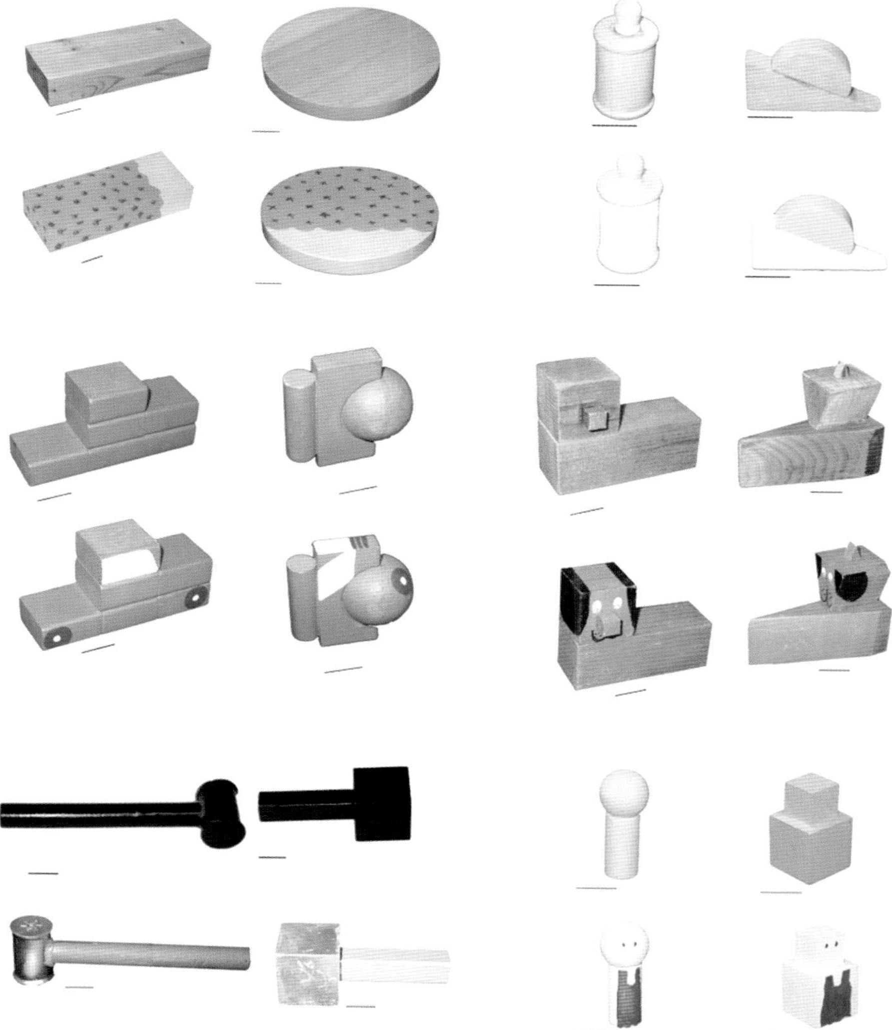

Figure 6.4 Photos of the stimuli used in Pereira and Smith's (2009) experiment 2. Each set of four pictures contains clockwise from the upper left: (–Local Details, +Shape Caricature), (–Local Details, –Shape Caricature), (+Local Details, –Shape Caricature), (+Local Details, +Shape Caricature). The black line close to each object is one inch in length.

representations of global shape. In brief, there is increasing recognition of the shape caricatures with increasing vocabulary size and a greater dependence on local features earlier in their vocabulary development. These results add to the growing number of findings suggesting significant changes in visual object recognition in the second year of life (Rakison & Lupyan, 2008; Smith, 2003; Son, Smith, & Goldstone, 2008).

The very idea that object recognition may change substantially during this developmental period is not commonly considered in studies of categorization and concepts in infancy and early childhood. This is so even though we know that there is at last one domain in which recognition undergoes significant changes as a function of development and experience. Specifically, face recognition is characterized

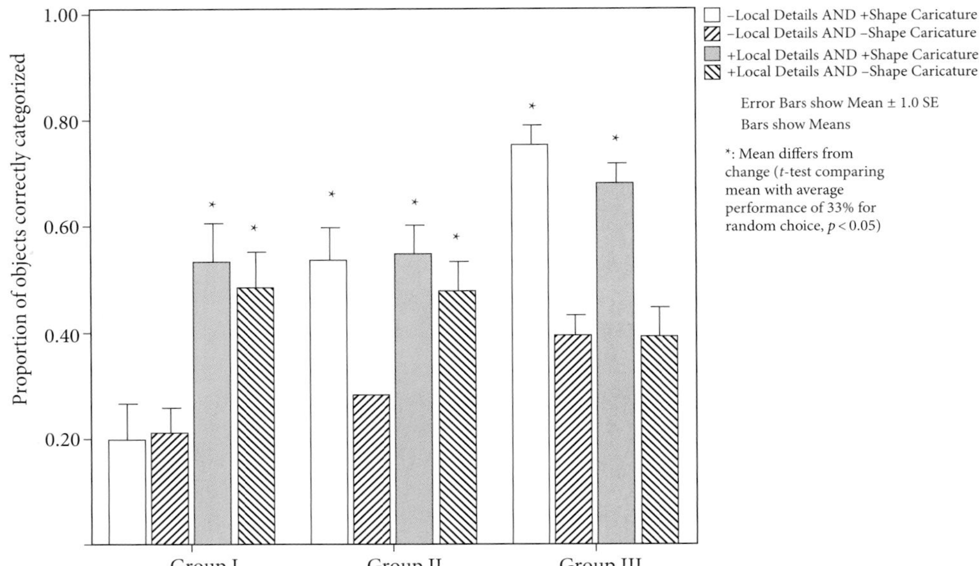

Figure 6.5 Mean proportion of number of objects correctly categorized (out of 6 trials) across the three groups of vocabulary level for the Local Details × Shape Caricature interaction (Pereira & Smith, 2009). Between-subjects conditions –Local Details and +Local Details are shown in white and black bars, respectively. Within-subjects conditions +Shape Caricature and –Shape Caricature are shown in solid and patterned bars, respectively.

by strong early sensitivities in infancy yet also shows a slow and protracted course of development with adult-like expertise not achieved until adolescence (e.g., Mondloch, Le Grand, & Maurer, 2002). In this context, the idea of significant changes in object recognition and a possibly protracted course of development seem less surprising (as also suggested by Abecassis, Sera, Yonas, & Schwade, 2001).

It seems likely that the visual system develops the kinds of representations that support the task that needs to done (Biederman & Kalocsai, 1997; Nelson, 2001). The task of object recognition for *many* different categories with *many* different potential instances in each category may demand a more abstract and geometric description of object shape—–one in which, for example, a chair is a horizontal surface (to sit on) and a vertical surface (to support one's back). The period in which children learn the names for many different categories of things could be a driving force behind these developments. And certainly, more abstract representations of object shape may foster more rapid category learning and generalization (see especially, Son, Smith, & Goldstone, 2007).

At the very least, there is growing evidence for significant changes in visual object recognition during the developmental period in which children's object name learning is rapidly expanding. Multiple kinds of information may be used to recognize objects and it appears that very young children, at the start of a period of rapid category learning, mostly rely on detailed local information to recognize instances of common categories but not more abstract information about geometric structure. Children who are only slightly more advanced, however, do recognize common objects from such shape caricatures. This period of rapid developmental change seems crucial to understanding the nature of human object recognition and may also provide a crucial missing link in our understanding of the developmental trajectory in early object name learning, a trajectory of vocabulary growth that begins slow but

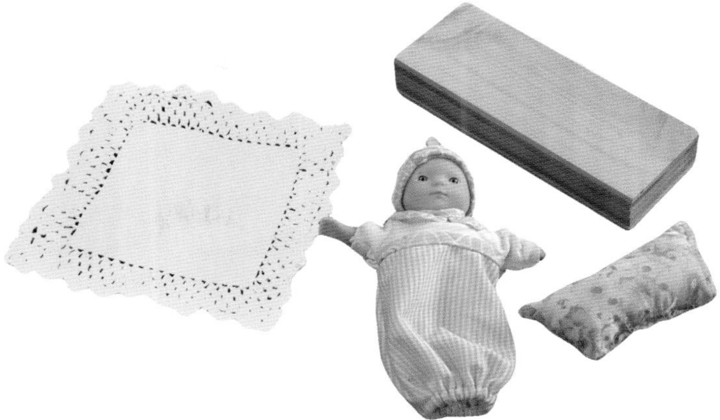

Figure 6.6 Sample stimulus set from Smith and Pereira (2008) for the symbolic play task.

progresses to quite rapid learning characterized by the fast-mapping of object names to categories of things alike in shape.

Unexpected Connections—Symbolic Play

These changes in visual object recognition raise a new hypothesis about the developmental origins of object substitutions in play. Although these inventive actions seem likely to involve many interacting processes (including wanting to engage in thematic play), they may also depend critically on abstract descriptions of object shape. Using a banana as a phone, a shoe as a car, a stick as a bottle, and a pot as a hat all suggest sensitivity to high-level structural properties of shape. Accordingly, in a recently completed study, we examined whether children's recognition of shape caricatures might predict the likelihood of object substitutions in play (Smith & Pereira, 2008). The participants were children 17 to 22 months of age. There were three dependent measures: (1) the number of nouns in the children's productive vocabulary (by MCDI parent report, see Fenson et al., 1993), (2) children's recognition of common categories from shape caricatures (given that they could recognize richly detailed instances of the same thing), and (3) performance in a symbolic play task.

To encourage children to engage in symbolic play, they were given a set of toys organized around a theme but with one key object missing. A sample set is shown in Figure 6.6. For this set, the child was given a doll, a blanket, and a pillow—three objects suggesting a "going to bed" theme—but no bed. Instead the fourth object was block. The question was whether the child would engage in thematic play, using the block as a bed. There were four such sets, the bed theme, an eating theme (doll, plate, spoon, pompoms to be potentially used as food), a car theme (road, bridge, stoplight, wooden shoe to be potentially used as car), and a house theme (house, table, chair, and stick to be potentially used as a person). Because children might inadvertently use the object in a way consistent with its targeted role, we required that children do two successive acts involving the target object in thematic play (e.g., laid the doll on the block then immediately put the blanket on the doll) to score it as an instance of symbolic play.

Figure 6.7 shows the performances of children with fewer and greater than 100 object names in their vocabulary: the proportion of shape caricatures they recognized (given they recognized the richly detailed instances) and the proportion of trials on which they engaged in symbolic play (as defined above). Children with fewer than 100 object names in their productive vocabulary were much less likely to use the target objects in thematic play and also much less likely to recognize the shape caricatures for

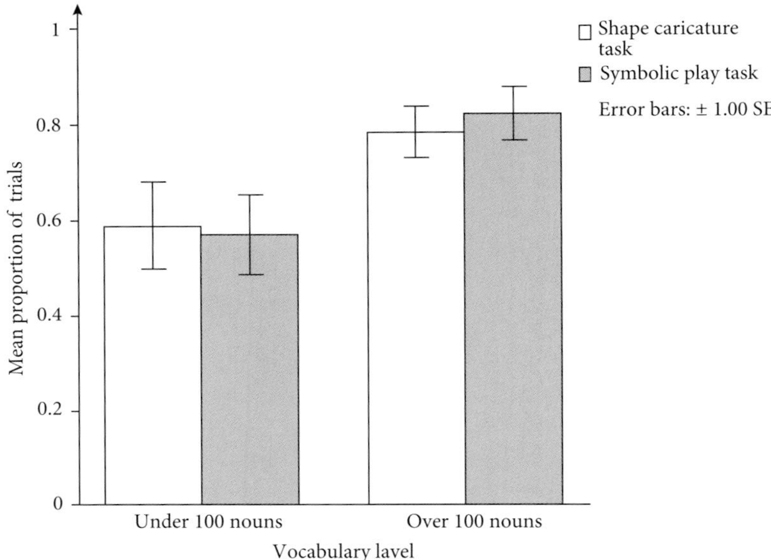

Figure 6.7 Mean proportion of trials on which children with fewer and with more than 100 object names in productive vocabulary recognized the shape caricatures in the caricature recognition task and used the target object for the missing object in the symbolic play task (Smith & Pereira, 2008).

common nouns. In contrast, children with over 100 object names in their productive vocabulary both used the target object for the missing object and also readily recognized the shape caricatures for common categories. Across the 36 children who participated in this study, there was a strong correlation between recognition of shape caricatures and symbolic play (r =.66, p < .001). Further a control study, which replaced the target object with richly detailed instances (e.g., replaced the block with a toy bed, the stick with a person), did not yield vocabulary-related differences in symbolic play nor a reliable correlation with shape caricature recognition. Finally, although vocabulary and age are correlated, size of the object name vocabulary is a better predictor of both symbolic play and shape caricature recognition than is age (see also, Pereira & Smith, 2009).

Although many abilities seem likely to be important to the development of thematic play and children's inventive object substitutions in that play, these results suggest that these object substitutions may be, at least in part, linked to language through developmental changes in visual object recognition, which are influenced by learning names for things.

Loop 3: Action and Shape Perception

The link between object substitution in play and the recognition of three-dimensional caricatures of the geometric structure of common objects suggests that an abstract and sparse description of object structure invites the generalization of actions and potentially classes of actions. This makes sense as there is a strong causal link between the shape of things, how they are held, how they feel while being held, and the actions those objects afford.

Contemporary research in cognitive neuroscience also indicates a coupling between brain regions involved in visually recognizing objects and in producing action that may be particularly relevant to an understanding of the developmental relationship between the abstraction of sparse descriptions of object structure and action. In particular, perceptual-motor interactions have been shown in behavioral paradigms and in recordings of brain activation (Christou

& Bulthoff, 1999; Craighero et al., 1996; Freyd, 1983; Harman, Humphrey, & Goodale, 1999; James, Humphrey, & Goodale, 2001; James et al., 2002; Tong et al., 1995; Wexler & von Boxtel, 2005; A. Wohschlager & A. Wohlschlager, 1998). Specifically, there appear to be automatic links among visual systems used for object perception and recognition, and motor systems used to act on objects (Arbib, 1981; Chao & Martin, 2000; Grezes & Decety, 2002; James et al., 2006; Longcamp, Boucard, Gilhodes, & Vely, 2005; Paillard, 1991; Vivani & Stucchi, 1992) such that, upon visual perception of an object, motor areas are automatically activated. These studies have demonstrated that activation in motor cortices emerges upon visual presentation of manipulable objects such as tools (Chao & Martin, 2000) and kitchen utensils (Gerlach et al., 2000 ; Grezes & Decety, 2002; Grezes et al., 2003; Mecklinger, Gruenewald, Besson, Magnie, & Cramon, 2002); and manually created objects such as letters (James & Gauthier, 2006; Longcamp et al., 2005). That is, visual presentations of objects with which we have had extensive motor interactions appear to automatically activate the motor areas responsible for those actions.

There are several open questions about these links, including why and how they are constructed, and whether they play a role in visual recognition (James & Gauthier, 2006; Mecklinger et al., 2002; Wexler & van Boxtel, 2005). One possibility is that such links are neural correlates of mere associations, so that although the motor regions are activated in response to visual stimuli, perhaps as preparation for action, they play no role in the visual recognition of the objects. A second possibility is that these motor activations feed back on and actually influence and help select activations in visual regions. More radically, a third possibility is that a developmental history of the dynamic coupling of visual and motor activations constitutes the stored representation of the object, with the history of activations in visual regions influencing stored representations in motor regions, and with the history of activations in motor regions influencing stored representations in visual regions.

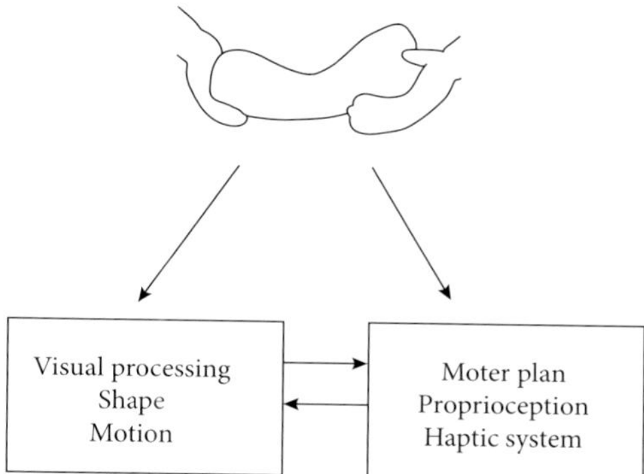

Figure 6.8 A schematic representation of the inter-relating of multiple simultaneous representations across modalities.

Figure 6.8 provides a schematic representation of this possibility—of what Edelman (1987) calls *re-entry*, the explicit interrelating of multiple simultaneous representations across modalities. For example, when a child is given a toy to hold and look at, both the visual and motor systems are simultaneously engaged. Together, they yield a constellation of sensations and movements associated with various actions on the toy and their consequences. Importantly, these multimodal experiences are time-locked and correlated. Changes in the way the hand feels when it moves the toy are time-locked with the changes the infant sees as the toy is moved. The time-locked correlations potentially create a powerful learning mechanism, as illustrated in the figure, which shows five related mappings. One map is between the physical properties of the toy and the neuronal activity in the visual system. Another map is between the physical properties of the toy and neuronal activity in the motor planning, proprioceptive, and haptic systems. A third map is between the motor systems and actions on the object. The fourth and fifth maps are what Edelman calls the re-entrant maps: activity in the visual system is mapped to the motor (and haptic and proprioceptive) systems, and activity in the motor system is mapped to the visual system. Thus independent mappings of the stimulus—the sight of it and the action on it—provide qualitatively different takes on the world.

By being correlated in real time, these different takes can potentially educate each other. At the same time as the visual system is activated by time-varying changes in visual information about shape and collinear movement of points on the toy, the motor and proprioceptive system is activated by action and felt movements. At every step in real time, the activities in these heterogeneous processes are mapped to each other, potentially enabling the coupled systems through their own activity to discover higher-order regularities that transcend the individual systems considered alone. Again, developmental relations may be bidirectional—changes in the perception of object shape may foster the generalizations of actions, and action, in turn, may promote attention to or the representation of relevant geometric properties of shape.

As a first step in considering how action may educate a sparse structural description shape—the kind of category encompassing description that enables one to recognize the sameness in shape across all varieties of shape—we have concentrated on two structural properties that are related to each other, commonly considered important across a wide variety of different theories of human and machine visual object recognition and potentially informed by action: (1) planar and nonplanar views and (2) the major axes of an object. We consider each of these in turn, presenting background on why they are likely structural properties for seeking a relation between action and object recognition and also new evidence suggesting marked developmental change during the period between 18 to 24 months.

Preferred Views

There is ample evidence that not all viewpoints of objects are equal in terms of the ease with which an object is recognized from that viewpoint. Two views—off-axis versus on-axis views—have generated considerable interest in the adult object recognition literature. These two perspectives, illustrated in Figure 6.9 are often called the "3/4" and "planar" (front on and side on) views. These are the terms we will use here. With familiar objects, adults can recognize an object faster from a single image if that image is a 3/4 or off-axis view than if it is a planar view (Blanz, Tarr, & Bulthoff, 1999; Humphrey & Jolicouer, 1993; Lawson & Humphreys, 1998; Newell & Findlay, 1997; Palmer, Rosch, & Chase, 1981). In addition, when asked to pick the "best" view of an object, adults will usually pick a 3/4 view (Blanz et al., 1999; Palmer et al., 1981). Critically, these results are specific to the

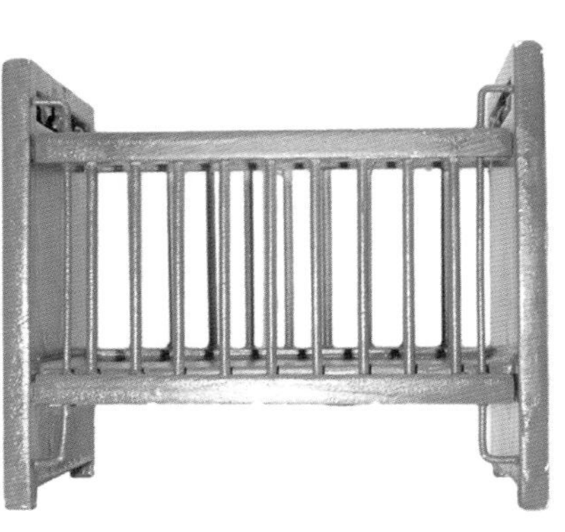

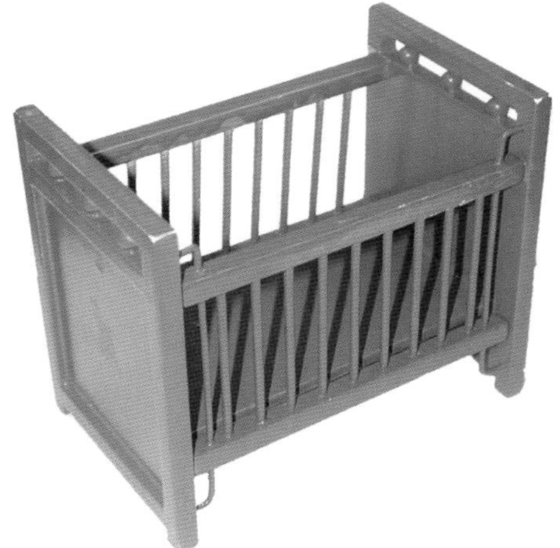

Figure 6.9 A planar and nonplanar view of an object.

recognition of pictures of well-known category instances. When adults are asked to pick the "best" view of a novel object, the planar views are picked as often as the 3/4 views (Blanz et al., 1999), perhaps because these views are less likely to occlude relevant object features that cannot be inferred for novel things. Similarly, when adults dynamically explore novel objects prior to visual recognition tasks, they actually prefer planar over 3/4 views. That is, during active exploration, adults spend a significantly greater amount of time looking at views of objects where axes are foreshortened (front) or elongated (side) (Harman et al., 1999; James et al., 2001, 2002; Perrett & Haries, 1988; Perrett et al., 1992). The suggestion from the above work is that the preferred view of an object depends upon whether the task is one of recognition (retrieval of information) or exploration (encoding of information), on whether the object in question is highly familiar or novel, and on whether it is a static, two-dimensional representation versus an actively perceived three-dimensional thing.

In a series of studies particularly relevant to our developmental work, James and colleagues asked the adult subjects to view, for later tests of recognition, computer rendered, virtual 3-D objects on a computer monitor by rotating them using a trackball device (Harman et al., 1999; James et al., 2001). Subjects rotated the objects in any dimension (*x*, *y*, and *z*) for a total of 20 s. The subjects spent most of their viewing time on the planar views (see also James et al., 2002; Perrett & Harries, 1988; Perrett, Harries, & Looker, 1992). In a separate experiment, James et al. (2001) also showed that dynamically viewing mostly planar views facilitated subsequent recognition when compared with the dynamic viewing of mostly 3/4 views. Thus, not only do adults prefer to study planar views of novel objects, but also when these views are controlled experimentally, dwelling on and around the planar views promotes the formation of more robust memories of object shape.

When and how do these preferences emerge developmentally? We have new results (Pereira, James, Smith, & Jones, 2007) that suggest that this preference emerges between 18 and 24 months, the very same period in which children learn many object names, in which the shape bias emerges, in which children begin to recognize objects from sparse representations of geometric structure, and in which they first show shape-based object substitutions in thematic play. One cannot ask 18- to 24-month-old children to manipulate computer-rendered images with a trackball (the method used by James et al.). What we did instead was that we asked children to manually and visually explore objects while wearing a head-camera, a methodology for tapping the first-person view developed by Yoshida and Smith (2008). Children were given novel and familiar objects to explore as they sat in a chair with no table so that each object could only be held by one or two hands. The child was given one object at a time to look at and explore for up to 20 s.

The data were coded using a custom-made software application that allowed a coder to compare an image taken from the camera to an image of a computer-rendered object. Here, we will report two analyses. The first is at a coarser grain, and just asked whether the view was "near planar" (within 15°) for each of the 6 possible planar views compared to a random object manipulation. The second analysis yields a detailed continuous presentation of the actual *x*, *y*, and *z* coordinates, a map of dwell times. The 18-month-old children showed no preference for the planar compared to baseline when they explored either the novel or the familiar objects. In contrast, the 24-month-old children showed marked preferences for the planar views for known but not for novel objects as shown in Figure 6.10. These results suggest an emerging preference for planar views in the active exploration of objects that begins with known object shapes and thus potentially may develop from experience with those particular objects. An important detail to consider here is that in the James et al. study, adults spent around 70% of their dwell time around planar views. This is considerably higher that the values here, even for the older group, so it seems that we have identified the beginning of this phenomenon.

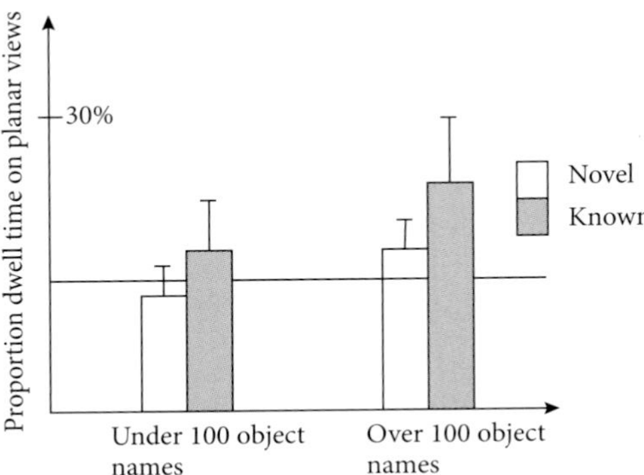

Figure 6.10 Dwell times on planar views given exploration of novel and known objects for children with fewer and with more than 100 object names in productive vocabulary as compared to that expected (the solid line) by random object rotations (Pereira et al., 2007).

To the best of our knowledge, there are no prior developmental studies directly comparing children's recognition of objects from 3/4 and planar views and no prior studies of the views of objects that children actively generate for themselves as they explore objects. This is a critical gap in our understanding of the development of visual object recognition. Children's first-hand views of objects are the visual experiences on which they must build their object recognition systems and their representations of specific objects (see chapter by Johnson in this volume). That these views change with development—that younger children present different views to themselves than do older children—suggest a link between perceptual development and action, with developmental changes in object representations perhaps driving changes in the views that children present themselves. These self-generated views, in turn, seem likely to be driving forces in the development of object representations. Although we have not made the direct link yet, the fact that these changes in preferred views begin at the same time when children learn many object category names, begin to build abstract and category encompassing representations of object structure, and engage in shape-based object substitutions in play suggest that they may be connected. At the very least, all the results reviewed thus far suggest that fundamentally important changes in visual object recognition—evident in a variety of task domains—are occurring between 18 and 24 months.

Axes of Elongation

Planar and 3/4 views are defined by the relation of the object's axis of elongation to the viewer; that is, in the planar view, the axis of elongation is parallel or perpendicular to the viewer's line of sight. Many theorists of visual object recognition have posited that axes of elongation (and/or symmetry, which is often correlated with the axis of elongation) play a particularly critical role in a current input's activation of stored object representations (Biederman, 1987; Marr & Nishihara, 1992). This is because the object's major axes are proposed to play an important role in parsing objects into their main parts and for the comparison of sensory inputs to stored representations (Biederman, 1987; Jolicoeur, 1985, 1990; Marr & Nishihara, 1992; Ullman, 1996). This makes sense: the principal axes are enduring characteristics of objects and provide a systematic means for transforming and comparing images by defining a common reference frame for alignment. Axes of elongation and their relation to the body are also important determiners of how objects are picked up, held, viewed, and used (Goodale & Humphrey, 1998; Jeannerod, 1988, 1997; Jones & Lederman, 2006; Milner & Goodale, 1995; Turvey, Park, Dumais, & Carello, 1998).

Studies of the influence of axes of elongation in adult object recognition mainly involve the presentation of objects from various viewpoints that differ in the relation of the axes of elongation to the viewer. Put together, these studies have yielded mixed results. Studies that have used pictures of highly familiar objects rotated in the picture plane typically find, at best, small effects (Large, McMullen, & Hamm, 2003; Sekuler, 1996). As Large et al. note, strong top-down effects in adults' recognition of prototypical pictures of things may overwhelm any role for variations in the main axes. Consistent with this idea, Liu and Cooper (2001) found strong axis of symmetry effects in judgments about nonsense objects. Thus, the principal axes may be particularly important in setting up one's initial representations of an object, and perhaps in integrating multiple images into a coherent whole. In support of this idea, Jolicoeur (1985) found that axes of elongation were important in recognizing novel objects, but played a decreasing role with increasing object familiarity.

There is also evidence that object shape, and perceived axes of elongation and symmetry, depend on (and also influence) the perceived frame of reference (Quinlan & Humphrey, 1993; Rock, 1973; Sekuler, 1996; Sekuler & Swimmer, 2000). For example, the same pattern can be seen as a square or a diamond, depending on how one assigns the reference frame and the main axis of symmetry (Rock, 1973). Particularly relevant to our interest in the relation between action and perception, the perceived axes of elongation and symmetry in adults are also influenced by motion (Bucher & Palmer, 1985; Rock 1973; Sekuler & Swimmer, 2000). Adults are biased to see both the main axis of symmetry and the main axis of elongation as parallel to the path of movement (Morikawa, 1999; Sekuler & Swimmer, 2000).

There is almost no evidence on how children perceive axes of elongation, on how principle axes relate to the development of object recognition or on how action—holding and moving objects—may be related to the perceptual definition of the principle axes of an object (but see E.J. Gibson, 1969; Turvey et al., 1998) even though object shape and axes of elongation strongly influence not only how we hold and grasp objects, but also how objects may be used functionally (Goodale & Humphrey, 1998; Jeannerod, 1988; Jones & Lederman, 2006; Milner & Goodale, 1995). However, if the axes of elongation are important for setting up frames of reference for the perception of shape, as many theories of visual object recognition suggest, and if axes of elongation determine how we hold, grasp, and use objects, then children's actions on objects may play an important developmental role in their discovery and representation of these axes, and thus in visual object recognition. There are many well-documented demonstrations of how action organizes perceptual development in other domains (e.g. Amso & Johnson, 2006; Bushnell & Bourdreau, 1993; Gibson, 1969; Needham, Barrett, & Peterman, 2002; Ruff & Rothbart, 1996). Two recent developmental studies in our laboratory suggest that this may also be the case in children's representation of the major axes of an object.

The first relevant study (Smith, 2005) demonstrates how action may promote the discovery of deeper regularities concerning three-dimensional object structure, particularly, the definition of an object's axes of elongation and symmetry. The participants were 24- to 30-month-old children. In the first experiment, the children were given a three-dimensional object to hold in one hand that is shown in Figure 6.11A. This nearly sphere-like exemplar object did not have a single main axis of elongation. In one condition, children moved the object up and down along a 1-m vertical path. In a second condition, they moved the object back and forth on a 1-m horizontal path. Immediately following, children were asked to group the exemplar object with other like things. No movement was involved in this categorization task. Children who had acted on the exemplar by moving it vertically grouped it with objects elongated on their vertical axes (Figure 6.11B), but children who had moved the exemplar horizontally grouped it with objects elongated on their horizontal axes. These categorization choices emerged only as a consequence of action and not when children merely observed someone else move the exemplar along the same path. The path of action thus selected or highlighted the corresponding visual axis, altering the perceived similarity of the exemplar to the test objects.

The second experiment in this study used an exemplar like that shown in figure, part C, an exemplar not quite symmetrical around its center axis. The actions are illustrated in the figure, part D. Children who held the exemplar in one hand by one part and moved it back and forth subsequently grouped the exemplar with test objects (part E) that were less symmetrical in shape than the exemplar itself, as if they saw the exemplar as composed of two unequal parts. Children who held the exemplar in the two

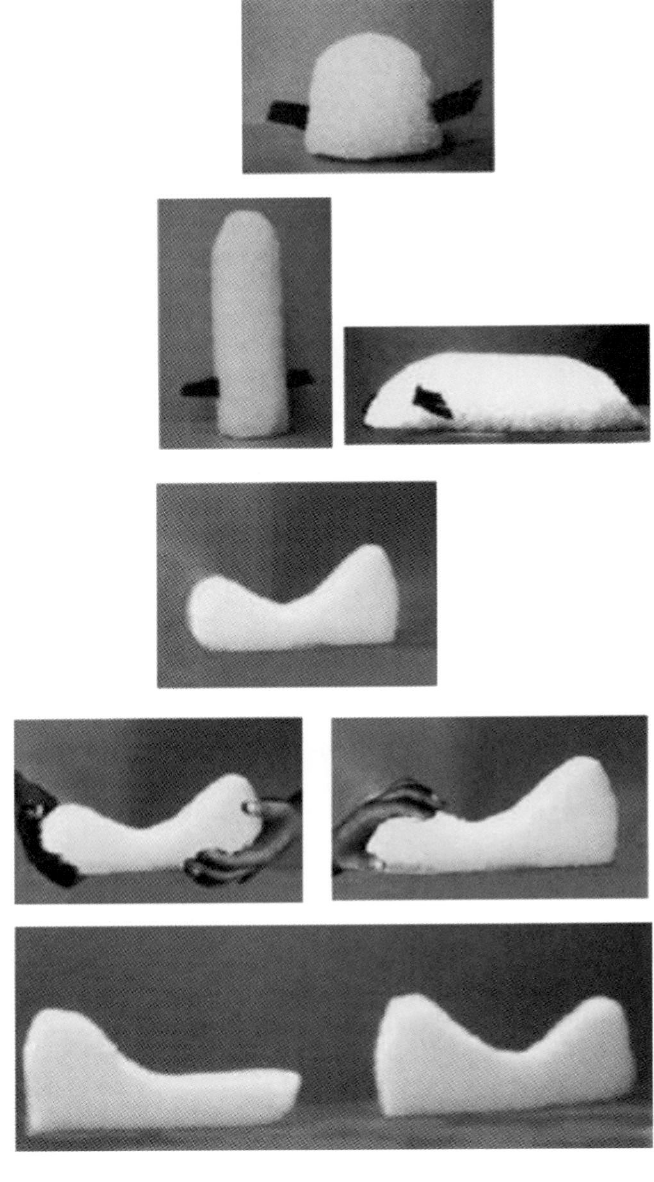

Figure 6.11 Exemplars and test objects used in Smith (2005).

hands and rotated it about a central axis subsequently grouped the exemplar with objects more symmetrical in shape than the exemplar, as if they saw the exemplar as composed of two comparable and symmetric parts. Again, these results only obtained when children acted on the objects, not when they watched someone else do the action. The enacted action appears to have selected compatible visual descriptions of object shape.

Axes of elongation and symmetry are higher-order dimensions of object shape fundamental to processes of human object recognition (e.g., Marr, 1982). These results suggest that they may be developmentally defined not by vision alone but by the in-task coordination of visual and motor processes. This is potentially of considerable importance. Theories of object recognition are for the most part theories of static object recognition (see also, Liu & Cooper, 2003). Yet how we act on objects is intimately related to their shapes, and may even developmentally be defining of them. Every time the child lays a doll in a doll bed, or perhaps on top of a block as a pretend bed, the child acts in ways that may help define the major axes of an object and the frame of reference for comparing one shape to another. There are physical and biological constraints on how we can hold and move objects of different shapes and thus highly constrained associations between symmetry, elongation, and paths of movement that may bootstrap these developments. Related to this idea is Morikawa's (1999) proposal that adults are biased to perceive movement parallel to an object's long axis and this bias derives from a regularity in the world, that objects in general move on paths parallel to their long axis (there are obvious exceptions: people, e.g., move orthogonally to their long axis). Still, a person's movements of objects (rather than, or as well as, how objects move on their own) may well be systematically related to shape in ways that matter to the development of object recognition. And critically, the visual information young learners receive about objects varies systematically with their own actions on those objects. Thus it seems likely that changes in visual object recognition support developmental changes in action (including object substitution in play) and that those activities in turn help define and refine structural descriptions of shape. This, then, is another potential loop of codeveloping processes, of causes as consequences and consequences as causes. At the very least, the present results show that action has a strong influence on the range of shapes 2-year-olds take as being similar and appears to do so by defining axes of elongation and symmetry.

Our most recent work on this topic (Street, Smith, James, & Jones, 2008) uses a task that is commonly used to diagnose developmental delays and is included in many assessment procedures. This is a shape-sorting task in which children are presented with objects of various shapes and asked to fit them into a container through holes specific to those shapes (Wyly, 1997). Although there are normative standards for preschool children's success in these tasks (and their perseveration in the task), there is remarkably little empirical study of the processes and skills that underlie success. We have preliminary evidence in a version of a shape-sorting task designed to measure children's ability to abstract the axis of elongation of shapes of various complexities.

Our approach is based on the "posting" studies of Efron (1969) with adults and neuropsychological patients (see also Goodale & Milner, 1992; Milner, Perrett, & Johnston., 1991; Warrington 1985). In these studies, subjects were given a range of "Efron rectangles": flat, simple, plaques that differ in their height–width ratio. Their task was to insert them in a slot aligned at a particular orientation. The critical dependent measure was whether subjects oriented the handheld object to match the slot. We use a much simpler version of this "posting task" to ask whether—given the goal of inserting an object in a slot—children align that object's axis of elongation to the axis of elongation of the slot. This task thus provides a good measure of children's ability to abstract the axis of elongation and to make use of that information in action. The participants are 30 children in two age groups, 17–18 and 23–24 months of age. Children are presented with a box with a quite large slot (7 by 21 cm) oriented either horizontally or vertically. They are then given objects, one at a time, and asked to put them into the slot. All the objects can be easily fit into the slot–either by aligning the axis of orientation or by tilting the object so that the foreshortened end goes in first. The key independent variables were: the Orientation of the objects on the table (that were Matching or Mismatching the orientation of the slot); and the Complexity of the objects. Complexity of shape was manipulated in three ways: Shape Matches, solid rectangular blocks whose shape matched the slot; Simple Shapes, novel forms with height–width ratios comparable to the rectangular blocks); and Known Shapes, complex real objects with height–width ratios comparable to the rectangular blocks but with multiple parts and a canonical axis of orientation (e.g., a tiger versus a rocket). Children wear the head-camera in this study so that we can record the alignment of object and slot from their point of view.

This is a highly enjoyable and engaging task and on virtually every trial the children inserted the object into the slot in one way or another. The first main result, however, is that this skill undergoes considerable developmental change in this period. Eighteen-month-old children struggle in this task, often making many wrong attempts (see Figure 6.12). In contrast, 24-month-old children are nearly perfect, aligning and inserting the object rapidly and almost without error. Our main dependent measure is degree of alignment, measured from the head-camera view as shown in Figure 6.12. For the younger children, this angle averages 33° across all objects, that is, these children were typically off the mark, and their error was greater for complex than for simple objects. In contrast, older children's alignment error was less 10° for all objects. How the objects were presented did not matter, perhaps because the children held and rotated them, exploring them, before attempting insertion. These results again suggest marked growth during this developmental period in children's representation and use of the structural dimensions of three-dimensional shape.

From Visual Object Recognition to Symbolic Play to Word Learning and Back

This chapter began with a phenomenon often known as symbolic play, an extremely interesting behavior that has been strongly linked to language learning, to social interactions in collaborative play, and to developing tool use (see Rakoczy, Tomasello, & Striano, 2006). The program of research reviewed in this chapter in no way explains symbolic play, since that explanation will likely consist of a cascade of interacting processes beyond those involved in perceiving and representing object shape. The findings reviewed here, however, do suggest that one component of that larger developmental story will be changes in fundamental processes of visual object recognition, which is the main focus of this chapter. The entire pattern of results reviewed here strongly suggests that there are significant and consequential changes

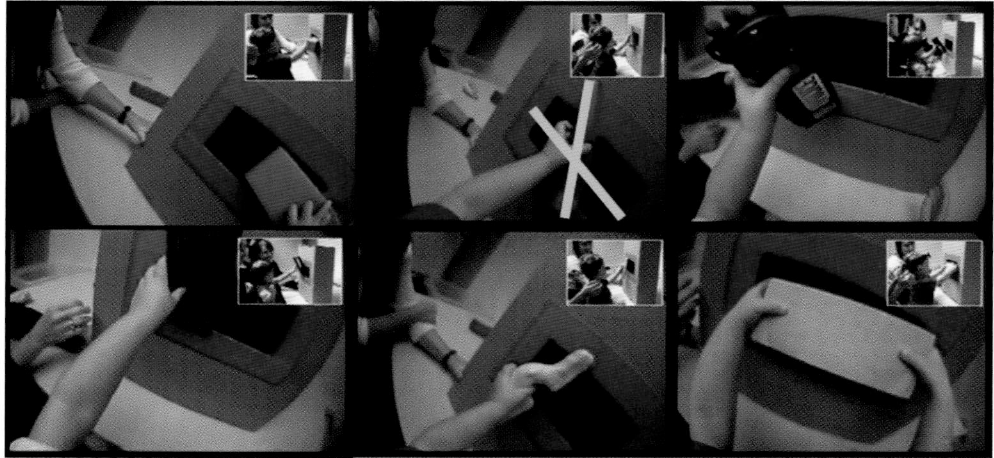

Figure 6.12 **Head-camera views from Street et al. (2008) of a 18-month-old infant inserting objects into slots. The smaller images show the view was an additional camera. As shown in the third image, alignment at first attempt is measured by the angle between the major axis of the slot and the major axis of the object to be inserted.**

in how children perceive, represent, and compare three-dimensional object shape, a shift from more piecemeal emphasis on local details to a sparse, and thus category encompassing, description of shape in terms of global geometric structure. These changes are seen in (1) the recognition of instances of common categories, (2) in object substitution in pretend play, (3) in active exploration of objects, and (4) in actions that make use of structural properties.

From this first set of studies, we cannot know with any certainty what causes what, but it may well be, as suggested by the opening Figure 6.1, that there are causal influences in all directions. Development, after all, occurs in real time, in incremental steps, across a number of interleaved real-time experiences. The child hears a new object named (say an oddly shaped mug), uses it to drink from, sees and imitates his older brother pretend to use it as a hat. All these experiences influence what the child sees, what the child feels, and how this one experience is connected to other experiences. The inventiveness of human cognition, its adaptability and power, may, quite literally, be constructed from the overlapping, mutually influencing, interactions of many different tasks involving and educating the same component processes.

Acknowledgments

This research was supported by National Institute for Child Health and Development (R01HD 28675); Portuguese Ministry of Science and Higher Education PhD scholarship SFRH/BD/13890/2003 and a Fulbright fellowship to AF.P.

References

Abecassis, M., Sera, M. D., Yonas, A., & Schwade, J. (2001). What's in a shape? Children represent shape variability differently than adults when naming objects. *Journal of Experimental Child Psychology, 78*, 213–239.

Amso, D., & Johnson, S. P. (2006). Learning by selection: Visual search and object perception in young infants. *Developmental psychology, 42*(6), 1236–1245.

Arbib, M. A. (1981). Visuomotor coordination: From neural nets to schema theory. *Cognition and Brain Theory, 4*, 23–39.

Biederman, I. (1987). Recognition-by-components: A theory of human image understanding. *Psychological Review, 94*(2), 115–147.

Biederman, I., & Gerhardstein, P. C. (1993). Recognizing depth-rotated objects: Evidence and conditions for three-dimensional viewpoint invariance. *Journal of Experimental Psychology, 19*(6), 1162–1182.

Biederman, I., & Kalocsai, P. (1997). Neurocomputational bases of object and face recognition. *Philosophical Transactions of the Royal Society of London B: Biological Sciences, 352*(1358), 1203–1219.

Blanz, V., Tarr, M. J., & Bulthoff, H. H. (1999). What object attributes determine canonical views? *Perception, 28*(5), 575–599.

Bucher, N. M., & Palmer, S. E. (1985). Effects of motion on perceived pointing of ambiguous triangles. *Perception and Psychophysics, 38*(3), 227–236.

Bushnell, E. W., & Bourdreau, J. P. (1993). Motor development and the mind: The potential role of motor abilities as a determinant of aspects of perceptual development. *Child Development, 64*(4), 1005–1021.

Cerella, J. (1986). Pigeons and perceptrons. *Pattern Recognition, 19*, 431–438.

Chao, L. L., & Martin, A. (2000). Representation of manipulable man-made objects in the dorsal stream. *NeuroImage, 12*(4), 478–484.

Christou, C. G., & Bulthoff, H. H. (1999). View dependence in scene recognition after active learning. *Memory and Cognition, 27*(6), 996–1007.

Colunga, E. (2003, April). *Where is the cow hiding? A new method for studying the development of features.* Paper presented at the Biennial meeting of the Society for Research on Child Development, Tampa, FL.

Colunga, E., & Smith, L. B. (2005). From the lexicon to expectations about kinds: A role for associative learning. *Psychological Review, 112*(2), 342–382.

Cooper, E. E., Biederman, I., & Hummel, J. E. (1992). Metric invariance in object recognition: A review and further evidence. *Canadian Journal of Psychology, 46*(2), 191–214.

Craighero, L., Fadiga, L., Umilta, C. A., & Rizzolatti, G. (1996). Evidence for visuomotor priming effect. *Cognitive Neuroscience and Neuropsychology, 8*(1), 347–349.

Edelman, G. (1987) *Neural darwinism. The theory of neuronal group selection*. New York: Basic Books.

Edelman, S. (1995). Representation, similarity, and the chorus of prototypes. *Minds and Machines. 5*(1), 45–68.

Edelman, S., & Duvdevani-Bar, S. (1997). Similarity, connectionism, and the problem of representation in vision. *Neural Computation, 9*(4), 701–720.

Edelman, S., & Intrator, N. (1997). Learning as extraction of low-dimensional representations. In R. L. Goldstone, D. L. Medin, & P. G. Schyns (Eds.), *Perceptual learning. The psychology of learning and motivation,* (pp. 353–380): San Diego, CA: Academic Press.

Edelman, S., & Intrator, N. (2003). Towards structural systematicity in distributed, statically bound representations. *Cognitive Science, 27*, 73–109.

Efron, R. (1969). What is perception? *Boston Studies of the Philisophical Society, 4*, 137–173.

Fenson, L. Marchman, V. A., Thal, D. J., Dale, P. S., Reznick, S., & Bates, E. (1993). *MacArthur-Bates communicative development inventories* (2nd ed.). Baltimore, MD: Brookes Publishing.

Fize, D., Fabre-Thorpe, M. I., Richard, G., Doyon, B., & Thorpe, S. J. (2005). Rapid categorization of foveal and extrafoveal natural images: Associated ERPs and effects of lateralization. *Brain and Cognition, 59*(2), 145–158.

Freyd, J. J. (1983). Representing the dynamics of static form. *Memory & Cognition, 11*, 342–346.

Gathercole, V. C. M., & Min, H. (1997). Word meaning biases or language-specific effects? Evidence from English, Spanish and Korean. *First Language, 17*, 31–56.

Gerlach, C., Law, I., Gade, A., & Paulson, O. B. (2000). Categorization and category effects in normal object recognition: A PET study. *Neuropsychologia, 38*, 1693–1703.

Gershkoff-Stowe, L., & Smith, L. B. (2004). Shape and the first hundred nouns. *Child Development, 75*(40), 1098–1114.

Gibson, E. J. (1969). *Principles of perceptual learning and development*. New York: Appleton Century Crofts.

Gibson, J. J. (1979). *The ecological approach to visual perception*. Hillsdale, NJ: Erlbaum.

Goodale, M. A., & Milner, A. D. (1992) Separate visual pathways for perception and action, *Trends in Neurosciences, 15*, 2025.

Goodale, M. A., & Humphrey, G. K. (1998) The objects of action and perception. *Cognition, 67*, 181–207.

Grezes, J., & Decety, J. (2002). Does visual perception of object afford action? Evidence from a neuroimaging study. *Neuropsychologia, 40*, 212–222.

Hayward, W. G. (2003). After the viewpoint debate: where next in object recognition? *Trends in Cognitive Science, 7*(10), 425–427.

Harman, K. L., Humphrey, G. K., & Goodale, M. A. (1999). Active manual control of object views facilitates visual recognition. *Current Biology, 9*(22). 1315–1318.

Hummel, J. E. (2000). Where view-based theories break down: The role of structure in shape perception and object recognition. In E. Dietrich & A. Markman (Ed.), *Cognitive dynamics: Conceptual change in humans and machines* (pp. 157–185). Hillsdale, NJ: Erlbaum.

Hummel, J. E., & Biederman, I. (1992). Dynamic binding in a neural network for shape recognition. *Psychological Review, 99*(3), 480–517.

Humphrey, G. K., & Jolicoeur, P. (1993). An examination of the effects of axis foreshortening, monocular depth cues, and visual field on object identification. *The Quarterly Journal of Experimental Psychology, 46*(1), 137–159.

Imai, M., Gentner, D., & Uchida, N. (1994). Children's theories of word meaning: The role of shape similarity in early acquisition. *Cognitive Development, 9*(1), 45–75.

James, K. H., Humphrey, G. K., & Goodale, M. A. (2001). Manipulating and recognizing virtual objects: Where the action is. *Canadian Journal of Experimental Psychology, 55*(2), 111–120.

James, K. H., Humphrey, G. K., Vilis, T., Baddour, R., Corrie, B., & Goodale, M. A. (2002). Learning three-dimensional object structure: A virtual reality study. *Behavioral Research Methods, Instruments and Computers, 34*(3), 383–390.

James, K. H., & Gauthier, I. (2006). Letter processing automatically recruits a sensory-motor brain network. *Neuropsychologia, 44*, 2937–2949.

Jeannerod, M. (1988) *The neural and behavioral organization of goal-directed movements*. New York: Oxford University Press.

Jeannerod, M. (1997). *The cognitive neuroscience of action*. Cambridge, MA: Blackwell.

Jolicoeur, P. (1985). The time to name disoriented natural objects. *Memory and Cognition, 13*(4), 289–303.

Jolicoeur, P. (1990). Identification of disoriented objects: A dual-systems theory. *Mind and Language, 5*(4), 387–410.

Jones, S. S. (2003). Late talkers show no shape bias in object naming. *Developmental Science, 6*(5), 477–483.

Jones, L. A., & Lederman, S. J. (2006). *Human hand function*. New York: Oxford University Press.

Jones, S. S., & Smith, L. B. (2005). Object name learning and object perception: A deficit in late talkers. *Journal of Child Language, 32*(1), 223–240.

Keil, F. C. (1994). The birth and nurturance of concepts by domains: The origins of concepts of living things. In L. A. Hirschfeld & S.A. Gelman (Eds.), *Mapping the mind: Domain specificity in cognition and culture* (pp. 234–254). New York: Cambridge University Press.

Kellman, P. J. (2001). Separating processes in object perception. *Journal of Experimental Child Psychology. Special Issue: Reflections, 78*(1), 84–97.

Landau, B., Smith, L., & Jones, S. (1988). The importance of shape in early lexical learning. *Cognitive Development, 3*, 299–321.

Large, M. E., McMullen, P. A., & Hamm, J. P. (2003). The role of axes of elongation and symmetry in rotated object naming. *Perception and Psychophysics, 65*(1). 1–19.

Lawson, R., & Humphreys, G. W. (1998). View-specific effects of depth rotation and foreshortening on the initial recognition and priming of familiar objects. *Perception and Psychophysics, 60*(60), 1052–1066.

Longcamp, M., Boucard, C., Gilhodes, J. C., & Vely, J. L. (2005). Remembering the orientation of newly learned characters depends on the associated writing knowledge: A comparison between handwriting and typing. *Human Movement Science, 25*(4–5), 646–656.

Liu, T., & Cooper, L. A. (2003). Explicit and implicit memory for rotating objects. *Journal of Experimental Psychology: Learning, Memory, and Cognition, 29*, 554–562.

Marr, D. (1982) *Vision: A computational investigation into the human representation and processing of visual information*. New York, NY: Henry Holt and Co., Inc.

Marr, D. & Nishihara, H. K. (1978). Representation and recognition of the spatial organization of three-dimensional shapes. *Proceedings Royal Society of London, Series B, 200*(1140): 269–94

McCune-Nicolich, L. (1981). Toward symbolic functioning: Structure of early pretend games and potential parallels with language. *Child Development, 52*(3), 785–797.

McCune, L. (1995). A normative study of representational play in the transition to language. *Developmental psychology, 31*(2), 198–206.

Mecklinger, A., Gruenewald, C., Besson, M., Magnie, M. N., & Cramon, D. Y. (2002). Seperable neuronal circuitries for manipulable and non-manipulable objects in working memory. *Cerebral Cortex, 12*(11), 1115–1123.

Milner, D., & Goodale, M. (1995) *The visual brain in action*. New York: Oxford University Press.

Milner, A. D., Perrett, D. I., & Johnston, R. S. (1991). Perception and action in 'visual form agnosia'. *Brain, 114*, 405–428.

Mondloch, C. J., Le Grand, R., & Maurer, D. (2002). Configural face processing develops more slowly than featural face processing. *Perception, 31*(5), 553–566.

Morikawa, K. (1999). Symmetry and elongation of objects influence perceived direction of translational motion. *Perception and Psychophysics, 61*, 134–143.

Namy, L. (2002) *Symbol use and symbolic representation: Developmental and Comparative Perspectives*: New York: Rutledge

Needham, A., Barrett, T., & Peterman K. (2002). A pick-me-up for infants' exploratory skills: Early simulated experiences reaching for objects using "sticky mittens" enhances young infants' object exploration skills. *Infant Behavior and Development, 25*(3), 279–295.

Nelson, C. A. (2001). The development and neural bases of face recognition. Infant and *Child Development. Special Issue: Face Processing in Infancy and Early Childhood, 10*(1–2), 3–18.

Newell, F. N., & Findlay, J. M.(1997). The effect of depth rotation on object identification. *Perception, 26*(10), 1231–1257.

Paillard, J. (1991). *Brain and space*. New York: Oxford University Press.

Palmer, S. E., Rosch, E., & Chase, P. (1981). Canonical perspective and the perception of objects. In J. Long & A. Baddeley (Eds), *Attention and performance* (pp. 135–151) Hillsdale, NJ: Erlbaum.

Pegna, A. J., Khateb, A., Michel, C. M., & Landis, T. (2004). Visual recognition of faces, objects, and words using degraded stimuli: Where and when it occurs. *Human Brain Mapping, 22*(4), 300–311.

Pereira, A. & Smith, L. B. (2009). Developmental changes in visual object recognition between 18 and 24 months of age. *Developmental Science, 12*(4), *67–80*.

Pereira, A., James, K. H., Smith, L. B., & Jones, S. S. (2007). Preferred views in children's active exploration of objects, *Society for Research in Child Development, Annual Meeting*, Boston, MA.

Perner, J. (1991). *Understanding the representational mind*. Cambridge, MA: MIT Press.

Perrett, D. I., & Harries, M. H. (1988). Characteristic views and the visual inspection of simple faceted and smooth objects: Tetrahedra and potatoes. *Perception, 17*(6), 703–720.

Perrett, D. I., Harries, M. H., & Looker, S. (1992). Use of preferential inspection to define the viewing sphere and characteristic views of an arbitrary machined tool part. *Perception, 21*, 497–515.

Peissig, J. J., & Tarr, M. J. (2007). Visual object recognition: Do we know more now than we did 20 years ago? *Annual Review of Psychology, 58*(1), 75–96.

Peterson, M. (Ed.) (1999) *The MIT encyclopedia of the cognitive sciences*. Cambridge, MA: The MIT Press.

Piaget, J. (1962). *Play, dreams, and imitation in childhood*. New York: Norton.

Quinlan, P. T. & Humphreys, G. W. (1993). Perceptual frames of reference and two-dimensional shape recognition: further examination of internal axes. *Perception. 22*(11):1343–64.

Rakison, D. H., & Butterworth, G. E. (1998a). Infants' attention to object structure in early categorization. *Developmental Psychology, 34*(6), 1310–1325.

Rakison, D. H., & Butterworth, G. E. (1998b). Infant's use of object parts in early categorization. *Developmental Psychology, 34*(1), 49–62.

Rakison, D. H., & Cicchino, J. B. (2008). Induction in infancy. in S. Johnson (Ed.), *A neo-constructivist approach to early development*. New York: Oxford University Press.

Rakison, D. H., & Cohen, L. B. (1999) Infants' use of functional parts in basic-like categorization. *Developmental Science, 2*, 423–431.

Rakison, D. H., & Lupyan, G. (2008). Developing object concepts in infancy: An associative learning perspective. *Monographs of the SRCD, 73*(1).

Rakoczy, H., Tomasello, M., & Striano, T. (2006). The role of experience and discourse in children's developing understanding of pretend play actions. *British Journal of Developmental Psychology, 24*(2), 305–335.

Rock, I. (1973). *Orientation and form*. New York, NY: Academic Press.

Rosch, E., Mervis, C. B., Gray, W. D., Johnson, D. M., & Boyes-Braem, P. (1976). Basic objects in natural categories. *Cognitive Psychology, 8*, 382–439.

Ruff, H. A., & Rothbart, M. K. (1996). *Attention in early development*. New York: Oxford University Press.

Samuelson, L. K. (2002). Statistical regularities in vocabulary guide language acquisition in connectionist models and 15–20-month-olds. *Developmental Psychology, 38*(6), 1016–1037.

Samuelson, L. K., & Smith, L. B. (1999). Early noun vocabularies: Do ontology, category structure and syntax correspond? *Cognition, 73*, 1–33.

Sekuler, A. B. (1996) Axis of elongation can determine reference frames for object perception. *Canadian Journal of Experimental Psychology, 50*(3), 270–279.

Sekuler, A. B., & Swimmer, M. B. (2000). Interactions between symmetry and elongation in determining reference frames for object perception. *Canadian Journal of Experimental Psychology*, 54(1), 42–56.

Sekuler, E. B. (1996). Perceptual cues in pure alexia. *Cognitive Neuropsychology, 13*(7), 941–974.

Shore, C., O'Connell, B., & Bates, E. (1984). First sentences in language and symbolic play. *Developmental Psychology, 20*(5), 872–880.

Smith, L. B. (2003). Learning to recognize objects. *Psychological Science, 14*(3) 244– 251.

Smith, L. B. (2005). Action alters perceived shape. *Cognitive Science, 29*, 665–679.

Smith, L. B., Jones, S. S., Landau, B., Gershkoff-Stowe, L., & Samuelson, S. (2002). Early noun learning provides on-the-job training for attention. *Psychological Science, 13*, 13–19.

Smith, L. B., & Pereira. A. F. (2008) *Symbolic play links to language through object recognition*. Unpublished manuscript, Department of Psychological and Brain Sciences, Indiana University Bloomington, Bloomington, IN.

Soja, N. N. (1992). Inferences about the meanings of nouns: The relationship between perception and syntax. *Cognitive Development, 7*, 29–45.

Son, J.Y., Smith, L.B., & Goldstone, R.L. (2008). Simplicity and generalization: Short-cutting abstraction in children's object categorizations. *Cognition, 108*, 626–638.

Stankiewicz, B. J. (2003). Just another view. *Trends in Cognitive Science, 7*, 526.

Street, S., Smith, L. B., James. K. H., & Jones, S. S. (2008). *Posting ability and object recognition in 18–24 month old children.* Unpublished manuscript, Department of Psychological and Brain Sciences, Indiana University Bloomington, Bloomington, IN.

Tarr, M., & Vuong, Q. C. (2002). Visual object recognition. In S. Yantis (Ed.), *Steven's Handbook of Experimental Psychology: Vol. 1. Sensation and Perception* (Vol. 1). New York, NY: John Wiley & Sons, Inc.

Tong, F. H., Marlin, S. G., & Frost, B. J. (1995). *Cognition map formation in a three-dimensional visual virtual world.* Poster presented at the IRIS/PRECARN Workshop,Vancouver, BC.

Turvey, M. T., Park, H., Dumais, S. M., & Carello, C. (1998). Nonvisible perception of segments of a hand-held object and the attitude spinor. *Journal of Motor Behavior, 30*(1), 3–19.

Ullman, S. (1996). *High level vision.* Cambridge, MA: MIT Press.

Ullman, S. (2000). *High-level vision: Object recognition and visual cognition.* Cambridge, MA: MIT Press.

Ullman, S., & Bart, E. (2004). Recognition invariance obtained by extended and invariant features. *Neural Networks, 17*(5/6), 833–848.

Ullman, S., Vidal-Naquet, M., & Sali, E. (2002). Visual features of intermediate complexity and their use on classification. *Nature Neuroscience, 5*(7), 682–687.

Vivani, P., & Stucchi, N. (1992). Biological movements look uniform: Evidence for motor-perceptual interactions. *Journal of Experimental Psychology, 18*, 603–623.

Warrington, E. K. (1985). Agnosia: the impairment of object recognition. In P. J. Vinken, G. W. Bruyn, & H. L. Klawans (Eds.), *Handbook of clinical neurology.* Amsterdam: Elsevier.

Weismer, S. E. (2007). *Typical talkers, late talkers, and children with specific language impairment: A language endowment spectrum?* Mahwah, NJ: Lawrence Erlbaum Associates.

Wexler, M., & van Boxtel., J. (2005). Depth perception by the active observer. *Trends in Cognitive Science*, 9, 431–8. s

Wohlschlager, A., & Wohlschlager, A. (1998). Mental and manual rotation. *Journal of Experimental Psychology, Human Perception and Performance, 24*(2), 397–412.

Wyly, M. V. (1997). *Infant assessment.* Boulder, CO: Westview Press.

Yoshida, H., & Smith, L. B. (2003). Shifting ontological boundaries: How Japanese- and English-speaking children generalize names for animals and artifacts. *Developmental Science, 6*, 1–34.

Yoshida, H. & Smith, L.B. (2008). What's in view for toddlers? Using a head camera to study visual experience. *Infancy, 13*(3), 229–248.

CHAPTER 7
Musical Enculturation: How Young Listeners Construct Musical Knowledge through Perceptual Experience

Erin E. Hannon

Human musical capacities have recently become the focus of an exploding quantity of theoretical and empirical contributions in the psychological and brain sciences (Avanzini Lopez, Koelsch, & Majno, 2006; Compston, 2006; Peretz, 2006; Spiro, 2003; Wallin, Merker, & Brown, 2000; Zatorre & Peretz, 2003). This marks a significant change in the status of musical behavior and cognition as the topic of empirical investigation. Until recently, it was widely assumed that musical skills and knowledge were only possessed by an elite, highly trained minority, a view bolstered by characterizations of music as frivolous, devoid of adaptive significance, and subject to insurmountable individual and cross-cultural variability (Pinker, 1997, 2002). Current approaches refute this view by emphasizing biological substrates of music (i.e., Zatorre & Peretz, 2003), potential survival advantages of music (Huron, 2003; Miller, 2000), and the ubiquity of many basic musical skills. For example, most adults have sufficient musical knowledge to sing a familiar tune (Dalla Bella, Giguere, & Peretz, 2007), detect "wrong notes" in a musical sequence (Drayna et al., 2001; Hyde & Peretz, 2004; Trainor & Trehub, 1992), recognize and experience emotions communicated by music (Grewe, Kopiez, & Altenmüller, 2005; Juslin & Laukka, 2003), and move or dance in synchrony with music (Large, Fink, & Kelso, 2002; McAuley, Jones, Holub, Johnstone, & Miller, 2006; Snyder & Krumhansl, 2001). Thus, just as most children eventually learn to understand their native language, every member of a particular culture—with or without formal musical training—can be expected to acquire basic musical competence and a working knowledge of familiar musical structures (Bigand & Poulin-Chourronnat, 2006; Hannon & Trainor, 2007).

The question of exactly how this musical knowledge is structured and acquired during development is of great interest but as of yet unanswered. One proposal is that such knowledge arises from a "music faculty" that is modular and built from innate, "core" capacities (Hauser & McDermott, 2003; Peretz & Coltheart, 2003; Peretz & Morais, 1989). Proponents of the modular approach have cited evidence of music-specific neural circuitry in adults (Janata et al., 2002; Koelsch & Siebel, 2005), cases of double-dissociations between music and other cognitive or linguistic abilities in patients with brain damage (Peretz et al., 1994; Vignolo, 2003), and parallels between the musical abilities of adults and young infants (Trehub, 2003). According to the modular view, musical knowledge and behavior arise from an innate set of music-specific evolutionary adaptations.

An alternative to the modular approach, embraced here, is that highly specialized knowledge of music in adulthood arises through simple perceptual learning mechanisms that build increasingly specific representations from domain-general capacities (Trehub & Hannon, 2006). According to this view, the appearance of domain-specificity and even encapsulation in adult music processing does not necessarily signify the existence of modularity in the initial state—rather, such specialization could be the result of developmental processes (Karmiloff-Smith, 1992; McMullen & Saffran, 2004). Thus, observed parallels between adult and infant performance in music cognition tasks may arise from general properties of the nervous system that are not necessarily specific to music or even to humans. Such initial abilities constrain musical enculturation, the process through which everyday exposure to the statistics of music drives the acquisition of culture-specific musical knowledge.

This chapter explores the question of how infants and children build musical representations, with particular focus on perception and knowledge of temporal structure in music, such as rhythm and meter. Rhythm and meter are fundamental to most socially significant and universal musical behaviors, such as synchronous dancing or ensemble performance (Brown, 2003). In this chapter, I will review published and new evidence that infants can perceive rhythm and meter by attending to the same statistical properties that underlie adults' perception, that representations of rhythm and meter undergo reorganization as a result of culture-specific perceptual experience, and that infants and adults share some basic temporal processing constraints despite infants' initial flexibility. In addition to examining development of music-specific knowledge, a parallel goal is to understand the emergence of domain-specific representations in auditory cognition. If we assume that early representations of music are primarily domain-general and become culture-specific through perceptual experience, then a question of great interest is whether overlapping structures are present and detected in the musical and linguistic input available to infants and children. I will briefly review some new evidence suggesting that this is may be the case.

Statistical learning and musical time

Numerous studies suggest that infants and adults use domain-general statistical learning mechanisms to infer structure across a number of domains (Conway & Christiansen, 2006; Kirkham, Slemmer, & Johnson, 2002; Saffran, Aslin, & Newport, 1996; see Kirkham, Saffran, and Gomez chapters, this volume). Statistical learning depends on the perceiver's simple capacity to track the frequency with which certain units or combinations of units occur. Many examples of statistical learning have been documented in the language domain. For instance, infants infer phonemic distinctions between syllables only when the prototypical speech sounds occur more frequently than nonprototypical sounds (Maye, Werker, & Gerken, 2002). Transitional probabilities between units (i.e., the likelihood that one unit will be preceded or followed by another) enable infants to segment unfamiliar sequences of syllables or tones into groups or "words" after brief exposure (Saffran, Johnson, Aslin, & Newport, 1999). Multiple and correlated statistical cues provide a powerful means by which infants can rapidly build increasingly complex representations from simple learning mechanisms (Christiansen, Allen, & Seidenberg, 1998; Christiansen, Dale, & Reali, this volume; Thiessen & Saffran, 2007).

Relatively little is known about the role of statistical learning in the development of musical representations. Transitional probabilities and frequency of occurrence likely provide information about the hierarchical pitch organization of Western music or tonality, since tonally prominent pitches tend to occur more frequently than do other pitches, and the sequential structure of pitch sequences is often highly constrained by harmonic cadences (Krumhansl, 2004). When presented with an unfamiliar pitch sequence, adults can use frequency of occurrence to infer tonal prominence (Creel & Newport, 2002), and a self-organizing neural network exposed to the statistics of Western music can simulate tonal expectations (Tillman, Bharucha, & Bigand, 2000). Despite the presence of such statistical information, however, it does not appear that tonality is learned during infancy. On the contrary, most evidence suggests that adult-like knowledge of tonality does not emerge until after at least 5 years of age (Cuddy & Badertscher, 1987; Koelsch, Fritz, Schulze, Alsop, & Schlaug,

2005; Krumhansl & Keil, 1982; Schellenberg, 2005; Trainor & Trehub, 1992). By contrast, statistical information about temporal structure in music is available and used by infants and adults alike.

Musical meter is the hierarchical temporal structure of music. The ability to dance or move in synchrony with music depends on a listener's ability to infer the underlying meter in the auditory input, which in turn guides temporal expectations and gives rise to the subjective experience of a primary pulse and alternating patterns of strong and weak beats. Although the pulse of a simple metronomic or isochronous sequence is obvious from the acoustic input (i.e., every tone onset corresponds to a pulse), real music presents a greater challenge to the listener because any number of amplitude peaks or event onsets could mark multiple and sometimes conflicting primary pulse rates. It is nevertheless trivial for most adults to perceive and move in synchrony with music. Evidence suggests that adult listeners infer the meter by attending to periodically occurring statistics. For example, in Western music (both classical and children's), event onsets tend to occur more frequently at strong than at weak metrical positions (Palmer & Krumhansl, 1990; Palmer & Pfordresher, 2003). Events that are accented or made salient through changes in amplitude, length, pitch, or grouping also tend to occur more frequently at strong metrical positions in music (Huron & Royal, 1996). Frequencies of event and accent occurrence predict when adults will tap to music (Snyder & Krumhansl, 2001) and their perception of meter in unfamiliar melodic patterns (Hannon, Snyder, Eerola, & Krumhansl, 2001). Figure 7.1 illustrates how a given set of events and accents might support duple or triple meters by virtue of their frequency distribution at metrically weak or strong locations over time.

Infants use frequency of occurrence to infer the meter in simple rhythmic patterns. In Hannon and Johnson (2005), 7-month-old infants were habituated to three unique rhythms containing events and accents that were more likely to occur every three units (i.e. "triple" meter) or every two and four units (i.e., "duple" meter) (see Figure 7.1). After habituation, they were presented with two novel rhythms that were otherwise matched but differed only in the extent to which the frequency distribution of events and accents supported the meter induced during habituation. Infants dishabituated to the stimulus with a novel meter, which demonstrates that they not only detected changes in the temporal statistics of the rhythms but that they categorized rhythms on the basis of the underlying meter. Interestingly, a third experiment suggested that infants could also learn to associate particular pitches with strong and weak metrical positions. Because tonally prominent pitches tend to occur at strong metrical positions in music (Järvinen & Toivianien, 2000; Meyer, 1973; Palmer & Pfordresher, 2003), this finding suggests that at least in principle infants' ability to infer meter could provide a foundation for learning about tonality through similar statistical learning processes.

Not only do infants infer meter from statistics in auditory input, but recent findings suggest they also integrate metrically relevant information across sensory modalities. When presented with an ambiguous rhythm in which events and accents support either triple or duple meter, 7-month-old infants use movement cues to infer the meter (Phillips-Silver & Trainor, 2005). In this set of experiments, infants were familiarized with an ambiguous rhythm while being bounced or while watching an experimenter bounce on every two or three beats. After familiarization, infants preferred listening to a version of the rhythm containing disambiguating cues that matched the meter to which they were bounced, but showed no preference when they had only watched someone bouncing. Thus, infants use information from their own movement patterns to structure their metrical interpretations. This result underscores the importance of movement for meter perception, and it converges with numerous adult studies documenting robust associations between movement and time perception using behavioral measures (Ivry & Hazeltine, 1995; Meegan, Aslin, & Jacobs, 2000; Phillips-Silver & Trainor, 2007; Todd, Cousins, & Lee, 2007; Trainor, 2007) and brain responses (Platel

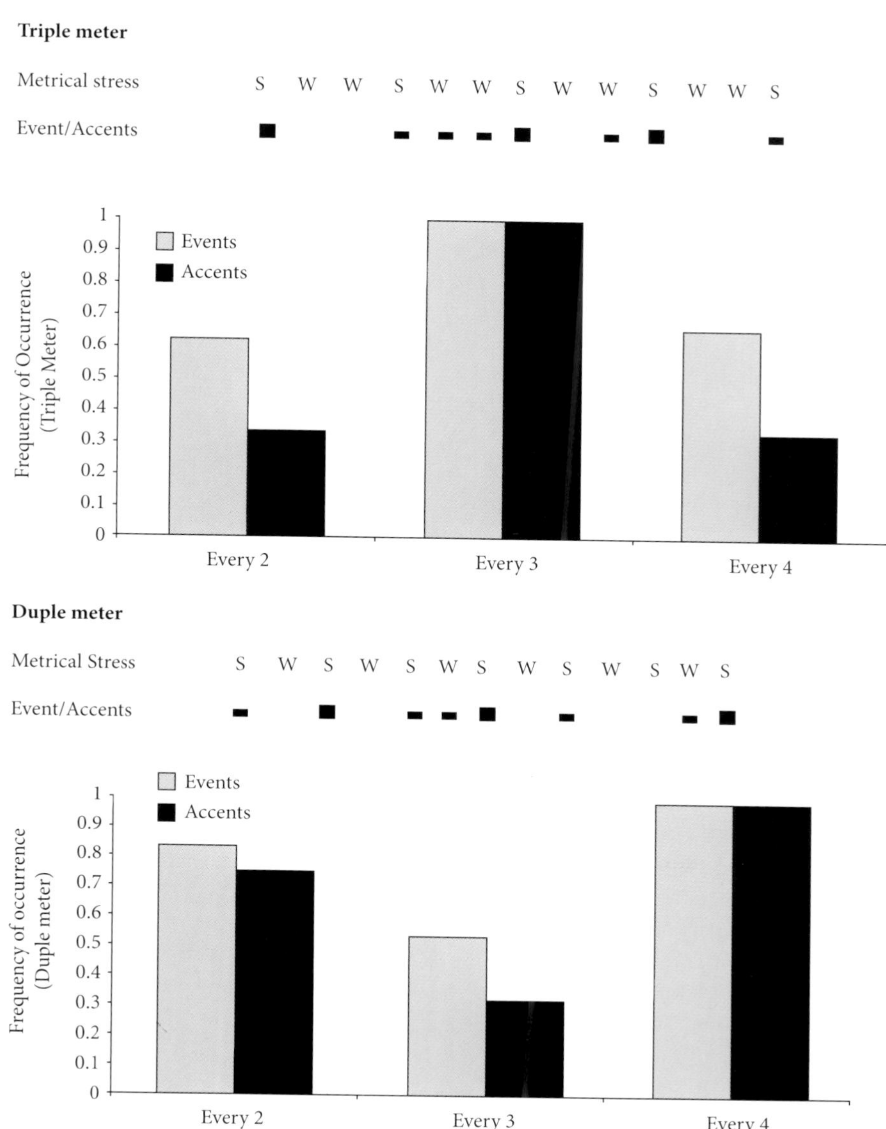

Figure 7.1 Patterns that support duple and triple meters. Both rhythmic patterns have potentially 13 temporal units during which events could occur, but the frequency distribution of event onsets (depicted by squares) and accents (depicted by larger squares) differs dramatically depending on whether the rhythm supports a triple meter (i.e., sww or strong weak weak) or a duple meter (i.e., swsw or strong weak strong weak). Specifically, events and accents occur most frequently every three units in the triple-meter rhythm but every two or four units in the duple-meter pattern. The bar graphs represent the average frequency of events and accents for duple- and triple-meter rhythms used in Hannon and Johnson (2005).

et al., 2007; Schubotz, Friederici, & Yves von Cramon, 2000).

Do infants ignore visual information related to meter? Although infants in Phillips-Silver and Trainor (2005) were not able to use visual information to infer meter in an ambiguous rhythm, infants may nevertheless perceive congruence of metrical information across auditory and visual modalities and use this information to further their music learning. In a recent experiment (Hannon, in preparation-a), 10-month-old infants were habituated to a movie of a woman dancing to a fast or a slow song. After habituation, infants saw two movies containing a novel segment of the same song they had already heard, but the visual stimulus (i.e. the dancing) that accompanied that segment differed for each movie. For the synchronous movie, the dancing matched the song and for the asynchronous movie the dancing matched a separate song with a contrasting tempo. Infants dishabituated only to the asynchronous video, presumably because they noticed that the dancing did not match the music. In a control condition, infants showed no preference after habituation to the same visual stimuli presented without sound, suggesting that discrimination in the experimental condition was based on true intersensory perception. Although previous studies have shown that infants perceive audiovisual synchrony when both auditory and visual stimuli contain discrete events, such as the sight and sound of a ball bouncing (Lewkowicz, 1996), the above task requires inference of metrical structure from rich and complex information in both modalities. Thus, infants may be sensitive to visual temporal information that is correlated with musical meter. Future studies will investigate the relative contributions of both vestibular/movement and visual cues in infants' music learning.

To summarize, the findings described above strongly support the claim that infants can infer temporal structure in music from the same basic statistics that are known to influence adults' perception of such structures. Moreover, they do this not only in the auditory modality, but also make use of multiple and redundant cues available through movement and vision.

Building musical knowledge through enculturation

Throughout first several months after birth, exposure to the statistics of the environment begins to alter infants' basic perceptual processes in a number of seemingly disparate domains. One well-documented example of this comes from speech perception, where infants develop language-specific biases during the second half of the first year after birth. At only a few months of age, infants discriminate speech sounds from virtually all spoken languages, even languages they have never heard (Eimas, 1974, 1975; Eimas, Siqueland, Jusczyk, & Vigorito, 1971; Trehub, 1976). These early abilities change dramatically by the end of the first year, when infants only discriminate speech sounds that demarcate meaning in their native language, presumably because of their exposure to linguistic input containing disproportionately frequent exemplars of native-language categories (Kuhl, Williams, Lacerda, Stevens, & Lindblom, 1992; Kuhl et al., 2006; Maye et al., 2002; Werker & Lalonde, 1988; Werker & Tees, 1984). Other recent findings suggest that a similar progression occurs for face identification, where accurate discrimination of individual monkey and human faces is robust early in infancy (i.e., before 6 months) but declines between 6 and 9 months, when infants continue to accurately discriminate only individuals of their own species (Pascalis, de Haan, & Nelson, 2002) or race (Kelly et al., 2007). Even intersensory perception may undergo comparable developmental changes, such as discriminating the visual head and lip movements of one's native language from those of a foreign language, an ability that declines between 4 and 8 months of age (Weikum et al., 2007).

The above examples demonstrate perceptual tuning for socially significant, frequently encountered stimuli in multiple domains. Given the prominence of music in early caregiving contexts (Trehub & Trainor, 1998), it is not surprising that enculturation to musical structures is also characterized by a similar developmental trajectory, where young infants discriminate musical structures that elude their parents but begin to exhibit culture-specific declines by the end of the first year.

Developmental Changes in Perception of Meter

It is widely assumed that when listeners infer the meter in music, they not only experience a primary pulse that is isochronous (i.e. composed of equal duration intervals), but they also perceive additional isochronous levels that are subdivisions or multiples of the primary pulse, all of which are integral to the metrical hierarchy (Lerdahl & Jackendoff, 1983; Palmer & Krumhansl, 1990). Figure 7.2 (top) illustrates a typical Western, isochronous metrical hierarchy, with three levels of isochronous structure giving rise to weak, strong, and stronger metrical positions. Because perception of meter is dependent on the regular occurrence of events at strong metrical positions, isochronous metrical hierarchies tend to constrain the pattern of interonset intervals in music by requiring primarily simple-integer duration ratios. For example, in order for the rhythm depicted in Figure 7.2 (top) to support an isochronous metrical hierarchy, its event onsets must occur primarily at strong metrical positions, which naturally leads to 1:1 and 2:1 duration ratios.

The challenge of inferring a primary pulse in music seems particularly daunting when one considers the fact that live music is rarely isochronous but instead tends to contain interonset intervals that vary continuously as a function of the performer's expressive intentions (Repp, 1992). For example, when a performer begins to slow down at the end of a phrase, the interonset intervals will become incrementally longer, but this does not necessarily lead the listener to reinterpret the meter. Rather, the listener ignores the subtle differences in interval size and consequent interval ratios, and categorizes intervals according to the metrical hierarchy that he or she has inferred (Desain & Honing, 2003).

Abundant evidence of metrical categorization can be found in studies of perception and

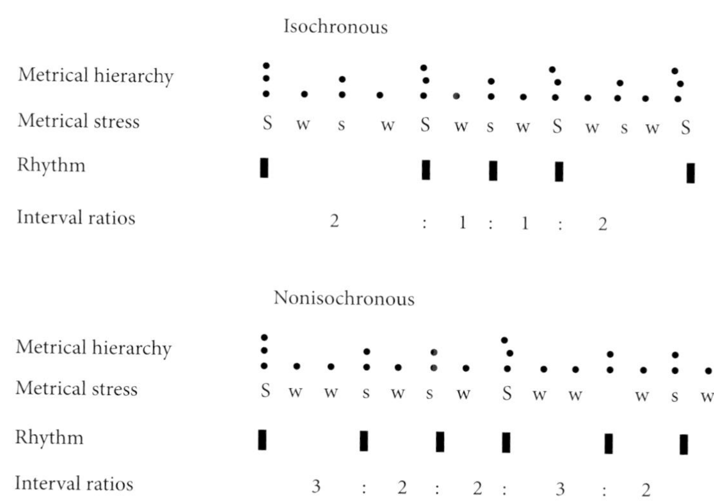

Figure 7.2 Metrical hierarchies for isochronous Western (top) and nonisochronous Balkan (bottom) meters. In an isochronous metrical hierarchy, typical of Western music, multiple levels of isochronous structure can be felt simultaneously, giving rise to simple duration ratios in the set of interonset intervals comprising the rhythm. In a nonisochronous metrical hierarchy, typical in Balkan music, multiple levels can also be felt but the intermediate level, which tends to be the primary pulse for dancing and movement, is made up of alternating long and short intervals having a 3:2 ratio. These ratios are also evident in the rhythm that supports that meter.

production of rhythms. In spontaneous rhythm production tasks, French adults tend to produce exclusively 1:1 and 2:1 ratios (Fraisse, 1978) even when asked to tap irregularly (Fraisse, 1982). When attempting to reproduce or synchronize with target rhythms containing complex interonset interval ratios, most adults ignore instructions and instead tend to produce 2:1 and 1:1 ratios (Cummins & Port, 1998; Essens, 1986; Essens & Povel, 1985; Povel, 1981; Repp, London, & Keller, 2005; Snyder, Hannon, Large, & Christiansen, 2006). Likewise, the brain activity that accompanies rhythmic reproduction tasks is qualitatively different for simple- versus complex-ratio sequences, with more automatic processing associated with simple ratios (Sakai et al., 1999). In perception tasks, listeners will label or transcribe (i.e. put into musical notation) a rhythm according to a simple-ratio category despite a continuous range of interval ratios in the physical stimulus (Clarke, 1987; Desain & Honing, 2003; Large, 2000). These findings probably reflect listeners' tendency to assume that rhythms fit into metrical hierarchies and thus assimilate complex-integer ratios toward simple-integer ratios that support familiar Western meters (the section "Constraints on Music Learning" will discuss additional explanations of simple-ratio biases).

If biases toward simple-integer ratios arise from a tendency to assimilate patterns to isochronous metrical hierarchies, then a listener's musical experience and knowledge would be expected to exert at least some influence on performance. In particular, listeners who are accustomed to nonisochronous meters should not have difficulty reproducing or identifying ratios other than 2:1 or 1:1 if such ratios exist in the music of their culture. Both isochronous *and* nonisochronous meters are very common in traditional music from throughout the world, such as Africa, the Middle East, Eastern Europe, and South Asia (Clayton, 2000; London, 1995, 2004). Figure 7.2 (bottom) provides an example of a typical Balkan rhythm and its metrical hierarchy. Note that in addition to having frequent 1:1 ratios, the rhythm also contains 3:2 ratios that are usually challenging for Western listeners to perceive and produce (Essens, 1986). This is reflected in the performance of North American adults ("Western Adults"), who notice superthreshold temporal disruptions of a folk tune only when that tune has an isochronous meter (with 2:1 ratios) but not when it has a nonisochronous meter (with 3:2 ratios, see Figure 7.3) (Hannon & Trehub, 2005a). By contrast, adults from Macedonia and Bulgaria ("Balkan Adults") perform equally well in both isochronous and nonisochronous conditions, presumably because both are equally familiar to these subjects.

Western adults may fail to detect disruptions to nonisochronous meters because their encoding of the original stimulus is compromised by a strong tendency to assimilate all patterns toward a familiar metrical template. The tendency to assimilate can thus be interpreted as evidence of acquired culture-specific knowledge of meter, which may begin to emerge as early as infancy. After familiarization with the same folk tunes described above, 6-month-old infants exhibit a novelty preference for disrupted versions, regardless of whether the familiarization stimulus was isochronous or nonisochronous (Figure 7.3) (Hannon & Trehub, 2005a). By 12 months, however, this pattern changes, and Western infants fail to discriminate rhythmic variations in the nonisochronous condition, even though they continue showing a novelty preference in the isochronous condition (Hannon & Trehub, 2005b). Thus, enculturation to musical rhythms, more specifically acquisition of culture-specific metrical categories, rapidly changes infants' behavior and closely parallels trends observed in other domains, where initial discrimination abilities are maintained for familiar structures but decline for unfamiliar structures by the end of one year.

The Role of Everyday Music Listening in Perceptual Reorganization

The observed developmental changes in Western infants' musical rhythm perception are presumably driven by exposure to Western music, where simple ratios are much more frequent than complex ratios. Thus, infants may build their culture-specific musical representations by simply listening to music, in the same way

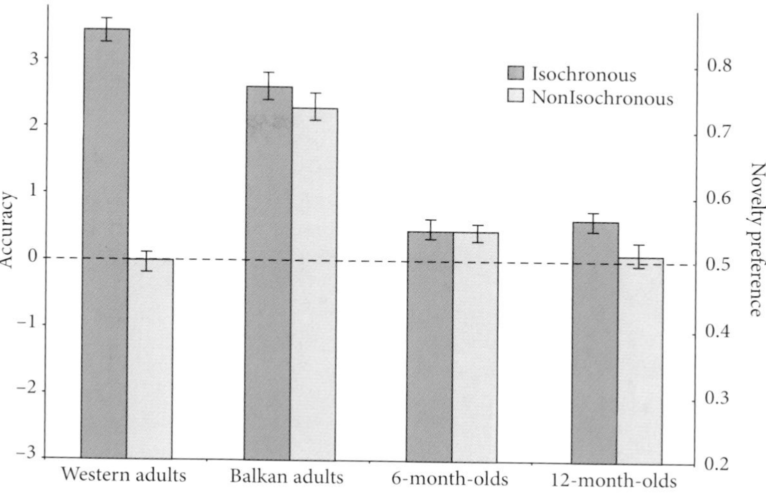

Figure 7.3 Perception of isochronous and nonisochronous meters by infants and adults. Adults' accuracy for the perceptual judgment task (i.e., tendency to state that a disrupted version of a folk tune is dissimilar relative to a standard) is on the left *y*-axis, while infants' novelty preference (amount of orienting to the disrupted variation divided by total looking time) is on the right *y*-axis. Dashed line indicates chance performance. Balkan adults and 6-month-old infants accurately differentiate rhythmic variations in isochronous and nonisochronous contexts, while Western adults and 12-month-olds only perform accurately in the isochronous metrical context. Data replotted from Hannon and Trehub (2005a, 2005b).

that listening to native language and watching familiar faces leads to declines in perception of unfamiliar speech and faces (Kelly et al., 2007; Pascalis, et al., 2002; Werker & Tees, 1984). Simple training paradigms have been used to demonstrate the effects of perceptual experience, by testing discrimination in older infants after exposure to unfamiliar structures. For example, after American 9-month-old infants are exposed to Mandarin Chinese through a series of interactions with native speakers over a 4- to 6-week period, they successfully discriminate Mandarin speech contrasts that their age-matched American counterparts do not (Kuhl, Tsao, & Liu, 2003). Similarly, when 9-month-old infants are sent home with picture books containing monkey faces, they subsequently discriminate individual monkey faces, unlike 9-month-olds without such exposure (Pascalis et al., 2005).

A brief period of at-home exposure to foreign music also reverses the decline in the performance of older infants in the nonisochronous condition (Hannon & Trehub, 2005b). In this study, parents of 12-month-old infants were sent CDs containing 10 minutes of Balkan folk dance music having nonisochronous meters, which they were asked to play for their infants twice per day for 2 weeks prior to coming into the laboratory. During testing, infants were then presented with the same stimuli as described above. Importantly, the specific recordings heard at home were completely different from the stimuli presented in the laboratory aside from sharing nonisochronous meters. Nevertheless, after exposure to the Balkan music, 12-month-old infants successfully discriminate nonisochronous rhythms on the basis of metrical disruptions. As can be seen from Figure 7.4, novelty preferences in the nonisochronous condition after exposure are indistinguishable from those obtained from Western 12-month-olds in the isochronous condition.

It is tempting to conclude from these results that by 12 months of age, infants have achieved adult-like knowledge of meter. However,

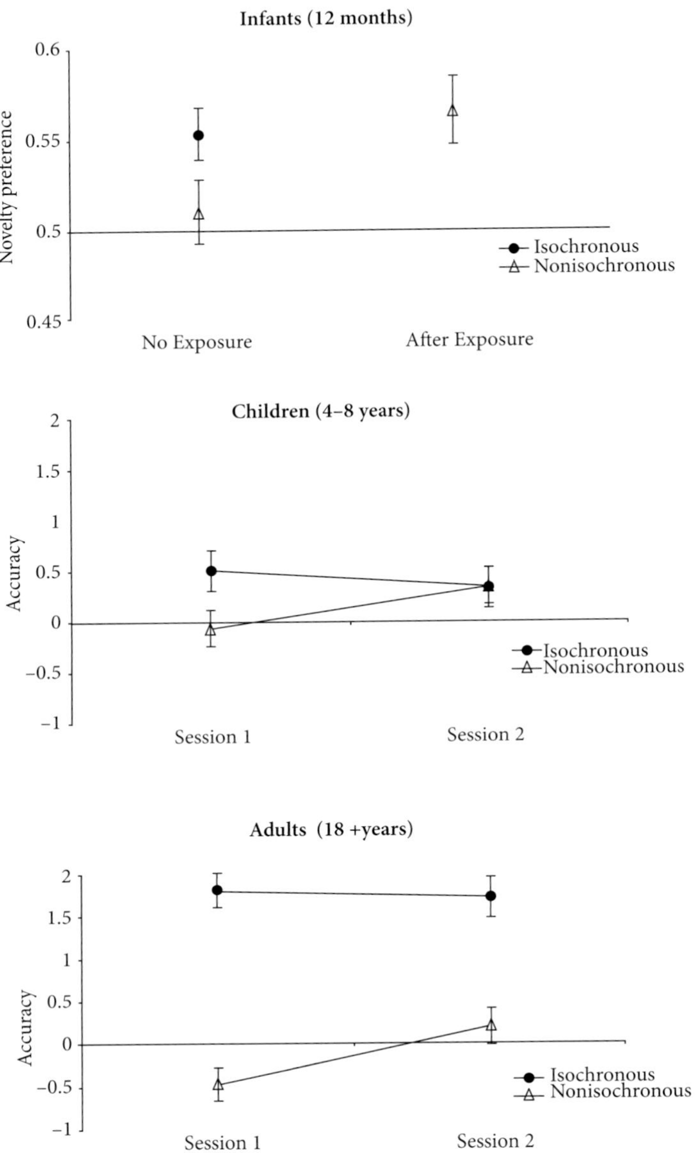

Figure 7.4 Effects of perceptual experience at different ages. For 12-month-old infants (top), at-home exposure to nonisochronous meters results in significant improvement in discrimination performance, where a novelty preference is only obtained in the non-isochronous condition after exposure. For children (middle), comparable results are obtained using a perceptual judgment paradigm. Preexposure performance reflects accurate performance in the isochronous condition but chance performance in the nonisochronous condition. After exposure, children's performance in the nonisochronous condition is above chance and indistinguishable from performance in the isochronous condition. By contrast, the performance of adults (bottom) in the nonisochronous condition does change after at-home exposure, but never reaches above-chance levels or levels of accuracy obtained in the isochronous condition. Infant and adult data are replotted from Hannon and Trehub (2005b). Child data are from Hannon and Soley (in preparation).

exposure to foreign music does not have the same effect on adults, who improve after the same amount of exposure but do not discriminate nonisochronous rhythms above chance levels off after 2 weeks of at-home exposure (Figure 7.4) (Hannon & Trehub, 2005b). It is not clear exactly why the effects of training differ across ages, but such disparities may indicate that infants' musical representations have greater flexibility and are more susceptible to being influenced by perceptual experience than are those of adults. In particular, it should be possible to document developmental changes not only in a listener's tendency to assimilate unfamiliar rhythms to culture-specific categories, but also in the extent to which those assimilative tendencies can be modified by passive exposure to unfamiliar music.

Recent research on this topic (Hannon & Soley, in preparation) suggests that adult-like representations of musical meter may not emerge until after age 8. North American children aged 4–8 undertook the same basic training regimen as described above for adults. Testing occurred at repeated sessions 2 weeks apart, using a game-like procedure adapted from the adult task in which they judged the similarity of two musical stimuli by adjusting the position of a game piece. During the 2-week training period, children listened at home to 10-min recordings of Balkan folk music twice every day. Figure 7.4 shows that data from children replicate the classic findings obtained with Western adults and 12-month-olds prior to exposure; 4- to 8-year-old children successfully distinguish rhythms in the isochronous condition but perform at chance levels in the nonisochronous condition. Importantly, performance in the isochronous and nonisochronous conditions differs significantly. After exposure, however, children perform at above-chance levels in both isochronous and nonisochronous conditions and their performance in the two conditions is indistinguishable. As can be seen in Figure 7.4, children's accuracy is lower than that of adults in all conditions, but it is nevertheless striking that passive exposure to foreign music gives rise to native-like levels of performance in children (and 12-month-olds) but not in adults. Despite the fact that Western adults do improve in the nonisochronous condition, a considerable gap remains between performance in isochronous versus nonisochronous contexts even after exposure. Thus, by investigating the extent to which a representation is susceptible to modification, we learn that culture-specific representations of musical rhythm and meter may continue to undergo developmental change throughout childhood.

Mechanisms of Perceptual Development and Reorganization

Across speech, face, and music perception, we see a strikingly similar developmental picture. What drives these developmental changes during infancy and why are similar patterns observed across such disparate domains? One proposal is that repeated exposure to particular sounds and sights leads neural circuits underlying perception to become increasingly committed to the statistics of the input (Kuhl, 2004). Thus, initial abilities to discriminate unfamiliar structures arise from immature, uncommitted circuitry, which is then "warped" by experience, whereby representations of more frequently encountered stimuli expand as prototypes. These modified representations in turn influence the extent to which future learning is possible because novel stimuli will tend to be assimilated toward the prototype if they share its properties.

This account is generally consistent with patterns of early brain development. Infancy is characterized by a proliferation of synapses followed by pruning, a process driven by Hebbian learning through which repeated use (i.e., exposure to particular types of faces) leads to a strengthening of neural circuits and disuse (i.e., lack of exposure to other-species or other-race faces) leads to deterioration (Huttenlocher & Dabholkar, 1997; Scott, Pascalis, & Nelson, 2007). It is also consistent with studies of second language learning, in which adult learners have greater difficulty perceiving and producing foreign speech contrasts than do younger learners, especially when the target contrasts interfere with the phonology of the subjects' native language (Flege, Yeni-Komshian, & Liu,

1999; Iverson et al., 2003; McCandliss, Fiez, Protopapas, Conway, & McClelland, 2002). Such a model might also describe the formation of culture-specific metrical categories, where frequent exposure to simple ratios and isochronous meters leads to the formation of metrical prototypes that subsequently influence how listeners interpret events and form expectations while listening to music.

Importantly, the observed declines in discrimination across modalities have not been interpreted as signifying a loss of ability. Rather, they are seen to reflect an enhancement of representations that code familiar structures and a rise in the ability to ignore irrelevant information. In the speech domain, recent evidence suggests that declines in discrimination of nonnative contrasts are accompanied by improvements in perception of native contrasts (Kuhl et al., 2005, 2006). Similarly, individual variability in discrimination of native and nonnative speech contrasts is correlated with language skills during childhood, such as language production, comprehension, and reading (Burnham, 2004; Kuhl et al., 2005; Tsao, Liu, & Kuhl, 2004). Thus, declines in discrimination of foreign meters are probably not due to a worsening of music perception, but rather the result of strengthened culture-specific music knowledge.

Moreover, despite showing poor discrimination of unfamiliar structures in behavioral tasks, paradigms using eye-tracking or event-related brain potentials reveal that adults and older infants do in fact, at a preattentive level, respond to subtle distinctions in foreign speech and in nonhuman faces (McMurray & Aslin, 2005; Rivera-Gaxiola, Csibra, Johnson, & Karmiloff-Smith, 2000; Rivera-Gaxiola, Silva-Pereyra, & Kuhl, 2005; Scott, Shannon, & Nelson, 2006). At some level, older infants, children, and adults must also remain sensitive to complex ratios and meters in music despite their poor performance in the behavioral task, otherwise it would not be possible for discrimination to improve as a result of exposure. Thus, developmental declines across all modalities may be less indicative of perceptual deterioration and more indicative of a reorganization in which the system automatically overcomes or suppresses perceptual distinctions that are not relevant to a particular individual's experience (Rivera-Gaxiola et al., 2000).

Consistent with this view is the notion that developmental changes across these multiple domains arise from domain-general aspects of cognitive development, such as the ability to inhibit irrelevant information. Indeed, when 8- to 10-month-old infants' nonnative consonant discrimination is compared with their performance in object search (A not B) and visual categorization tasks, developmental changes across tasks appear to occur in synchrony (Werker & Lalonde, 1995). In other words, infants who perform most accurately in a nonspeech task are also poorest at nonnative consonant discrimination. It is not currently known whether performance on nonmusical cognitive tasks would correlate with perception of unfamiliar musical structures.

Maturational changes in neural plasticity and cognitive control may account for the occurrence of similar patterns of perceptual development across music, speech, and face perception, and may explain why adults have greater difficulty learning unfamiliar, culture-specific structures than do infants. It is also worth considering, however, the ways in which perceptual experience itself could function to change the nature of the learner, independent of maturation. One possibility is that age-related changes in the ability to learn novel structures arise from the amount of interference between culturally unfamiliar and familiar structures (Flege et al., 1999). As representations of familiar structures become more elaborate and more entrenched, whether for own-species faces, native language speech contrasts, or familiar musical meters, the impact of unfamiliar structures on the existing representation will diminish because the unfamiliar structures will be perceptually assimilated or ignored. Studies of second language learning are largely consistent with this account (Iverson et al., 2003; McCandliss et al., 2002), but controlled studies are made difficult by the fact that age and acquisition of knowledge are typically confounded throughout development. Evidence from animal models suggests that after being deprived of patterned input to sensory cortex, cortical organization in deprived but older animals closely resembles that of younger animals (Chang & Merzenich, 2003). This strongly supports the notion that by preventing experience-related tuning from occurring, we can reverse or postpone expected developmental changes independent of age or maturation.

To summarize, multiple mechanisms may account for parallel developmental changes across the music, face, and language domains, ranging from brain maturation and pruning to cognitive control to experience-based interference. An important goal for future research will be to describe in more detail the developmental trajectory of culture-specific knowledge in multiple domains and to compare individual development across domains to understand why such change occurs. For example, if experience-based changes are solely responsible for developmental change, we should see little correlation across domains and individual differences that vary according to amount of exposure in a specific domain. If, however, more general maturational factors also play a role, we would expect to see more congruence across domains and relatively small individual differences as a function of specific experience. Music may provide a particularly unique opportunity to address these questions, because exposure to music even within a culture is subject to much greater individual variability (i.e., different listening practices across families and individuals) than exposure to other structures such as speech and faces.

Constraints on Music Learning

The above sections focus on the role of perceptual experience and learning mechanisms in acquiring music knowledge. It is also important, however, to understand the constraints that define the starting point for learning and limit what can be learned. Because newborns are faced with a virtual cacophony of structures across all sensory modalities, we might expect the learning process to be easily derailed as infants voraciously and indiscriminately absorb all information encountered. Yet infants somehow manage to focus on the statistics that lead to mastery of appropriate structures in appropriate domains. In this section, I will discuss possible constraints for learning musical rhythm and meter.

What are the starting points for music learning? It is sensible to assume that all learning will be constrained to some extent by intrinsic properties of the nervous system, such as the structure of sensory organs. The phenomenon of musical consonance and dissonance provides a classic example of this in the auditory domain. Simultaneous pitches that stand in simple integer ratios (such as 2:1, 3:2, and 4:3, corresponding to the octave, fifth, and fourth) are termed *consonant,* while pitches standing in more complex ratios (such as 11:12 or 45:32, corresponding to the minor second and the tritone) are termed *dissonant.* Throughout the world and over the course of history, consonant intervals tend to occur more frequently in music and give rise to positive affective responses, whereas the opposite is true of dissonant intervals (Cross, 2001; Dowling & Harwood, 1984; Kilmer, Crocker, & Brown, 1976; Koelsch, Fritz, Cramon, Müller, & Friederici, 2006). The distinction between consonance and dissonance likely originates in the structure of the ear—the frequencies of dissonant intervals tend to be too close to be resolved on the basilar membrane so their resulting vibration patterns give rise to beating and perception of roughness (Fishman et al., 2001; Tramo, Cariani, Koh, Makris, & Braida, 2003). It is presumably for this reason that human infants and even nonhuman animals are able to discriminate and categorize sounds on the basis of consonance and dissonance (Schellenberg & Trainor, 1996; Watanabe, Uozumi, & Tanaka, 2005).

Humans not only discriminate consonance and dissonance, but they find beating and roughness aversive, which is probably why robust listening preferences to consonant over dissonant intervals have been observed in very young infants, including hearing newborns of deaf mothers who may have reduced prenatal exposure to musical intervals (Masataka, 2006; Trainor & Heinmiller, 1998; Trainor, Tsang, & Cheung, 2002; Zentner & Kagan,

1996). Interestingly, encoding and memory for musical patterns can be compromised by dissonance. For example, adults and 6-month-old infants have greater difficulty detecting subtle frequency changes in patterns containing dissonant intervals than in patterns containing consonant intervals (Acker, Pastore, & Hall, 1995; Schellenberg & Trehub, 1994, 1996). The phenomenon of consonance and dissonance thus illustrates how peripheral properties (i.e., frequency resolution in the ear) can give rise to a cascade of effects shaping discrimination, esthetic preferences, and efficiency of encoding in infants and adults, which may ultimately determine which structures humans prefer in music throughout the world.

Do similar constraints affect temporal structures in music? Although the ear is not a likely candidate for constraining perception of rhythm and meter, domain-general mechanisms in the nervous system—such as those underlying prediction and movement—may give rise to intrinsic biases for temporal regularity. Unpredictable auditory sequences result in more anxiety-like behavior and sustained amygdala activity than do predictable sequences, suggesting that at some level, listeners find temporal irregularity aversive and may therefore seek out regularity (Herry et al., 2007). Adult listeners also have greater difficulty discriminating temporal intervals, patterns, or individual pitches when the preceding context is unpredictable than when it is predictable (Barnes & Jones, 2000; Drake & Botte, 1993; Jones, Johnston, & Puente, 2006; Jones, Moynihan, Mackenzie, & Puente, 2002). As reviewed above, the simplicity of serial interval ratios predicts how well adults can reproduce, identify, remember, and synchronize with rhythmic patterns (Collier & Wright, 1995; Desain & Honing, 2003; Essens, 1986; Essens & Povel, 1985; Hannon & Trehub, 2005a; Large, 2000; Povel, 1981; Repp et al., 2005; Snyder et al., 2006). Abundant evidence also suggests that production and perception of parallel ratios (i.e., the ratios between two simultaneous periodic patterns, such as polyrhythms) is affected by ratio simplicity (Deutsch, 1983; Klapp, 1981; Klapp et al., 1985; Peper, Beek, & van Wieringen, 1995; Treffner & Turvey, 1993).

Biological Basis for Biases toward Regularity?

Why are irregular rhythms so challenging for listeners? Most explanations rely on the assumption that internal timekeeping mechanisms, such as a grid, clock, or bank of oscillators, constrain rhythmic perception and behavior such that regular sequences are more efficiently processed than irregular sequences. Clock or grid models assume that the listener deduces a maximally efficient description of rhythmic patterns where individual events line up with the period of one or more internal clocks (Povel, 1984). Rhythms containing event onsets that do not consistently support a single clock (or when they simultaneously support many clocks) are not easily described, and thus force the listener to rely on explicit memory of each interval instead of iterated interval categories (Janata & Grafton, 2003; Povel, 1984; Semjen & Ivry, 2001).

Dynamical systems approaches describe rhythmic pattern coordination using the mathematics of nonlinear oscillators (Large, 2001; Treffner & Turvey, 1993). One model of musical meter proposes that temporal patterns are represented by a bank of internal oscillators that entrain to periodicities in the stimulus and compete for activation through inhibition (Large, 2001; Large & Jones, 1999). The intrinsic dynamics of oscillators give rise to greater stability for simple ratios and greater instability for complex ratios. Importantly, the behavioral output of coupled oscillators need not rely on complex or highly specialized neural substrates. The ratios that are most stable for human interlimb coordination (Peper et al., 1995) are also most stable for synchronous behavior in singing birds (Laje & Mindlin, 2003) and courting fireflies (Buck, 1988), suggesting that in principle, similar mechanisms could be responsible for movement coordination across species. Thus, basic human interlimb coordination, such as walking, running, and other forms of movement, may give rise to temporal processing mechanisms that bias listeners toward regularity (Summers, 2001).

By claiming that simple-integer temporal ratios are intrinsically easier for timekeeping mechanisms to represent, the above accounts are seemingly at odds with findings reviewed in the section "Building Musical Knowledge through Enculturation," which underscore the role of culture and experience by showing that one's prior exposure to nonisochronous musical structures dramatically shapes the extent to which irregularity disrupts performance (Hannon & Trehub, 2005a, 2005b). Learning and experience are also implicated by individual differences in production of complex-ratio sequences, because 3:2 ratios can pose great difficulty for most subjects (Povel, 1981) but pose minimal difficulty for subjects with extensive music training (Collier & Wright, 1995; although this was not found by Hannon & Trehub, 2005a or Repp et al., 2005). Training studies also show that practice can dramatically improve the production of complex-ratio polyrhythms (Krampe, Kliegl, Mayr, Engbert, & Vorbert, 2000; Zanone & Kelso, 1992). Any explanation of intrinsic biases toward regularity must therefore account for the effects of experience and learning.

The Importance of Temporal Regularity for Infants

To the extent that basic timing mechanisms of the nervous system are responsible for biases toward temporal regularity in adults, we should expect infants and adults to have equal difficulty processing irregular patterns. Instead, as described above, 6-month-olds outperform adults at discriminating patterns containing 3:2 ratios, suggesting that either (1) infants in these experiments are not processing rhythmic patterns in an entirely adult-like fashion but are using some alternative strategy such as remembering interval sequences or (2) infants and adults process patterns using the same mechanisms, which can accommodate slightly complex ratios such as 3:2 but not highly complex ratios—enculturation processes during infancy then suppress ratios not used in familiar musical styles. The mechanisms underlying infants' perception of rhythm and meter are not yet understood, but recent findings lend support to the latter hypothesis.

Like adults, young infants exhibit listening preferences for simple over complex rhythmic patterns (Nakata & Mitani, 2005; Soley & Hannon, submitted), and they appear to have difficulty in processing and remembering patterns having unconventional rhythmic structure (Trehub & Hannon, 2009). In this study, adults listened to a corpus of rhythmic arrangements of a 12-note pitch sequence and labeled each arrangement as either "good" or "bad." The arrangement most frequently labeled bad and the one labeled good were selected for use in a detection task, where adults and 6-month-old infants were trained to respond to subtle disruptions of either the good or bad arrangement (adults responded by raising a hand while infants made a head-turn). Although changes were successfully detected in all conditions, both infants and adults were significantly better at detecting a 260-ms rhythmic change to the good arrangement than to the bad arrangement, even though the serial position and size of the change was identical in both conditions. Thus, some aspect of rhythm in the sequence most preferred by adults may have afforded better perceptual processing regardless of experience and culture. The basis for this processing advantage is difficult to determine, however, because the good and bad arrangements were unique and thus differed from each other in multiple ways. One potential explanation is that the good rhythm implied a consistent underlying pulse whereas the bad rhythm implied multiple pulses at different points in the pattern. Without controlled manipulation of specific structures, however, it is impossible to know why the good arrangement gave rise to superior performance.

The above finding implies that infants' rhythm perception is not infinitely flexible, but might instead be constrained by at least some of the limitations that apply to adults. If infants and adults rely on the same basic temporal mechanisms, we should see even very young infants struggle with highly complex ratios that are relatively rare in music. If, however, infants use an alternative strategy to discriminate rhythmic patterns, such as memorizing a sequence of specific intervals, then the complexity of interval ratios should not matter as long as the serial structure of rhythms is simple.

Hannon (in preparation-b) recently addressed this question by examining how 4- to 6-month-old infants perceive rhythmic patterns having varying levels of ratio complexity. Three rhythmic variations of the same folk tune were created containing simple Western (2:1), complex Balkan (3:2) and highly complex "Alien" (7:4) ratios (see Figure 7.5). In all three conditions, the song cycled through a sequence of Long–Short–Short intervals with the duration of the long interval set at 756 ms; the only difference between conditions was the size of the short interval and the resulting ratio. After habituation to the standard version of one of the three variations, infants were alternately presented with the standard and a changed version containing a 200-ms increase in the duration of the long interval. Thus, across the three conditions, the absolute size of the target interval and the change were held constant. Infants showed a novelty preference for the disrupted stimulus in the simple and complex conditions, but showed no preference in the highly complex condition, suggesting that ratio complexity does influence how listeners perceive rhythms even prior to enculturation.

In summary, although young infants are culture-general music listeners, they are nevertheless influenced by the regularity of rhythmic patterns and the simplicity of temporal interval ratios, presumably because there is some continuity between infants and adults in the nature and limitations of basic temporal processing mechanisms. Although such mechanisms are not fully understood, they may derive from dynamic behaviors such as anticipatory attending and the coordination of various types of movement. Models of rhythmic timing suggest that perfectly isochronous meters are optimal, but they also suggest that there is a continuum of complexity with ratios such as 3:2 positioned at the simpler end. In this light, it is interesting to consider features of non-isochronous musical meters throughout the world, such as those common in India, the Balkans, and throughout Africa, which tend to be restricted, at least in practice, to alternating patterns of 2 and 3 (London, 2004; Powers & Widdess, 2001). By better understanding early temporal processing constraints, future research can develop more thorough and complete accounts of musical rhythm learning.

Culture-specific rhythmic structures in music and speech

Music and speech unquestionably depend on specialized perceptual processes that are often associated with distinct and separable brain areas (Binder et al., 2000; Narain et al., 2003; Peretz et al., 1994; Vouloumanos, Kiehl, Werker & Liddle, 2001), a fact that has contributed to

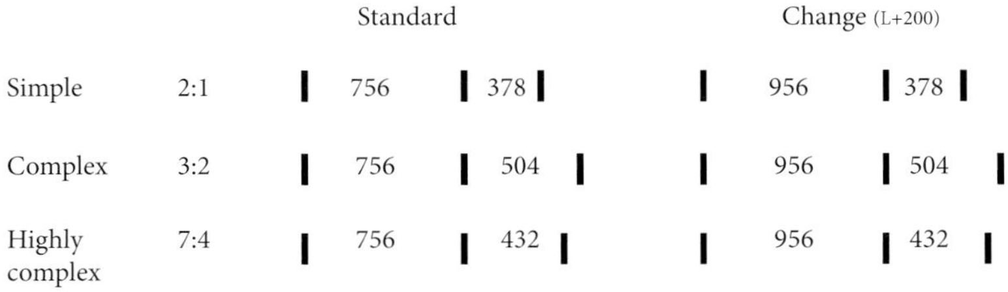

		Standard		Change (L+200)	
Simple	2:1	756	378	956	378
Complex	3:2	756	504	956	504
Highly complex	7:4	756	432	956	432

Figure 7.5 Simple, complex, and highly complex versions of a folk tune used in three conditions of a habituation experiment with young infants (Hannon, in preparation-b). The standard rhythm in the simple condition contained a repeating cycle of long and short intervals having a 2:1 ratio. The complex Balkan rhythm contained 3:2 ratios, whereas the highly complex rhythm contained a 7:4 ratio, which is relatively rare in music. In all three conditions, the standard and a changed version were presented after habituation. The change consisted of a 200-ms increase in the duration of the long interval. Note that the absolute size of the long interval was identical across conditions for the standard and change stimulus.

the widely held assumption that music and language abilities arise from modular, innate adaptations (Fodor, 1983; Liberman & Mattingly, 1985; Peretz & Coltheart, 2003; Peretz & Hyde, 2003). However, these assumptions have been challenged by evidence that individuals with music-specific deficits also exhibit impairments in speech perception (Patel, Foxton, & Griffiths, 2005) and that individuals with language-specific deficits also show impairment on music tasks (Alcock, Passingham, Watkins, & Vargha-Khadem, 2000). Studies using brain-imaging in normal adult listeners have provided additional evidence that purportedly language-specific brain regions, such as Broca's area, are also involved in music processing (Maess, Koelsch, Gunter, & Friederici, 2001). Thus, evidence of at least some shared processes for music and speech contradicts a strictly modular account.

Nevertheless, there are undoubtedly many speech- and music-specific structures in the adult brain, although the origins of such specialization are not clear. Some behavioral evidence suggests that speech-specific processes may be functional very early—for example, 2-month-old infants prefer speech to nonspeech stimuli, even when the acoustic structure of speech and nonspeech is very similar (Vouloumanos & Werker, 2004) and infants may employ a type of rule-learning that is optimally suited to language (Marcus, Fernandes, & Johnson, 2007, but see Saffran, Pollak, Seibel, & Shkolnik, 2007 for an example of rule-learning in vision). It is not clear, however, that fully lateralized, language- and music-specific structures exist in the brain of the newborn (Dehaene-Lambertz, 2000). In fact, recent studies suggest that language-specific brain areas do not emerge until late in infancy or after infancy (Imada et al., 2006; Minagawa-Kawai, Mori, Naoi, & Kojima, 2007). Thus, it is worth considering the possibility that domain-specificity develops—that infants might initially approach both speech and music with one set of basic auditory perceptual skills and learning mechanisms.

As representations of music become increasingly culture-specific, so too might representations of sound become increasingly domain-specific. Enculturation is defined here as the process through which culture-specific knowledge is built through everyday listening experiences, as infants and children attempt to actively predict and interpret patterns that unfold over time. Because speech and music are both complex and dynamic acoustic structures, young listeners likely build music- and language-specific representations in parallel. Thus, if the culture-specific structures of child-directed music and speech contain a high degree of overlap, this might have implications for early representations of music and speech.

Rhythm is not unique to music. Rhythmic structure is also fundamental for speech comprehension and in fact probably plays a vital role in infants' early responses to language. Within days of birth, newborn infants can discriminate native from foreign utterances of speech (Bahrick & Pickens 1988; Mehler et al., 1988; Moon, Cooper, & Fifer, 1993). The preference is maintained even when utterances are low-pass filtered, preserving only the rhythmic properties of speech and mimicking the quality of sound in utero (Abrams et al., 2000; Mehler et al., 1988).

Language-specific rhythmic structures probably form the basis for these early native-language preferences. The speech rhythm of a language has historically been defined by linguists as arising from the way languages divide time; *syllable-timed* languages such as French and Spanish use the syllable to mark equal time units whereas *stress-timed* languages such as English and Dutch use stressed syllables to mark equal units of time (Cutler, 1994; Jusczyk, 2002). These rhythm-based classifications also map onto newborn's discrimination of languages—newborns fail to discriminate languages from the same rhythmic class but easily discriminate languages from separate rhythmic classes (Nazzi, Bertoncini, & Mehler, 1998). Acoustic measures have been identified that can classify languages based on the amount of variability that characterizes adjacent vocalic and intervocalic intervals (Grabe & Low, 2002; Ramus, Nespor, & Mehler, 1999). One such measure, the normalized pairwise variability index (nPVI), has been successfully used to distinguish stress-timed languages such as English and German, which have higher vocalic interval variability, from syllable-timed languages such as French and Spanish, which have lower vocalic interval variability.

Recent evidence suggests that there may be a link between rhythmic structure in language and music. Inspired by musicologists' speculations that a culture's language influences its music, Patel and Daniele (2003) used nPVI to examine the variability of musical note durations in the themes of instrumental art music written by English- and French-speaking composers. They discovered that, like actual utterances of English and French speech, English musical themes contained higher durational contrast than did French themes. Subsequent studies have further verified a relationship between speech prosody and musical structures (Huron & Ollen, 2003; Patel, Iverson, & Rosenberg, 2006; Sadakata, Desain, Honing, Patel, & Iversen, 2004). Given that culture-specific differences in rhythmic structure appear to exist in both speech and music, a natural question to ask is whether such differences exist in musical input directed toward young listeners and if so whether the differences can be perceived.

To address the first question, 140 songs from French- and English-speaking cultures were selected from children's music anthologies and analyzed for their rhythmic properties (Hannon, in preparation-c). Consistent with prior findings, English-language songs contained higher nPVI values than did French-language songs (see Figure 7.6). Interestingly, the magnitude of the difference in children's music was somewhat larger than has been obtained in prior studies using instrumental (Huron & Ollen, 2003; Patel & Daniele, 2003) and popular music (Sadakata et al., 2004). This could arise if child-directed musical input exaggerates culture-specific rhythmic properties, but it could also result from the presence of words in all children's songs examined, which might have maximized the influence of the native language on musical rhythm over more

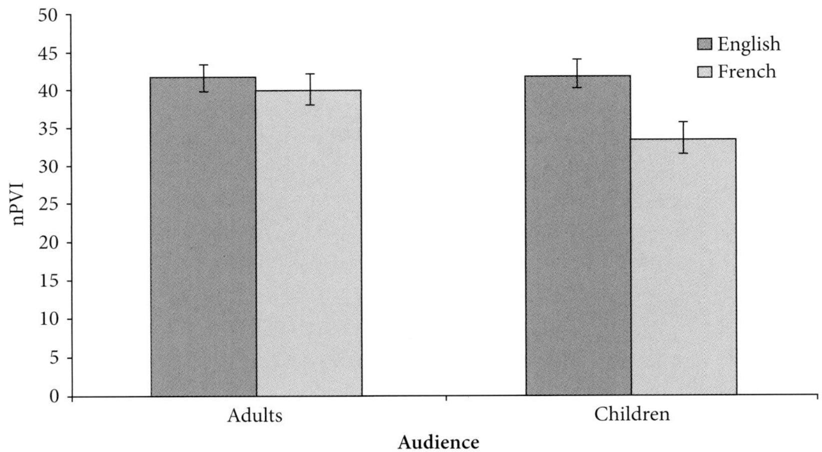

Figure 7.6 Analysis of rhythmic variability in French and English songs for children and adults (Hannon, in preparation-c). The normalized pairwise variability index (nPVI) for adjacent musical notes represents the *y*-axis, and the compilation from which songs were selected as children's or adult's (i.e., traditional folk songs with text) is on the *x*-axis. Dark bars represent English songs and light bars represent French songs. For songs taken from adult compilations, the nPVI for English was slightly higher ($M = 41.6$, $N = 70$) than for French ($M = 40.01$, $N = 70$). For songs taken from children's compilations, the nPVI for English was much higher ($M = 42.03$, $N = 70$) than for French ($M = 33.54$, $N = 70$). Error bars represent standard error.

instrumental samples. To test this possibility, a second set of 140 French and English songs with text were selected from traditional folk and popular music anthologies. This analysis revealed the same trend but much more modest differences (see Figure 7.6). Future research will further explore differences between child- and adult-directed songs, but these initial findings point toward the presence of culture-specific rhythm differences in music directed toward young listeners.

In order for such differences to affect infants' learning of music and speech, speech-based rhythmic structures must actually be meaningful to listeners in the context of music. Although it is clear that infants and adults can perceive and categorize utterances of spoken language on the basis of nPVI (Nazzi et al., 1998; Ramus et al., 1999), comparable structures in music may simply exist as a by-product of setting text to music and not necessarily be perceived by listeners. To address this question, adult listeners were required to categorize instrumental versions of French and English children's songs as belonging to one of two fictional languages (Hannon, in press). During the training phase, they received feedback following every trial, but during the test phase, they had to categorize an entirely novel set of French and English children's songs. Results showed that listeners were highly accurate (77% correct) in their categorization of novel songs after training. Moreover, performance was unchanged after pitch information was removed from the songs, suggesting that rhythm was the primary cue and not culture-specific pitch structure or familiarity. Thus, adult listeners were able to perceive and use language-based rhythmic differences to categorize novel songs, suggesting that in principle, infants may also be sensitive to these structures.

In summary, a burgeoning research area is beginning to explore similarities in music and language processing from a developmental perspective. By examining the nature of auditory input in the environment of the young listener, we may better understand developmental changes in culture-specific representations across music and speech domains.

SUMMARY

This chapter has outlined a research program that aims to understand how individuals build musical representations throughout development. Instead of framing the question of musical knowledge and behavior in terms of modular and unique capacities evolved through natural selection, this approach emphasizes the role of perceptual experience and statistical learning that is domain-general, operating in tandem with simple constraints that arise from properties of the sensory organs and the nervous system. Infants learn about music as they actively attempt to predict and interpret musical events that unfold over time, and these experiences in turn influence the nature of subsequent perception and learning. Investigations of musical knowledge acquisition therefore have the potential not only to shed light on the nature and origins of human musical behavior but also may inform our understanding of perceptual development across a number of domains.

REFERENCES

Abrams, R. M., Gerhardt, K. J., Huang, X., Peters, A. J. M., & Langford, R. G. (2000). Musical experiences of the unborn baby. *Journal of Sound and Vibration, 231*, 253–258.

Acker, B. E., Pastore, R. E., & Hall, M. D. (1995). Within-category discrimination of musical chords: Perceptual magnet or anchor? *Perception & Psychophysics, 57*, 863–874.

Alcock, K. J., Passingham, R. E., Watkins, K., & Vargha-Khadem, F. (2000). Pitch and timing abilities in inherited speech and language impairment. *Brain and Language, 75*, 34–46.

Avanzini, G., Lopez, L., Koelsch, S., & Majno, M. (Eds.). (2006). *The neurosciences and music II: From perception to performance.* New York: The New York Academy of Sciences.

Bahrick, L. E., & Pickens, J. N. (1988). Classification of bimodal English and Spanish passages by infants. *Infant Behavior and Development, 11*, 277–296.

Barnes, R., & Jones, M. R. (2000). Expectancy, attention, and time. *Cognitive Psychology, 41*, 254–311.

Bigand, E., & Poulin-Charronnat, B. (2006). Are we "experienced listeners"? A review of the musical capacities that do not depend on formal music training. *Cognition, 100,* 100–130.

Binder, J. R., Frost, J. A., Hammeke, T. A., Bellgowan, P. S. F., Springer, J. A., Kaufman, J. N., et al. (2000). Human temporal lobe activation by speech and nonspeech sounds. *Cerebral Cortex, 10,* 512–528.

Brown, S. (2003). Biomusicology, and three biological paradoxes about music. *Bulletin of Psychology and the Arts, 4,* 15–17.

Buck, J. (1988). Synchronous rhythmic flashing of fireflies. II. *The Quarterly Review of Biology, 63,* 265–289.

Burnham, D. (2004). Language specific speech perception and the onset of reading. *Reading and Writing, 16,* 573–609.

Chang, E., & Merzenich, M. (2003). Environmental noise retards auditory cortical development. *Science, 300*(5618), 498–502.

Christiansen, M. H., Allen, J., & Seidenberg, M. S. (1998). Learning to segment speech using multiple cues: A connectionist model. *Language and Cognitive Processes, 13,* 221–268.

Clarke, E. F. (1987). Levels of structure in the organization of musical time. *Contemporary Music Review, 2,* 211–239.

Clayton, M. (2000). *Time in Indian music.* New York: Oxford University Press.

Collier, G. L., & Wright, C. E. (1995). Temporal rescaling of simple and complex ratios in rhythmic tapping. *Journal of Experimental Psychology: Human Perception and Performance, 21,* 602–627.

Compston, A. (Ed.). (2006). Music and the brain [Special Issue]. *Brain, 129.*

Conway, C. M., & Christiansen, M. H. (2006). Statistical learning within and between modalities: Pitting abstract against stimulus specific representations. *Psychological Science, 17,* 905–912.

Creel, S. C., & Newport, E. L. (2002). Tonal profiles of artificial scales: Implications for music learning. In C. Stevens, D. Burnham, G. McPherson, E.Schubert, & J. Renwick (Eds.), *Proceedings of the 7th International Conference on Music Perception and Cognition*, Sydney. Adelaide: Causal Productions.

Cross, I. (2001). Music, cognition, culture and evolution. *Annals of the New York Academy of Sciences, 930,* 28–42.

Cuddy, L. L., & Badertscher, B. (1987). Recovery of the tonal hierarchy: Some comparisons across age and levels of musical experience. *Perception & Psychophysics, 41,* 609–620.

Cummins, F., & Port, R. (1998). Rhythmic constraints on stress timing in English. *Journal of Phonetics, 26,* 145–171.

Cutler, A. (1994). Segmentation problems, rhythmic solutions. *Lingua, 92,* 81–104.

Dalla Bella, S., Giguere, J., & Peretz, I. (2007). Singing proficiency in the general population. *Journal of the Acoustical Society of America, 121,* 1182–1189.

Deutsch, D. (1983). The generation of two isochronous sequences in parallel. *Perception & Psychophysics, 34,* 331–337.

Dehaene-Lambertz, G. (2000). Cerebral specialization for speech and non-speech stimuli in infants. *Journal of Cognitive Neuroscience, 12,* 449–460.

Desain, P., & Honing, H. (2003). The formation of rhythmic categories and metric priming. *Perception, 32,* 341–365.

Dowling, W. J., & Harwood, D. L. (1986). *Music cognition.* Orlando, FL: Academic Press.

Drake, C. & Botte, M. (1993). Tempo sensitivity in auditory sequences: Evidence for the multiple look model. *Perception and Psychophysics, 54,* 277–286.

Drayna, D., Manichaikul, A., de Lange, M., Snieder, H., & Spector, T. (2001). Genetic correlates of musical pitch recognition in humans. *Science, 291,* 1969–1972.

Eimas, P. D. (1974). Auditory and linguistic processing of cues for place of articulation by infants. *Perception & Psychophysics, 16,* 513–521.

Eimas, P. D. (1975). Auditory and phonetic coding of the cues for speech: Discrimination of the [r-l] distinction by young infants. *Perception & Psychophysics, 18,* 341–347.

Eimas, P. D., Siqueland, E. R., Jusczyk, P. W., & Vigorito, J. (1971). Speech perception in infants. *Science, 171,* 303–306.

Essens, P. (1986). Hierarchical organization of temporal patterns. *Perception & Psychophysics, 40,* 69–73.

Essens, P., & Povel, D. (1985). Metrical and nonmetrical representations of temporal patterns. *Perception & Psychophysics, 37,* 1–7.

Fishman, Y. I., Volkov, I. O., Noh, M. D., Garell, P. C., Bakken, H., Arezzo, J. C., et al. (2001). Consonance and dissonance of musical chords: Nural correlates in auditory cortex of monkeys and humans. *The Journal of Neurophysiology, 86,* 2761–2788.

Flege, J. E., Yeni-Komshian, G. H., & Liu, S. (1999). Age constraints on second-language acquisition. *Journal of Memory and Language, 1,* 78–104.

Fodor, J. A. (1983). *The modularity of mind: An essay on faculty psychology.* Cambridge, MA: MIT Press.

Fraisse, P. (1978). Time and rhythm perception. In E. C. Carterette & M. P. Friedman (Eds.), *Handbook of perception* (Vol. 8, pp. 203–254). New York: Academic Press.

Fraisse, P. (1982). Rhythm and tempo. In D. Deutsch (Ed), *The psychology of music* (pp. 149–180). New York: Academic Press.

Grabe, E., & Low, E. L. (2002). Durational variability in speech and the rhythm class hypothesis. In C. Gussenhoven & N. Warner (Eds.), *Laboratory phonology* (pp. 515–546). Berlin: Mouton de Gruyter.

Grewe, O., Kopiez, R., & Altenmüller, E. (2005). How does music arouse "chills"? Investigating strong emotions, combining psychological, physiological, and psychoacoustic methods. *Annals of the New York Academy of Sciences, 1060,* 446–449.

Hannon, E. E. *Infants know bad dancing when they see it: Audiovisual synchrony perception of dancing to music in 10-month-old infants.* Manuscript in preparation-a.

Hannon, E. E. *Infants' perception of musical rhythm is culture-general but constrained by ratio simplicity.* Manuscript in preparation-b.

Hannon, E. E. *Speech rhythms are exaggerated in children's music.* Manuscript in preparation-c.

Hannon, E. E., & Soley, G. *Children learn to perceive foreign musical structures after passive listening experience.* Manuscript in preparation.

Hannon, E. E. (in press). Perceiving speech rhythm in music: Listeners categorize instrumental songs according to language of origin. *Cognition.*

Hannon, E. E., & Johnson, S. P. (2005). Infants use meter to categorize rhythms and melodies: Implications for musical structure learning. *Cognitive Psychology, 50,* 354–377.

Hannon, E. E., Snyder, J. S., Eerola, T., & Krumhansl, C. L. (2004). The role of melodic and temporal cues in perceiving musical meter. *Journal of Experimental Psychology: Human Perception and Performance, 30,* 956–974.

Hannon, E. E., & Trainor, L. J. (2007). Music acquisition: Effects of enculturation and formal training on development. *Trends in Cognitive Sciences, 11,* 466–472.

Hannon, E. E., & Trehub, S. E. (2005a). Metrical categories in infancy and adulthood. *Psychological Science, 16,* 48–55.

Hannon, E. E., & Trehub, S. E. (2005b). Tuning in to rhythms: Infants learn more readily than adults. *Proceedings of the National Academy of Sciences (USA), 102,* 12639–12643.

Hauser, M. D., & McDermott, J. (2003). The evolution of the music faculty: A comparative perspective. *Nature Neuroscience, 6,* 663–668.

Herry, C., Bach, D. R., Esposito, F., Di Salle, F., Perrig, W. J., Scheffler, K., et al. (2007). Processing of temporal unpredictability in human and animal amygdala. *The Journal of Neuroscience, 27,* 5958–5966.

Huron, D. (2003). Is music an evolutionary adaptation?. In I. Peretz & R. J. Zatorre (Eds.), *The cognitive neuroscience of music* (pp. 57–75). New York: Oxford University Press.

Huron, D., & Ollen, J. (2003). Agogic contrasts in French and English themes: Further support for Patel and Daniele (2003). *Music Perception, 21,* 267–271.

Huron, D., & Royal, M. (1996). What is melodic accent? Converging evidence from musical practice. *Music Perception, 13,* 489–516.

Huttenlocher, P. R., & Dabholkar, A. S. (1997). Regional differences in synaptogenesis in human cerebral cortex. *Journal of Comparative Neurology, 387,* 167–178.

Hyde, K. & Peretz, I. (2004). Brains that are out of tune but in time. *Psychological Science, 15,* 356–360.

Imada, T., Zhang, Y., Cheour, M., Taulu, S., Ahonen, A., & Kuhl, P. K. (2006). Infant speech perception activates Broca's area: A developmental magnetoencephalography study. *Neuroreport, 17,* 957–962.

Iverson, P., Kuhl, P. K., Akahane-Yamada, R., Diesch, E., Tohkura, Y., Kettermann, A., et al. (2003). A perceptual interference account of acquisition difficulties for non-native phonemes. *Cognition, 87,* B47–B57.

Ivry, R. B., & Hazeltine, R. E., (1995). Perception and production of temporal intervals across a range of durations: Evidence for a common timing mechanism. *Journal of Experimental Psychology: Human Perception and Performance, 21,* 3–18.

Janata, P., Birk, J. L., Van Horn, J. D., Leman, M., Tillman, B., & Bharucha, J. J. (2002). The cortical topography of tonal structures underlying western music. *Science, 298,* 2167–2170.

Janata, P., & Grafton, S. T. (2003). Swinging in the brain: Shared neural substrates for behaviors related to sequencing and music. *Nature Neuroscience, 6*, 682–687.

Järvinen, T., & Toivianien, P. (2000). The effect of metre on the use of tones in jazz improvisation. *Musicae Scientiae, 4*, 55–74.

Jones, M. R., Johnston, H. J., & Puente, J. (2006). Effects of auditory pattern structure on anticipatory and reactive attending. *Cognitive Psychology, 53*, 59–96.

Jones, M. R., Moynihan, H., Mackenzie, N., & Puente, J. (2002). Temporal aspects of stimulus-driven attending in dynamic arrays. *Psychological Science, 13*, 313–319.

Juslin, P. N., & Laukka, P. (2003). Communication of emotions in vocal expression and music performance: Different channels, same code? *Psychological Bulletin, 129*, 770–814.

Jusczyk, P. W. (2002). How infants adapt speech-processing capacities to native-language structure. *Current Directions in Psychological Science, 11*, 15–18.

Karmiloff-Smith, A. (1992). *Beyond modularity: A developmental perspective on cognitive science.* Cambridge, MA: MIT Press.

Kelly, D. J., Quinn, P. C., Slater, A. M., Lee, K., Ge, L., & Pascalis, O. (2007). The other-race effect develops during infancy: Evidence of perceptual narrowing. *Psychological Science, 18*, 1084–1089.

Kilmer, A. D., Crocker, R. L., & Brown, R. R. (1985). *Sounds from silence: Recent discoveries in ancient Near Eastern music.* Berkeley, CA: Bit Enki Publications.

Kirkham, N. Z., Slemmer, J. A., & Johnson, S. P. (2002). Visual statistical learning in infancy: Evidence for a domain general learning mechanism. *Cognition, 83*, B35–B42.

Koelsch, S., Fritz, T., Cramon, Y., Müller, K., & Friederici, A. D. (2006). Investigating emotion with music: An fMRI study. *Human Brain Mapping, 27*, 239–250.

Koelsch, S., Fritz, T., Schulze, K., Alsop, D., & Schlaug, G. (2005). Adults and children processing music: An fMRI study. *NeuroImage, 25*, 1068–1076.

Koelsch, S., & Siebel, W. A. (2005). Towards a neural basis of music perception. *Trends in Cognitive Sciences, 9*, 578–584.

Klapp, S. T. (1981). Temporal compatibility in dual motor tasks II: Simultaneous articulation and hand movements. *Memory & Cognition, 9*, 398–401.

Klapp, S. T., Hill, M. D., Tyler, J. G., Martin, Z. E., Jagacinski, R. J., & Jones, M. R. (1985). On marching to two different drummers: Perceptual aspects of the difficulties. *Journal of Experimental Psychology: Human Perception and Performance, 11*, 814–827.

Krampe, R., Kliegl, R., Mayr, R., Engbert, R., & Vorbert, D. (2000). The fast and the slow of skilled bimanual rhythm production: Parallel vs. integrated timing. *Journal of Experimental Psychology: Human Perception and Performance, 26*, 206–233.

Kuhl, P. K. (2004). Early language acquisition: Cracking the speech code. *Nature Reviews Neuroscience, 5*, 831–843.

Kuhl, P. K., Conboy, B. T., Padden, D., Nelson, T., & Pruitt, J. (2005). Early speech perception and later language development: Implications for the "critical period." *Language Learning and Development, 3–4*, 237–264.

Kuhl, P. K., Stevens, E., Hayashi, A, Deguchi, T., Kiritani, S., & Iverson, P. (2006). Infants show a facilitation effect for native language phonetic perception between 6 and 12 months. *Developmental Science, 9*, F13–F21.

Kuhl, P. K., Tsao, F-M., & Liu, H-M. (2003). Foreign-language experience in infancy: Effects of short-term exposure and social interaction on phonetic learning. *Proceedings of the National Academy of Sciences (USA), 100*, 9096–9101.

Kuhl, P. K., Williams, K. A., Lacerda, F., Stevens, K. N., & Lindblom, B. (1992). Linguistic experience alters phonetic perception in infants by 6 months of age. *Science, 255*, 606–608.

Krumhansl, C. L. (2004). The cognition of tonality: As we know it today. *Journal of New Music Research, 33*, 253–268.

Krumhansl, C. L., & Keil, F. C. (1982). Acquisition of the hierarchy of tonal function in music. *Memory & Cognition, 10*, 243–251.

Laje, R., & Mindlin, G. B. (2003). Highly structure duets in the song of the South American Hornero. *Physical Review Letters, 91*, 1–4.

Large, E. W. (2000). Rhythm categorization in context. In C. Woods, G. B. Luck, R. Brochard, S. A. O'Neill, & J. A. Sloboda (Eds.), *Proceedings of the 6th International Conference on Music Perception and Cognition.* Keele, Staffordshire, UK: Department of Psychology.

Large, E. W. (2001). Periodicity, pattern formation, and metric structure. *Journal of New Music Research, 30*, 173–185.

Large, E. W., Fink, P., & Kelso, J. A. (2002). Tracking simple and complex sequences. *Psychological Research, 66*, 3–17.

Large, E. W., & Jones, M. R. (1999). The dynamics of attending: How we track time varying events. *Psychological Review, 106*, 119–159.

Lerdahl, F., & Jackendoff, R. (1983). *A generative theory of tonal music*. Cambridge, MA: MIT Press.

Lewkowicz, D. (1996). Perception of auditory-visual temporal synchrony in human infants. *Journal of Experimental Psychology: Human Perception and Performance, 22*, 1094–1106.

Liberman, A. M., & Mattingly, I. G. (1985). The motor theory of speech perception revised. *Cognition, 21*, 1–36.

London, J. (1995). Some examples of complex meters and their implications for models of metric perception. *Music Perception, 13*, 59–77.

London, J. (2004). *Hearing in time: Psychological aspects of musical meter*. New York: Oxford University Press.

Maess, B., Koelsch, S., Gunter, T. C., & Friederici, A. D. (2001). Musical syntax is processed in Broca's area: An MEG study. *Nature Neuroscience, 4*, 540–545.

Marcus, G. F., Fernandes, K. J., & Johnson, S. P. (2007). Infant rule learning facilitated by speech. *Psychological Science, 18*, 387–391.

Masataka, N. (2006). Preference for consonance over dissonance by hearing newborns of deaf parents and of hearing parents. *Developmental Science*, 9: 46–50.

Maye, J., Werker, J. F., & Gerken, L. (2002). Infant sensitivity to distributional information can affect phonetic discrimination. *Cognition, 82*, B101–B111.

McAuley, D., Jones, M. R., Holub, S., Johnstone, H. M., & Miller, N. S. (2006). The time of our lives: Life span development of timing and event tracking. *Journal of Experimental Psychology: General, 135*, 348–367.

McCandliss, B. D., Fiez, J. A., Protopapas, A., Conway, M., & McClelland, J. L. (2002). Success and failure in teaching the [r]-[l] contrast to Japanese adults: Tests of a Hebbian model of plasticity and stabilization in spoken language perception. *Cognitive, Affective, and Behavioral Neuroscience*, 2, 89–108.

McMullen, E., & Saffran, J. R. (2004). Music and language: A developmental comparison. *Music Perception, 21*, 1–23.

McMurray, B., & Aslin, R. D. (2005). Infants are sensitive to within-category variation in speech perception. *Cognition, 95*, B15–B26.

Mehler, J., Jusczyk, P. W., Lambertz, G., Halsted, N., Bertoncini, J., & Amiel-Tison, C. (1988). A precursor of language acquisition in young infants. *Cognition, 29*, 143–178.

Meegan, D. V., Aslin, R. N., & Jacobs, R. A. (2000). Motor timing learned without motor training. *Nature Neuroscience, 3*, 860–862.

Meyer, L. B. (1973). *Explaining music*. Chicago: University of Chicago Press.

Miller, G. F. (2000). Evolution of human music through sexual selection. In N. L. Wallin, B. Merker, & S. Brown (Eds.), *The origins of music* (pp. 329–360). Cambridge, MA: MIT Press.

Minagawa-Kawai, Y., Mori, K., Naoi, N., & Kojima, S. (2007). Neural attunement processes in infants during the acquisition of a language-specific phonemic contrast. *The Journal of Neuroscience, 10*, 315–321.

Moon, C., Cooper, R. P., & Fifer, W. P. (1993). Two-day-olds prefer their native language. *Infant Behavior and Development, 16*, 495–500.

Nakata, T. & Mitani, C. (2005). Influences of temporal fluctuation on infant attention. *Music Perception, 22*, 401–409.

Narain, C., Scott, S. K., Wise, R. J. S., Rosen, S., Leff, A., Iversen, S. D., et al. (2003). Defining a left-lateralized response specific to intelligible speech using fMRI. *Cerebral Cortex, 13*, 1362–1368.

Nazzi, T., Bertoncini, J., & Mehler, J. (1998). Language discrimination by newborns: Toward an understanding of the role of rhythm. *Journal of Experimental Psychology: Human Perception and Performance, 24*, 756–766.

Palmer, C., & Krumhansl, C. L. (1990). Mental representations for musical meter. *Journal of Experimental Psychology: Human Perception and Performance, 16*, 728–741.

Palmer, C., & Pfordresher, P. Q. (2003). Incremental planning in sequence production. *Psychological Review, 110*, 683–712.

Pascalis, O., de Haan, M., & Nelson, C. A. (2002). Is face-processing species-specific during the first year of life? *Science, 296*, 1321–1323.

Pascalis, O., Scott, L. S., Kelly, D. J., Shannon, R. W., Nicholson, E., Coleman, M., et al. (2005). Plasticity of face processing in infancy. *Proceedings of the National Academy of Sciences, USA, 102*, 5297–5300.

Patel, A. D., & Daniele, J. R. (2003). An empirical comparison of rhythm in language and music. *Cognition, 87,* B35–B45.

Patel, A. D., Foxton, J. M., & Griffiths, T. D. (2005). Musically tone-deaf individuals have difficulty discriminating intonation contours extracted from speech. *Brain and Cognition, 59,* 310–333.

Patel, A. D., Iversen, J. R., & Rosenberg, J. C. (2006). Comparing the rhythm and melody of speech and music: The case of British English and French. *Journal of the Acoustical Society of America, 119,* 3034–3047.

Phillips-Silver, J. & Trainor, L. J. (2005). Feeling the beat: Movement influences infant rhythm perception. *Science, 308,* 1430.

Phillips-Silver, J., & Trainor, L. J. (2007). Hearing what the body feels: Auditory encoding of rhythmic movement. *Cognition, 105,* 533–546.

Peper, C. E., Beek, P. J., van Wieringen, P. C. W. (1995). Multifrequency coordination in bimanual tapping: Asymmetrical coupling and signs of supercriticality. *Journal of Experimental Psychology: Human Perception and Performance, 21,* 1117–1138.

Peretz, I. (Ed.). (2006). The nature of music [Special Issue]. *Cognition, 100.*

Peretz, I., & Coltheart, M. (2003). Modularity of music processing. *Nature Neuroscience, 7,* 688–691.

Peretz, I., & Hyde, K. L. (2003). What is specific to music processing? Insights from congenital amusia. *Trends in Cognitive Sciences, 7,* 362–367.

Peretz, I., Kolinsky, R., Tramo, M., Labrecque, R., Hublet, C., Demeurisse, G. et al. (1994). Functional dissociations following bilateral lesions of auditory cortex. *Brain, 117,* 1283–1301.

Peretz, I., & Morais, J. (1989). Music and modularity. *Contemporary Music Review, 4,* 277–291.

Pinker, S. (1997). *How the mind works.* New York: Norton.

Pinker, S. (2002). *The blank slate: The modern denial of human nature.* New York: Penguin.

Platel, H., Price, C., Baron, J., Wise, R., Lambert, J., Frackowiak, R. S. J., et al. (1997). The structural components of music perception: A functional anatomical study. *Brain, 120,* 229–243.

Povel, D. (1981). Internal representation of simple temporal patterns. *Journal of Experimental Psychology: Human Perception and Performance, 7,* 3–18.

Povel, D. (1984). A theoretical framework for rhythm perception. *Psychological Research, 45,* 315–337.

Powers, H. S., & Widdess, R. (2001). Theory and practice of classical music: Rhythm and tala. In S. Sadie & J. Tyrrell, (Eds.), *The new Grove dictionary of music and musicians* (2nd ed., pp. 195–202). London: MacMillan.

Ramus, F., Nespor, M., & Mehler, J. (1999). Correlates of linguistic rhythm in the speech signal. *Cognition, 73,* 265–292.

Repp, B. H. (1992). Diversity and commonality in music performance: An analysis of timing microstructure in Schumann's "Träumerei". *Journal of the Acoustical Society of America, 92,* 2546–3568.

Repp, B. H., London, J., & Keller, P. E. (2005). Production and synchronization of uneven rhythms at fast tempi. *Music Perception, 23,* 61–78.

Rivera-Gaxiola, M., Csibra, G., Johnson, M. H., & Karmiloff-Smith, A. (2000). Electrophysiological correlates of cross-linguistic speech perception in native English speakers. *Behavioral and Brain Research, 111,* 11–23.

Rivera-Gaxiola, M., Silva-Pereyra, J., & Kuhl, P. K. (2005). Brain potentials to native and nonnative speech contrast in 7- and 11-month-old American infants. *Developmental Science, 8,* 162–172.

Sadakata, M., Desain, P., Honing, H., Patel, A. D., & Iversen, J. R. (2004). A cross-cultural study of the rhythm in English and Japanese popular music. *Proceedings of the International Symposium on Musical Acoustics (ISMA),* 41–44. Nara.

Saffran, J. R., Aslin, R. N., & Newport, E. L. (1996). Statistical learning by 8-month-old infants. *Science, 274,* 1926–1928.

Saffran, J. R., Johnson, E. K., Aslin, R. N., & Newport, E. L. (1999). Statistical learning of tone sequences by human infants and adults. *Cognition, 70,* 27–52.

Saffran, J. R., Pollak, S. D., Seibel, R. L., & Shkolnik, A. (2006). Dog is a dog is a dog: Infant rule learning is not specific to language. *Cognition, 105,* 669–680.

Sakai, K., Hikosaka, O., Miyauchi, S., Takino, R., Tamada, T., Iwata, N., et al. (1999). Neural representation of a rhythm depends on its interval ratio. *The Journal of Neuroscience, 15,* 10074–10081.

Schellenberg, E. G. (2005). Children's implicit knowledge of harmony in Western music. *Developmental Science, 8,* 551–566.

Schellenberg, E. G., & Trainor, L. J. (1996). Sensory consonance and the perceptual similarity of complex-tone harmonic intervals: Tests of adult and infant listeners. *Journal of the Acoustical Society of America, 100*, 3321–3328.

Schellenberg, E. G. & Trehub, S. E. (1994). Frequency ratios and the discrimination of pure tone sequences. *Perception & Psychophysics, 56*, 472–478.

Schellenberg, E. G., & Trehub, S. E. (1996). Natural musical intervals: Evidence from infant listeners. *Psychological Science, 7*, 272–277.

Schubotz, R. I., Friederici, A. D., & Yves von Cramon, D. (2000). Time perception and motor timing: A common cortical and subcortical basis revealed by fMRI. *NeuroImage, 11*, 1–12.

Scott, L. S., Pascalis, O., & Nelson, C. A. (2007). A domain-general theory of the development of perceptual discrimination. *Current Directions in Psychological Science, 16*, 197–201.

Scott, L. S., Shannon, R. W., & Nelson, C. A. (2006). Neural correlates of human and monkey face processing by 9-month-old infants. *Infancy, 10*, 171–186.

Semjen, A., & Ivry, R. B. (2001). The couled oscillator model of between-hand coordination in alternate-hand tapping: A reappraisal. *Journal of Experimental Psychology: Human Perception and Performance, 27*, 251–265.

Snyder, J. S., Hannon, E. E., Large, E. W., & Christiansen, M. H. (2006). Synchronization and continuation tapping to complex meters. *Music Perception, 24*, 135–146.

Snyder, J. S., & Krumhansl, C. L. (2001). Tapping to ragtime: Cues to pulse-finding. *Music Perception, 18*, 445–489.

Soley, G. & Hannon, E.E. Infants prefer music of their own culture: A cross-cultural comparison. Manuscript submitted for publication.

Spiro, J. (Ed.). (2003). Music and the brain [Special Issue]. *Nature Neuroscience, 6*.

Summers, J. (2001). Practice and training in bimanual coordination tasks: Strategies and constraints. *Brain and Cognition, 48*, 1–13.

Thiessen, E. D., & Saffran, J. R. (2007). Learning to learn: Infants' acquisition of stress-based strategies for word segmentation. *Language Learning and Development, 3*, 73–100.

Tillman, B. A., Bharucha, J. J., & Bigand, E. (2000). Implicit learning of tonality: A self-organized approach. *Psychological Review, 107*, 885–913.

Todd, N. P. M., Cousins, R., & Lee, C. S. (2007). The contribution of anthropometric factors to individual differences in the perception of rhythm. *Empirical Musicology Review, 2*, 1–13.

Trainor, L. J., & Heinmiller, B. M. (1998). The development of evaluative responses to music: Infants prefer to listen to consonance over dissonance. *Infant Behavior and Development*, 21, 77–88.

Trainor, L. J. & Trehub, S. E. (1992). A comparison of infants' and adults' sensitivity to Western musical structure. *Journal of Experimental Psychology: Human Perception and Performance, 18*, 394–402.

Trainor, L. J., Tsang, C. D., & Cheung, V. H. W. (2002). Preference for sensory consonance in 2- and 4-month-old infants. *Music Perception*, 20, 187–194.

Tramo, M. J., Cariani, P. A., Koh, C. K., Makris, N., & Braida, L. D. (2003). Neurobiology of harmony perception. In I. Peretz and Zatorre, R.J. (Eds.), *The cognitive neurosciences of music* (pp. 121–151). Oxford: Oxford University Press.

Treffner, P. J., & Turvey, M. T. (1993). Resonance constraints on rhythmic movement. *Journal of Experimental Psychology: Human Perception and Performance, 19*, 1221–1237.

Trehub, S. E. (1976). The discrimination of foreign speech contrasts by infants and adults. *Child Development, 47*, 466–472.

Trehub, S. E. (2003). The developmental origins of musicality. *Nature Neuroscience, 6*, 669–673.

Trehub, S. E., & Hannon, E. E. (2006). Infant music perception: Domain-general or domain-specific mechanisms? *Cognition, 100*, 73–99.

Trehub, S. E., & Hannon, E. E. (2009). Conventional rhythms enhance infants' and adults' perception of musical patterns. *Cortex, 45*, 110–118.

Trehub, S. E., & Trainor, L. J. (1998). Singing to infants: Lullabies and play songs. *Advances in Infancy Research, 12*, 43–77.

Tsao, F.-M., Liu, H.-M., & Kuhl, P. K. (2004). Speech perception in infancy predicts language development in the second year of life: A longitudinal study. *Child Development, 75*, 1067.

Vignolo, L. A. (2003). Music agnosia and auditory agnosia. *Annals of the New York Academy of Sciences, 999*, 50–57.

Vouloumanos, A., Kiehl, K. A., Werker, J. F., & Liddle, P. F. (2001). Detection of sounds in the auditory stream: Event-related fMRI evidence for differential activation to speech and nonspeech. *Journal of Cognitive Neuroscience, 13*, 994–1005.

Vouloumanos, A., & Werker, J. F. (2004). Tuned to the signal: The privileged status of speech for young infants. *Developmental Science, 7,* 270–276.

Wallin, N. L., Merker, B., & Brown, S. (2000). *The origins of music.* Cambridge, MA: MIT Press.

Watanabe, S., Uozumi, M., & Tanaka, N. (2005). Discrimination of consonance and dissonance in Java sparrows. *Behavioural Processes, 70,* 203–208.

Weikum, W. M., Vouloumanos, A., Navarra, J., Soto-Faraco, S., Sebastian-Galles, N., & Werker, J. F. (2007). Visual language discrimination in infancy. *Science, 316,* 1159.

Werker, J. F., & Lalonde, C. E. (1988). Cross-language speech perception: Initial capabilities and developmental change. *Developmental Psychology, 24,* 672–683.

Werker, J. F. & Lalonde, C. E. (1995). Cognitive influences on cross-language speech perception in infancy. *Infant Behavior and Development, 18,* 459–475.

Werker, J. F., & Tees, R. C. (1984). Cross-language speech perception: Evidence for perceptual reorganization during the first year of life. *Infant Behavior and Development, 7,* 49–63.

Zanone, P. G., & Kelso, J. A. S. (1992). Evolution of behavioral attractors with learning: Nonequilibrium phase transitions. *Journal of Experimental Psychology: Human Perception and Performance, 18,* 403–421.

Zatorre, R. J., & Peretz, I. (Eds.). (2003). *The neurosciences and music.* New York: The New York Academy of Sciences.

Zentner, M. R., & Kagan, J. (1996). Perception of music by infants. *Nature, 383,* 29.

PART III

Learning Mechanisms

CHAPTER 8
Integrating Top-down and Bottom-up Approaches to Children's Causal Inference

David M. Sobel

Several chapters in this volume are dedicated to describing how children learn conceptual structure from the data available to them (e.g., Kirkham, this volume; Rakison & Cicchino, this volume; Sloutsky, this volume). My plan for this chapter is to focus this discussion on a particular piece of conceptual knowledge: understanding the causal relations among events. Piaget, on whom the constructivist approach to cognitive development is based, recognized the importance of causality in children's cognitive development (Piaget, 1929, 1930). However, he failed to attribute significant causal reasoning abilities to young children, with preoperational children often receiving the label "precausal" based on their verbal explanations of behaviors in the world. The first goal of this chapter is to highlight young children's sophisticated causal reasoning abilities.

There are two approaches to causal learning that are critical to the present discussion in this volume. First, there is a long tradition of research in causal learning and inference that has focused on how causal knowledge is acquired from observing events—algorithms that construct a mental model of causal knowledge from patterns of correlational information. One might consider such a tradition more "bottom-up." But there is a second tradition of research in cognitive development—dating back to Piaget—describing how children using their prior knowledge or contextual information in the environment to learn new causal information. One might consider this tradition more "top-down." The second goal of this chapter is to consider how to integrate these two approaches for describing children's causal reasoning abilities.

In particular, following a set of proposals developed by Josh Tenenbaum and Tom Griffiths (Griffiths & Tenenbaum, 2005, 2007; Sobel, Tenenbaum, & Gopnik, 2004; Tenenbaum & Griffiths, 2001, 2003), I will suggest a description of children's causal inference. This approach offers a way of considering how causal principles are acquired from data to learn representations of causal structure. I will first present some background information, then some empirical work consistent with this description as well as what might be developing. Finally, I will consider some limitations of this mechanism, focusing on other information that might be available to the child to facilitate their causal inference and learning.

Causal learning from "bottom-up" mechanisms

There have been numerous accounts of causal learning in which a representation of causal structure is built from observing data in the environment. On these accounts, children use little prior knowledge to learn about causal relations. Often, they only have the ability to translate associations among events into a causal representation. The simplest such account is that children associate causes and effects in the same way that animals associate conditioned and unconditioned stimuli in classical conditioning (e.g., Mackintosh, 1975; Rescorla & Wagner, 1972).

But since associative models only output strength relations, they do not appear to make predictions about how learners use causal knowledge to generate interventions to elicit effects. It appears that even rats are capable of causal reasoning in a manner that reflects more than just an associative mechanism (Blaisdell, Sawa, Leising, & Waldmann, 2006). As a result, several independent research programs have suggested that to generalize an associative approach, causal learning occurs by transforming a measure of associative strength into a measure of causal strength. Measures of causal strength are then used to make inferences or generate interventions. Some of these models were based on the Rescorla-Wagner equation (see e.g., Cramer et al., 2002). Other accounts emerged as researchers discovered a set of learning paradigms that this model has trouble explaining (e.g., Krushke & Blair, 2000; Van Hamme & Wasserman, 1994; Wasserman & Berglan, 1998). One advantage of these accounts is that they allow a way to describe how a learner might generate interventions on the world—actions (usually intentional) that change the value of an event exogenously (without affecting other variables in the model directly). To use a traditional example, some associative mechanisms were designed to describe classical conditional paradigms, in which the learner passively observed the environment. These accounts of human learning also take operant paradigms into account, in which the learner also generates actions, which have varying degrees of efficacy, and must learn the strength of the existing causal relation (see e.g., Dickinson & Shanks, 1995, for a detailed discussion).

Still other endeavors have considered more complex relations among events beyond stimulus, response, and reinforcement (e.g., Allan, 1980; Cheng, 1997; Shanks, 1995). These models estimate the strength of a particular causal model using the probability that an effect occurs given a cause and some background information. The critical difference between these models and the ones mentioned above is that they estimate the strength of a fixed representation of causal structure, and do so accurately only given sufficiently large quantities of data (see Tenenbaum & Griffiths, 2001, for further discussion of this issue). Most of these models, however, are agnostic as to how that causal structure is fixed, with a potential exception being the Power PC model (Cheng, 1997; Novick & Cheng, 2004), which suggests ways of discerning cause from effect (see e.g., Cheng & Novick, 1990).

Causal structure learning

The models described above focus on deriving the strength of a set of known causal relations. Informally, here is the first way in which traditionally bottom-up accounts of causal learning can be integrated with prior knowledge: If the learner is determining the strength of a known cause and effect, then there must be some knowledge in addition to the data that identifies cause from effect. While there are several theories of causal inference that place such mechanistic information central to understanding causality (Ahn, Kalish, Medin, & Gelman, 1995; Shultz, 1982), such knowledge might also be entirely minimal, perhaps limited to only priority, contiguity, and contingency (e.g., Hume, 1978/1739; Michotte, 1962).

However, there are some contemporary accounts of causal learning that consider how causal structure is learned: How do children (and adults) recognize that an event is a cause or effect of another event (in addition to considering the strength of that causal relation)? Most of the psychological investigation on this approach has concentrated on adult causal learning (Griffiths & Tenenbaum, 2005; Lagnado & Sloman, 2004; Steyvers, Tenenbaum, Wagenmakers, & Blum, 2003; Tenenbaum & Griffiths, 2001; Waldmann & Hagmayer, 2005; see Lagnado, Waldmann, Hagmayer, & Sloman, 2007, for a review). There are also investigations that suggest that children construct an abstract representation of the causal structure among a set of variables (Gopnik, Sobel, Schulz, &

Glymour, 2001; Schulz & Gopnik, 2004; Sobel, Tenenbaum, & Gopnik, 2004; see Gopnik et al., 2004, for a review).

This description of causal learning and inference has been grounded in the literature on causal graphical models, which have been developed in computer science and statistics (Pearl, 2000; Spirtes, Glymour, & Scheines, 2001). Causal graphical models are representations of a joint probability distribution: the probability that each possible combination of events occurs. These representations embody conditional probability information among events. Events are represented as nodes, and causal relations are represented as edges between nodes.

Making inferences from this account relies on a set of assumptions. One assumption is that any vertex represents a causal relation between two nodes, specifically in the form of a mechanism that can be either observed or unobserved (following Pearl, 2000). As such, any graph is consistent with a set of probabilistic models that specify the nature of the relation among the variables. A unique causal structure is formed by defining the probability distribution for each variable conditioned on its parents (called *parameterizing* a graph). Parameterizing a graph can be thought of as assigning weights to each edge that represent the strength of the corresponding causal relations. A graph's parameterization can reflect the nature of the mechanism(s) by which causes produce effects.

Causal graphical models support reasoning about interventions—actions that change the value of variables in the graph (without directly influencing those other variables, see Pearl, 2000). Consider the simple graph $X \rightarrow Y$. In this graph, the probability that event Y takes a particular value given that event X takes a particular value is the same when you observe that X has that value as when you act to make X have that value. Such interventions are represented by Pearl (2000) and others as the $do(X)$ operator. Note that the opposite is not true in this graph: The probability that X has a particular value given that you observe Y has a particular value is not necessarily the same as the probability that X has that value given that you force Y to take on the same value. To use a classic philosophical example, if I make the rooster to crow at 2 am, I should not expect the sun to rise; the causal relation between sunrises and roosters crowing runs in the opposite direction (see Woodward, 2003, for further discussion). Children clearly learn causal structure from observing (and generating) these interventions (see e.g., Schulz, Gopnik & Glymour, 2007).

A second assumption that underlies causal graphical models is the faithfulness assumption. Faithfulness specifies that data are indicative of the causal structure in the world. Suppose that three events are related in the following manner: $X \rightarrow Y \leftarrow Z$ and that X has a generative relation with Y (i.e., the occurrence of X raises the probability that Y will occur) and that Z has a preventative relation with Y (i.e., the occurrence of Z lowers the probability that Y will occur). Faithfulness states that the causal relations among X, Y, and Z will never be such that X and Z exactly cancel each other's effects on Y, so that the three events appear independent. I do not know of a psychological investigation dedicated to faithfulness; however, most psychologists investigating children's causal learning assume this to be true.

A third assumption is the Markov assumption, which is a way of translating between causal relations and conditional probability information (Pearl, 2000). The Markov assumption states that the value of an event (i.e., a node in the graph) is independent of all other events except its children (i.e., its direct effects) conditional on its parents (i.e., its direct causes). For example, consider the causal model $A \rightarrow B \rightarrow C$. In this model, the values of events A and C are dependent. The Markov assumption states that these values become independent conditional on the value of event B. C has no children, and B is its only parent. If you want to predict the value of C and know the value of B, additional knowledge about the value of A does not help: the only influence that A has on C is through B.

In the next section, I will consider evidence that suggests children engage in causal reasoning in a manner consistent with the Markov assumption. Specifically, this evidence suggests that young children can recognize dependencies among events as well as when events are independent based on the presence of a third event. Such inference is tantamount to recognizing the difference between correlations due to causal relations and correlations due to spurious associations.

Learning causal structure using structure learning: Data from young children

In order to investigate whether children recognize the difference between dependence and conditional independence information, we need a method that presents a novel causal property to children wherein researchers can control the amount of prior knowledge they possess. Much of the research I will describe uses a blicket detector (shown in Figure 8.1), a machine that lights up and plays music (controlled by the experimenter) when certain objects are placed upon it. The blicket detector presents a novel, nonobvious causal property, which any object might possess.

Gopnik et al. (2001) trained 3- and 4-year-olds that objects that activated the detector were labeled, "blickets." Children quickly learned this relation. Then, children observed a set of trials in which objects either independently activated the machine, or did so only in the presence of another object. Specifically, on the one-cause trials, children were shown two objects. Children observed one object (A) activate the detector by itself. Then, they saw that the other object (B) did not activate the detector by itself. Finally, they saw objects A and B activate the detector twice together. Children were asked whether each object was a blicket. Three- and 4-year-olds labeled only object A as a blicket (although this was more likely for the older children), recognizing that object B only activated the detector in the presence of the object A.

Performance on these trials were compared with performance on two-cause trials, in which the same children were shown two objects that activated the detector individually with the same frequency as the objects in the one-cause trials. Specifically, children saw two new objects (C and D). Object C was placed on the machine three times and activated it all three times. Object D was placed on the machine three times, and activated two out of three times. Children categorized both objects as blickets. Both objects individually activated the detector; they just did so with different frequencies.

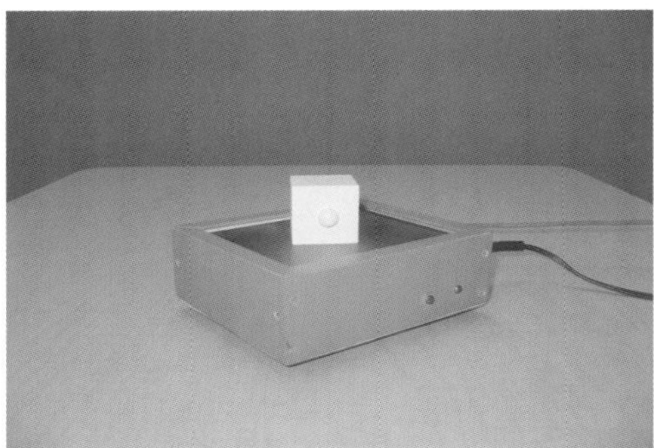

Figure 8.1 A blicket detector (specifically the detector used in Gopnik and Sobel, 2000, and elsewhere). In this case, an object is placed on the detector, and it is enabled, so that the object is activating the detector. This particular detector lights up red and plays *fur elise*.

These data suggest that children recognize the difference between two events that are dependent because of a causal relation and two events that are dependent because of the presence of a third (causal) event.[1] This procedure generalizes beyond reasoning about physical events: Schulz and Gopnik (2004) demonstrated that 3- and 4-year-olds make similar inferences across a variety of domains. Using some slight manipulations to the procedure, Gopnik et al. (2001) demonstrated that 30-month-olds also made these inferences.

The trouble with simply concluding that children reason according to the Markov assumption is that the data presented above are analogous to *blocking*, a phenomenon from the animal conditioning literature (Kamin, 1969). In a blocking

[1] This kind of inference has often been called "explaining away." It is consistent with the Markov assumption, but is a different inference from the example provided in the previous section (in which an individual reasons about a causal chain). There is evidence that under some conditions, children can learn causal chains from these patterns of data (Sobel & Sommerville, 2009), but most of the evidence suggesting children reason according to the Markov assumption asks them to make this "explaining away" inference.

procedure, a learner is shown an association between a conditioned and unconditioned stimulus (e.g., that a tone predicts the occurrence of food). This association is trained until asymptote, and then the learner is shown a novel stimulus, which presented in compound with the established conditioned stimulus will predict the same unconditioned stimulus (e.g., that the same tone paired with light will predict food). In most cases, learners do not learn that the second stimulus is predictive. Various models of associative reasoning (e.g., Rescorla & Wagner, 1972) were designed to explain this phenomenon. In the blicket detector paradigm described above, one might consider object A to be analogous to the first stimulus, object B the second stimulus, and the detector's activation the unconditioned stimulus. Children's performance, thus, is analogous to that of animal learners.

It is necessary to consider alternate procedures that models of associative reasoning have difficulty explaining. One such example involves considering how children reason retrospectively about ambiguous events (following Shanks, 1985, 1995). Sobel et al. (2004) introduced 3- and 4-year-olds to the blicket machine in the same manner as Gopnik et al. (2001), and then presented them with two types of trials. In their one-cause trials, children saw that two objects (A and B) activated the machine together, and then that object A did not activate the machine by itself. In their backwards blocking trials, children saw two new objects (C and D) activate the machine together, and then that one of those objects (C) did activate the machine by itself (note that this procedure is analogous to the reverse of Kamin's blocking procedure described above, hence its name). Children were asked whether each of these objects were blickets.

The blicket status of objects A and C are unambiguous given these data, but one's intuitions about objects B and D should differ. Object B should be a blicket in the one-cause trial; this is consistent with the Markov assumption: object A only activates the machine dependent on the presence of object B, so object B must be the causal factor. Object D's status is uncertain; the data (under a few assumptions, which I will make clear in subsequent sections) are equally consistent with it being a blicket and not being one. However, these intuitions differ from the associative relations that objects B and D have with the machine's activation. In both cases, children observe the object activate the machine in conjunction with another object. That other object (A or C) then activates or fails to activate the machine, but this piece of information should not change the associative relation between objects B and D and the machine's activation. If children were responding on the basis of these associative calculations, they should treat these objects the same. Three- and 4-year-olds responded in a manner consistent with the intuitions, not the associative relations: object B was almost always judged to be a blicket, while object D was judged to be so approximately 35% of the time. Preschoolers reasoned in a manner consistent with the Markov assumption, and less consistent with at least some models of causal reasoning based on calculations of associative strength (e.g., Rescorla & Wagner, 1972).

An Aside: Data from Infants

An open question raised by the previous section is whether younger children would reason in a similar manner. A variety of researchers have suggested that children's causal reasoning abilities develop during the preschool years (e.g., Bullock, Gelman, & Baillargeon, 1982; Das Gupta & Bryant, 1989; Goswami & Brown, 1990; Gottfried & Gelman, 2005). Further, children's ability to relate causal inferences to perceptions of time develops after the preschool years (e.g., McCormack & Hoerl, 2005).

But these findings are mostly concerned with how children understand causal mechanisms—how events are related to each other in a causal manner. In subsequent sections, I will outline a description of a domain-general causal learning mechanism, and then demonstrate how domain-specific knowledge influences children's use of this mechanism. But before we consider those ideas, the issue of whether younger children's causal reasoning is consistent with the Markov assumption is still open.

Sobel and Kirkham (2006) considered this question by investigating 19- and 24-month-olds' inferences using a similar procedure to the one-cause and backwards blocking trials described above. In their one-cause condition, they placed two objects (A and B) on the machine together, which activated, and then showed the children that object A failed to activate the machine by itself. The objects and detector were slid over to the child, who was asked to "make it go." In their backwards blocking condition, they placed three objects on the table (C, D, and E). Objects C and D made the machine go together, and then object C made the machine go by itself. Object C was removed, and the child was given objects D and E with the detector to "make it go." Twenty-four-month-olds used object B to activate the machine in the one-cause trial, more often than they used object D to do so in the backwards blocking trial. However, the younger children responded at chance levels, and did not discriminate between objects B and D.

A difficulty with asking children this young to make manual responses consistent with their causal knowledge (i.e., put objects on the detector to make it go), is that there are cases in which 18-month-olds fail to engage in simple imitative "means–ends" behaviors (e.g., Uzgiris & Hunt, 1975; see also Gopnik & Meltzoff, 1992). In the one-cause trial, children had to inhibit an event they observed activate the machine (placing both objects on it) in favor of a novel intervention (placing only object B on it). The demand characteristics of this experiment might have overwhelmed the toddlers, and prevented them from producing the appropriate responses.

There is reason to believe that 18-month-olds, and even younger infants, have the ability to detect conditional probabilities among events. Saffran, Aslin, and colleagues found that 8-month-old infants could parse a stream of auditory stimuli based solely on the transitional probabilities within and between syllables (i.e., the likelihood that one syllable would predict the next syllable; Aslin, Saffran, & Newport, 1998; Saffran, Aslin, & Newport, 1996). Infants' statistical learning abilities extend beyond learning word boundaries. Infants are capable of recognizing and discriminating between complex grammars relating words together (e.g., Gomez & Gerken, 1999). They also parse auditory streams based on statistical probabilities even when the stimuli are tones (Saffran, Johnson, Aslin, & Newport, 1999). This suggests that the ability to perceive statistical structure is perhaps not language-specific.

Further evidence for this position comes from work on infants' parsing of visuospatial sequences of events. Using a procedure analogous to Saffran et al. (1996), Kirkham, Slemmer, and Johnson (2002) demonstrated that infants as young as 2 months old register statistical relations among sequences of visual events (see Kirkham, this volume, for a detailed description of this literature). Similarly, Fiser and Aslin (2002) demonstrated that 9-month-olds can recognize conditional probability relations between the spatial positions of visual events. Both of these projects have their origins with work by Haith and colleagues (Haith, 1993; Wentworth, Haith, & Hood, 2002), who demonstrated that young infants (3–4-month-olds) learn simple, two-location spatial sequences of events. Haith and colleagues used a visual expectation paradigm, in which infants' eye gaze to a particular spatial location represented where the infants thought an event would appear.

Sobel and Kirkham (2006) modified this technique to investigate whether infants reasoned about sequences of events in a manner similar to preschoolers' causal inference. Eight-month-olds were shown a video screen similar to what is seen in Figure 8.2. Four frames were always

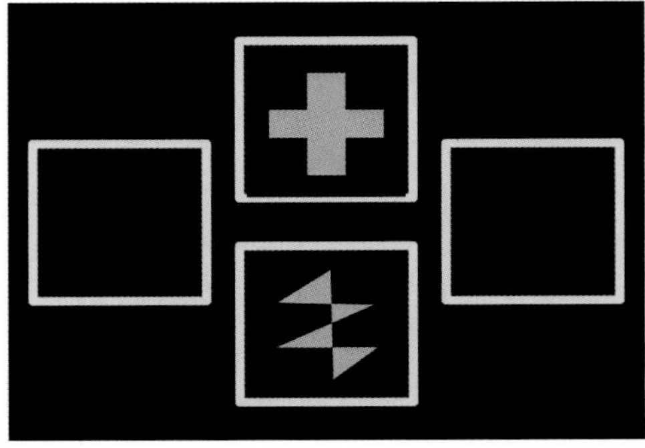

Figure 8.2 A screenshot shown to infants in Sobel and Kirkham (2006, 2007). In this shot, events A and B are presented together.

present on the screen. I will refer to the top center frame as A and the bottom center frame as B, the right frame as C and the left frame as D, but this was counterbalanced in the experiment. Infants observed sequences of events appear in their respective frames. During familiarization, infants saw a sequence of three types of events (the first event was randomly chosen from the three). One was that the A and B events could appear in their respective frames together. These were two grayscale events that silently rotated in space for 8 s. The AB compound predicted the occurrence of the C event (which occurred in the C frame) with 100% certainty. The C event was a more interesting color event, which moved around in the frame and was accompanied by a piece of cartoonish music. It also lasted for 8 s. The C event, however, did not predict any event. Half of the time it was followed by the AB compound (in which case, the subsequent event would again be C), and half of the time it was followed by the D event, which was the same color event occurring in the D frame for 8 s accompanied by the same music. The D event also did not predict anything. Half of the time it was followed by the AB compound, and half of the time it was followed by C.

Infants observed this sequence of events until they saw four occurrences of the AB→C pairing (usually 11 events total). Immediately after the last AB→C pairing, infants who had been assigned to the indirect screening-off condition observed only the A event appear on the screen by itself, followed by the D event. This sequence was shown twice. Infants in the backwards blocking condition observe only the A event followed by the C event (twice). Immediately after this, infants were shown the B event, and then the screen went blank. The music that had accompanied the C and D events began to play, and at this point infants' eye gaze was measured for 8 s.

One might think of this sequence of events in a manner similar to objects being placed on a blicket detector. Events A and B correspond to the two objects being placed on the detector, and events C and D correspond to the detector activating or not, respectively. In the indirect screening-off condition (analogous to the one-cause condition in the previous experiments described above), events A and B together predict C, and then A alone does not. Events A and C are dependent in the presence of B, but independent, conditioned on the absence of B; this makes B predictive of C. The expectation is that infants will look more to the C frame, expecting an event to appear there. In the backwards blocking condition, the associative relation between events B and C is the same as in the indirect screening-off condition, but since A and C are not independent, conditioned on the absence of B, B is not necessarily predictive of C. We would expect to find an interaction between the amount of time spent looking at each frame and the condition the infant was assigned to. This was exactly what was found (see Figure 8.3). Eight-month-olds spent more time looking

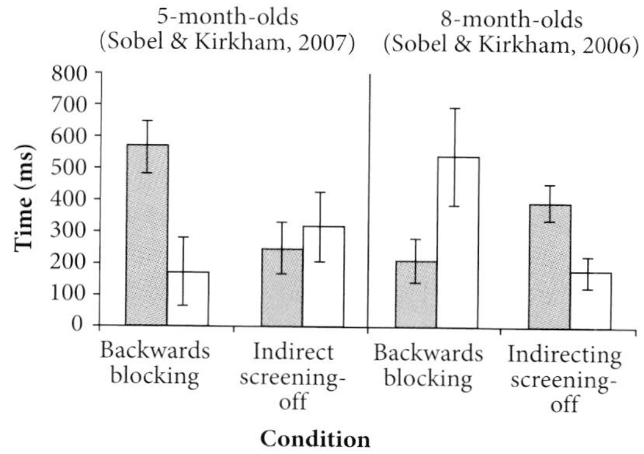

Figure 8.3 Amount of time spent looking to the C and D frames in the indirect screening-off and backwards blocking conditions by 8-month-olds (Sobel & Kirkham, 2006) and 5-month-olds (Sobel & Kirkham, 2007).

in the C frame in the indirect screening-off condition than the D frame, and more time looking in the D frame than the C frame in the backwards blocking condition. Moreover, they spent more time looking in the C frame in the indirect screening-off condition than backwards blocking condition.

These data suggest that infants' statistical learning abilities appear to be consistent with the Markov assumption. However, this inferential ability may not be available to younger infants. In a follow-up, Sobel and Kirkham (2007) found that 5-month-olds' pattern of looking time in response to the same procedure was quite different (see Figure 8.3). Five-month-olds looked longer at the C frame in the backwards blocking condition, and equally long at the two frames in the indirect screening-off condition, inconsistent with the Markov assumption. One interpretation of these data is that infants might be developing a mechanism for causal and statistical reasoning that moves from recognizing associations among events to one that incorporates the Markov assumption. However, the 5-month-olds' responses were inconsistent with an associative mechanism as well. An alternative interpretation is that when events A and B occur together, younger infants might simply treat them as the same event. If infants are treating event A alone, event B alone, and the AB compound as the same event, then their pattern of performance is consistent with both associative reasoning mechanisms and reasoning mechanisms consistent with the Markov assumption. More research is necessary to discriminate between these possibilities.

Second, the research on infancy presented so far has focused on infants' statistical reasoning, and not necessarily their understanding of cause and effect. These data do not demonstrate that 8-month-olds register that event B causes event C in the indirect screening-off condition. Rather, they suggest that infants' statistical reasoning is consistent with the Markov assumption, and may form the building block for a representation of causal knowledge. An open question is to consider how to convert this procedure to one in which infants' causal reasoning can be measured.

Natasha Kirkham and I have begun several investigations focused on this question. One involves infants watching videos of objects placed on a blicket detector, consistent with the data shown in the one-cause and backwards blocking conditions described above. Using a violation-of-expectation procedure, we should be able to discern infants' expectations about the causal efficacy of individual objects. Further, using the anticipatory eye-gaze paradigm, we are attempting to train children that looks to particular locations of a screen actually cause events to occur. Using eye gaze to allow infants to generate interventions might allow them to respond in a causal manner to sequences similar to the one used in our previous work. These investigations are currently underway.

Bayesian Inference as a Description of Causal Structure Learning

An objection that one might have to the lines of research described above is that the difference between responses in the indirect screening-off or one-cause condition and responses in the backwards blocking condition is problematic for certain models of associative reasoning (e.g., Rescorla & Wagner, 1972), but not others. Several contemporary accounts of associative reasoning were designed with the backwards blocking paradigm in mind (e.g., Kruschke & Blair, 2000; Van Hamme & Wasserman, 1994; Wasserman & Berglan, 1998). For instance, Wasserman and Berglan (1998) use a derivative of the Rescorla-Wagner equation, in which the strength of a relation changes positively when a potential cause and effect occur and negatively when the effect occurs without a potential cause. Similarly, models of causal reasoning that rely on the estimation of causal parameters based on the frequency with which events co-occur also explain the backwards blocking data (e.g., Cheng, 1997; Shanks, 1995). These models categorize events as causes or effects and then calculate the probability that an effect occurs given a cause and some background information. For example, Cheng's (1997) Power PC model makes a clear prediction about the causal efficacy of the objects in the one-cause conditions, but generates an undefined value in the backwards blocking case, which can be interpreted as consistent with the present findings.

Is there a method of distinguishing among all of these competing options as explanations of children's causal reasoning? One difficulty with considering the majority of these algorithms is that they rely on multiple pieces of data (i.e., large sample sizes) in order to make rational inferences. What we have observed in children's causal reasoning is that they appear capable of making such inferences based on small amounts of data. Following researchers in adult cognition and cognitive science (e.g., Griffiths & Tenenbaum, 2005; Steyvers et al., 2003; Tenenbaum & Griffiths, 2001, 2003), Sobel et al. (2004, see also Griffiths, Sobel, Tenenbaum, & Gopnik, submitted) proposed that children's causal learning and inference was better described by a model that relies on Bayesian inference.

On this view, causal reasoning can best be described by inference over a set of hypotheses (H). Hypotheses take the form of a causal graphical model with a particular parameterization. Each hypothesis ($h_1, h_2, \ldots h_n$) is assigned a prior probability, $p(h)$ before observing any data. These priors reflect the learner's causal knowledge about possible causal structures as well as any other information the learner gleams from the environment before observing the data. Given the data, d (values for the variables in the hypotheses), the learner computes the posterior probability that each hypothesis is the actual causal structure of the system, $p(h \mid d)$. This is done using Bayes' rule:

$$p(h|d) = \frac{p(d|h)p(h)}{\sum_{h' \in H} p(d|h')p(h')} \qquad (1)$$

The prior $p(h)$ is the probability that each hypothesis is the hypothesis that actually generated the data. The value $p(d \mid h)$ is the likelihood of the observed data being generated if that particular hypothesis was the actual causal structure in the world. For example, if A→B with a deterministic parameterization (i.e., A always causes B) is one of the hypotheses, and the data consists of trials of A occurring in the absence of B, then the $p(d|h) = 0$ for this particular hypothesis. This hypothesis requires B to occur whenever A occurs, and that is not the case.

To see this computational description in action, consider the backwards blocking sequences in which two objects activate the blicket detector together and then one of those two objects activates the detector by itself. There are four hypotheses potentially consistent with these data:

h_1: that neither object is a blicket
h_2: that only the first is a blicket
h_3: that only the second is a blicket
h_4: that both are blickets

The data are equally inconsistent with hypotheses h_1 and h_3 (i.e., $p(d \mid h) = 0$), since the first object has to be a blicket (it activates the machine by itself, but more on this in the subsequent sections). The data, however, are equally consistent with the other two hypotheses (h_2 and h_4), and as such the $p(d \mid h) = 1$ for both. But this description allows for another piece of information to influence causal inference, namely the prior probabilities, and these priors might affect children's inferences.

A rational way in which these priors might be assigned is through observing the base rate of objects with causal efficacy—the frequency of blickets in the world. If there are few blickets in the world, then the prior probability of hypothesis h_2 should be higher than that of h_4, since h_2 posits fewer blickets. Similarly, if blickets are relatively common, then the reverse should be true. Using this logic, Sobel et al. (2004) presented 3- and 4-year-olds with a version of the backwards blocking procedure in which they initially manipulated the base rate of blickets. Children were shown the blicket detector, and taught that blickets make the machine go. The experimenter then brought out a box of identical blocks. In one condition (the rare condition), 2 out of the first 12 blocks shown to the child activated the detector, and were categorized as blickets. In the other condition (the common condition), 10 out of the first 12 blocks activated the detector, and were blickets. Then the experimenter brought out two more blocks (A and B), and proceeded with the backwards blocking demonstration: these blocks together activated the detector, and then that object A activated the detector by itself.

The causal status of object A is unambiguous— it is a blicket—and all of the children categorized it as such. The causal status of object B is ambiguous given the data, but if children relied on the observed base rates, they should treat this object differently between the rare and common conditions. In the common condition, both 3- and 4-year-olds claimed that object B was a blicket, consistent with children recognizing prior probabilities when evaluating ambiguous data. In the rare condition, the 4-year-olds claimed that object B was not a blicket, again consistent with recognizing priors, but the 3-year-olds did not. They judged that the B object was a blicket regardless of the base rate of blickets in the environment.

There are two conclusions from these data. The first is that 4-year-olds' inferences were consistent with the Bayesian description in so far as they could recognize priors from the environment and use that information to make rational inferences about ambiguous data. The second is that there was a developmental difference between 3- and 4-year-olds' inferences. It is possible that a system for causal inference develops between these ages. However, there is another possibility, which involves considering what information is necessary for the child to possess in order to formulate a hypothesis space accurately.

Children's developing knowledge about blicket detectors

In the previous section, I asserted that there were four hypotheses consistent with the backwards blocking data. What knowledge was necessary to form this hypothesis space? Do children possess this knowledge?

Some spatiotemporal knowledge appears necessary. First, placing an object on the blicket detector activates it; the detector's activation should not cause the experimenter to place an object on it. Second, an object's location in space should be independent of another object's locations in space. Given research on infants' causal perception (e.g., Leslie & Keeble, 1987; Oakes & Cohen, 1990), and preschoolers' causal knowledge (e.g., Bullock et al., 1982; Sophian & Huber, 1984), it seems reasonable to assume that young children reason according to these two principles. Such knowledge limits the hypothesis space to the four models described above.

But children also need to understand that there is a particular parameterization between objects and the detector activating—what Tenenbaum and Griffiths (2003) and Sobel et al. (2004) called the *activation law*. Do children recognize that there is something about a blicket that makes the machine go? The activation law specifies that children recognize that there is some mechanism that relates blickets to the detector's activation in a deterministic (or near-deterministic) manner. This information allows the learner to recognize that the data in the backwards blocking procedure are ambiguous. Without this information (i.e., if children believed that blickets only sometimes made the machine go), the data are more consistent with object B having the capacity to activate the detector than not. To illustrate this, suppose that blickets only activated the detector 80% of the time. Even though object A clearly is a blicket (by virtue of activating the machine alone), it might have failed to be responsible for activating the machine when it was placed together with object B on the machine; there would be a nontrivial chance that the detector's activation was uniquely caused by object B having the efficacy to activate the machine.

While there is some good evidence that suggests 4-year-olds treat causal relations, including causal relations involving the blicket detector, as deterministic (Bullock et al., 1982; Schulz & Sommerville, 2006), it is not clear whether younger children do so as well. Further, even this work does not suggest that children recognize that deterministic data are related to particular causal mechanisms. As such, in a series of investigations, my colleagues and I considered how 3- and 4-year-olds reasoned about the relation between the causal properties of artifacts and nonobvious, internal properties. Our question was whether 3- and 4-year-olds recognized that insides of objects could act as mechanisms for those objects' causal properties, and whether children might understand such mechanisms differently across domains of knowledge.

In one set of experiments (Sobel, Yoachim, Gopnik, Meltzoff, & Blumenthal, 2007), we presented children with the blicket detector (although we simply labeled it as a machine, so that children were not influenced by object label information) and a set of objects such as those shown in Figure 8.4. Two objects were externally identical, and another was unique in appearance. All three objects had holes drilled into them, covered by dowels, which could reveal whether each contained an internal part. Four-year-olds were shown the insides of each toy: one of the identical objects and the unique object contained an internal part (a white map pin), while the third member of the set was empty inside. Children were then shown that the member of the pair with the internal part activated the detector, and they were asked to show the experimenter another object that would activate the machine. The majority of children chose the other object with the internal part (66% of the time), significantly more often than chance. Four-year-olds also claimed that objects that shared internal parts were more likely to share causal properties (i.e., activate the detector) than objects that shared external parts (e.g., had stickers on them).

This inference also worked in the other direction. In another experiment 3- and 4-year-olds were shown the same sets of objects and the blicket detector (again, without it being labeled as such), and were shown the causal efficacy of the three objects. One member of the pair and the unique object activated the detector, while the other member of the pair did not. The

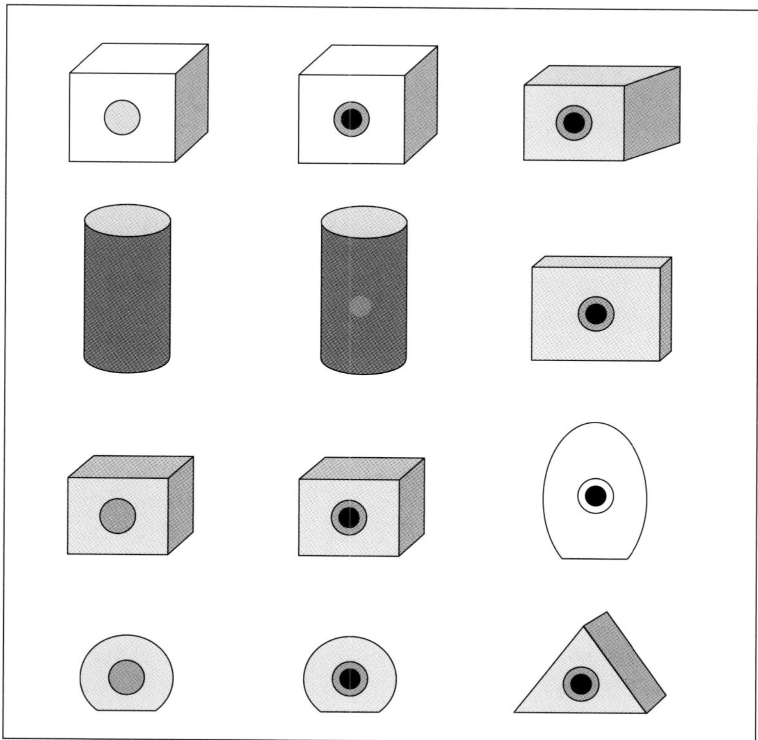

Figure 8.4 Stimulus set used to measure whether children appreciated the relation between objects causal properties and insides (Sobel et al., 2007).

member of the pair that activated the detector was opened to reveal that it contained an internal part, and children were asked which other object also contained such an inside. A striking developmental difference was found: 3-year-olds chose the other object that activated the detector 31% of the time, significantly lower than what would be expected by chance. Four-year-olds chose this object with significantly greater frequency (72%), and more often than chance responding. Importantly, Sobel et al. (2007) also ran a condition in which the association between the detector's activation and each object was held constant, but the object was not causally related to the machine. Each object was held over the detector, and the experimenter pressed a button on the detector for the objects that would have activated the machine. Here, both 3- and 4-year-olds made causal responses less than 30% of the time, significantly lower than what would be expected by chance.

What these data suggest is that 4-year-olds, but not 3-year-olds, recognize that there is a relation between an object's causal and internal properties. However, these data do not demonstrate that 4-year-olds understand an activation law—that there is something about the internal part that is responsible for activating the detector. Four-year-olds do integrate some amount of correlational information together when making inferences about causal mechanisms: they only respond on the basis of the machine's activation when the spatiotemporal connection between the object and machine warrants a causal relation. A stronger argument would be to demonstrate that 4-year-olds, but not younger children, interpret an object's internal parts as being necessary and sufficient for the detector's activation.

To test this, Emily Blumenthal and I introduced 3- and 4-year-olds to the blicket detector and provided children with (what we thought was) the strongest possible information about its efficacy. We told children that the machine was a "blicket machine" and "things with blickets inside made the machine go." We then showed children that a set of objects with internal parts (labeled blickets) all activated the machine, and that a set of objects without internal parts did not. We also showed children that the detector activated if at least one object with a blicket inside was on it. After receiving this training, children were shown two objects (A and B), which activated the machine together. The door on object A was opened to reveal it was empty. Children had no trouble inferring whether each object contained an internal part. The critical question was an intervention question—children were asked to make the machine go. The child has observed the experimenter generate an intervention that activates the machine—placing both objects on it. But this imitative response is not the most efficient way of activating the machine. If children recognize that the internal part is responsible for the object's causal property, then they should recognize there is no need to put object A on the detector, and when asked to generate an intervention that activates the machine, place only object B on the machine. This was the response generated by the majority of 4-year-olds, significantly more often than the younger children. The younger children were more likely to imitate, and place A and B on the machine together (Sobel & Blumenthal, in preparation).

These data suggest that 4-year-olds tie together the correlational information they observe between each object and the detector's activation, and mechanism information about what is necessary for each object to activate the detector: namely, a nonobvious property. Three-year-olds have a harder time integrating this information. This development might relate to children's developing use of a Bayesian mechanism of causal inference. Correlational information is reflected in how the data generate posterior probabilities of each hypothesis being correct. Mechanism information is reflected in how those hypotheses are formed: what causal structures come under consideration and how those causal structures are parameterized.

Specifically, what we would like to show is that children who recognize the activation law, by virtue of connecting objects' causal and internal parts together, are more likely to engage in inferences consistent with recognizing the prior probability information they observe. The 3-year-olds who failed to discriminate between the rare and common conditions in Sobel et al.'s (2004) procedure might have lacked the understanding that the way an object can produce its causal properties can be related to its insides. Lacking this knowledge might indicate that they lacked an activation law relating objects with the detector, which would make their failure to respond like the older children rational.

That's Mr. Blicket to you: Causal Mechanisms Across Domains

In order to test this hypothesis, we need to consider how we might facilitate 3-year-olds' understanding of an activation law. One possibility is to consider how children reason about such causal relations in another domain of knowledge; all of the experiments mentioned so far have been exclusive to the domain of blicket detectors and aspects of physical causality. Can similar manipulations be performed in another domain? There is some reason to suspect that some causal inference abilities, such as inferences consistent with the Markov assumption, appear to be domain-general (e.g., Schulz & Gopnik, 2004). However, these inferences involved general logical principles, not specific pieces of causal mechanism information.

Research in theory of mind tells us that young children understand a particular mental state—the results of an agent's desires—at very young ages. Eighteen-month-olds recognize that others can have desires different from their own (Repacholi & Gopnik, 1997). Two- and 3-year-olds have a good understanding of the outcomes of fulfilled and unfulfilled desires (Wellman & Woolley, 1990). Three-year-olds can also keep track of their own and other's desires over time and changes in the environment (e.g., Gopnik & Slaughter, 1991). Fawcett and Markson (2005) asked 2-year-olds to make inferences about their own preferences based on another's desires. They showed children that one person consistently played with toys that matched the child's preferences, and that another person consistently played with toys that did not match the child's preferences. They then presented two novel (equally preferential) toys, and each person played with one. When those two toys were given to the children, they preferred to play with the toy associated with the first person. This suggests that children infer a nonobvious property to the toy based on another's desires, since that property must be responsible for those desires (see also Perner, 1991; Yuill, 1984).

Sobel and Munro (2009) manipulated the blicket detector to attempt to introduce it to 3-year-olds as a psychological agent. They placed a set of cardboard eyes on the machine (shown in Figure 8.5) and introduced it to children as "Mr. Blicket." The experimenter conducted a dialogue with the machine, which activated spontaneously in response to questions and comments (this procedure was modeled after Johnson, Slaughter, and Carey (1998) and Johnson, Booth, and O'Hearn (2001), who used a similar procedure to study agent gaze-following in infants). The children were then told that they were going to play a game in which Mr. Blicket would tell them whether he liked an object. They then repeated the procedure used by Sobel et al. (2007) to study whether 3-year-olds linked the internal parts of objects with their causal property (in this case, whether Mr. Blicket liked the object). Three-year-olds did link the causal property with the object's insides in this condition, significantly more often than in another condition, in which the same procedure was performed with a machine that spontaneously activated during the warm-up of the procedure, with the same temporal contiguity as Mr. Blicket's activation (70% vs. 41% of the time).

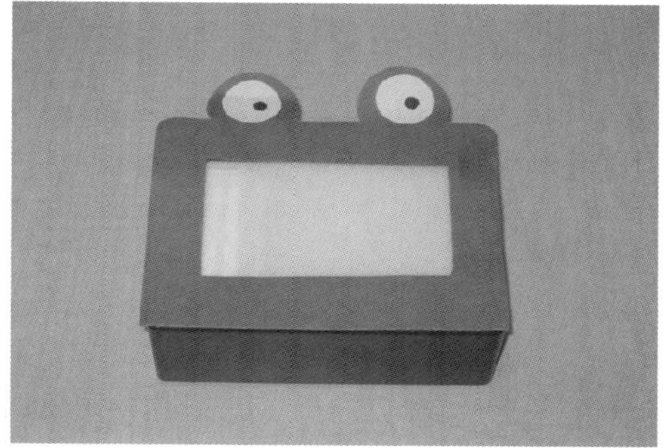

Figure 8.5 Mr. Blicket.

These data suggest that 3-year-olds might integrate the correlational data they observe about agent's desires toward objects with mechanism information—that there must be something about those particular objects responsible for Mr. Blicket's desires. If this is the case, then 3-year-olds might have an activation law about Mr. Blicket's desire, and reason more consistently with the Bayesian description than they do in the physical domain. To test this, we (Sobel & Munro, 2009) introduced 3-year-olds to Mr. Blicket in the same manner as described above, and then gave them the same rare or common training as in Sobel et al. (2004), followed by the same backwards blocking trial. Two new objects (A and B) were placed on Mr. Blicket together, and he activated. Then object A alone was placed on him with the same result. All children claimed that Mr. Blicket liked object A, and the question was how they categorized object B.

Three-year-olds claimed that Mr. Blicket liked object B 44% of the time when trained that he liked relatively few things (recall that the base rate in this condition was 1/6). By contrast, when Mr. Blicket liked many things (a base rate of 5/6), children responded that he liked object B 93% of the time, a significant difference between the conditions. Performance in the rare condition, however, could have been influenced by a number of factors. One possibility is that children were influenced by the spontaneous activation of the box, and would respond in a similar manner to a blicket machine that they observed spontaneously activate. This was not the case. Another group of 3-year-olds were shown a blicket machine that spontaneously activated during the initial part of the procedure. They were trained that objects that activate the machine (and hence, are blickets) were rare, and were given the same procedure. In this condition, 3-year-olds categorized object B as a blicket 72% of the time, more often than in the desire condition.

Similarly, another possibility is that children were simply more interested in Mr. Blicket than when it was a blicket machine. There are cases where children's interest level clearly mediates their cognition (e.g., Renninger & Wozniak, 1985). To consider this possibility, we gave another group of 3-year-olds the same Mr. Blicket procedure, except that we labeled his activation as indicating what he was thinking about, instead of what he liked. Unlike desire, 3-year-olds have little knowledge of other's belief states (e.g., Wellman, Cross, & Watson, 2001), the role of thinking in other mental activities (Flavell, Green, & Flavell, 1995; Johnson & Wellman, 1982; Lillard, 1996), or the possibility that thoughts could be related to objects or other thoughts (Eisbach, 2004). It seemed likely that only a few 3-year-olds would recognize that an agent's thoughts could be based on an internal property of objects, which would provide them with a causal mechanism equivalent to the activation law. This also appeared to be the case. In this condition, 3-year-olds categorized object B as something Mr. Blicket was thinking about 72% of the time, more often than in the desire condition.

Further, in the three conditions in which children were trained that the causal power (Mr. Blicket's desire, thoughts, or the activation of a spontaneous machine) was rare, we also gave children a set of unrelated cognitive measures as well as a measure in which they were asked to relate the causal power of objects to those objects insides (analogous to the procedure used in Sobel et al., 2007). Across all of these conditions, the ability to relate the causal property of objects to those objects' insides predicted whether children claimed that object B did not have causal efficacy (i.e., a response consistent with the Bayesian description), even when age and other measures of general cognition were considered.

These data indicate that children are not specifically developing causal inference abilities between the ages of 3 and 4. Rather, children appear to have such an inferential mechanism in place at the age of three, and lack the particular domain-specific knowledge necessary to use that mechanism appropriately. The Bayesian description I am suggesting here (following similar proposals by Griffiths & Tenenbaum, 2005; Griffiths et al., submitted; Tenenbaum & Griffiths, 2001, 2003; Tenenbaum, Griffiths, & Niyogi, 2007) offers a rational way of considering how children's developing prior knowledge influences their causal reasoning abilities.

An open question is how such causal knowledge might be acquired. In the final sections, I want to consider two possibilities. The first is an extension of the Bayesian mechanism. The second attempts to integrate other pieces of information from the environment.

LEARNING CAUSAL MECHANISMS

So far we have considered how children recover a representation of the causal environment based on the data they observe. This learning mechanism is guided by a particular set of causal principles, which potentially constrain the hypothesis space children consider and the parameterization of those hypotheses. An open question is how children develop knowledge of these causal principles.

Consider the mechanism that underlies the blicket detector. The previous sections argued that preschoolers develop a conception that the mechanism that underlies the detector's activation is deterministic. This knowledge is what allows us (and young children) to make inferences based on small samples of data. In almost all of the experiments described above, children are never shown data that contradict a deterministic mechanism. What happens if this is the case?

In Gopnik et al. (2001), children were shown cases in which objects sometimes made the machine go and sometimes did not. In their two-cause trials, children inferred that an object that activated the blicket detector two out of three times was a blicket most of the time. This trial provides evidence that the detector is not deterministic and might activate based on a more probabilistic mechanism. How might seeing this trial first affect children's inferences on other trials, in which a deterministic mechanism is required?

Like the backwards blocking procedure, Gopnik et al.'s (2001) one-cause procedure relies on children understanding that there is a deterministic mechanism that relates blickets to the blicket detector (recall that on a one-cause trial, object A activates the machine by itself, object B does not by itself, then both objects activated the machine together twice). If the detector is probabilistic, then there should be the possibility that object B is a blicket; object B might have failed to be effective when it was placed on the machine alone, but demonstrated its efficacy when placed on the machine with object A. If the detector is deterministic, then this is not the case: object A should be a blicket, and object B should not be by virtue of it failing to activate the detector independently. Gopnik et al. (2001) found that overall, children (particularly 4-year-olds) who were shown these data responded consistently with the deterministic interpretation. Tom Griffiths and I reanalyzed performance on the one-cause trials as a function of whether they observed a two-cause trial first (recall that in the two-cause trial, one object activates the detector probabilistically; it fails to activate the machine the first time it is placed on it, and does so the next two times). Four-year-olds were more likely to say that object B was a blicket in the one-cause trial if they saw a two-cause trial first.

Griffiths et al. (submitted) considered more systematically whether children and adults can extract mechanism information from the data they observe. Specifically, if learners first observe evidence that the detector is deterministic will they make different inferences about the same data than if they first observe evidence that the detector is not deterministic? This question can also be formulated as one of Bayesian inference, although the hypotheses are about the principles that govern how hypotheses about causal models are formulated. In this example, the hypotheses include the nature of the activation law—the mechanism that relates objects to the detector—in addition to the specific causal structures (following Tenenbaum, Griffiths, & Kemp, 2006; Tenenbaum et al., 2007). For purposes of space, I will only describe the psychological investigation with young children, but we have done similar investigations on adults.

Griffiths et al. (submitted) showed 4-year-olds the blicket detector, and trained them that the detector was either deterministic or probabilistic. In the deterministic condition, children were introduced to the detector as in Gopnik et al. (2001). They then observed six objects, each placed on the machine three times. Five of the six objects activated the machine all three times, and were labeled blickets; the other object failed to activate the machine all three times, and was labeled as not a blicket. In the probabilistic condition, children received the same introduction, and saw the same six objects. But here, the objects that activated the machine perfectly in the previous condition did so with some noise. Objects either activated the machine perfectly (one object), two out of three times (two objects) or one out of three times (two objects), and any of the objects that activated the machine was labeled a blicket. The object that failed to activate the machine all three times was still labeled as not a blicket, keeping the base rate of blickets the same across the conditions.

Children then observed a set of trials similar to the one-cause condition in Gopnik et al. (2001). The critical part of the trial involved them observing two new objects (A and B). Object A activated the machine by itself once. Object B failed to activate the machine by itself once, and then A and B together activated the machine twice. Children were asked whether each was a blicket. In the deterministic condition, performance paralleled Gopnik et al. (2001): children stated that object A was a blicket (100% of the time), and object B was not (only 9% of the time). In the probabilistic condition, children stated that object A was a blicket (92% of the time), but were significantly more likely to state that object B was as well (79% of the time).

These data offer preliminary evidence that 4-year-olds not only can recover information about causal models from the data that they observed, but that they also recover the principles necessary to learn causal structure from those data. Given the same correlational information, their inferences were different depending on the nature of the mechanism they were exposed to. Children's understanding of these mechanisms might not be terribly deep; they might not have explicit understanding of the mechanism, but rather just be aware that some kind of mechanism exists, which constrains inference in certain ways. This seems consistent with the work on relating causes and insides: the internal parts of the objects in Sobel et al. (2007) are dummy mechanisms, but the older children treat them as if they were the mechanism for the detector's activation, without (apparently) a real conception of how such mechanisms function.

Integrating Top-Down and Bottom-Up Learning

Appealing to a Bayesian description of a causal learning mechanism—specifically one that might be able to extract such mechanism knowledge from observed data—does not imply that all causal learning is "bottom-up." Instead, the Bayesian description seems more integrative: "top-down" principles for constraining causal learning can be derived from data, but this should not be considered the only way causal learning works. Below, I suggest several additional ways children might be able to acquire information about the principles for causal learning.

Testimony

More likely than not, the best way in which children learn new causal structures (or new causal principles) is through direct instruction—what Harris and Koenig (2006) call learning from "testimony." Harris, Pasquini, Duke, Asscher, and Pons (2006), for example, demonstrated that children made strong ontological commitments about different nonobservable scientific and endorsed entities (e.g., vitamins vs. Santa Claus). Further, the degree of their commitment in these entities varied with the exposure that they received about them.

More generally, one could imagine that children learn a great deal of causal structure simply by being told about that structure (something that might be particularly important in learning science, see Klahr & Nigam, 2004). This is evident in the introduction to most blicket detector experiments, in which children are told that the machine is a "blicket machine," and that objects that make it go are "blickets." The fact that children learn this readily (established in the pretests of almost all of these experiments), suggests that they can learn causal principles directly from the language they hear, but this is a topic for further investigation.

Analogy

Numerous investigations suggest that young children can make inferences from analogies (e.g., Brown & Kane, 1988; Gentner, 1977), and this is especially true when reasoning about causal relations (e.g., Goswami & Brown, 1989; Goswami, Leevers, Pressley, & Wheelwright, 1998; Ratterman & Gentner, 1998). This suggests that children can come to make new causal inferences from analogous information, or learn new information faster/more accurately if the analogy is mapped out for them. Emily Hopkins and I (Hopkins & Sobel, 2007; Sobel & Hopkins, submitted) have recently considered this possibility by looking at a particular type of causal inference: reasoning about enabling condition. Specifically, we found that 4-year-olds struggled to understand enabling conditions in a decontextualized environment (where the part of an object that acted as the enabling condition was labeled an "inside"). However, young children do appear to understand enabling conditions in a particular setting: a Child Language Data Exchange System (CHILDES; MacWhinney, 2000) analysis revealed that children talk about how batteries are necessary to make machines and toys function. Four-year-olds were able to make proper inferences about enabling conditions in a condition in which the part that acted in this manner was labeled as a battery.

Contextual Information in Data

A potential limitation of the causal graphical model framework is that it does not easily describe a way in which contextual cues can influence learning. For example, active construction of knowledge in the world is a hallmark of both classic (e.g., Montessori, 1912; Piaget, 1952) and certain contemporary (e.g., Gopnik & Meltzoff, 1997) approaches to cognitive development. The computational approaches described here do not consider whether the child has an active hand in constructing its knowledge as opposed to recovering causal structure from simply observing the environment.

The ability to control what data one observes, and generate interventions consistent with those data appear to facilitate learning over observing similar data in adult participants (Lagnado & Sloman, 2004; Steyvers et al., 2003; Waldmann & Hagmayer, 2005), in child participants (Schulz et al., 2007), and in animals (Blaisdell et al., 2006). Moreover, young children appear to treat their own data as more informative than if the same data were generated by another person (Kushnir & Gopnik, 2005).

Jessica Sommerville and I investigated how young children's causal learning was affected by particular contextual demands (Sobel & Sommerville, in preparation). We found that 4-year-olds whose free play with a system allowed them to discover causal structure learned that structure better than children whose free play with a system came after they observed an experimenter generate a small number of interventions on the system (enough to discover the structure). Further, when children were shown identical intervention data, which was sufficient to learn a causal structure, children who were given an inappropriate rationale for why the experimenter has generated those data failed to learn the system; children given an appropriate rationale learned above chance values (Sobel & Sommerville, 2009). These contextual factors are not part of the computational description I have described so far, and must be accounted for therein.

Conclusions

In this chapter, I have suggested a description of causal inference based on Bayesian inference, which illustrates how children engage in causal learning (for a more detailed description of this model, see e.g., Griffiths & Tenenbaum, 2007). This description is meant at the computational level of analysis (followed Marr, 1982), which means that an obvious limitation of this approach is that it should not be taken for the actual algorithm by which children learn causal knowledge, nor should it be considered how the brain instantiates such inference. However, in describing the way in which children learn causal knowledge, we provide insight into these questions.

I want to conclude by emphasizing that computational models are a good way to focus an investigation, but a psychological description of human causal learning should not be completely model-dependent (whether that model be bottom-up, top-down, or something in between). One should integrate model with human workings to describe psychological accounts of reasoning (what Lagnado et al., 2007, calls a "heuristic-based" approach). Here, it should be emphasized that young children possess considerable causal reasoning abilities, starting at a very young age. The goal of future research is to describe these abilities, and potentially develop an algorithmic and implementational level of children's causal inference—in more detail.

Acknowledgments

I was supported by NSF (DLS-0518161 to D.M.S.) during the writing of this chapter. I would like to thank all of the parents and children who participated in the research described here. I would also like to thank Scott Johnson, David Buchanan, Claire Cook, Tom Griffiths, Natasha Kirkham and the members of the NYBUG workshop for helpful discussions about material in this chapter.

References

Ahn, W., Kalish, C. W., Medin, D. L., & Gelman, S. A. (1995). The role of covariation versus mechanism information in causal attribution. *Cognition, 54*, 299–352.

Allan, L. G. (1980). A note on measurement of contingency between two binary variables in judgment tasks. *Bulletin of the Psychonomic Society, 15*, 147–149

Aslin, R. N., Saffran, J. R., & Newport, E. L. (1998). Computation of conditional probability statistics by 8-month-old infants. *Psychological Science*, 9, 321–324.

Blaisdell, A. P., Sawa, K., Leising, K. J., & Waldmann, M. R. (2006). Causal reasoning in rats. *Science, 311*, 1020–1022.

Blumenthal, E. J., & Sobel, D. M. (2008). *Preschoolers' developing knowledge of causal and internal properties of artifacts.* Manuscript in preparation, Brown University.

Brown, A. L., & Kane, M. J. (1988). Preschool children can learn to transfer: Learning to learn and learning from example. *Cognitive Psychology, 20*, 493–523.

Bullock, M., Gelman, R., & Baillargeon, R. (1982). The development of causal reasoning. In W. J. Friedman (Ed.), *The developmental psychology of time* (pp. 209–254). New York: Academic Press.

Cheng, P. W. (1997). From covariation to causation: A causal power theory. *Psychological Review, 104*, 367–405.

Cheng, P. W., & Novick, L. R. (1990). A probabilistic contrast model of causal induction. *Journal of Personality and Social Psychology, 58*, 545–567.

Cramer, R. E., Weiss, R. F., Williams, R., Reid, S., Nieri, L., & Manning-Ryan, B. (2002). Human agency and associative learning: Pavlovian principles govern social process in causal relationship detection. *Quarterly Journal of Experimental Psychology: Comparative and Physiological Psychology, 55B*, 241–266.

Das Gupta, P., & Bryant, P. E. (1989). Young children's causal inferences. *Child Development, 60*, 1138–1146.

Dickinson, A., & Shanks, D. (1995). Instrumental action and causal representation. In D. Sperber, D. Premack, & A. J. Premack (Eds.), *Causal cognition: A multidisciplinary debate* (pp. 5–25). New York: Clarendon Press/Oxford University Press.

Eisbach, A. O. D. (2004). Children's developing awareness of diversity in people's trains of thought. *Child Development, 75*, 1694–1707.

Fawcett, C., & Markson, L. (2005). *Developing ideas about other's preferences.* Poster presented at the 2005 meeting of the Cognitive Development Society, San Diego, CA.

Fiser, J., & Aslin, R. N. (2002). Statistical learning of new visual feature combinations by infants. *Proceedings of the National Academy of Sciences, USA*, 99, 15822–15826.

Flavell, J. H., Green, F. L., & Flavell, E. R. (1995). *Young children's knowledge about thinking.* Monographs of the Society for Research in Child Development, *60*(1, Serial No. 243).

Gentner, D. (1977). Children's performance on a spatial analogies task. *Child Development, 48*, 1034–1039.

Gomez, R. L., & Gerken, L. A., (1999). Artificial grammar learning by 1-year-olds leads to specific and abstract knowledge. *Cognition, 70*, 109–135.

Gopnik, A., Glymour, C., Sobel, D. M., Schulz, L. E., Kushnir, T., & Danks, D. (2004). A theory of causal learning in children: Causal maps and Bayes nets. *Psychological Review, 111*, 3–32.

Gopnik, A., & Meltzoff, A. N. (1992). Categorization and naming: Basic-level sorting in eighteen-month-olds and its relation to language. *Child Development, 63*, 1091–1103.

Gopnik, A., & Meltzoff, A. N. (1997). *Words, thoughts, and theories*. Cambridge, MA: MIT Press.

Gopnik, A., & Slaughter, V. (1991). Young children's understanding of changes in their mental states. *Child Development, 62*, 98–110.

Gopnik, A., & Sobel, D. M. (2000). Detecting blickets: How young children use information about novel causal powers in categorization and induction. *Child Development, 71*, 1205–1222.

Gopnik, A., Sobel, D. M., Schulz, L., & Glymour, C. (2001). Causal learning mechanisms in very young children: Two, three, and four-year-olds infer causal relations from patterns of variation and co-variation. *Developmental Psychology, 37*, 620–629.

Goswami, U., & Brown, A. L. (1989). Melting chocolate and melting snowmen: Analogical reasoning and causal relations. *Cognition, 35*, 69–95.

Goswami, U., & Brown, A. L. (1990). Higher-order structure and relational reasoning: Contrasting analogical and thematic relations. *Cognition, 36*, 207–226.

Goswami, U., Leevers, H., Pressley, S., & Wheelwright, S. (1998). Causal reasoning about pairs of relations and analogical reasoning in young children. *British Journal of Developmental Psychology, 16*, 553–569.

Gottfried, G. M., & Gelman, S. A. (2005). Developing domain-specific causal-explanatory frameworks: The role of insides and immanence. *Cognitive Development, 20*, 137–158

Griffiths, T. L., Sobel, D. M., Tenenbaum, J. B., & Gopnik, A. (2008). *Bayesian reasoning in adults' and children's causal inferences*. Manuscript in preparation, University of California at Berkeley.

Griffiths, T. L., & Tenenbaum, J. B. (2005). Structure and strength in causal induction. *Cognitive Psychology, 51*, 334–384.

Griffiths, T. L., & Tenenbaum, J. B. (2007). Two proposals for causal grammars. In A. Gopnik & L. E. Schulz (Eds.), *Causal learning: Psychology, Philosophy, and Computation* (pp. 323–346). New York: Oxford University Press.

Haith, M. M. (1993). Future-oriented processes in infancy: The case of visual expectations. In C. Granrud (Ed.), *Visual perception and cognition in infancy* (pp. 235–264). Hillsdale, NJ: Erlbaum.

Harris, P. L., & Koenig, M. A. (2006). Trust in testimony: How children learn about science and religion. *Child Development, 77*, 505–524.

Harris, P. L., Pasquini, E. S., Duke, S., Asscher, J. J., & Pons, F. (2006).Germs and angels: The role of testimony in young children's ontology. *Developmental Science, 9*, 76–96.

Hopkins, E. J., & Sobel, D. M. (2007, March). *Children's causal inferences about enabling conditions in the physical and psychological domains*. Poster presented at the 2007 Biennial meeting of the Society for Research in Child Development, Boston, MA.

Hume, D. (1978). *A treatise of human nature*. Oxford: Oxford University Press. (Original work published 1739)

Johnson, C. N., & Wellman, H. M. (1982). Children's developing conceptions of the mind and brain. *Child Development, 53*, 222–234.

Johnson, S., Slaughter, V., & Carey, S. (1998). Whose gaze will infants follow? The elicitation of gaze-following in 12-month-olds. *Developmental Science, 1*, 233–238.

Johnson, S. C., Booth, A., & O'Hearn, K. (2001). Inferring the goals of a nonhuman agent. *Cognitive Development*, 16, 637–656.

Kamin, L. J. (1969). Predictability, surprise, attention, and conditioning. In B. A. Campbell & R. M. Church (Eds.), *Punishment and aversive behavior* (pp. 279–296). New York: Appleton-Century-Crofts.

Kirkham, N. Z., Slemmer, J. A., & Johnson, S. P. (2002). Visual statistical learning in infancy. *Cognition, 83*, B35–B42.

Klahr, D., & Nigam, M. (2004). The equivalence of learning paths in early science instruction. *Psychological Science, 15*, 661–667.

Kruschke, J. K., & Blair, N. J. (2000). Blocking and backward blocking involve learned inattention. *Psychonomic Bulletin and Review, 7*, 636–645.

Kushnir, T., & Gopnik, A. (2005). Young Children Infer Causal Strength from Probabilities and Interventions. *Psychological Science, 16*, 678–683.

Lagnado, D. A., & Sloman, S. (2004). The advantage of timely intervention. *Journal of Experimental Psychology: Learning, Memory, and Cognition, 30*, 856–876.

Lagnado, D. A., Waldmann, M. R., Hagmayer, Y., & Sloman, S. A. (2007). Beyond covariation: Cues to causal structure. In A. Gopnik & L. E. Schulz (Eds.), *Causal learning: Psychology, philosophy, and computation* (pp. 154–172). New York: Oxford.

Leslie, A. M., & Keeble, S. (1987). Do six-month-old infants perceive causality? *Cognition, 25*, 265–288.

Lillard, A. S. (1996). Body or mind: Children's categorizing of pretense. *Child Development, 67*, 1717–1734.

Mackintosh, N. J. (1975). A theory of attention: Variations in the associability of stimuli with reinforcement. *Psychological Review, 82*, 276–298.

MacWhinney, B. (2000). *The CHILDES project: Tools for analyzing talk* (3rd ed.). Mahwah, NJ: Lawrence Erlbaum Associates.

Marr, D. (1982). *Vision*. New York: Henry Holt.

McCormack, T., & Hoerl, C. (2005). Children's reasoning about the causal significance of the temporal order of events. *Developmental Psychology, 41*, 54–63.

Michotte, A. (1962).*Causalite, permanence et realite phenomenales*. Oxford, England: Publications Universitaires.

Montessori, M. (1912/1964). *The montessori method*. New York: Schocken.

Novick, L. R., & Cheng, P. W. (2004). Assessing interactive causal influence. *Psychological Review, 111*, 455–485.

Oakes, L. M., & Cohen, L. B. (1990). Infant perception of a causal event. *Cognitive Development, 5*, 193–207.

Pearl, J. (2000). *Causality: Models, reasoning, and inference*. New York: Cambridge University Press.

Perner, J. (1991). *Understanding the representational mind*. Cambridge, MA: MIT Press.

Piaget, J. (1929). *The child's conception of the world*. London: Routledge and Kegan Paul.

Piaget, J. (1930). *The child's conception of physical causality* (M. Gabain, Trans.). London: Lund Humphries.

Piaget, J. (1952). *The origins of intelligence in children* (M. Cook, Trans.). Madison, WI: International Universities Press.

Ratterman, M. J., & Gentner, D. (1998). More evidence for a relational shift in the development of analogy: Children's performance on a causal-mapping task. *Cognitive Development, 13*, 453–478.

Renninger, K. A., & Wozniak, R. H. (1985). Effect of interest on attentional shift, recognition, and recall in young children. *Developmental Psychology, 21*, 624–632.

Repacholi, B. M., & Gopnik, A. (1997). Early reasoning about desires: Evidence from 14- and 18-month-olds. *Developmental Psychology, 33*, 12–21.

Rescorla, R. A., & Wagner, A. R. (1972). A theory of Pavlovian conditioning: Variations in the effectiveness of reinforcement and nonreinforcement. In A. H. Black & W. F. Prokasy (Eds.), *Classical Conditioning II: Current theory and research* (pp. 64–99). New York: Appleton-Century-Crofts.

Saffran, J. R., Aslin, R. N., & Newport, E. L. (1996). Statistical learning by 8-month-old infants. *Science, 274*, 1926–1928.

Saffran, J. R., Johnson, E. K., Aslin, R. N., & Newport, E. L. (1999). Statistical learning of tone sequences by human infants and adults. *Cognition, 70*, 27–52.

Schulz, L. E., & Gopnik, A. (2004). Causal learning across domains. *Developmental Psychology, 40*, 162–176.

Schulz, L. E., Gopnik, A., & Glymour, C. (2007). Preschool children learn causal structure from conditional independence. *Developmental Science, 10*, 322–332.

Schulz, L. E., & Sommerville, J. (2006). God does not play dice: Causal determinism and children's inferences about unobserved causes. *Child Development, 77*, 427–442.

Shanks, D. R. (1985). Forward and backward blocking in human contingency judgment. *Quarterly Journal of Experimental Psychology, 37B*, 1–21.

Shanks, D. R. (1995). Is human learning rational? *Quarterly Journal of Experimental Psychology A, 48*, 257–279.

Shultz, T. R. (1982). Rules of causal attribution. *Monographs of the Society for Research in Child Development, 47*(1, Serial No. 194).

Sobel, D. M. & Blumenthal, E. J. (2009). *Children's causal inferences about ambiguous evidence reflect their developing understanding of mechanisms*. Manuscript in preparation, Brown University.

Sobel, D. M., & Hopkins, E. (2009). *Batteries not included: Children's causal inferences about enabling conditions*. Manuscript in preparation, Brown University.

Sobel, D. M., & Kirkham, N. Z. (2006). Blickets and babies: The development of causal reasoning in toddlers and infants. *Developmental Psychology, 42*, 1103–1115.

Sobel, D. M., & Kirkham, N. Z. (2007). Bayes nets and blickets: Infants developing representations of causal knowledge. *Developmental Science, 10*, 298–306.

Sobel, D. M., & Munro, S. A. (2009). Domain generality and specificity in children's causal inferences about ambiguous data. *Developmental Psychology, 45*, 511–524.

Sobel, D. M., & Sommerville, J. A. (2009a). Rationales in children's causal learning from other's actions. *Cognitive Development, 24*, 70–79.

Sobel, D. M. & Sommerville, J. A. (2009b). *The importance of discovery for children's causal learning from interventions.* Manuscript in preparation, Brown University.

Sobel, D. M., Tenenbaum, J. B., & Gopnik, A. (2004). Children's causal inferences from indirect evidence: Backwards blocking and Bayesian reasoning in preschoolers. *Cognitive Science, 28*, 303–333.

Sobel, D. M., Yoachim, C. M., Gopnik, A., Meltzoff, A. N., & Blumenthal, E. J. (2007). The blicket within: Preschoolers' inferences about insides and causes. *Journal of Cognition and Development, 8*, 159–182.

Sophian, C., & Huber, A. (1984). Early developments in children's causal judgments. *Child Development, 55*, 512–526.

Spelke, E. S., Breinlinger, K., Macomber, J., & Jacobson, K. (1992). Origins of knowledge. *Psychological Review, 99*, 605–632.

Spirtes, P., Glymour, C., & Scheines, R. (2001). *Causation, prediction, and search (Springer Lecture Notes in Statistics, 2nd ed., Rev.).* Cambridge, MA: MIT Press.

Steyvers, M., Tenenbaum, J. B., Wagenmakers, E. J., & Blum, B. (2003). Inferring causal networks from observations and interventions. *Cognitive Science, 27*, 453–489.

Tenenbaum, J. B., & Griffiths, T. L. (2001). *Structure learning in human causal induction.* Proceedings of the 13th Annual Conference on the Advances in Neural Information Processing Systems.

Tenenbaum, J. B., & Griffiths, T. L. (2003). *Theory-based causal inference.* Proceedings of the 14th Annual Conference on the Advances in Neural Information Processing Systems.

Tenenbaum, J. B., Griffiths, T. L., & Kemp, C. (2006). Theory-based Bayesian models of inductive learning and reasoning. *Trends in Cognitive Science, 10*, 309–318.

Tenenbaum, J. B., Griffiths, T. L., & Niyogi, S. (2007). Intuitive theories as grammars for causal inference. In A. Gopnik & L. E. Schulz (Eds.), *Causal learning; Psychology, philosophy and computation* (pp. 301–322). New York: Oxford.

Uzgiris, I. C., & Hunt, J. M. V. (1975). *Assessment in infancy: Ordinal scales of psychological development.* Oxford, England: University of Illinois Press.

Van Hamme, L. J., & Wasserman, E. A. (1994). Cue competition in causality judgments: The role of nonpresentation of compound stimulus elements. *Learning and Motivation, 25*, 127–151.

Waldmann, M. R., & Hagmayer, Y. (2005). Seeing versus doing: Two modes of accessing causal knowledge. *Journal of Experimental Psychology: Learning Memory and Cognition, 31*, 216–227.

Wasserman, E. A., & Berglan, L. R (1998). Backward blocking and recovery from overshadowing in human causal judgment: The role of within-compound associations. *Quarterly Journal of Experimental Psychology: Comparative & Physiological Psychology, 51*, 121–138.

Wellman, H. M., Cross, D., & Watson, J. K. (2001). A meta-analysis of theory of mind: The truth about false belief. *Child Development*, 72, 655–684.

Wellman, H. M., & Woolley, J. D. (1990). From simple desires to ordinary beliefs: The early development of everyday psychology. *Cognition*, 35, 245–275.

Wentworth, N. Haith, M. M., & Hood, R. (2002). Spatiotemporal regularity and interevent contingencies as information for infants' visual expectations. *Infancy*, 3, 303–321.

Woodward, J. (2003). *Making things happen: A theory of causal explanation.* New York: Oxford.

Yuill, N. (1984). Young children's coordination of motive and outcome in judgments of satisfaction and morality. *British Journal of Developmental Psychology*, 2, 73–81.

CHAPTER 9
What Is Statistical Learning, and What Statistical Learning Is Not

Jenny R. Saffran

Over the past decade, researchers in developmental cognitive science and psycholinguistics have become increasingly interested in the role that statistical learning may play in perceptual and cognitive development. Despite the term being weighty, the idea is quite simple. To the extent that structure in the environment is patterned, learners with appropriate learning mechanisms can make use of that patterning to discover underlying structure. This idea has a long history, across myriad domains. For example, linguists in the first half of the twentieth century routinely examined the distribution of sounds, words, and categories of words in novel languages to infer the structures that generated those distributions, including phonemes, words, morphemes, and rudimentary syntax (e.g., Bloomfield, 1933; Harris, 1955). Similarly, researchers studying the behavior of nonhuman animals, both in the laboratory and in their natural habitats, discovered that nonhuman animals skillfully track environmental regularities to increase the probabilities of reward (for an extensive review, see Gallistel, 1990).

The term "statistical learning" itself originated in the area of computer science. Statistical learning algorithms are typically used for pattern recognition processes and are applied across numerous domains from face recognition to speech processing. In this field, statistical learning is sometimes used to refer to algorithms that themselves learn from data. In the subfield of computer science known as natural language processing, statistical learning typically refers to a set of processes or procedures for parsing, part-of-speech tagging (e.g., discovering lexical categories), or induction of grammatical structures using such procedures as Hidden Markov Models (e.g., Charniak, 1993). The broad idea behind this body of research is that bottom-up processes tracking joint frequencies, conditional probabilities, prior probabilities, mutual information, and/or entropy (among many other possible computations) may efficiently discover structure in complex domains, at least given relatively constrained search spaces.

Consistent with but largely separate from these developments, computational modelers in cognitive science were developing novel techniques for learning via 'dumb' algorithms operating en masse, intended to mimic the operation of neural structures (e.g., Hebbian learning). Again, working within relatively constrained domains and/or toy corpora, researchers demonstrated discovery procedures using neural network models that essentially capitalized on statistical properties of the input to parse sentences, discover lexical categories, and discern structure via learning (e.g., Allen & Seidenberg, 1999; Chater & Redington, 1999; Curtin et al., 2001; Mintz, Newport, & Bever, 2002; Reali & Christiansen, 2005; Seidenberg & MacDonald, 2001). These models have been highly effective in demonstrating the information content available in various types of input, as they permit researchers to determine what types of cues are, in principle, available to actual human learners and to test specific hypotheses concerning how learning might operate (e.g., the debate between proponents of rules vs. statistics: cf. Altmann, 2002; Christiansen & Curtin, 1999; Marcus, 1999a, 1999b, 2001; McClelland, McClelland, & Plaut, 1999; Rohde & Plaut, 1999; Seidenberg & Elman, 1999).

Connectionist models have had a tremendous impact on theoretical and empirical work in the cognitive sciences. Interestingly, because these are learning models, they are arguably more relevant to developmental psychology than to any other branch of cognitive science. Perhaps because of this fact, connectionist models have been especially vulnerable to the kinds of critiques and concerns raised most prominently by developmentalists. For example, each model is typically tailored to handle just one type of task. That is, a model trained to learn the past tense of English verbs cannot turn around and do object segregation as well (the input/output representations are wrong; even given overlapping representations, new learning would lead to catastrophic interference, erasing the prior learning). These kinds of observations raise questions about how domain-specific such models need to be. What is "innate" or prespecified in the representations and/or architectures of individual models? What about types of learning—e.g., more abstract structures—that do not appear to be captured by statistical models? Perhaps most importantly, do developing humans really learn this way?

Perhaps because of these developments and debates, the initial findings that infants can track the probabilities of sequential elements (syllables and/or phonemes) in speech received a great deal of attention (Aslin, Saffran, & Newport, 1998; Goodsitt, Morgan, & Kuhl, 1993; Hauser, Newport, & Aslin, 2001; Saffran, Aslin, & Newport, 1996), both positive and negative. On the positive side, these results unambiguously demonstrated that infants can track regularities in rapid speech, without the benefit of added linguistic cues, social cues, or external reinforcement; learning itself appears to be reinforcing in these tasks. This is not to say that other sorts of information are not beneficial—indeed they are, as discussed below. These data were intended to provide an existence proof that infants can, at least under certain circumstances, track types of information that are relevant to linguistic structure (according to the computational and linguistic literatures). Importantly, the initial claims never suggested that statistical learning could account for *all* of language acquisition, or even all of any subset of language (e.g., discovering words in fluent speech). The intent was to develop methods, using artificial languages, which would allow subsequent researchers to test specific hypotheses concerning the role of statistical learning in language acquisition in infancy and beyond. And to a large extent, this is exactly what has happened.

However, perhaps because of its relatively simple beginnings, the area of statistical language learning has been caricatured as focusing on a single computation (pairwise transitional probabilities) performed between physically observable entities (syllables) in a highly artificial language. Given this view of statistical language learning, it is indeed the case that the theoretical oomph of statistical learning is extremely limited. To acquire natural languages, learners need to detect more complex relationships between more abstract entities in a far richer set of input. The insufficiency of statistical learning is even true for a task like detecting word boundaries in fluent speech. While tracking sequential probabilities is demonstrably useful, given corpus analyses (Swingley, 2005), other sources of information are absolutely necessary to achieve good learning outcomes. These might range from tracking additional regularities in speech, such as the degree of stress carried by a syllable (Curtin, Mintz, & Christiansen, 2005), to potential innate knowledge concerning universal phonological regularities (Yang, 2004).

Importantly, the initial reports concerning statistical learning attempted to be very explicit on this point, repeatedly pointing out the fact that sequential statistics alone are not enough to fully solve any real language learning problems. For example, Saffran et al. (1996) noted that "although experience with speech in the real world is unlikely to be as concentrated as it was in these studies, infants in more natural settings presumably benefit from other types of cues correlated with statistical information" (p. 1928). In an adult study of this phenomenon also published in 1996, these investigators explicitly manipulated an additional cue to word boundaries, vowel lengthening, to investigate additive effects of multiple cues (Saffran, Newport, & Aslin, 1996). It has become increasingly clear that sequential statistical cues (such as transitional probabilities) operate in tandem with other types of regularities in the service of infant word segmentation, including lexical stress (e.g., Curtin et al., 2005; Johnson & Jusczyk, 2001; Jusczyk, 1999; Jusczyk, Houston, & Newsome, 1999; Thiessen & Saffran, 2003, 2007), known words (Bortfeld, Morgan, Golinkoff, & Rathbun, 2005), and other relevant cues in speech to infants (for a recent review, see Saffran, Werker, & Werner, 2006). Moreover, use of sequential statistics appears to be enhanced by the presence of attention-grabbing infant-directed speech (Thiessen, Hill, & Saffran, 2005).

It is thus very much not the case that sequential statistics operate in a vacuum; this point is both implicitly and explicitly made throughout this burgeoning literature. Moreover, it is important to note that many of the types of information usually considered in opposition to statistics are themselves nondeterministic. For example, the lexical stress information upon which English-learning 9-month-olds rely to segment bisyllabic words (first syllable stress) is itself probabilistic (Cutler & Carter, 1987). An issue for the field, then, is to decide what "counts" as statistical. Are probabilistic regularities that are not sequential still statistical? It seems that the logical answer is yes, in which case the question becomes how to characterize the myriad different types of statistical regularities in the input, including phonological and social cues (Goldstein, King, & West, 2003; Kuhl, 2007; Kuhl, Tsao, & Liu, 2003).

With these considerations in mind, let us return to the caricature: statistical learning consists of a single computation (pairwise transitional probabilities, either adjacent or nonadjacent) over simple elements (e.g., phonemes or syllables) in a highly artificial language. To the extent that this caricature is accurate, the potential role for statistical learning in language acquisition is limited at best. For the remainder of this chapter, I will focus on three issues that are implicit in this characterization of statistical learning: the nature of the computations, the complexity of the learning problem, and the role of artificial languages.

Which Statistics Are Computed During Statistical Learning?

The short answer to this question is that we do not yet know. There are (at least) three different ways to approach this problem. The first is to analyze language corpora to determine which statistics, in principle, might be useful/necessary to capture language structure. The second is to create carefully designed experiments to determine whether appropriately aged learners can make use of the statistics in question. These two approaches, in tandem, have been quite useful, in that they have shown that infants can keep track of, at minimum, the adjacent pairwise probabilities (e.g., Aslin et al., 1998) that corpus analyses suggest would be useful for word segmentation (e.g., Swingley, 2005), nonadjacent pairwise probabilities (e.g., Gomez, 2002), and histogram frequencies (e.g., Maye, Werker, & Gerken, 2002). The latter case is particularly interesting, as it suggests that infants not only track the individual frequencies of occurrence of elements, but the distribution of those frequencies, distinguishing unimodal and bimodal functions from one another. Importantly, these functions are useful for discovering speech categories given the statistics of real speech samples (Vallabha, McClelland, Pons, Werker, & Amano, 2007; Werker et al., 2007). These sorts of statistics, along with others currently described in the adult literature—e.g., clustering words into categories (Mintz, 2002); tracking probabilities of individual word pairs (Thompson & Newport, 2007)—suggest that infants may have access to a powerful tool set for exploiting the distributional regularities of human languages. The exact nature of this tool set, however, remains underspecified.

The third approach is somewhat different and is perhaps best exemplified by connectionist models. Rather that trying to specify which statistics are used by infant learners, the problem can be turned on its head by asking what *task* infants are attempting to perform. Computational models such as simple recurrent networks (SRNs) take as their task the problem of trying to predict what is coming up downstream in the input (Elman, 1990). This idea—learning by predicting—is consistent with a body of recent work in adult language comprehension that has focused on predicting during skilled language processing (for a recent review, see MacDonald & Seidenberg, 2006). For example, event-related potential (ERP) evidence suggests that adults use the phonology of a determiner (e.g., *a* versus *an*) to generate expectations concerning what noun will come next: consonant-initial nouns follow *a*, while vowel-initial nouns follow *an* (DeLong, Urbach, & Kutas, 2005). Semantic information in the verb (e.g., *eats*) constrains adults' anticipatory eye movements, such that listeners look toward object pictures that are consistent with the verb (e.g., *cake*) well before the noun itself occurs (Altmann & Kamide, 1999; Kamide, Altmann, & Haywood, 2003); this effect is maintained even when the noun pictures are removed (Altmann, 2004). Similarly, adults and young children can use the gender of a determiner (e.g., *le* vs. *la* in French) to generate expectations concerning the following noun (Dahan, Swingley, Tanenhaus, & Magnuson, 2000; Lew-Williams & Fernald, 2007).

It is thus possible that infants, along with adults and children, exploit patterns in their linguistic environment—including statistics—to make predictions about what will come next, as well as to interpret what has already occurred (which is necessary given the vast amount of ambiguity in natural language). The question then is not which statistics do infants compute, but which statistics inform infants' expectations about subsequent input? Efficient tracking of relevant regularities would allow infants to become skilled at rapid language processing, as observed occurs over the course of typical language development (in the absence of language disorders). Making use of expectations is even more critical in language production, where decisions about future speech acts constantly inform current motor actions.

We can thus consider statistical learning as a component of language processing and use. By anticipating what will come next, infants can potentially increase the efficiency of their language comprehension—which is necessary given the amazing rapidity of speech. Patterns in the input thus can serve to influence this comprehension, by biasing perceivers toward likely outcomes. Sequential patterns at numerous grains of analysis could be construed as providing such biasing information. For example, predicting which syllable will come next provides information about where a word might end, facilitating word segmentation and, eventually, lexical access. Predicting which word will come downstream facilitates lexical access and subsequent sentence-level parsing. Category-level predictions (e.g., that nouns follow adjectives, or that certain types of verbs are followed by the complementizer "*that*") are likely to be particularly germane to syntactic structure; that is, predicting which word class should follow another word class.

Moreover, such predictions might serve as an important learning signal. Connectionist networks frequently take this approach, learning by predicting the next element in the input and assessing the match between the prediction and what actually occurs. Differences between predicted input and actual input serve as an implicit error signal, such that weights can be updated to reflect actual occurrences (e.g., Elman, 1990). Note that this idea is quite different from the classic concept of "negative evidence," wherein learners are provided with explicit corrections; such evidence is argued to be rarely available to children, and often not useful even when it does occur (Brown, Hanlon, & 1970; Marcus, 1993; Morgan & Travis, 1989). Implicit negative evidence, based on prediction, could provide corrective information at far more time points, facilitating learning relative to explicit negative evidence. This intuition is supported by modeling results contrasting different approaches to learning a toy grammar (Spivey-Knowlton & Saffran, 1995).

Despite extensive evidence suggesting that adults generate predictions while comprehending language, and a few exciting studies showing similar abilities in early childhood, no studies have yet tested the hypothesis that infants generate predictions concerning sequences of sound. We know that infants are of course highly attuned to sequential information in language, including the statistical knowledge described above. However, these tasks are essentially off-line, with measurement after learning has already occurred. We also know that in nonlinguistic tasks, infants appear to generate on-line predictions. For example, infants generate anticipatory eye movements when exposed to patterns of shapes (e.g., Canfield & Haith, 1991; Canfield, Smith, Brezsnyak, & Snow, 1997; Haith, Hazan, & Goodman, 1988; Haith, Wass, & Adler, 1997), and can even do so when the patterns are removed and the screen is blank (Richardson & Kirkham, 2004). Infants compute trajectories, anticipating where objects will appear (e.g., Johnson, Amso, & Slemmer, 2003), and their hand movements suggest computation of expectancies (e.g., von Hofsten, Vishton, Spelke, Feng, & Rosander, 1998). However, to date, the only infant studies examining on-line anticipation in a linguistic task have involved speech perception (McMurray & Aslin, 2004): infants who have learned an arbitrary sound/object correspondence can use the sound to predict the object's location, as indexed by their anticipatory eye movements.

We have recently begun to develop a methodology to ask whether infants generate anticipations on-line during *sequential* linguistic events. To do so, we have borrowed from prior studies that use eye movements to interrogate infant predictions. As a starting point, we began by examining infant processing of extremely simple grammatical structures: determiner–adjective–noun sequences. Of course, our studies concern spoken language, but the dependent variable concerns infants' eyes, so the method requires that the infant link spoken words with visually presented objects. In our first study, we decided to simply ask whether infants show different levels of anticipation from word to word when the word sequence is deterministic—that is, 100% probability from one word to the next—than when the word sequence is probabilistic—50% probability from one word to the next (Romberg & Saffran, 2009). The targets were names of animals that our 16-month-old participants would already likely know; the names were paired with pictures shown on a large computer screen. These noun targets were preceded by adjectives. Our principal manipulation concerned the distribution of the adjective/noun pairs. Some pairs were deterministic: e.g., *pretty* always preceded *doggie*. Other pairs were probabilistic: e.g., *little* preceded *kitty* on half the trials and *fish* on the other half; the specific pairing of nouns and adjectives was counterbalanced. Infants listened to several minutes of speech in which this distributional information was provided: e.g., "*This little kitty and one pretty doggie and one little fish and …*". During this training phase, infants also watched pictures of animals on the screen. Each of the animals always appeared in the same position—right or left—on the screen and flashed when it was spoken in the accompanying audio stream. This gave the infants the opportunity to learn the positions of the animal pictures while also learning about the adjective/noun distributions.

Following this brief training, infants were tested to see if they generated anticipatory looks as a function of the distributions of the adjective/noun pairs. Unlike the visual stimuli presented during training, the screen was blank during the test until the onset of the noun when the matching picture would flash on the screen. However, the auditory materials were the same as those presented during exposure. We hypothesized that if infants were using the adjectives to predict the upcoming nouns, we should see anticipatory looks to the position where the noun picture would occur, *prior* to the noun/picture event. In particular, we predicted a difference between deterministic pairs and probabilistic pairs. In the deterministic pairs, infants could—in principle—generate an expectation regarding the upcoming noun based on the adjective. However, in the probabilistic pairs, no information was available to tell the infant which noun would follow the adjective. Indeed, as hypothesized, infants only made reliable anticipatory eye movements to the target location (on the blank screen) for the deterministic pairs using the adjective as a cue to the upcoming target noun. For the probabilistic pairs, infants did not reliably fixate the target location until the onset of the noun itself. These results suggest that the statistics of the input influenced infants' eye movements in response to sequential linguistic stimuli, as we would expect if infants generate on-line expectations about upcoming linguistic events.

While this is just an initial study, and the methodology is still under development, these results suggest that like adults and young children, infants can use distributional information in speech to generate expectations about what might come next. On the basis of this view, infants are not static computers, using a set of algorithms to perform some set of computations. Instead, infants may be engaged in a dynamic process of using whatever information they can amass that might help to generate informative predictions, thereby facilitating comprehension and, eventually, production. The goal of our ensuing research will be to determine how infants assess which aspects of linguistic input are informative and which are not, and to test the related hypothesis that part of the learning process entails input-driven error correction.

Are statistics used in higher-level language tasks?

The initial reports about statistical learning in infants concerned word segmentation; tracking the probabilities of syllable co-occurrences. At the time of the Saffran et al. (1996) *Science* paper, it was unclear how broad the claims should be. While the paper itself restricted the claims to the domain of word segmentation, an accompanying "Perspective" piece broadened the implications to include critiques of nativist approaches to syntax acquisition (Bates & Elman, 1996), and a furor erupted in the "Correspondence" pages of subsequent issues. Was the claim simply that statistical learning played a role in word segmentation—a relatively uncontroversial idea, given that on any theory, word boundary information must be learned. Or was the intent to argue that statistical learning functioned for tasks up the linguistic food chain, including the acquisition of syntax?

At the time, we viewed this to be rightly an empirical question and the decade that followed has seen the publication of numerous adult studies focusing on the role of statistics in syntax learning (Lany, Gomez, & Gerken, 2007; Saffran, 2001a, 2002; Thompson & Newport, 2007). The broad claim is that, analogous to the work in segmentation and other phonological processes, learners can track statistical regularities across words and/or word classes that afford detection of syntactic patterns. Importantly, the presence of multiple correlated cues, such as prosodic or phonological regularities, appears to facilitate this process (Gerken, Wilson, & Lewis, 2005; Gomez & Lakusta, 2004; Kaschak & Saffran, 2006; Morgan, Meier, & Newport, 1987), just as observed in word segmentation.

Nevertheless, much remains unknown about the manner in which these regularities are learned. Some of these issues revolve around the long-standing rules versus statistics debates, whose roots lie in the fracas that emerged following the publication of the original Parallel Distributed Processing volume (Pinker & Prince, 1988; Rumelhart & McClelland, 1987). More recent incarnations of this debate have surrounded artificial language learning studies involving different types of syllable-level computations tracked over streams of speech. To what extent do generalizations in these tasks require rule-level processes (Pena, Bonatti, Nespor, & Mehler, 2002) as opposed to statistical processes (Perruchet, Tyler, Galland, & Peereman, 2004; Seidenberg, MacDonald, & Saffran, 2002)? That is, can statistical learning operate over primitives that are more abstract than physically available syllables or words, or is this necessarily the purview of algebraic rules (Marcus, 2000, 2001)?

In order to be useful for grammar acquisition, the relevant computation(s) must be able to operate over classes or categories. As observed 50 years ago by Chomsky (1959), the acceptability of nonsensical sentences like "Colorless green ideas sleep furiously" means that our representations must supercede word-to-word transitions to include transitions between categories of words (e.g., nouns, verbs, adverbs, etc.). The question, again, becomes what "counts" as statistical. On some views, only observable elements can be tracked in this fashion (Marcus & Berent, 2003). There are many ways to address these representational questions, ranging from computational models designed to implement one process or another to adult studies that carefully manipulate structures in artificial grammars. Our approach has largely involved studies of infant learners, in an attempt to ascertain which sorts of regularities they detect.

In one set of studies, we exposed 12-month-old infants to two types of grammatical structures (Saffran et al., 2008). One grammar structure contained statistical cues to phrase structure, providing infants with information concerning the types of words that typically co-occurred together. In the other grammar structure, these particular cues were absent, though the grammar was otherwise equally complex. Across several experiments manipulating the size of the grammar structure, we consistently found the same result: learning only occurred when statistical dependencies within phrases were present. These findings mirrored previous results with adults and children (Saffran, 2002), which suggested that learners' focus on these statistical regularities was not specific to language.

In infant artificial grammar studies, the critical test contrasts compare infants' responses to familiar (grammatical) versus novel (ungrammatical) sentences, which violate one or more of the regularities in the language. In the case of infant artificial grammar learning studies, while it is clear that infants have learned something about the patterns that differ between the grammatical and ungrammatical sentences, the nature of this knowledge remains unclear. One possibility is that infants have learned the rules of the language, which are then violated in the ungrammatical sentences. Another possibility is that infants have learned the (high) probability sequences of the language, which differ from the low probability sequences in the ungrammatical sentences. A third possibility is a hybrid system, in which infants learn the probabilities with which rules occur, and detect violations as a function of the rules' likelihood.

These possibilities are extremely challenging to disentangle empirically, particularly given the relatively simple structures typically used in infant language studies—and also given that patterns can be tracked across various levels of representation, from individual exemplars (e.g., words) to categories (e.g., grammatical classes). In a recent study, we began to investigate this issue by manipulating the types of ungrammatical sentences used at test (Saffran, 2009). Twelve-month-old infants were first exposed to a small grammar, written over small lexical categories. Critically, some of the transitions in the grammar were high probability (100%) while others were not (50%). Infants were then tested on grammatical sentences versus two different types of ungrammatical sentences (between-subjects manipulation); all test sentences were novel. In one group, infants were tested on grammatical sentences versus ungrammatical sentences that violated a high-probability transition. In the second group, infants were tested on grammatical sentences versus ungrammatical sentences that violated a low-probability transition. Importantly, both types of transitions were equally frequent in the exposure corpus. We hypothesized that if infants were responding solely to grammaticality, then discrimination performance should be equivalent across the two groups, as the ungrammatical sentences both violated the same number of transitions and were matched for frequency of transitions. However, if infants were attuned to the probability of the transitions presented during training, we hypothesized that violations of the high-probability transitions should be more readily detected than the violations of the low-probability transitions.

The data were consistent with the latter prediction: only those infants tested on violations of high-probability transitions discriminated between the grammatical and ungrammatical sentences. Importantly, data from a no-exposure control group confirmed that these results were due to language exposure, not idiosyncratic features of the test items. These data thus support the hypothesis that at least when learning artificial grammars, infants are sensitive to the probabilities with which words (or possibly word classes) co-occur. To the extent that infant language learning is subserved by the same mechanisms as adult language processing, these results are consistent with myriad results from sentence processing, suggesting that adult comprehenders are attuned to the statistical properties of syntactic structures at multiple grains of analysis, from concrete to abstract (e.g., MacDonald & Seidenberg, 2006; Seidenberg & MacDonald, 2001).

Moving beyond artificial languages

One major critique of studies focused on statistical learning is the artificial nature of the experimental tasks. These methods originated from a tradition in cognitive psychology and experimental psycholinguistics, which involved the use of artificial language materials (Gomez & Gerken, 2000). Dating back to the 1970s, researchers used these miniature languages to test specific hypotheses—with adults—concerning the types of information used by language learners (Braine, 1987; Moeser & Bregman, 1973; Morgan et al., 1987; Morgan, Meier, & Newport, 1989; Morgan & Newport, 1981; Smith, 1966). While these methods were clearly very artificial, like those used throughout cognitive psychology at the time, they permitted researchers to isolate particular cues hypothesized to influence language learning, while controlling other potential confounding variables. At the same time, the field of implicit learning developed parallel methodologies using artificial grammars, but with a focus primarily on learning and memory rather than on the acquisition of structures found in natural languages (Allen & Reber, 1980; Reber, 1967, 1993). Despite largely separate literatures during the 1980s and 1990s, these two literatures are beginning to converge in an exciting way, generating testable predictions that constrain theories of both implicit learning and language acquisition (Perruchet & Pacton, 2006).

Nevertheless, one can critique both literatures—artificial language learning and implicit learning—for their use of highly artificial, simplified materials. This issue is gaining attention; indeed, a summer workshop in 2007 was dedicated to the topic of "Current Issues in Language Acquisition: Artificial and Statistical Language Learning." The question is whether the mechanisms that appear to subserve learning in simplified laboratory tasks are also operating "in the wild"; that is, given more naturalistic types of language input. Again, it is necessarily the case that infant language learners exploit cues beyond sequential statistics. Indeed, it may be the case that sequential statistics *help* learners to discover other cues in the input, which may be specific to an individual language and thus require some initial learning. For example, infants in a word segmentation task can use transitional probability statistics to discover an additional word boundary cue in the input, even one that is entirely novel, which can then be used for subsequent segmentation (e.g., Sahni, Seidenberg, & Seidenberg, 2009).

Across several lines of research, we have begun to ask whether statistical learning in these artificial tasks translates into actual language learning skill. We know that infants do appear to be sensitive to natural language statistics, at least in some limited domains. For example, infants are known to track phonotactic probability information in their native language: the likelihood that certain phonemes will co-occur in particular positions within a word (Friederici & Wessels, 1993; Jusczyk, Friederici, Wessels, & Svenkerud, 1993; Jusczyk, Luce, & Charles-Luce, 1994). Laboratory tasks have demonstrated that infants can make use of these phonotactic probabilities when segmenting novel words from fluent speech (Mattys & Jusczyk, 2001; Mattys, Jusczyk, Luce, & Morgan, 1999) and when mapping novel labels to objects (Graf Estes, Edwards, & Saffran, 2009). Do artificial language statistics operate in a similar way?

To date, we have pursued three different approaches to this question. The first approach has involved experiments in which we ask whether the "words" from our artificial speech streams are treated in a word-like fashion by infants. For example, 8-month-old infants appear to integrate the nonsense words from our speech streams into English test sentences

(Saffran, 2001b). In related work, we found that 18-month-olds more readily mapped these nonsense words to novel meanings (objects) than part-words, which violated the statistics of the artificial speech stream (Graf Estes, Evans, Alibali, & Saffran, 2007). Infants can also go from segmentation to syntax, first finding nonsense words in fluent speech and then learning about their order, as required for natural language learning (Saffran & Wilson, 2003). Across all these studies, the results support the hypothesis that infants are doing the very things with these sound sequences that we would expect infants acquiring language to do.

The second line of research is focused on individual differences in natural language acquisition. Approximately 5%–10% of elementary school-aged children are diagnosed with specific language impairment (SLI): despite nonverbal IQ in the normal range, their language skills lag significantly behind their peers. We hypothesized that if individual differences in statistical learning abilities are related to the emergence of SLI, individuals with SLI should find our artificial tasks more challenging than an age- and nonverbal IQ-matched comparison group (Evans, Saffran, & Robe-Torres, 2009). We compared two groups of grade-school children, those with a diagnosis of SLI and those with age-appropriate language skills, on an incidental artificial language word segmentation task previously used with children (Saffran et al., 1997). As predicted, the children with SLI evinced poorer performance on this task, though they caught up with additional exposure. Interestingly, given the language focus of this diagnosis, the children with SLI also performed more poorly than comparison children on an analogous statistical learning task using nonlinguistic tone sequences (Saffran, Johnson, Aslin, & Newport, 1999). Thus, school-aged children with a diagnosed language disorder found both linguistic and nonlinguistic statistical learning tasks particularly challenging. This finding is consistent with prior research testing adolescents with SLI on a different nonlinguistic implicit learning task, visual serial reaction time (Tomblin, Mainela-Arnold, & Zhang, 2007). Moreover, we found that even within our typical sample, performance on the artificial language task was correlated with standardized measures of English vocabulary, providing an additional link between statistical learning skill and native language proficiency (Evans et al., 2009).

The third source of evidence required us to move away from artificial language methodologies. To what extent is statistical learning performance tied to the use of these highly unnatural structures? The statistical learning studies performed in our laboratory and elsewhere typically entail speech that is monotone, isochronous (that is, devoid of variations in rhythm), and synthesized. We have manipulated these features to some extent, but always within the purview of artificially devised systems. For example, we manipulated the pitches of our artificial speech streams to mimic infant-directed pitch contours versus adult-directed pitch contours; the results suggested that statistical learning was facilitated by the expansive pitch contours of infant-directed speech, likely due to enhanced attention (Thiessen et al., 2005). Related work suggests that infants show better memory for sung word sequences than for spoken word sequences (Thiessen & Saffran, 2009). Multiple studies have also examined the interaction between sequential statistics and lexical stress cues in artificial language segmentation tasks, showing that the importance of sequential statistical cues varies as a function of the availability of other cues and the age of the learner (e.g., Johnson & Jusczyk, 2001; Thiessen & Saffran, 2003). We have also used natural speech produced like a synthesizer in various studies (e.g., Graf Estes et al., 2007). However, these studies all used artificial languages, in the sense that the words are nonsense and the materials were created without all the variability inherent in natural speech. Can infants make use of statistics in *natural* language segmentation tasks?

We are currently addressing this question using a hybrid natural/artificial language design, in which the materials are spoken naturally and the words are all from Italian, but the words were chosen to exemplify specific statistical distributions (Pelucchi, Hay, & Saffran, 2009). In this study, 8-month-old infants were exposed to sentences produced by a native Italian speaker, with natural infant-directed prosody. Critically, the sentences were carefully designed to contain: (1) target words that contained high-probability syllable sequences (relative to the exposure corpus) and (2) foil words that occurred equally often but which contained low-probability syllable sequences. Importantly, unlike our prior studies, these materials were naturally produced, with all the variability inherent in Italian speech—which is of course foreign to our monolingual Wisconsin infants. Nevertheless, infants successfully discriminated the target words from novel Italian words, replicating Jusczyk and Aslin's (1995) seminal study with a cross-language design (English learners, Italian speech). Most germane to the issue of statistical learning in natural languages, infants also successfully discriminated the high-probability target words from low-probability foil words, despite the fact that both types of words occurred equally often in the speech stream. These results provide a conceptual replication of the infant results from the artificial language learning literature, but with natural language materials. We can now continue on to examine how other cues (e.g., lexical stress) interact with sequential statistical cues in natural language segmentation tasks.

What is Statistical Learning, and What Statistical Learning is Not: Looking Ahead

The answer to the question of what statistical learning is and what it is not remains in the eye of the beholder. Empirical results are rapidly rolling in, and these should serve to disambiguate the myriad views concerning these learning mechanisms. If one thing is clear, it is this: statistical learning is not just a single computation over a single set of primitives. Learners, including infants, appear to be capable of tracking multiple levels of regularities in complex input. Some of these regularities are the types of sequential patterns we traditionally think of as "statistical"; others are still statistical, but are more correlational (e.g., phonological regularities, such as placement of stress cues as a function of syllable position within a word). Infants can make use of such regularities on-line and given natural language input.

Is this interest in statistical learning an indicator of the return of flat-earth empiricism? The answer, we believe, is very much no. In order to make use of all of this information, infants must come to the task of language learning with learning mechanisms that are "factory-installed"; such learning is likely part and parcel of neural systems. In this sense, these mechanisms—including both statistical learning mechanisms and other types of learning mechanisms—are innate. Rather than a nativism of specific knowledge, however, this claim concerns the nativism of learning mechanisms, including categorization abilities and perceptual systems that are a good fit to incoming linguistic information. Notably, the linguistic information may be structured to provide this good fit. Human learning abilities potentially play a role in structuring human languages, as suggested by studies contrasting the acquisition of possible versus impossible languages, and human versus nonhuman learners (e.g., Newport & Aslin, 2004; Newport, Hauser, Spaepen, & Aslin, 2004; Saffran, 2002, 2003; Saffran et al., 2008; Saffran & Thiessen, 2003). To the extent that this is the case, we might expect learning mechanisms to operate over stimuli that are not solely linguistic, but which are similarly structured across important stimulus attributes (e.g., Kelly & Martin, 1994; Kirkham, this volume; Kirkham, Slemmer, & Johnson, 2002; Saffran et al., 1999; Saffran, Pollak, Seibel, & Shkolnik, 2007; Saffran & Thiessen, 2007).

To better address these issues, I would expect future research to focus on a few specific questions. One is the nature of generalization. Under which circumstances do infants generalize, and what data do infants take as relevant for their generalizations (for two recent elegant examples, see Gerken, 2004, 2006). A related question concerns categorization: when do infants group linguistic elements into categories, and what kinds of computations can be performed across these categories? Dynamic learning systems should cascade, such that the output of one learning process serves as input to another—or to itself. Exciting new work has begun to focus on how these newly identified learning processes work together in this fashion (for a recent review, see Gómez, 2006; this volume).

I would also anticipate continued interest in studying individual differences in statistical learning processes, both as a way to better understand how typical learning unfolds and to examine potential causes for language delays and disorders. There have been numerous recent studies that have taken a longitudinal approach, predicting native language outcomes from language learning and processing tasks in infancy (Fernald, Perfors, & Marchman, 2006; Newman, Bernstein Ratner, A. M. Jusczyk, P. W. Jusczyk, & Dow, 2006; Tsao, Liu, & Kuhl, 2004). These, in concert with emerging studies using language-disordered children and adults (Evans et al., 2009; Plante, Gomez, & Gerken, 2002; Tomblin et al., 2007), hold great potential for uncovering the manner in which language learning actually unfolds across development, and, eventually, possible hope for novel interventions that target the learning process.

Acknowledgments

Preparation of this manuscript was supported by a grant to J.R.S. from NICHD (R01HD37466). I am grateful to Julia Evans, Katie Graf Estes, Jessica Hay, Bruna Pelucchi, Alexa Romberg, Sarah Sahni, and the members of the UW-Madison Infant Learning Lab for many helpful discussions about these issues.

References

Allen, J., & Seidenberg, M. S. (1999). *The emergence of grammaticality in connectionist networks.* Mahwah, NJ: Lawrence Erlbaum Associates.

Allen, R., & Reber, A. S. (1980). Very long term memory for tacit knowledge. *Cognition, 8*(2), 175–185.

Altmann, G. T. M. (2002). Statistical learning in infants. *Proceedings of the National Academy of Sciences USA, 99*(24), 15250–15251.

Altmann, G. T. M. (2004). Language-mediated eye movements in the absence of a visual world: The 'blank screen paradigm'. *Cognition, 93*(2), B79–B87.

Altmann, G. T. M., & Kamide, Y. (1999). Incremental interpretation at verbs: Restricting the domain of subsequent reference. *Cognition, 73*(3), 247–264.

Aslin, R. N., Saffran, J. R., & Newport, E. L. (1998). Computation of conditional probability statistics by 8-month-old infants. *Psychological Science, 9,* 321–324.

Bates, E., & Elman, J. (1996). Learning rediscovered. *Science, 274*(5294), 1849–1850.

Bloomfield, L. (1933). *Language.* New York: Holt.

Bortfeld, H., Morgan, J. L., Golinkoff, R. M., & Rathbun, K. (2005). Mommy and me: Familiar names help launch babies into speech-stream segmentation. *Psychological Science, 16*(4), 298–304.

Braine, M. D. S. (1987). What is learned in acquiring word classes—A step toward an acquisition theory. In B. MacWhinney (Ed.), *Mechanisms of language acquisition* (pp. 65–87). Hillsdale, NJ: Lawrence Erlbaum.

Brown, R., & Hanlon, C. (1970). Derivational complexity and order of acquisition in child speech. In J. R. Hayes (Ed.), *Cognition and the development of language* (pp. 11–54). New York: Wiley.

Canfield, R. L., & Haith, M. M. (1991). Young infants' visual expectations for symmetric and asymmetric stimulus sequences. *Developmental Psychology, 27,* 198–208.

Canfield, R. L., Smith, E. G., Brezsnyak, M. P., & Snow, K. L. (1997). Information processing through the first year of life: a longitudinal study using the visual expectation paradigm. *Monographs of the Society for Research in Child Development, 62*(2), 1–145.

Charniak, E. (1993). *Statistical language learning.* Cambridge, MA: MIT Press.

Chater, N., & Redington, M. (1999). Connectionism, theories of learning, and syntax acquisition: Where do we stand? *Journal of Child Language, 26*(1), 226–232.

Chomsky, N. (1959). Review of B. F. Skinner's *Verbal learning. Language,* 35, 26–58.

Christiansen, M. H., & Curtin, S. (1999). Transfer of learning: Rule acquisition or statistical learning? *Trends in Cognitive Sciences, 3*(8), 289–290.

Curtin, S., Mintz, T. H., Byrd, D., Do, A. H. J., Dominguez, L., & Johansen, A. (2001). Coarticulatory cues enhance infants' recognition of syllable sequences in speech. *Proceedings of the Boston University Conference on Language Development*. Somerville, MA: Cascadilla Press.

Curtin, S., Mintz, T. H., & Christiansen, M. H. (2005). Stress changes the representational landscape: Evidence from word segmentation. *Cognition, 96*(3), 233–262.

Cutler, A., & Carter, D. M. (1987). The predominance of strong initial syllables in the English vocabulary. *Computer Speech and Language, 2*, 133–142.

Dahan, D., Swingley, D., Tanenhaus, M. K., & Magnuson, J. S. (2000). Linguistic gender and spoken-word recognition in French. *Journal of Memory and Language, 42*(4), 465–480.

DeLong, K. A., Urbach, T. P., & Kutas, M. (2005). Probabilistic word pre-activation during language comprehension inferred from electrical brain activity. *Nature Neuroscience, 8*(8), 1117–1121.

Elman, J. L. (1990). Finding structure in time. *Cognitive Science, 14*(2), 179–211.

Evans, J., Saffran, J. R., & Robe-Torres, K. (2009). Statistical learning in children with Specific Language Impairments. *Journal of Speech, Language, & Hearing Research, 52*, 321–335.

Fernald, A., Perfors, A., & Marchman, V. A. (2006). Picking up speed in understanding: Speech processing efficiency and vocabulary growth across the 2nd year. *Developmental Psychology, 42*(1), 98–116.

Friederici, A. D., & Wessels, J. M. (1993). Phonotactic knowledge of word boundaries and its use in infant speech perception. *Perception & Psychophysics, 54*(3), 287–295.

Gallistel, C. R. (1990). *The organization of learning*. Cambridge, MA: MIT Press.

Gerken, L. (2004). Nine-month-olds extract structural principles required for natural language. *Cognition, 93*(3), B89–B96.

Gerken, L. (2006). Decisions, decisions: Infant language learning when multiple generalizations are possible. *Cognition, 98*(3), B67–B74.

Gerken, L., Wilson, R., & Lewis, W. (2005). Infants can use distributional cues to form syntactic categories. *Journal of Child Language, 32*(2), 249–268.

Goldstein, M. H., King, A. P., & West, M. J. (2003). Social interaction shapes babbling: Testing parallels between birdsong and speech. *Proceedings of the National Academy of Science USA, 100*(13), 8030–8035.

Gomez, R. (2002). Variability and detection of invariant structure. *Psychological Science, 13*(5), 431–436.

Gómez, R. (2006). Dynamically guided learning. In Y. Munakata & M. H. Johnson (Eds.), *Processes of change in brain and cognitive development: Attention and performance XXI*. Oxford: University Press.

Gomez, R. L., & Gerken, L. (2000). Infant artificial language learning and language acquisition. *Trends in Cognitive Science, 4*(5), 178–186.

Gomez, R. L., & Lakusta, L. (2004). A first step in form-based category abstraction by 12-month-old infants. *Developmental Science, 7*(5), 567–580.

Goodsitt, J. V., Morgan, J. L., & Kuhl, P. K. (1993). Perceptual strategies in prelingual speech segmentation. *Journal of Child Language, 20*(2), 229–252.

Graf Estes, K., Edwards, J., & Saffran, J. R. (2009). Phonotactic constraints on infant word learning. Manuscript submitted for editorial review.

Graf Estes, K., Evans, J. L., Alibali, M. W., & Saffran, J. R. (2007). Can infants map meaning to newly segmented words? Statistical segmentation and word learning. *Psychological Science, 18*(3), 254–260.

Haith, M. M., Hazan, C., & Goodman, G. S. (1988). Expectation and anticipation of dynamic visual events by 3.5-month-old babies. *Child Development, 59*(2), 467–479.

Haith, M. M., Wass, T. S., & Adler, S. A. (1997). Infant visual expectations: Advances and issues. *Monographs of the Society for Research in Child Development, 62*(2), 150–160.

Harris, Z. S. (1951). *Methods in structural linguistics*. Chicago: University of Chicago Press.

Hauser, M. D., Newport, E. L., & Aslin, R. N. (2001). Segmentation of the speech stream in a non-human primate: statistical learning in cotton-top tamarins. *Cognition, 78*(3), B53–B64.

Johnson, E. K., & Jusczyk, P. W. (2001). Word segmentation by 8-month-olds: When speech cues count more than statistics. *Journal of Memory and Language, 44*(4), 548–567.

Johnson, S. P., Amso, D., & Slemmer, J. A. (2003). Development of object concepts in infancy: Evidence for early learning in an eye-tracking paradigm. *Proceedings of the National Academy of Sciences, 100*(18), 10568–10573.

Jusczyk, P. W. (1999). How infants begin to extract words from speech. *Trends in Cognitive Science, 3*(9), 323–328.

Jusczyk, P. W., & Aslin, R. N. (1995). Infants' detection of the sound patterns of words in fluent speech. *Cognitive Psychology, 29*, 1–23.

Jusczyk, P. W., Friederici, A. D., Wessels, J. M., & Svenkerud, V. Y. (1993). Infants' sensitivity to the sound patterns of native language words. *Journal of Memory and Language, 32*(3), 402–420.

Jusczyk, P. W., Houston, D. M., & Newsome, M. (1999). The beginnings of word segmentation in English-learning infants. *Cognitive Psychology, 39*(3–4), 159–207.

Jusczyk, P. W., Luce, P. A., & Charles-Luce, J. (1994). Infants' sensitivity to phonotactic patterns in the native language. *Journal of Memory and Language, 33*(5), 630–645.

Kamide, Y., Altmann, G. T. M., & Haywood, S. L. (2003). The time-course of prediction in incremental sentence processing: Evidence from anticipatory eye movements. *Journal of Memory and Language, 49*(1), 133–159.

Kaschak, M. P., & Saffran, J. R. (2006). Idiomatic syntactic constructions and language learning. *Cognitive Science, 30*(1), 43–63.

Kelly, M. H., & Martin, S. (1994). Domain-general abilities applied to domain-specific tasks: Sensitivity to probabilities in perception, cognition, and language. *Lingua, 92*, 105–140.

Kirkham, N. Z., Slemmer, J. A., & Johnson, S. P. (2002). Visual statistical learning in infancy: Evidence for a domain general learning mechanism. *Cognition, 83*(2), B35–B42.

Kuhl, P. K. (2007). Is speech learning 'gated' by the social brain? *Developmental Science, 10*(1), 110–120.

Kuhl, P. K., Tsao, F. M., & Liu, H. M. (2003). Foreign-language experience in infancy: Effects of short-term exposure and social interaction on phonetic learning. *Proceedings of the National Academy of Sciences, 100*(15), 9096–9101.

Lany, J., Gomez, R. L., & Gerken, L. (2007). The role of prior experience in language acquisition. *Cognitive Science, 31*(3), 481–507.

Lew-Williams, C., & Fernald, A. (2007). Young children learning Spanish make rapid use of grammatical gender in spoken word recognition. *Psychological Science, 18*(3), 193–198.

MacDonald, M. C., & Seidenberg, M. S. (Eds.). (2006). *Constraint satisfaction accounts of lexical and sentence comprehension*. London: Elsevier.

Marcus, G. F. (1993). Negative evidence in language acquisition. *Cognition, 46*(1), 53–85.

Marcus, G. F. (1999a). Connectionism: With or without rules? Response to J.L. McClelland and D.C. Plaut (1999). *Trends in Cognitive Sciences, 3*(5), 168–170.

Marcus, G. F. (1999b). Reply to Seidenberg and Elman. *Trends in Cognitive Sciences, 3*(8), 289–289.

Marcus, G. F. (2000). Pabiku and Ga Ti Ga: Two mechanisms infants use to learn about the world. *Current Directions in Psychological Science, 9*(5), 145–147.

Marcus, G. F. (2001). *The algebraic mind: Integrating connectionism and cognitive science*. Cambridge, MA: The MIT Press.

Marcus, G. F., & Berent, I. (2003). Are there limits to statistical learning? *Science, 300*(5616), 53–55.

Mattys, S. L., & Jusczyk, P. W. (2001). Phonotactic cues for segmentation of fluent speech by infants. *Cognition, 78*(2), 91–121.

Mattys, S. L., Jusczyk, P. W., Luce, P. A., & Morgan, J. L. (1999). Phonotactic and prosodic effects on word segmentation in infants. *Cognitive Psychology, 38*(4), 465–494.

Maye, J., Werker, J. F., & Gerken, L. (2002). Infant sensitivity to distributional information can affect phonetic discrimination. *Cognition, 82*(3), B101–B111.

McClelland, J. L., McClelland, J. L., & Plaut, D. C. (1999). Does generalization in infant learning implicate abstract algebra-like rules? *Trends in Cognitive Sciences, 3*(5), 166.

McMurray, B., & Aslin, R. N. (2004). Anticipatory eye movements reveal infants' auditory and visual categories. *Infancy, 6*(2), 203–229.

Mintz, T. H. (2002). Category induction from distributional cues in an artificial language. *Memory & Cognition, 30*(5), 678–686.

Mintz, T. H., Newport, E. L., & Bever, T. G. (2002). The distributional structure of grammatical categories in speech to young children. *Cognitive Science, 26*(4), 393–424.

Moeser, S. D., & Bregman, A. S. (1973). Imagery and language acquisition. *Journal of Verbal Learning and Verbal Behavior, 12*, 91–98.

Morgan, J. L., Meier, R. P., & Newport, E. L. (1987). Structural packaging in the input to language learning: Contributions of prosodic and morphological marking of phrases to the acquisition of language. *Cognitive Psychology, 19*(4), 498–550.

Morgan, J. L., Meier, R. P., & Newport, E. L. (1989). Facilitating the acquisition of syntax with cross-sentential cues to phrase structure. *Journal of Memory and Language, 28*(3), 360–374.

Morgan, J. L., & Newport, E. L. (1981). The role of constituent structure in the induction of an artificial language. *Journal of Verbal Learning & Verbal Behavior, 20*(1), 67–85.

Morgan, J. L., & Travis, L. L. (1989). Limits on negative information in language input. *Journal of Child Language, 16*, 531–552.

Newman, R., Bernstein Ratner, N., Jusczyk, A. M., Jusczyk, P. W., & Dow, K. A. (2006). Infants' early ability to segment the conversational speech signal predicts later language development: A retrospective analysis. *Developmental Psychology, 42*(4), 643–655.

Newport, E. L., & Aslin, R. N. (2004). Learning at a distance I: Statistical learning of non-adjacent dependencies. *Cognitive Psychology, 48*(2), 127–162.

Newport, E. L., Hauser, M. D., Spaepen, G., & Aslin, R. N. (2004). Learning at a distance II: Statistical learning of non-adjacent dependencies in a non-human primate. *Cognitive Psychology, 49*(2), 85–117.

Pelucchi, B., Hay, J. F., & Saffran, J. R. (2009). Statistical learning in a natural language by 8-month-old infants. *Child Development*, manuscript in press.

Pena, M., Bonatti, L. L., Nespor, M., & Mehler, J. (2002). Signal-driven computations in speech processing. *Science, 298*(5593), 604.

Perruchet, P., & Pacton, S. (2006). Implicit learning and statistical learning: one phenomenon, two approaches. *Trends in Cognitive Science, 10*(5), 233–238.

Perruchet, P., Tyler, M. D., Galland, N., & Peereman, R. (2004). Learning nonadjacent dependencies: No need for algebraic-like computations. *Journal of Experimental Psychology—General, 133*(4), 573–583.

Pinker, S., & Prince, A. (1988). On language and connectionism: Analysis of a parallel distributed processing model of language acquisition. *Cognition, 28*(1), 73–193.

Plante, E., Gomez, R., & Gerken, L. (2002). Sensitivity to word order cues by normal and language/learning disabled adults. *Journal of Communicative Disorders, 35*(5), 453–462.

Reali, F., & Christiansen, M. H. (2005). Uncovering the richness of the stimulus: Structure dependence and indirect statistical evidence. *Cognitive Science, 29*(6), 1007–1028.

Reber, A. S. (1967). Implicit learning of artificial grammars. *Journal of Verbal Learning & Verbal Behavior, 6*, 855–863.

Reber, A. S. (1993). *Implicit learning and tacit knowledge: An essay on the cognitive unconscious.* New York: Oxford University Press.

Richardson, D. C., & Kirkham, N. Z. (2004). Multimodal events and moving locations: Eye movements of adults and 6-month-olds reveal dynamic spatial indexing. *Journal of Experimental Psychology: General, 133*(1), 46–62.

Rohde, D. L., & Plaut, D. C. (1999). Simple recurrent networks can distinguish non-occurring from ungrammatical sentences given appropriate task structure: Reply to Marcus. *Cognition, 73*(3), 297–300.

Romberg, A. R., & Saffran, J. R. (2009). Statistical regularities influence on-line processing in infancy. Manuscript under editorial review.

Rumelhart D. E., & McClelland J. L. (1986). On learning past tenses of English verbs. In McClelland, J. L. and Rumelhart, D. E. (Eds), *Parallel Distributed Processing: Vol. 2: Psychological and Biological Models.* Cambridge, MA: MIT Press.

Saffran, J. R. (2001a). The use of predictive dependencies in language learning. *Journal of Memory and Language, 44*(4), 493.

Saffran, J. R. (2001b). Words in a sea of sounds: the output of infant statistical learning. *Cognition, 81*(2), 149–169.

Saffran, J. R. (2002). Constraints on statistical language learning. *Journal of Memory and Language, 47*(1), 172–196.

Saffran, J. R. (2003). Statistical language learning: Mechanisms and constraints. *Current Directions in Psychological Science, 12*(4), 110–114.

Saffran, J. R. (submitted). Weighing their words: Infants track statistics in artificial grammars. Manuscript under editorial review.

Saffran, J. R., Aslin, R. N., & Newport, E. L. (1996). Statistical learning by 8-month-old infants. *Science, 274*(5294), 1926–1928.

Saffran, J. R., Hauser, M., Seibel, R., Kapfhamer, J., Tsao, F., & Cushman, F. (2008). Cross-species differences in the capacity to acquire language: Grammatical pattern learning by human infants and monkeys. *Cognition, 107*, 479–500.

Saffran, J. R., Johnson, E. K., Aslin, R. N., & Newport, E. L. (1999). Statistical learning of tone sequences by human infants and adults. *Cognition, 70*(1), 27–52.

Saffran, J. R., Newport, E. L., & Aslin, R. N. (1996). Word segmentation: The role of distributional cues. *Journal of Memory and Language, 35*(4), 606–621.

Saffran, J. R., Newport, E. L., Aslin, R. N., Tunick, R. A., & Barrueco, S. (1997). Incidental language learning: Listening (and learning) out of the corner of your ear. *Psychological Science, 8*(2), 101–105.

Saffran, J. R., Pollak, S. D., Seibel, R. L., & Shkolnik, A. (2007). Dog is a dog is a dog: Infant rule learning is not specific to language. *Cognition, 105,* 669–680.

Saffran, J. R., & Thiessen, E. D. (2003). Pattern induction by infant language learners. *Developmental Psychology, 39*(3), 484–494.

Saffran, J. R., & Thiessen, E. D. (2007). Domain-general learning capacities. In E. Hoff & M. Shatz (Eds.), *Blackwell handbook of language development.* (pp. 68–86). Malden, MA: Blackwell Publishing.

Saffran, J. R., Werker, J. F., & Werner, L. A. (2006). The infant's auditory world: Hearing, speech, and the beginnings of language. In D. Kuhn & R. S. Siegler (Eds.), *Handbook of child psychology: Vol. 2, Cognition, perception, and language* (6th ed., pp. 58–108). Hoboken, NJ: John Wiley & Sons.

Saffran, J. R., & Wilson, D. P. (2003). From syllables to syntax: Multilevel statistical learning by 12-month-old infants. *Infancy, 4*(2), 273–284.

Sahni, S. D., Seidenberg, M. S., & Saffran, J. R. (2009). Connecting cues: Overlapping regularities support cue discovery in infancy. Manuscript submitted for publication.

Seidenberg, M. S., & Elman, J. L. (1999). Networks are not 'hidden rules.' *Trends in Cognitive Sciences, 3*(8), 288–289.

Seidenberg, M. S., & MacDonald, M. C. (2001). *Constraint satisfaction in language acquisition and processing.* Westport, CT: Ablex Publishing.

Seidenberg, M. S., MacDonald, M. C., & Saffran, J. R. (2002). Does grammar start where statistics stop? *Science, 298*, 553–554.

Smith, K. H. (1966). Grammatical intrusions in the recall of structured letter pairs: Mediated transfer or position learning? *Journal of Experimental Psychology, 72*, 580–588.

Spivey-Knowlton, M., & Saffran, J. R. (1995). *Inducing a grammar without an explicit teacher: Incremental distributed prediction feedback.* In Proceedings of the 17th Annual Conference of the Cognitive Science Society. Hillsdale, NJ: Erlbaum.

Swingley, D. (2005). Statistical clustering and the contents of the infant vocabulary. *Cognitive Psychology, 50*(1), 86–132.

Thiessen, E. D., Hill, E. A., & Saffran, J. R. (2005). Infant-directed speech facilitates word segmentation. *Infancy, 7*(1), 53–71.

Thiessen, E. D., & Saffran, J. R. (2003). When cues collide: Use of stress and statistical cues to word boundaries by 7- to 9-month-old infants. *Developmental Psychology, 39*(4), 706–716.

Thiessen, E. D., & Saffran, J. R. (2007). Learning to learn: Infants' acquisition of stress-based strategies for word segmentation. *Language Learning and Development, 3*(1), 73–100.

Thiessen, E. D., & Saffran, J. R. (2009). How the melody facilitates the message, and vice versa, in infant learning and memory. *Proceedings of the New York Academy of Sciences,* manuscript in press.

Thompson, S. P., & Newport, E. L. (2007). Statistical learning of syntax: The role of transitional probability. *Language Learning and Development, 3*(1), 1–42.

Tomblin, J. B., Mainela-Arnold, E., & Zhang, X. (2007). Procedural learning in adolescents with and without specific language impairment. *Language Learning and Development, 3,* 269–293.

Tsao, F.-M., Liu, H.-M., & Kuhl, P. K. (2004). Speech perception in infancy predicts language development in the second year of life: A longitudinal study. *Child Development, 75*(4), 1067–1084.

Vallabha, G. K., McClelland, J. L., Pons, F., Werker, J. F., & Amano, S. (2007). Unsupervised learning of vowel categories from infant-directed speech. *Proceedings of the National Academy of Sciences USA, 104*(33), 13273–13278.

von Hofsten, C., Vishton, P., Spelke, E. S., Feng, Q., & Rosander, K. (1998). Predictive action in infancy: Tracking and reaching for moving objects. *Cognition, 67*(3), 255–285.

Werker, J. F., Pons, F., Dietrich, C., Kajikawa, S., Fais, L., & Amano, S. (2007). Infant-directed speech supports phonetic category learning in English and Japanese. *Cognition, 103*(1), 147–162.

Yang, C. (2004). Universal grammar, statistics, or both. *Trends in Cognitive Sciences*, 451–456.

CHAPTER 10
Processing Constraints on Learning

Rebecca Gómez

If research on infant cognition has taught us anything it is that very young infants are equipped with precocious abilities, ranging from their capacity to reason about physical events in the world (Baillargeon, 1987; Kellman & Spelke, 1983; Xu & Garcia, 2008), to their understanding of and ability to make inferences based on number (McCrink & Wynn, 2007; Wynn, 1992; Xu & Garcia, 2008) to their rational ability to attribute goals to agents (Bíró, Csibra, & Gergely, 2007; Gergely, Nádasdy, Csibra, & Bíró 1999) and in their understanding of intentions of others (Woodward, 2005). In the beginning of infancy work, the early onset of an ability was often associated with innately given expectations or constraints, but with increased study on what develops the picture is changing. For instance, the finding that infants can perceive the persistence of partly occluded objects at 4months of age was initially taken as evidence for innate knowledge of principles governing objects (Kellman & Spelke, 1983). However, research since then shows that the ability to perceive the unity of occluded objects is experientially driven (Johnson, Davidow, Hall-Haro, & Frank, 2008) and develops over time (e.g., Johnson & Aslin, 1995; Johnson et al., 2003). Thus, if there is a lesson to be learned, it is that the question of what develops is a complicated one. Determining the abilities with which infants come equipped, their mechanisms for obtaining and retaining knowledge, and whether and how these abilities change as a function of development is a challenging problem.

As with work on object perception, there has been a spate of recent work suggesting that infants are extremely facile learners (e.g., Gómez & Gerken, 2000; Kirkham, Slemmer, & Johnson, 2002; Saffran, Aslin, & Newport, 1996a). Though the evidence is persuasive, the story is not simple. Showing that infants are fast learners is an initial step, but we need to know more about the mechanics of learning. Challenges have to do with determining how learning is constrained—how learners home in on the "right" information, whether they can do so under noisy learning conditions, and how they build on prior knowledge to generalize to more complex forms. We also need to understand how learners use memory in generalizing to cases that are similar, but not identical, to previous learning experiences.

To this end, I will discuss three types of processing constraints on learning. The first type of constraint arises from the learning process itself. The other two constraints arise from two naturally occurring memory processes: consolidation and reconsolidation. With respect to learning constraints, I will discuss research from my laboratory suggesting that learning is a dynamically guided process, arising in the interaction of internal and external pressures, and one that is fairly robust with respect to noisy input. Moreover, learners, and the structure they can acquire, change as a function of experience. With respect to memory processes instrumental in learning, one set of findings I will describe demonstrates a type of memory consolidation occurring with sleep, one that results in generalization to novel cases. Another set of findings demonstrates how the process of memory reconsolidation enables memory change. Both memory processes are important for understanding how children sustain sensitivity to prior knowledge while incorporating new information. In contrast to "knowledge" constraints traditionally proposed in the literature on development and learning, the constraints discussed here arise naturally from the mechanics of learning and memory processes themselves.

Constraints Arising from the Learning Process

Choosing among Multiple Possibilities

A particularly vexing problem has to do with how infants choose among multiple types of structure. One proposal is that learners are constrained to prefer certain kinds of information over others. Although such biases may exist, it would be a mistake to ignore other constraints on the learning process, including information in the environment itself, or the possibility that learning may arise in the interaction of the joint pressures from internal *and* external constraints. For instance, there is good reason to think that the ability to track dependencies between adjacent elements in sequential structure may be a default in learning (adjacent dependencies hold between elements that occur next to each other in sequence, for example, in the sentence "The boy jumped off the rock," the words "The boy" and "boy jumped"). Many different species can track adjacent dependencies, including humans, nonhuman primates, birds, and rats (Christie & Dalrymple-Alford, 2004; Hauser, Newport, & Aslin, 2001; Terrace, Chen, & Jaswal, 1996; Terrace, Son, & Brannon, 2003; Toro & Trobalón, 2005). Adjacent dependencies are learned easily by infants and by adults (Saffran et al., 1996a; Saffran, Newport, & Aslin, 1996b). They also appear to be learned incidentally when their presentation is secondary to a primary task (Saffran, Newport, Aslin, Tunick, & Barrueco, 1997). However, immediate sequential dependencies are not the only ones language learners must acquire. Many dependencies occur across longer distances, especially in language. Some examples are dependencies between auxiliaries and inflectional morphemes (e.g., *is* quickly runn*ing*), and between nouns and verbs in number and tense agreement (The boy*s* in the tree *are* laughing). If the tendency to track adjacent structure is a default, what might tune learners into more remote dependencies in sequential structure such as those separated by intervening words?

My colleagues and I have investigated this question by familiarizing infants with an artificial language that can be learned only if infants detect nonadjacent dependencies (Gómez, 2002; Gómez & Maye, 2005). Infants were exposed to one of two versions of an artificial language and were tested with sentences from each language such that a grammatical sentence for one group of infants was ungrammatical for the other group (this two-version design is used in all of the artificial language studies discussed here). Version 1 sentences followed the patterns aXb or cXd (e.g., pel-wadim-jic, vot-kicey-rud). In Version 2, the relationship between the first and third elements was reversed such that pel sentences ended with rud, and vot sentences ended with jic (aXd : pel-wadim-rud, cXb: vot-kicey-jic) (see Figure 10.1). The a, b, c, d, and X elements were restricted to the same positions in the two languages and adjacent dependencies were identical (aX occurred in both languages as did Xd) so that sentences could only be distinguished by learning the relationships between the nonadjacent first and third words. We also manipulated the size of the pool from which the middle element was drawn (set-size = 3, 12, or 24) while holding frequency of exposure to the nonadjacent dependencies constant. The purpose of this manipulation was to determine whether high variability in the middle element would lead to better perception of nonadjacent dependencies even though these were equally frequent in all three set-size conditions. This manipulation captures a characteristic of

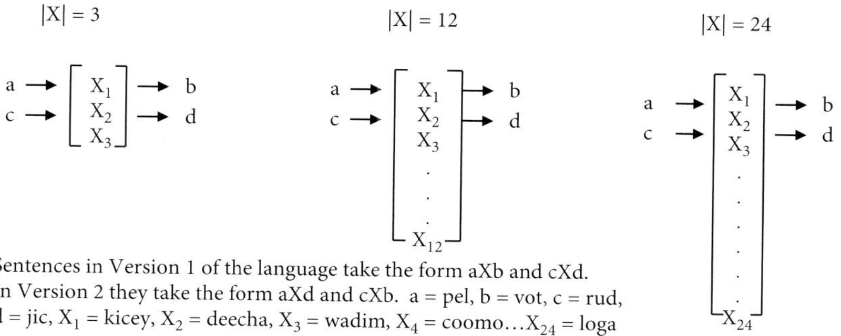

Figure 10.1 Depiction of the artificial language used in Gómez (2002) demonstrating the three variability conditions.

long-distance dependencies in natural language between frequent morphemes such as "is" and "-ing." These frequent morphemes occur in the context of verb stems that themselves belong to very large sets (e.g., "run" in "is running," "play" in "is playing," "sleep" in "is sleeping") potentially making the frequent morphemes more perceptible.

There were three possibilities for the outcome of this experiment according to three different learning models. In a statistics-driven model, learners could attend to multiple types of statistical information, weighing a type's importance by degree of statistical regularity. By this view, learners would be biased to track conditional probabilities between adjacent elements but learning should closely mirror the statistical probabilities in the stimulus set with learners increasingly more likely to track nonadjacent dependencies as conditional probabilities between adjacent elements decrease. Thus, this model predicts a monotonically increasing function such that nonadjacent dependency learning emerges gradually with increasing set size across the *X*-axis (and decreasing conditional probabilities).

In a constraints-driven model, learners will always attend more to a favored structure even if the less favored one has greater statistical certainty. This solution assumes no learning with our stimulus materials if learners have a tendency to stick to their bias of favoring conditional probabilities (because in our language knowledge of conditional probabilities will not distinguish the two versions of the language). Thus, the learning function will be flat with discrimination at chance.

A third possibility assumes some ordering of constraints in that conditional probabilities could be a default form of learning, but also that learners will only track a preferred structure to the extent that it occurs with some minimum degree of statistical certainty. Below that point, learners will track alternative sources of information. Although adjacent dependencies may have a more privileged status than nonadjacent ones (because of perceptual salience or ease of processing), statistical structure in the input plays a determining role in whether learners will focus on one type of structure or another. This model would predict a nonlinear function such that nonadjacent dependency learning does not emerge gradually with increasing set size, but instead emerges more abruptly. Figure 10.2 shows looking times to trained versus untrained strings after 3-min exposure to one of three variability conditions.

The results were consistent with the last proposed model, with learning occurring only under conditions of the greatest variability for infants and adults (see Gómez, 2002 and Gómez & Maye, 2005). One explanation for these findings is that learners focused on conditional probabilities between adjacent elements when these were relatively high (in the small set-size conditions), but when conditional probabilities between adjacent elements were sufficiently low (when set-size was 24) the adjacent dependencies

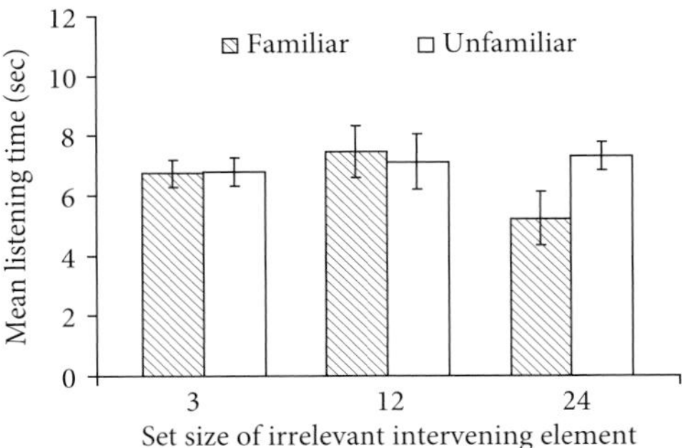

Figure 10.2 Mean listening times for 18-month-olds as a function of the variability manipulation from Gómez (2002). The middle word in the sentence comes from a set of 2, 6, or 24 possible elements. Discrimination only occurs in the set-size = 24 condition.

were no longer stable sources of structure, causing learners to instead track nonadjacent structure. Notably, learners did not show incremental increases in sensitivity to nonadjacent structure with incremental increases in variability of the middle element, a pattern we would expect if learners were responding primarily to the statistical structure. Instead, they seemed to focus on adjacent dependencies long after these ceased providing reliable information. In an experiment conducted with adults (where adults judged the acceptability of individual sentences and there were three nonadjacent dependencies to learn), the probability of the initial word being followed by a particular *X*-element was .33 (or 1 in 3) in a set-size 2 condition. This probability decreased to .17, .08, and .04 with set sizes of 6, 12, and 24, respectively. In contrast, in all conditions the probability of the initial element being followed by a third element was 1. If responses to changes in conditional probabilities had been veridical, we might have expected to see learning of nonadjacent structure in the set-size 6 condition (given the low conditional probability of .17). However, it was only after substantial variability was introduced in the middle element that learners appeared to rely on the nonadjacent structure (when set size was equal to 24). What appears to be critical for getting learners to notice the nonadjacent dependencies is sufficient variability in the middle element where what constitutes "sufficient" presumably varies as a function of the difficulty of the learning problem. In this way, the joint pressures of internal biases and external structure interact to result in dynamically guided learning. Thus, learning is constrained by the process itself without having to build in complex internal constraints for guiding the choices learners make.

Generalizing with Inconsistent Input

Consistent with the question of how learners choose among multiple possibilities in input is the issue of the degree to which children can learn in the face of inconsistent input. In the course of normal language acquisition, all children are exposed to inconsistencies of one type or another, in adults' informal speech, in children's own ungrammatical utterances, and in the ungrammatical utterances of other learners such as playmates and siblings. Inconsistencies also occur naturally in language, for instance, in English the degree to which verbs take the regular *-ed* ending for the past tense, or in Spanish the extent to which feminine nouns end in *-a*. Other instances of inconsistencies in linguistic input are less widespread, such as when a deaf child is exposed to American Sign Language through a hearing parent who has not achieved proficiency in this language and whose repertoire of grammatical forms is not only inconsistent, but limited. In all of these instances, children must distinguish grammatical from ungrammatical instances, and they must generalize beyond the data to which they are exposed, making it relevant to ask how well infants learn on exposure to inconsistent structure. This question is also important because critics of learning have cautioned that without strong internal constraints, learners would have no way to distinguish relevant from irrelevant structure and would acquire grammar indiscriminantly, even ungrammatical forms. But is this an issue of real concern?

Gómez and Lakusta (2004) investigated this question by familiarizing 12-month-olds with an artificial language with *aX* and *bY* strings (or *aY*/*bX* strings in Language 2). There were two each of the *a*- and *b*-words and 6 each of the *X*s

Language 1 (S→aXbY or bYaX)		Language 2 (S→bXaY or aYbX)	
a	**X**	**b**	**X**
ong	coomo	alt	coomo
erd	fengle	ush	fengle
	kicey		kicey
	loga		loga
	puser		puser
	wadim		wadim
b	**Y**	**a**	**Y**
alt	deech	ong	deech
ush	ghope	erd	ghope
	jic		jic
	skige		skige
	vabe		vabe
	tam		tam

Figure 10.3 Depiction of the Language 1 and Language 2 familiarization stimuli used in Gómez and Lakusta (2004). Sentences from Language 1 are ong-coomo ush-ghope, ush-jic erd-loga, alt-ghope ong-kicey, etc. Infants were tested on strings with new *X*- and *Y*-words to assess generalization.

and *Y*s, the latter of which were distinguishable by syllable number. Infants had to learn that *a*-elements went with *X*s and not *Y*s (and vice versa for *b*-elements). Three groups of infants were familiarized with one of three levels of probabilistic structure (see Figure 10.3). In a 100/0-condition, all of the training strings were from the infants' "predominant" training language. In this case, infants received strings of only the *aX* and *bY* forms. In an 83/17-condition, approximately 83% of the training strings were from the predominant *aX*/*bY* language, whereas the remaining 17% of the strings followed an *aY*/*bX* form such that one *Y*-word went with the two *a*-words as opposed the *b*s and an *X*-word went with the two *b*s as opposed to the *a*s. Thus these particular strings were inconsistent with the *aX*/*bY* structure. In the 67/33-condition, the split between the predominant and nonpredominant training languages was 67% and 33%. At test, infants had to discriminate strings from the predominant language with those from the nonpredominant one, but with novel *X*- and *Y*-elements to test generalization.

We were interested in knowing whether (a) infants could separate a predominant from a nonpredominant structure such that they would show learning in the presence of inconsistent input and (b) whether learning would break down at some point as it should if the predominant structure drops below a minimum level of predictability. As seen in the looking times

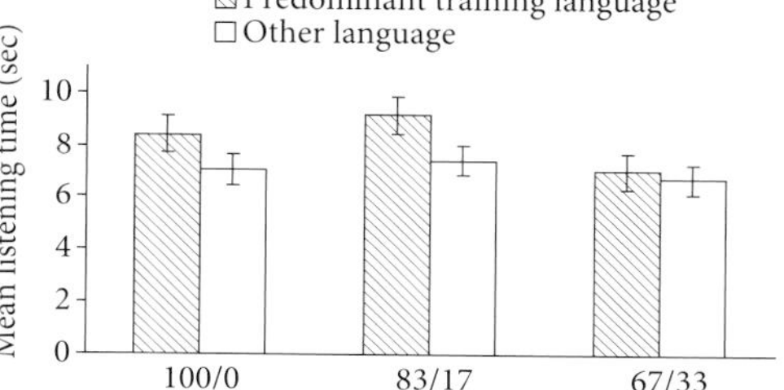

Figure 10.4 Mean listening times for 12-month-olds to novel test strings from the predominant or the nonpredominant familiarization language in one of three probability conditions in Gómez and Lakusta (2004). Infants show discrimination after familiarization with the 100/0 and 83/17 probability conditions.

shown in Figure 10.4, infants in the 100/0 and 83/17 conditions showed significant levels of learning and they learned equally well as reflected in longer looking times to strings instantiated in the predominant as opposed to the nonpredominant language, suggesting that they are able to track regularities in probabilistic input even when the regularities do not occur with perfect probability (as was the case with the 83/17 ratio). Thus fairly young infants appear able to track a regular structure even with some inconsistencies present. However, learning does need to be based on some minimum degree of consistency, as demonstrated by the fact that infants in the 67/33-condition failed to learn.

In sum, infants appear able to separate relevant from irrelevant structure, but such learning is dependent on the quality of the signal. Thus, learning appears to be constrained as a natural by-product in infants' processing of statistical structure.

Bootstrapping from Simpler to More Difficult Structure

A third way that learning is constrained by the learning process stems from prior learning. In the real world, and particularly during early development, learning is unlikely to result in an end state. Instead, learners encounter new examples with potential to build on, interfere with, or alter the type of generalizations they are able to make. Furthermore, the types of generalizations infants make are influenced by their prior experience. As such, it is important to begin to understand how prior knowledge supports or detracts from the learning of new or more complex forms.

There is precedent for the role of prior experience already in language acquisition in the work on infant speech perception showing that infants can discriminate speech sounds that occur in other languages early on in development but become more limited in the nonnative forms they can discriminate as they become more attuned to their native language input (Best, McRoberts, & Sithole, 1988; Polka & Werker, 1994; Werker & Tees, 1984). Presumably this change is a function of experience. Similar findings have been reported in the infant learning literature. Gerken and Bollt (2008) find that younger 7-month-olds are able to acquire an unnatural linguistic rule that older 9-month-olds cannot. Presumably increased tuning to the statistics of English helps older infants ignore unnatural generalizations in favor of linguistically natural ones. In this way, experience constrains the types of generalizations infants will make, but can prior experience also enable learning of forms that are normally too difficult to acquire?

Evidence for this comes from studies investigating how prior learning might bootstrap sensitivity to complex syntactic patterns, and specifically how prior learning impacts the acquisition of nonadjacent dependencies (Lany & Gómez, 2008). Infants in these studies were 12-month-olds who in previous studies have been unable to track nonadjacent structure (Gómez & Maye, 2005). Infants were familiarized with aX and bY strings, where *X*- and *Y*-elements were distinguishable by syllable number, and where infants had to learn that *a*-elements went with *X*s and not *Y*s (and vice versa for *b*-elements). After familiarization with the *aX*/*bY* structure infants were able to detect the *aX* and *bY* relationships in a more complex language involving long-distance dependencies (e.g., in *acX* and *bcY* sentences). See the results in Figure 10.5. This language was particularly challenging for this age group because the intervening *c*-element required the infants to track nonadjacent dependencies between *a*- and *X*- and *b*- and *Y*-words. A control group who did not receive prior experience with the simpler "adjacent" form of the language was not able to track the critical dependencies when they were nonadjacent. Thus, with prior exposure to simpler adjacent structure infants are able to detect the more difficult nonadjacent form. This finding is relevant for showing how infants might scaffold learning of more difficult structure from learning of more simple forms and for showing how prior experience can affect later learning. These findings also demonstrate how constraints can arise from the learning process itself, as opposed to being part of learners' knowledge beforehand.

In summary, the findings showing that (1) internal biases and external statistics interact to guide the choice of which structure is learned when multiple possibilities are available, (2) learning of a predominant form can persist in the face of inconsistent input but only to a point, and (3) prior experience can in some cases constrain and in others enable learning, are important for increasing our understanding of how learners negotiate complex statistical structure. They also shed light on how constraints and statistical structure both contribute to this process. Particularly important are the insights they provide into how the learning

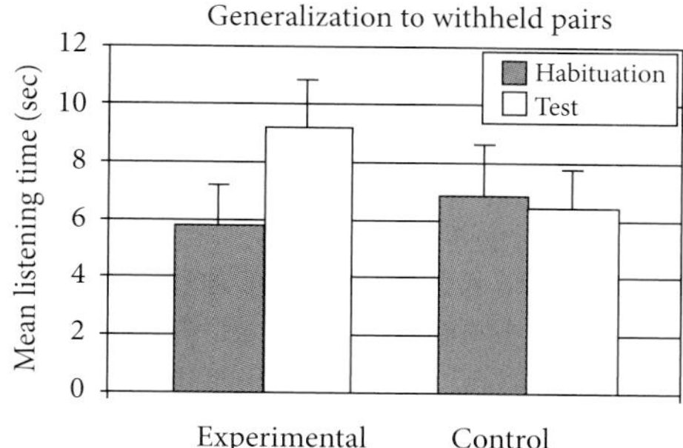

Figure 10.5 Twelve-month-olds' mean listening times to grammatical versus ungrammatical strings. Infants were familiarized with aX/bY (or aY/bX) phrases for which a subset of pairs were withheld. After habituation to acX/bcY (or acY/bcX) phrases, they were tested on phrases that were ungrammatical with respect to their familiarization language. From Lany and Gómez (submitted).

process itself constrains learning dynamically, such that learning arises in the interaction of preferences that may guide learning initially but that change in response to environmental pressure, in infants' ability to track predominant structure, and in the role of prior experience on constraining later learning. I will turn next to the role of memory in constraining children's generalizations.

The Role of Memory Processes in Constraining Learning

Most learning studies test performance immediately after training, but in fact newly encoded information undergoes a series of involuntary brain-dependent changes raising the possibility that what infants retain after memory consolidation is different in nature from what we see initially. Such changes include stabilization of the memory, enhancement of it, and integration of new information into what is already known. Thus, in addition to constraints that arise from the learning process itself, a second form of constraint arises in the transformation of new experiences into a more permanent form through a process of consolidation (or stabilization). Interestingly, although memories can stabilize across wake states, sleep is particularly instrumental in memory consolidation. Additionally, memories are updated with new information as a matter of course in learning. A candidate process for such updating is memory reconsolidation. Mounting evidence suggests that when memories are reactivated, they become labile and open to change. Retrieval can reinforce the reactivated memory, or update it through the incorporation of new information. Such transformed memories then undergo a time-dependent reconsolidation process. Although the idea that memories are malleable is not new in cognitive development (e.g., Loftus, 2005), the mechanism underlying such change has not been well understood. Work on memory reconsolidation has begun to define the critical determinants of episodic memory change and holds promise for identifying the conditions affecting the updating of prior knowledge in learning and cognitive development. Thus, memory consolidation and reconsolidation both have implications for constraining children's generalizations. These topics are addressed below.

Memory Consolidation

Memory consolidation is a process in which a newly formed memory trace is converted to a stable, less disruptable state over a period of days to years (McGaugh, 2000). In addition to stabilizing the memory, consolidation is thought to result in an enhancement of the remembered information in the form of greater accuracy and speed of execution, and better generalization. Memories are also thought to become more integrated with existing knowledge as a function of consolidation. Although there is evidence that memories become stabilized during wake states (Brashers-Krug, Shadmehr, & Bizzi, 1996, Muellbacher et al. 2002, Walker, Brakefield, Hobson, & Stickgold, 2003), memory enhancement appears to be a unique product of sleep (Fischer, Hallschmid, Elsner, & Born, 2002; Gais, Plihal, Wagner, & Born, 2000; Karni, Tanne, Rubenstein, Askenasy, & Sagi, 1994; Korman, Raz, Flash, & Karni, 2003; Stickgold, James, & Hobson, 2002a; Stickgold, Whidbee, Schirmer, Patel, & Hobson, 2002b; Walker et al. 2002a; Walker,

Brakefield, Hobson, & Stickgold, 2002b; Walker & Stickgold, 2006). Importantly, these improvements appear to arise from molecular, cellular, and systems-level processes that are specifically linked with sleep. For instance, there is some evidence that patterns of activation occurring during training reappear during rapid eye movement (REM) sleep (e.g., Maquet et al., 2000; Wilson & McNaughton, 1994; Euston, Tatsuno, & McNaughton, 2007) and immediate performance on a learning task can be shown to correlate with the magnitude of later brain activity during REM (Peigneux et al., 2003). While these findings suggest that brain activity during sleep is affected by training earlier in the day, brain activity during sleep also correlates with later memory performance and improvement, demonstrating a link not just between the original learning experience and sleep but also between sleep and memory consolidation as measured after sleep (Peigneux et al., 2004). The findings linking brain activity to earlier training, and brain activity to later consolidation, are important for ruling out explanations of memory stabilization and enhancement having to do with a decrease in sensory input (or a decrease in interference) during sleep.

How does sleep affect the consolidation of new learning? Research with adults shows that learners were faster and more accurate in tapping out a sequence with their fingers in a procedural learning task after sleep than before (Walker et al., 2003). Sleep also appears to be implicated in a type of memory consolidation that leads to generalization. Fenn, Nusbaum, and Margoliash (2003) found that adults were better able to recognize phonemes in new words after a night of sleep than after an equivalent interval of wake–time during the day. Learners were tested 12 h after training and either slept or not during this interval. Participants who did not sleep showed decreased levels of recognition whereas those who did sleep showed the same high levels of generalization on novel words as learners tested immediately after training. The time of day learning took place was not a factor. Groups who learned in the morning and in the evening had identical performance gains on novel words after a 24-h interval (during which both groups slept).

In addition to better performance and generalization, sleep has also been implicated in qualitative changes in memory having to do with gaining insight into a problem solution (Wagner, Gais, Haider, Verleger, & Born, 2004). Participants exposed to a problem that could be solved either in an iterative step-by-step fashion or according to a hidden rule were more likely to make the critical insight regarding the hidden rule after sleep than after an equivalent time awake. Two times as many of the participants in the sleep group detected the hidden rule as compared to the group who did not sleep, suggesting that sleep was implicated in a transformation in memory that made it easier for learners to discover the hidden rule. Sleep has also been implicated in memory transformations involving transitive inference of relations (Ellenbogen, Hu, Payne, Titone, & Walker, 2007), and learning of higher-order associations and their generalization (Cohen, Pascual-Leone, Press, & Robertson, 2005; Keele, Ivry, Mayr, Hazeltine, & Heuer, 2003; Spencer, Sunm, & Ivry, 2006). Ellenbogen et al. trained participants on visual stimuli of the form A>B (A precedes B), B>C, C>D, D>E, E>F then tested them for generalization to novel inference pairs (B>D, C>E, and B>E) after varying intervals that either did or did not contain sleep (20 min, 12 h wake, 12 h sleep, 24 h). Retention of the learned pairs was similarly high for all groups (85%), but generalization occurred only for groups tested 12 or more hours later, with sleep in the 12-h groups providing an additional boost for the most distant, and most difficult, inference pair (B>E, 69% wake, 93% sleep). Additionally, Cohen et al. (2005) found that transfer of goal-based versus movement-based skill in a serial reaction-time task improved differentially during wake and sleep with knowledge of movements themselves improving during wake and knowledge involving goals improving with sleep.

Although there is an established literature on patterns of infant sleep–wake states (Kleitman & Engelmann, 1953; Thoman, 1990), little is known about the role of sleep in infant learning with the exception that sleep–wake state organization is a predictor of cognitive development in infancy (Gertner et al., 2002), as well as the finding that sleep plays an instrumental role in brain development in animals (Frank, Issa, Stryker, & Keck, 2001). However, given the adult findings on the importance of sleep in memory consolidation, there is every reason to think that sleep is also implicated in infant memory. Indeed, recent research supports this view (Gómez, Bootzin, & Nadel, 2006).

In the first experiment designed to test the effects of sleep on learning, 15-month-old infants were exposed to a learning experience prior to a nap then were tested afterward. The infants were familiarized with the artificial language discussed in the first section on learning constraints detailed above. The artificial language required infants to track sequential dependencies between the first and third words in sentences such as pel-wadim-jic or vot-kicey-rud. Recall that previous research from our laboratory showed that the nonadjacent relationships between the first and third words are learned only when there is high variability in the middle position (created by selecting middle words from a large as opposed to a small set), making the flanking nonadjacent word-dependencies more salient perceptually (Gómez, 2002; Gómez & Maye, 2005). Because the two versions of the language were identical with respect to absolute position of words and dependencies between adjacent words, they can only be distinguished by noting the nonadjacent relationship between the first and third words. This feature of the language enabled us to ask whether sleep-enhanced memory of specific nonadjacent word-pairs (e.g. that pel predicted jic), or promoted learning of an abstract rule (that the first word predicts the last in an utterance, despite the specific words involved).

Infants were familiarized with the language in their homes by a research assistant who played the artificial language from a tape recorder while playing quietly with the infant. Familiarization lasted approximately 15 min. Infants were tested in the laboratory 4 h after familiarization. There were two groups of primary interest: infants who napped between familiarization and test and those who did not nap. Typically, infants this age look longer to familiar versus unfamiliar strings immediately after familiarization, reflecting memory of specific nonadjacent word-pairs (Gómez & Maye, 2005). However, if sleep induces a transformation in memory, infants might remember something more abstract involving a predictive relationship between the first and third words. If so, infants might show a preference for the nonadjacent word-pairs encountered on the first trial of the test even when they were not the exact nonadjacent words encountered earlier. If time alone plays a role in memory consolidation, infants in both the nap and no-nap groups should show the same pattern of effects. However, if sleep is the determining factor, then performance should differ between the two conditions. A nap-control group was also tested to determine whether sleep alone would alter learning. This group was exposed to the artificial language but the middle word came from a set of only three items, a condition that does not normally lead to nonadjacent dependency learning.

Infants were tested on sentences that both preserved the specific nonadjacent dependency encountered during familiarization and on sentences that contained violations of the specific nonadjacent dependency. The head-turn preference method was used to assess discrimination of the two stimulus types in the form of listening time differences (Kemler Nelson et al., 1995). The results are shown in Figure 10.6.

Infants in the no-nap group listened longer to familiar over unfamiliar trials consistent with veridical memory of specific nonadjacent word-pairs. In contrast, infants in the nap group listened longer to sentences consistent with the trial-type encountered on the first test trial, suggesting they had abstracted away from specific nonadjacent words such that they noticed particular nonadjacent dependencies on the first test trial (whether identical or not) and showed a greater tendency to listen to strings with the same nonadjacent dependencies in remaining trials. The control group showed no learning whatsoever, eliminating the possibility that sleep alone can alter memory apart from the learning manipulation.

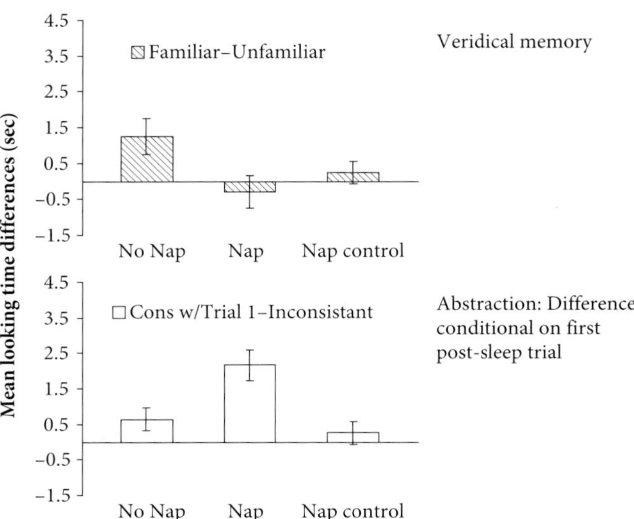

Figure 10.6 Fifteen-month-olds' mean listening times, 4 h after familiarization in Nap, No-Nap, and Nap-control conditions. Infants who napped in the interval between familiarization and test showed a significant difference on the abstraction measure. Infants who did not nap showed significant veridical memory. From Gómez, Bootzin, and Nadel (2006).

More recently, we have asked whether 15-month-olds need to nap fairly soon after learning or whether, like adults, any sleep later in the day will do (Hupbach, Gómez, Bootzin, & Nadel, in press). We familiarized two groups of infants with the artificial language used in Gómez (2002) and Gómez et al. (2006). One group was scheduled at a time of day when they were likely to nap in the 4-h interval after familiarization. Another group was scheduled when they were not likely to nap until at least 4 h later. Both groups were tested 24 h after familiarization. Thus, all infants slept during the night, but only the nap-group slept in the 4-h interval after familiarization. Interestingly, the nap group showed generalization 24 h later, whereas the no-nap group showed no learning of any kind. Thus, sleep fairly soon after a learning experience appears to be critical not only for memory retention, but for abstraction of the learned information.

These findings raise important questions about the role of sleep in memory change. For one, how do memories become more abstract? One possibility is that infants are sensitive to both specific and abstract information but weight these differentially before and after sleep. A second is that infants forget specific details of the stimulus with sleep. Although infants may indeed weight specific and abstract information differently immediately after learning, the idea that infants forget specific details of the stimulus with sleep seems more likely given that infants who did not sleep immediately after test showed no memory of the artificial language 24 h later.

Additionally, what kind of sleep is involved? Plihal and Born (1997) found that declarative learning in a paired-associates task was enhanced during slow-wave sleep (SWS) and procedural learning in a mirror-tracing task was linked with REM. It is not clear whether our artificial language studies engage declarative or procedural knowledge, however the naps of children this age contain components of both REM and SWS (Louis, Cannard, Bastuji, & Challamell, 1997). Thus, with testing of sleep architecture, it should be possible to determine which specific stage or stages of sleep are most involved.

Finally, the findings showing that sleep soon after learning is important for retention raises the question of when in childhood learning becomes less nap-dependent such that children, like adults (Gais et al., 2007), are able to consolidate memories with only nighttime sleep. It is tempting to assume that the rate at which children nap is sufficient and necessary for any given age, but differences in cultural practice and in individual families' schedules make it difficult to use existing napping norms to answer this question.

In sum, these findings suggest that the memory process itself is instrumental in constraining learning. In our particular studies, memory consolidation associated with sleep introduced flexibility into performance such that infants abstracted a pattern and detected it at test regardless of whether it was instantiated exactly as before. In this way, the process of memory consolidation gives rise to plasticity in learning by sustaining sensitivity to previously encountered information, while enabling children to generalize to similar but not identical cases. Memory change involving abstraction may be particularly important for developing infants who must retain key aspects of prior experience while generalizing in novel situations.

I turn next to the role of memory reconsolidation in learning, starting with a discussion of how the processes of memory consolidation and reconsolidation differ.

Memory Reconsolidation

Memory consolidation is a process that stabilizes a new memory trace. There are changes in the brain structures critical for memory storage and/or retrieval at both cellular and systems levels. At the cellular level, there are changes in synaptic efficacy and at the systems level, there are thought to be changes in memory expression such that it is no longer dependent on the hippocampus (Squire, Cohen, & Nadel, 1984). Two tenets of this process are that once complete, memories are stable and no longer subject to change. Additionally, consolidation is thought to involve strengthening of the memory as opposed to memory modification. How then does new information get incorporated? The answer lies in a phenomenon known as memory reconsolidation. Contrary to the view that memories become stable and resistant to change, reactivating a memory appears to make it labile and open to change. By this view, reactivation transfers memory from a passive to an active state during which it can be altered and/or disrupted (Lewis, 1979; Misanin, Miller, & Lewis, 1968; Nader, Schafe, & Le Doux, 2000; see also Sara, 2000). Altered memories must then undergo a time-dependent period of reconsolidation to register change.

Nader et al. (2000) showed that reactivation of a fear-response could bring a well-consolidated fear memory back to a labile state that could then be disrupted by inhibiting protein synthesis in the amygdala (the same treatment that disrupts initial consolidation), demonstrating that memories require de novo protein synthesis in order to survive. Importantly, impairment was not observed in the absence of reactivation. Reconsolidation has since been demonstrated in variety of species and learning situations and it appears to be distinct from consolidation in its neurobiological process (for a review, see Dudai, 2006).

Reconsolidation has also been recently demonstrated in two procedural memory tasks with humans. Walker et al. (2003) trained adult participants to tap out a visually presented sequence (e.g., 4-1-3-2-4) on a numeric keypad with their corresponding fingers. Twenty-four hours later, participants learned a second sequence (e.g., 2-3-1-4-2) in one of two conditions (one in which the first sequence was either briefly rehearsed, reactivating it, or one in which it was not rehearsed). Participants were then tested 24 h later for their accuracy and speed on the original sequence. Performance in the group that was reminded was significantly impaired in comparison to the group who did not rehearse the first sequence before learning the second one, demonstrating that reactivating a memory destabilizes it such that a competing motor pattern can then interfere. There is also evidence from a procedural learning task with 3-month-olds that reconsolidation occurs in very young infants. Galluccio (2005) and Galluccio and Rovee-Collier (2005) investigated the effects of reactivated memories on infants trained to kick their foot to activate a mobile. After a delay, the moving mobile was presented for a brief period during which it was no longer attached to the baby's foot (reminding the child of the original learning experience). After reactivation, infants were exposed a novel mobile. One day later, infants who were exposed to the novel mobile no longer recognized the original one—they responded solely with a kicking response to the novel mobile, suggesting that the experience with the new mobile had overwritten memory for the old one.

These findings were important for demonstrating how memories could be altered by new information, and thus are relevant to theories of learning and development, such as those having to do with the misinformation effect (Loftus, 2005). However, they also raised important questions. First, how broadly does reconsolidation apply to different forms of memory? The reconsolidation effects described thus far apply to tasks involving implicit memory, a form of memory that does not require conscious recollection. But does reconsolidation also apply to explicit memory, a form of memory that allows for the conscious recollection of events (episodic memory) and facts (semantic memory)? Additionally, previous demonstrations of reconsolidation have shown that new information interferes with previous learning, but can reconsolidation also be instrumental when learners have to incorporate new information into established memories?

These questions have been explored in the context of an explicit memory paradigm developed by Hupbach, Gómez, Hardt, and Nadel (2007). Adult participants learned a set of 20 common objects during a first session (e.g., bandaid, sunglasses, pencil, cup, sponge, etc.). The objects were contained in a yellow basket and were pulled out one-by-one and named. The participants were asked to recall the items immediately after exposure to the entire set. The procedure was then repeated until participants recalled at least 17 of the 20 objects or completed four rounds of recall trials. Forty-eight hours later. participants were reminded of the original learning experience or not. Reminding took the form of the same experimenter taking the participant back to the same location in the psychology building and asking them if they remembered what they had done previously with the yellow basket. Participants were encouraged to describe the procedure only. They were stopped if they began to recall any of the objects. Participants in the no-reminder group were taken by a different experimenter to a different location in the building and were not reminded of the yellow basket. All participants learned a second set of objects (in the case of the reminder group learning occurred immediately after reminding). Forty-eight hours later in a third session, participants were asked to recall the first set of objects only, the objects learned in the original session.

Reminded subjects showed a high number of intrusions from the second set of objects when recalling the first set, whereas participants who had not been reminded showed virtually no intrusions, demonstrating that the updating of preexisting memory is dependent on reactivation of that memory (Panel 1 in Figure 10.7). Importantly, the effect is not evident immediately after learning the second set of objects as would have been predicted if this were retroactive interference (Panel 2). Instead the effect took time to emerge. Therefore, as with animal fear conditioning (e.g., Nader et al., 2000) and human procedural memory (Walker et al., 2003), reactivated episodic memories appear to undergo a time-dependent reconsolidation process. However, our findings differ in an important way from previous ones in demonstrating constructive memory effects as opposed to interference of new information on old memories. Furthermore, the updating effect occurs only for the reactivated memory. When participants were asked to recall objects from the second training session, intrusions of objects from the original memory were rare, arguing against simple source-memory confusion (Panel 3).

Although conducted with adults, this memory-reconsolidation process is relevant for understanding memory updating generally in learning and development. Such a process appears to depend on reactivating memory through some form of reminding, providing new information at the time of reactivation, and allowing time for the new information to be incorporated with the old.

We have also tested 5- and 9-year-old children to see whether the updating effect occurs at earlier points in developmental time (Hupbach, Gómez, & Nadel, in preparation). It would be particularly informative to know whether 5-year-olds show the asymmetrical updating effect in the form of updating of the original memory because source memory errors are high in this age group relative to children 6 years of age and older (Drummey & Newcomb, 2002). Five-year-olds might be just as likely to intrude objects from the first learning

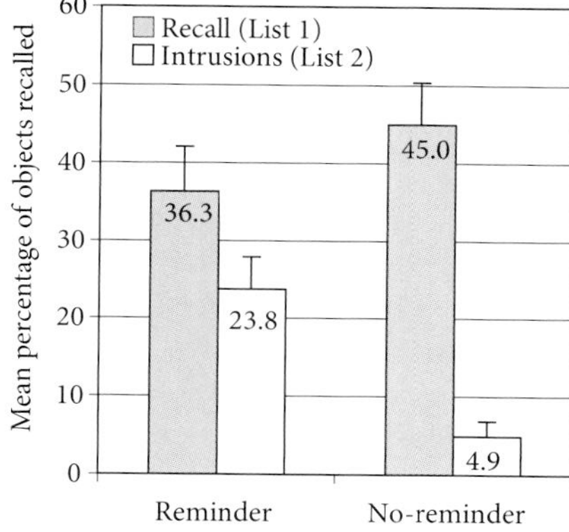

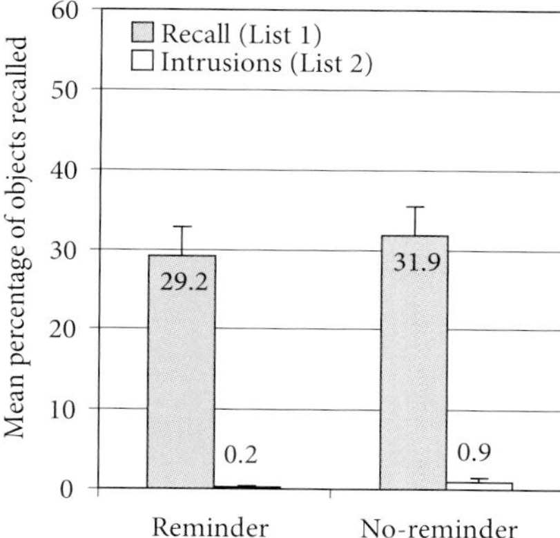

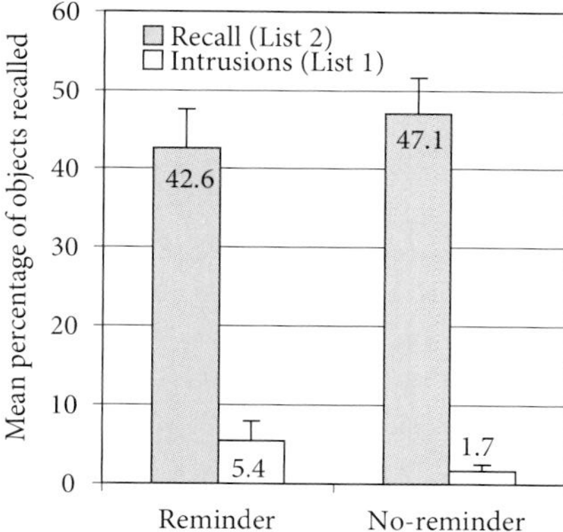

Figure 10.7 Mean number of objects correctly and falsely recalled in the reminder and the no-reminder groups. Panel 1: Recall of Set 1 in Session 3. Panel 2: Immediate recall of Set 1 in Session 2. Panel 3: Recall of Set 2 in Session 3. Error bars represent standard errors of means. Note in Panels 2 and 3 that there are no intrusions in the reminder conditions. From Hupbach, Gómez, Hardt, and Nadel (2007).

experience into their recall of the second set as they are to include the second set of objects into the original memory. Children were tested with a similar design as the adults with three exceptions: 9-year-olds were tested with 12 objects and 5-year-olds with 8, the children were tested in their homes instead of in the laboratory, and the delays between sessions were 24 h instead of 48 h in duration.

Children of both ages showed robust intrusion effects. Importantly, 5-year-olds showed the asymmetrical updating effect. Thus, although children this age tend to have difficulty monitoring the source of newly acquired information, they do not show such errors when a prior memory is reactivated at a later point in time. As with the adults, the effect is time-dependent. It does not appear when children are asked to recall the original list immediately after learning the second one. Instead, the effect only shows up 24 h later after memory reconsolidation has taken place.

One question has to do with the cues that trigger memory reconsolidation and updating. For adults and 5-year-old children, unfamiliar locations in themselves can serve as a reminder (updating occurs even when the experimenter is different and the reminder question is not asked, as long as the spatial context remains the same, Hupbach, Hardt, Gómez, & Nadel, 2008; Hupbach, Gómez, & Nadel, in preparation). However, not surprisingly, spatial context does not serve as a reminder when children are tested in a familiar spatial context such as when they are tested in their homes. In that case, the experimenter and reminder question together serve to reactivate memory (Hupbach, Gómez, & Nadel, in preparation). The importance of spatial context for determining whether memories of events are reactivated and updated makes sense given that the particulars of a current situation often determine which responses are appropriate (see Nadel, 2007). Other cues, may act as reminders for a different reason. Having an unknown person visit and interact with a child at home is an unusual and salient event, whereas an interaction with a new person is not so unusual when a child is in an unfamiliar location, as the data with children show. In that case, spatial location serves as the reminder

(Hupbach, Gómez, & Nadel, in preparation). Regardless of which reminders reactivate memory and why, the triggers demonstrated thus far are incidental in nature. They occur frequently in experience with potential to reactivate memories continually, resulting in a process of learning and memory that is fluid, as opposed to static, in nature, that may play a central role in cognitive development.

Summary

The central problem in cognitive development is understanding how cognition grows and changes over time. Research has had tended to focus on changes in the knowledge base itself in terms of documenting types of knowledge and abilities children exhibit at different ages, and asking how that knowledge constrains the choices children make. An example is children's tendency to extend labels to novel objects taxonomically, within the same category, as opposed to extending them to thematically related choices (e.g., extending a novel label for dog to a pig, but not to a bone; see Markman & Hutchison, 1984). Although children may well employ such constraints, it is important to ask whether and how they are learned. One possibility is that children note the consistency of the association between a label and objects of similar shape (e.g., cups come in a variety of colors and sizes, but they are similar in their shape), allowing them to generalize the principle that categories contain objects of similar shapes. This principle is consistent with children's taxonomic choices and is relevant for understanding how such choices come to be manifested in children's behavior (Colunga & Smith, 2004, 2005; Jones & Smith, 2002; Smith, Jones, Landau, Gershkoff-Stowe, & Samuelson, 2002). In this way, experience itself can lead to the formation of a general principle (see Lany & Gómez, in press, for a more thorough discussion of this idea).

In the tradition of emphasizing developmental processes, an aspect of development explored here is how learning and memory processes themselves might serve to constrain learning. There are processes that appear to guide learning dynamically, enabling infants to switch from learning of a simpler form of information (e.g., adjacent dependencies) when that source is not informative to other forms of structure that are not as simple (e.g., nonadjacent dependencies; Gómez, 2002). In this way, the choice of which structure to learn can arise naturally from the competing pressures of internal biases and information in the environment. We have also documented learning under noisy conditions showing that infant learners can track a predominant probabilistic structure despite irregularities in the input, and can even generalize on this basis (Gómez & Lakusta, 2004). Importantly learning diminishes, as it should, when the input contains higher levels of irregular structure, demonstrating that learning is constrained by the reliability of the information children encounter. Finally, we have seen how the information children acquire at one point in time can constrain what they are able to learn at older ages (Gerken & Bollt, in press) and can also enable learning of more difficult forms (Lany & Gómez, 2008). This work raises questions regarding the types of processing biases available to learners and which biases are likely to be employed in different learning situations. The findings also raise questions about the way learning changes as infants' cognitive processes are increasingly able to handle more difficult information. Do the learning processes themselves become more complex or are they able to execute over more difficult information?

We have also documented the role of memory processes in constraining learning, both the role of memory consolidation and sleep in transforming learned experiences into a more abstract form (Gómez et al., 2006) and the role of reconsolidation in constructive memory (Hupbach, Gómez, Hardt, & Nadel, 2007). Both memory processes are important for understanding how children sustain sensitivity to prior knowledge while incorporating new information. In addition to the role of memory processes in constraining learning, it is important to test memory to ensure that the behavioral effects seen immediately after a learning phase are not simply the result of short-term acclimatization to a stimulus as opposed to a more permanent change. That is, for the learning we observe in the laboratory to contribute in any meaningful way to development, it should result in some kind of memory change that is retained long enough to be reinforced or to be instrumental in later learning. Additionally, what is remembered after sleep or after a 24-h delay (Gómez et al., 2006; Hupbach et al., in press) may be very different than what is remembered immediately after learning. Importantly, adult work shows distinct processes of stabilization and enhancement in memory consolidation. As such, it will be important to fill in the developmental picture of how infant memories stabilize over wake and sleep states, whether this differs at different ages, and how this is linked to what we already know about infant memory.

With respect to the role of reconsolidation in memory change, additional research will be necessary for characterizing reconsolidation more fully, in terms of determining whether the effect is transient or long-lasting, whether the process is similar for older as compared to younger memories, how it is affected by sleep, and how it is affected by different kinds of reminders (e.g., what happens when learners are asked to recall an established memory as opposed to reactivating it implicitly?). Most importantly, how do these factors change across development and as children gain expertise in a particular domain, such as in language? The answers to these questions will be important for understanding the scope and limits of reconsolidation—and the implications for learning and development are far-reaching. In particular, the interference effects documented in the animal literature (Nader et al., 2000) and in human procedural memory (Walker et al., 2003) may explain how children recover from incorrect, or erroneous, generalizations. Presumably, if a generalization is activated, though incorrect, it will be overwritten in time by more statistically probable data. Furthermore, the memory updating effects that occur with reconsolidation of episodic memories are relevant to understanding how learners incorporate new information or experiences into prior memory. An important consideration is the fact that reconsolidation of episodic memory should be hippocampally mediated, but the hippocampus is not fully developed in humans until approximately 18–24 months (Nadel & Hupbach, 2008). Thus, reconsolidation involving episodic memory should not occur much before 18–24 months of age, but it should occur later. Further research will be necessary for understanding the exact nature of reactivation and reconsolidation of memories at younger ages, such as in the findings reported by Galluccio and Rovee-Collier (2005).

In sum, in contrast to "knowledge" constraints traditionally proposed in the literature on development and learning, the constraints proposed and discussed here arise naturally from the mechanics of learning and memory processes themselves.

References

Baillargeon, R. (1987). Object permanence in 3.5- and 4.5-month-old infants. *Developmental Psychology, 23,* 655–664.

Best, C. T., McRoberts, G. W., & Sithole, N. M. (1988). Examination of the perceptual reorganization for contrasts: Zulu click discrimination by English-speaking adults and infants. *Journal of Experimental Psychology: Human Perception and Performance, 14,* 245–360.

Bíró, S., Csibra, G., & Gergely, G. (2007). The role of behavioral cues in understanding goal-directed actions in infancy. *Progress in Brain Research, 164,* 303–322.

Brashers-Krug, T., Shadmehr, R., & Bizzi, E. (1996). Consolidation in human motor memory. *Nature, 382,* 252–255.

Christie, M. A., & Dalrymple-Alford, J. C. (2004). A new rat model of the human serial reaction time task: Contrasting effects of caudate and hippocampal lesions. *The Journal of Neuroscience, 24,* 1034–1039.

Cohen, D. A., Pascual-Leone, A., Press, D. Z., & Robertson, E. M. (2005). Off-line learning of motor skill memory: A double dissociation of goal and movement. *Proceedings of the National Academy of Sciences USA, 102,* 18237–18241.

Colunga, E., & Smith, L. B. (2003). The emergence of abstract ideas: Evidence from networks and babies. *Philosophical Transactions of the Royal Society, 358,* 1205–1214.

Colunga, E., & Smith, L.B. (2005). From the lexicon to expectations about kinds: A role for associative learning. *Psychological Review, 112,* 347–382.

Drummey, A., & Newcombe, N. (2002). Developmental changes in source memory. *Developmental Science, 5,* 502–513.

Dudai, Y. (2006). Reconsolidation: The advantage of being refocused. *Current Opinion in Neurobiology, 16,* 174–178.

Ellenbogen, J. M., Hu, P. T., Payne, J. D., Titone, D., & Walker, M. P. (2007). How relational memory requires time and sleep. *Proceedings of the National Academy of Sciences USA, 104,* 7723–7728.

Euston, D. R., Tatsuno, M., & McNaughton, B. L. (2007). Fast-forward playback of recent memory sequences in prefrontal cortex during sleep. *Science, 318,* 1147–1150.

Fenn, K., Nusbaum, H., & Margoliash, D. (2003). Consolidation during sleep of perceptual learning of spoken language. *Nature, 425,* 614–616.

Fischer, S., Hallschmid, M., Elsner, A. L., & Born, J. (2002). Sleep forms memory for finger skills. *Proceedings of the National Academy of Sciences USA, 99,* 11987–11991.

Frank, M., Issa, N., Stryker, M., & Keck, W. (2001). Sleep enhances plasticity of the developing visual cortex. *Neuron, 30,* 275–287.

Gais, S., Plihal, W.,Wagner, U., & Born, J. (2000). Early sleep triggers memory for early visual discrimination skills. *Nature Neuroscience, 3,* 1335–1339.

Gais, S., Albouy, G., Boly, M., Thien Thanh, D-V, Darsaud, A., Desseilles, M., et al. (2007). Sleep transforms the cerebral trace of declarative memories. *Proceedings of the National Academy of Sciences USA, 104,* 18778–18783.

Galluccio, L. (2005). Updating reactivated memories in infancy: I. Passive- and active-exposure effects. *Developmental Psychobiology, 47,* 1–17.

Galluccio, L., & Rovee-Collier, C. (2005). Updating reactivated memories in infancy: II. Time passage and repetition effects. *Developmental Psychobiology, 47,* 18–30.

Gergely, G., Nádasdy, Z., Csibra, G., & Bíró, S. (1999). Taking the intentional stance at 12 months of age. *Cognition, 56,* 165–193.

Gerken, L. A., & Bollt, A. (2008). Three exemplars allow at least some linguistic generalizations: Implications for generalization mechanisms. *Language Learning and Development, 4,* 228–248.

Gertner, S., Greenbaum, C., Sadeh, A., Dolfin, Z., Sirota, L., & Ben-Nun, Y. (2002). Sleep–wake patterns in preterm infants and 6 month's home environment: Implications for early cognitive development. *Early Human Development, 68,* 93–102.

Gómez, R. L. (2002). Variability and detection of invariant structure. *Psychological Science, 13,* 431–436.

Gómez, R. L., Bootzin, R., & Nadel, L. (2006). Naps promote abstraction in language learning infants. *Psychological Science, 17,* 670–674.

Gómez, R. L., & Gerken, L. A. (2000). Infant artificial language learning and language acquisition. *Trends in Cognitive Sciences, 4,* 178–186.

Gómez, R. L., & Lakusta, L. (2004). A first step in form-based category abstraction by 12-month-old infants. *Developmental Science, 7,* 567–580.

Gómez, R. L., & Maye, J. (2005). The developmental trajectory of nonadjacent dependency learning. *Infancy, 7,* 183–206.

Hauser, M. D., Newport, E. L., & Aslin, R. N. (2001). Segmentation of the speech stream in a non-human primate: Statistical learning in cotton-top tamarins. *Cognition, 78,* B53–B64.

Hupbach, A., Gómez, R. L., Bootzin, R., & Nadel, L. (in press). Nap-dependent learning in infants. *Developmental Science.*

Hupbach, A., Gómez, R., Hardt, O., & Nadel, L. (2007). Reconsolidation of episodic memories: A subtle reminder triggers integration of new information. *Learning & Memory, 14,* 47–53.

Hupbach, A., Hardt, O., Gómez, R., & Nadel, L.2008. The dynamics of memory: Context-dependent updating. *Learning & Memory, 15,* 574–579.

Hupbach, A., Gómez, R. L., & Nadel, L. *Memory capacity increases between 5- and 9-years of age, but memory reconsolidation is present at both ages.* Manuscript in preparation.

Johnson, S. P., & Aslin, R. N. (1995). Perception of object unity in 2-month-old infants. *Developmental Psychology, 31,* 739–745.

Johnson, S. P., Bremner, J. G., Slater, A., Mason, U., Foster, K., & Cheshire, A. (2003). Infants' perception of object trajectories. *Child Development, 74,* 94–108.

Johnson, S. P., Davidow, J., Hall-Haro, C., & Frank, M. C. (2008). Development of perceptual completion originates in information acquisition. *Developmental Psychology, 44,* 1214–1224.

Jones, S. S., & Smith, L. B. (2002). How children know the relevant properties for generalizing object names. *Developmental Science, 5,* 219–232.

Karni, A., Tanne, D., Rubenstein, B. S., Askenasy, J. J., & Sagi, D. (1994). Dependence on REM sleep of overnight improvement of a perceptual skill. *Science 265*, 679–82.

Keele, S. W., Ivry, R., Mayr, U., Hazeltine, E., & Heuer, H. (2003). The cognitive and neural architecture of sequence representation. *Psychological Review, 110*, 316–339.

Kellman, P., & Spelke, E. (1983). Perception of partly occluded objects in infancy. *Cognitive Psychology, 15*, 483–524.

Kemler Nelson, D. G., Jusczyk, P. W., Mandel, D. R., Myers, J., Turk, A., & Gerken, L. A. (1995). The head-turn preference procedure for testing auditory perception. *Infant Behavior and Development, 18*, 111–116.

Kirkham, N. Z., Slemmer, J. A., & Johnson, S. P. (2002). Visual statistical learning in infancy: Evidence for a domain general learning mechanism. *Cognition, 83*, B35–B42.

Kleitman, N., & Engelmann T. (1953). Sleep characteristics of infants. *Journal of Applied Physiolology, 6*, 263–282.

Korman, M., Raz, N., Flash, T., & Karni, A. (2003). Multiple shifts in the representation of a motor sequence during the acquisition of skilled performance. *Proceedings of the National Academy of Sciences USA, 100*, 12492–12497.

Lany, J. A., & Gómez, R. L.2008. Twelve-month-olds benefit from prior experience in statistical learning. *Psychological Science, 19*, 1247–1252.

Lany, J. A., & Gómez, R. L. (in press). Prior experience shapes abstraction and generalization in language acquisition. In M. Banich & D. Caccamise (Eds.), *Optimizing generalization of knowledge: Multidisciplinary perspectives*. Mahwah, NJ: Erlbaum.

Lewis, D. J. (1979). Psychobiology of active and inactive memory. *Psychonomic Bulletin, 86*, 1054–1083.

Loftus, E. F. (2005). Planting misinformation in the human mind: A 30-year investigation of the malleability of memory. *Learning & Memory, 12*, 361–366.

Louis, J., Cannard, C., Bastuji, H., & Challamell, M-J. (1997). Sleep ontogenesis revisited: A longitudinal 24-hour home polygraphic study on 15 normal infants during the first two years of life. *Sleep, 20*, 323–333.

Maquet, P., Laureys, S., Peigneux., P., Fuchs., S., Petiau, C., & Phillips, C. (2000). Experience-dependent changes in cerebral activation during human REM sleep. *Nature Neuroscience, 3*, 831–836.

McCrink, K., & Wynn, K. (2007). Ratio abstraction by 6-month-old infants. *Psychological Science, 18*, 740–745.

McGaugh, J. L. (2000). Memory—A century of consolidation. *Science, 287*, 248–251.

Misanin, J. R., Miller, R. R., & Lewis, D. J. (1968). Retrograde amnesia produced by electroconvulsive shock after reactivation of a consolidated memory trace. *Science, 160*, 554–555.

Markman. E. M., & Hutchison, J. E. (1984). Children's sensitivity to constraints on word meaning: Taxonomic vs. thematic relations. *Cognitive Psychology, 16*, 1–27.

Muellbacher, W., Ziemann, U., Wissel, J., Dang, N., Kofler, M., & Facchini, S. (2002). Early consolidation in human primary motor cortex. *Nature, 415*, 640–644.

Nader, K., Schafe, G. E., & Le Doux, J. E. (2000). Fear memories require protein synthesis in the amygdala for reconsolidation after retrieval. *Nature, 406*, 722–726.

Nadel, L. (2007). Hippocampus and context revisited. In S. J. Y. Mizumori (Ed.), *Hippocampal place fields: Relevance to learning and memory* (pp. 3–15). New York: Oxford University Press.

Nadel, L., & Hupbach, A. (2008). The hippocampus in infancy. In M. Haith & J. Benson (Eds.), *The encyclopedia of infant and early childhood development* (Vol. 2, pp. 89–96). San Diego: Academic Press.

Peigneux, P., Laureys, S., Fuchs, S., Collette, F., Perrin, F., & Reggers, J. (2004). Are spatial memories strengthened in the human hippocampus during slow wave sleep? *Neuron, 44*, 535–545.

Peigneux, P., Laureys, S., Fuchs, S., Destrebecqz, A., Collette, F., et al. (2003). Learned material content and acquisition level modulate cerebral reactivation during posttraining rapid eye-movements sleep. *Neuroimage 20*, 125–134.

Plihal, W., & Born, J. (1997). Effects of early and late nocturnal sleep on priming and spatial memory. *Psychophysiology, 36*, 571–582.

Polka, L., & Werker, J. F. (1994). Developmental changes in perception of nonnative vowel contrasts. *Journal of Experimental Psychology: Human Perception and Performance, 20*, 421–435.

Saffran, J. R., Aslin, R. N., & Newport, E. L. (1996a). Statistical learning by eight-month-old infants *Science, 274*, 1926–1928.

Saffran, J., Newport, E., & Aslin, R. (1996b). Word segmentation: The role of distributional cues. *Journal of Memory and Language, 35*, 606–621.

Saffran, J., Newport, E., Aslin, R., Tunick, R., & Barrueco, S. (1997). Incidental language learning: Listening (and learning) out of the corner of your ear. *Psychological Science, 8*, 101–05.

Sara, S. J. (2000). Retrieval and reconsolidation: Toward a neurobiology of remembering. *Learning & Memory, 7*, 73–84.

Squire, L. R., Cohen, N. J., & Nadel, L. (1984). The medial temporal region and memory consolidation: A new hypothesis. In H. Weingartner & E. Parker (Eds.), *Memory consolidation* (pp. 185–210). Hillsdale, NJ: Lawrence Erlbaum.

Smith, L .B., Jones, S. S., Landau, B., Gershkoff-Stowe, L., & Samuelson, L. (2002). Object name learning provides on-the-job training for attention. *Psychological Science, 13*, 13–19.

Spencer, R. M., Sunm, M., & Ivry, R. B. (2006). Sleep-dependent consolidation of contextual learning. *Current Biology, 16*, 1001–1005.

Stickgold, R., James, L., & Hobson, J. A. (2000a). Visual discrimination learning requires posttraining sleep. *Nature Neuroscience, 2*, 1237–1238.

Stickgold, R., Whidbee, D., Schirmer, B., Patel, V., & Hobson, J. A. (2000b). Visual discrimination task improvement: A multi-step process occurring during sleep. *Journal of Cognitive Neuroscience, 12*, 246–254.

Terrace, H. S., Chen, S., & Jaswal, V. (1996). Recall of three-item sequences by pigeons. *Animal Learning & Behavior, 24*, 193–205.

Terrace, H. S., Son, L. K., & Brannon, E. M. (2003). Serial expertise of rhesus macaques. *Psychological Science, 14*, 66–73.

Thoman, E. (1990). Sleeping and waking states in infants: A functional perspective. *Neuroscience of Biobehavioral Reviews, 14*, 93–107.

Toro, J. M., & Trobalón, J. B. (2005). Statistical computations over a speech stream in a rodent. *Perception & Psychophysics, 67*, 867–875.

Wagner, U., Gais, S., Haider, H., Verleger, R., & Born, J. (2004). Sleep inspires insight. *Nature, 427*, 352–355.

Walker, M. P., Brakefield, T., Morgan, A., Hobson, J. A., & Stickgold, R. (2002a). Practice with sleep makes perfect: Sleep-dependent motor skill learning. *Neuron 35*, 205–211.

Walker, M. P., Brakefield, T., Hobson, J. A., & Stickgold, R. (2003). Dissociable stages of human memory consolidation and reconsolidation. *Nature 425*, 616–620.

Walker, M. P., Liston, C., Hobson, J. A., & Stickgold, R. (2002b). Cognitive flexibility across the sleepwake cycle: REM-sleep enhancement of anagram problem solving. *Cognitive Brain Research, 14*, 317–324.

Walker, M. P., & Stickgold, R. (2006). Sleep, memory and plasticity. *Annual Review of Psychology, 57*, 139–166.

Werker, J. F., & Tees, R. C. (1984). Cross-language speech perception: Evidence for perceptual reorganization during the first year of life. *Infant Behavior and Development, 7*, 49–63.

Wilson, M., & McNaughton, B. (1994). Reactivation of hippocampal ensemble memories during sleep. *Science 265*, 676–679.

Woodward, A. L. (2005). The infant origins of intentional understanding. In R. V. Kail (Ed.), *Advances in child development and behavior* (Vol. 33, pp. 229–262). Oxford: Elsevier.

Wynn, K. (1992). Addition and subtraction by human infants. *Nature, 358*, 749–750.

Xu, F. & Garcia, V. (2008). Intuitive statistics by 8-month-old infants. *Proceedings of the National Academy of Sciences USA, 105, 5012–5015.*

CHAPTER 11
Mixing the Old with the New and the New with the Old: Combining Prior and Current Knowledge in Conceptual Change

Denis Mareschal and Gert Westermann

One of the greatest challenges facing the developing child is knowing how to combine new experiences with existing prior knowledge. Throughout infancy and childhood, the growing child continually explores the world. She soon discovers new objects, new events, and new situations that she has never been confronted with before. This raises an important conundrum. On the one hand, she will want to learn from the new experiences. She will therefore need to adjust her world model (or world knowledge) in response to the new events so that next time a similar event is encountered, she will be able to draw on her prior experiences to respond rapidly to this new situation. On the other hand, because of the stochastic nature of experiences in the world, she will not know how representative or important a new experience is, and thus to what extent it needs to be remembered and her world knowledge revised.

Consider the example of a young child learning about birds. Perhaps as a 2-year-old, she has encountered a dozen different bird types and has a clear idea that birds fly. Then, on an outing to the zoo, she is confronted with an ostrich that clearly does not fly. Should this child revise her beliefs about birds to remove the constraint that birds fly? The answer to this question will depend on how representative the ostrich is of the birds that she is likely to meet and how important it is to know that not all birds fly.

This tension between needing to hold on to your beliefs while at the same time updating and constructing a system of world knowledge is central to many theories of cognitive development. Indeed, Piaget's notions of assimilation, accommodation, and equilibration (e.g., Piaget, 1952) capture the idea that cognitive development consists of a balancing act between these two sources of information.

While many authors recognize this problem, few have tackled it straight on (see Keil, 1984 for one important exception). One reason for this dearth of research is that answers to this problem require researchers to be explicit about how knowledge is represented, how learning takes places, and how the learning of new knowledge affects previously stored knowledge. These are the questions that computational modeling can attempt to answer. Implemented computer models force the researcher to be explicit about such things as knowledge representations, learning mechanisms, and how one affects the other (Mareschal & Thomas, 2007; Mareschal et al. 2007a; Lewandowski, 1991).

In this chapter, we will examine two approaches to resolving the question of how prior knowledge and current knowledge interact in category learning. The first relies on mathematical models of statistical inference. The second is an implemented connectionist computational model. To illustrate the usefulness of these latter models, we will sketch out a possible connectionist model of how prior knowledge and on-line learning integrate during early concept learning.

The Bayesian proposal

One promising approach to the problem of how prior knowledge affects on-line learning directly during development draws on concepts taken from Bayesian statistical inference. The Bayesian approach has been adopted by a number of researchers with slightly different theoretical frameworks (e.g., Gopnik & Tenenbaum, 2007; Gopnik et al., 2004; Xu & Tenenbaum, 2007; see also chapter by Sobel in this volume) who explicitly ask how prior knowledge influences inferences that can be drawn from evidence acquired in the here and now. The basic idea is that the inferences that we make based on current events are modulated by our prior beliefs about the distribution of events in the world (see Box 11.1: Bayesian inference). So, for example, imagine that you are returning home from work to what you believe to be a safe low-crime neighborhood. As you turn into your street, you see a masked man running down the road past you. Masked men are often associated with burglaries so you could image that the most likely interpretation of this event is that there has been a burglary near by. However, suppose you now consider the fact that there has not been a burglary in your neighborhood for well over 10 years. Based on this prior experience, the likelihood that there has actually been a burglary seems reduced. In fact, in light of this information, it may seem more likely that there is some other (perhaps initially more complex or less frequent) explanation for why a masked man is running down your street (for example, that it is Halloween).[1]

The point of this example is to illustrate how often and how naturally we draw inferences not only on the basis of the events that we are experiencing right now, but also on the basis of probabilistic knowledge of the distribution of events that occurred before (see Oaksford & Chater, 2007, for a more detailed discussion of Bayesian inference and reasoning).

Bayesian stumbling blocks

At the heart of this Bayesian "revolution" in developmental research is the desire to understand how prior knowledge combines with on-line learning. However, as models of development, the current Bayesian proposals still have a number of obstacles to overcome (see Shultz, 2007). First, current developmental models never state where the prior distribution information comes from (e.g., Gopnik et al., 2004; Xu & Tennebaum, 2007—though see the Sobel chapter in this volume for an initial discussion of this issue). Without such information, the models are no longer developmental. Instead of explaining how a child or infant gets from one level of competence to the next, it becomes a model of how children at different ages (with different prior probability assumptions) function. This is certainly informative, but falls into the same trap that many rule-based models of cognitive development fell into in the 1970s and early 1980s (Sternberg, 1984; Shultz, Schmidt, Buckingham, & Mareschal, 1995). While theoreticians were able to come up with sets of rules that captured children's thinking at different ages (e.g., Klahr & Wallace, 1978; Young, 1979), they were never truly able to come up with a plausible learning algorithm that would enable a system to move from one set of rules describing a 3-year-old to a second set of rules describing a 5-year-old. Without explaining transitions, development has not been explained (Elman et al., 1996; Mareschal et al, 2007a; Sternberg, 1984; Simon, 1963; Simon & Halford, 1995; Thelen & Smith, 1994).

Fortunately, this is not the death knell for the Bayesian approach. Indeed, it is not in principle impossible to come up with a mechanism by which prior probability distributions would change with experience. In fact, this is a very active research question in machine learning (Mackay, 2003) but, as we shall see below, answering such questions may require researchers to commit a little more forcefully to the machinery that underlies learning and knowledge representation.

[1] This example is adapted from Anderson (1990).

Box 11.1 Bayesian Inference and Bayesian Belief Networks

Bayesian approaches are increasingly popular in Artificial Intelligence (MacKay, 2003; Mitchel, 1997), visual sciences (Kersten, Mamassian, & Yuille, 2003), and the human reasoning literature (Heit, 1998; Oaksford & Chater, 2007). All of these approaches share a set of fundamental principles derived from Bayesian statistics. More specifically, Bayesian theory is a branch of mathematical probability theory that allows one to model uncertainty about the world and outcomes of interest by combining commonsense knowledge and observational evidence. Bayesian inference involves starting with a predefined set of hypotheses about events in the world, then collecting evidence that is meant to be consistent or inconsistent with a given hypothesis. As evidence accumulates, the degree of belief in the hypotheses is changed. As a result of these changes, our belief in certain prior hypotheses will often become very high or very low.

This change in beliefs can be embodied mathematically using a simple theorem from probability theory. Bayes' theorem adjusts probabilities of hypotheses given new evidence in the following way:

$$\text{Prob}(H|E) = [\text{Prob}(E|H)]/[\text{Prob}(H) \times \text{Prob}(E)] \text{ where:}$$

- Prob(H) represents the probability (according to our prior beliefs) of a hypothesis before new evidence (E) became available. This is called the prior probability of hypothesis H.
- Prob(E | H) is the probability of seeing the evidence E if hypothesis H is indeed true. This is sometimes referred to as the conditional probability of observing E if H is true.
- Prob(E) is the probability of witnessing the new evidence (E) under all circumstances.
- P(H|E) is the probability that H is indeed true given that we have just observed E. This is sometimes called the posterior probability of H and reflects our belief that H is true after observing some new evidence E.

The factor [Prob(E|H)]/[Prob(E)] represents the impact that the evidence has on the belief (Prob(H)] that the hypothesis H0 is true. If it is likely that the evidence will be observed when the hypothesis under consideration is true, then this factor will be large. Multiplying the prior probability of the hypothesis by this factor would result in a large posterior probability of the hypothesis given the evidence. In a sense, Bayes' theorem reflects how much new evidence should alter a belief in a hypothesis. Such procedures are used in models of word and category learning (e.g., Xu & Tenenbaum, 2007).

A related but distinct set of formalisms are called Bayesian Belief Networks (Gopnik et al., 2004; Pearl, 2000). A belief network involves (1) a set of variables, (2) a graphical structure connecting the variables, and (3) a set of conditional distributions over the values of these variables.

A belief network is commonly represented as a graph, which is a set of vertices and edges. The vertices, or nodes, represent the variables and the edges, which represent the conditional dependencies in the model. The absence of an arc between two variables indicates conditional independence; that is, there are no situations in which the probabilities of one of the variables depend directly upon the state of the other. Prior causal knowledge about the relating between the variables is often used to guide the connections made in the graph to specify the initial conditional distributions between the variables. Bayesian statistics (such as that described above) can then be used to update the links in the graph as a function of new evidence.

A second problem with current Bayesian models of development is that they generally operate in "batch mode": when drawing inferences on the basis of currently available information, they compute the probability of events occurring over the whole set of available events (e.g., I observe 10 birds at the zoo and then calculate the frequency of observing wings by summing over all the birds I have encountered during my visit). This is unlikely to be plausible as (1) children have limited working memories and (2) in the real world, it is unlikely that we experience a whole clustered set of events like that. Therefore, while the Bayesian approach may work well for modeling inferences that are drawn on the basis of the complete set of information provided during a test session in an experiment, it seems implausible as an account of how the child learns in the real world. Again, this is not an insurmountable problem, but one that modelers and theoreticians need to address if their models are to be taken seriously as explaining cognitive development.

A third, and to our mind the greatest, problem with the Bayesian approach has to do with the fact that it is restricted to the computational level of description (Chater, Tenenbaum & Yuille, 2006; Gopnik & Tenenbaum, 2007). The computational level is one of the three levels of description proposed by Marr (1982). Marr argued that (cognitive) computational systems could be studied at three independent levels. The first (top) level was the computational level that specified what needed to be computed to solve a particular problem (e.g., when interpreting a visual scene, figure/ground segmentation must be computed to determine what are objects and what is background to make sense of the scene). The second level was the algorithmic level that specified how the computation was carried out (e.g., perhaps using an edge detection strategy). Finally, the implementational level specified how the algorithm was implemented in the particular hardware used (e.g., how edge detection would be implemented in a neural network). According to Marr, each of the levels could be studied independently because what happens at one level is not dependent on decisions made at another level.

Marr's approach has dominated much of cognitive science research since the 1980s (e.g., Fodor, 1983; Pylyshyn, 1984). It has been particularly influential (albeit indirectly) in developmental theorizing. Indeed, much theoretical work in the 1980s and early 1990s chose to focus only on the computational level, putting aside questions of how the cognitive processes proposed were carried out and how they might be implemented in the brain (Carey, 1985; Keil, 1989; Marcus, 2001; Gelman, 2003; Mandler, 2004). However, both in the adult and in the developmental literature, several groups of researchers have begun to argue that this artificial partitioning of levels cannot work (e.g., Elman et al., 1996; Mareschal et al., 2007a; Rumelhart & McClelland, 1986; Thelen & Smith, 1994).

There are two main reasons why we believe that the different levels of description cannot be studied independently (see Mareschal et al., 2007). The first is for reasons of computational efficiency. While it is true that different computations can be carried out in a multitude of different ways (thus, the computational and algorithmic levels may appear separate), these will have different resources costs. So, it may be possible to construct a rule-following system from a neural network (e.g., Touretzky & Pomerlo, 1994), but this is very computationally expensive. Similarly, while it may be possible to construct a context-sensitive parallel processing system from rules (Newell, 1990), this as well turns out to be very computationally expensive, requiring many rules and a complex control system. Thus, decisions made at the algorithmic and implementation levels do impinge on the computational level if resource constraints are taken into consideration.

In fact, resource constraints are particularly important in systems that are dynamically evolving such as the developing brain. The developing system only responds (adapts) to local pressures, without a global view of what it should be developing toward. Thus, at any point in development, it is likely to select the least computationally expensive (hence easiest to implement) computational solution. As a result, there will be a bias toward solutions emerging at each level that are most easily reconcilable with the constraints at work at the other levels.

The second reason is that models that focus only on the computational level (with no commitment to how the computations are carried out or how they are implemented in the brain) are generally unable to say anything about how the system goes wrong. In other words, they cannot predict the kind of errors children will make when cognitive load is exceeded or what kind of errors atypically developing children with developmental disorders will make. Indeed, recent research has found a host of different subtle behavioral patterns arising in children with a range of developmental disorders (Karmiloff-Smith, 1998). These patterns betray not only the different adaptations that have been made to altered constraints arising from an atypical genome, but also the kind of plasticity and compensation that is possible in a given system given the implementational constraints (Thomas & Karmiloff-Smith, 2002).

Thus, while current Bayesian accounts may provide us with a description of what children need to do to combine prior knowledge with current online learning, they do not provide us with a causal account of how this is done that will allow us to understand and predict the kinds of errors observed in typically and atypically developing children.

Connectionist solutions

So what is the solution? The solution is to consider cognitive computational models that take seriously constraints from at least the algorithmic level. Connectionist neural networks provide one such tool (Elman et al., 1994; Shultz, 2003; see also chapter by Christiansen, Dale & Reali in this volume), though other valid approaches also exist (see Mareschal et al., 2007a, 2007b).

Connectionist models are computer models loosely based on the principles of neural information processing (Elman, Bates, Johnson, Karmiloff-Smith, Parisi, & Plunkett, 1996; McLeod, Plunkett, & Rolls, 1998; Rumelhart & McClellend, 1986). However, they are not intended to be models of neurons in the brain. Instead, they attempt to strike the balance between importing some of the key ideas from the neurosciences while maintaining sufficiently discrete and definable components to allow questions about behavior to be formulated in terms of a high-level computational concepts.

Connectionist networks are an ideal tool for modeling development because they develop their own internal representations as a result of interacting with an environment (Plunkett & Sinha, 1991). However, these networks are not simply *tabula rasa* empiricist learning machines. The representations they develop can be strongly predetermined by initial constraints. These constraints can take the form of different associative learning mechanisms attuned to specific information in the environment (e.g., temporal correlation or spatial correlation), or they can take the form of architectural constraints that guide the flow of information in the system. Although connectionist modeling has its roots in associationist learning paradigms, it has inherited the Hebbian rather than the Hullian tradition. That is, what goes on *inside* the network is as important in determining the overall behavior of the networks as is the correlation between the inputs (stimuli) and the outputs (responses).

In the next section, we will illustrate how a connectionist system (Box 11.2) can be used to investigate how prior knowledge and online learning combine to explain behaviors both across developmental time and real time. We focus on the domain of concept learning because it typifies a domain were prior knowledge and current experience interact heavily.

Modeling infant category learning

How Do Infants Form Categories?

Forming categories is one of the most fundamental aspects of cognitive processing. Therefore, studying the development of this ability in infancy is vital for understanding the basics of cognitive processing as a whole. As infants cannot speak and communicate their knowledge verbally, nonlinguistic methods of probing early categorization have been developed. However,

Box 11.2 Connectionist Information Processing

Connectionist networks are made up of simple processing units (idealized neurons) interconnected via weighted communication lines (idealized synapses). Units are often represented as circles and the weighted communication lines, as lines between these circles. Activation flows from unit to unit via these connection weights. Figure B11.1 shows a generic connectionist network in which activation can flow in any direction. However most applications of connectionist networks impose constraints on the way activation can flow.

Figure B11.1 also shows a typical feed-forward network. Activation (information) is constrained to move in one direction only. Some units (those units through which information enters the network) are called *input units.* Other units (those units through which information leaves the network) are called *output units.* All other units are called *hidden units.* In a feed-forward network, information is first encoded as a pattern of activation across the bank

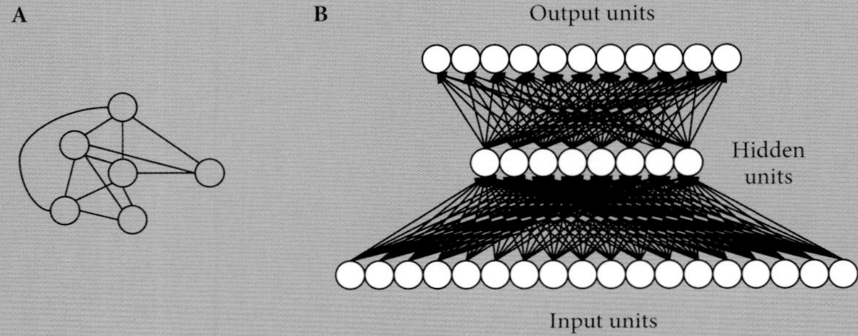

Figure B11.1 Schema of (A) a generic and (B) a feed-forward connectionist network.

of input units. That activation then filters up through a first layer of weights until it produces a pattern of activation across the band of hidden units. The pattern of activation produced across the hidden units constitutes an *internal re-representation* of the information originally presented to the network. The activation at the hidden units continues to flow through the network until it reaches the output unit. The pattern of activation produced at the output units is taken as the network's response to the initial input.

Each unit is a very simple processor that mimics the functioning of an idealized neuron. The unit sums the weighted activation arriving into it. It then sets it own level of activation according to some nonlinear function of that weighted input. The nonlinearity allows the units to respond differentially to different ranges of input values. The key idea of connectionist modeling is that of collective computations. That is, although the behavior of the individual components in the network is simple, the behavior of the network as a whole can be very complex. It is the behavior of the network as a whole that is taken to model different aspect of infant behaviors.

The network's global behavior is determined by the connection weights. As activation flows through the network, it is transformed by the set of connection weights between successive layers in the network. Learning (i.e., adapting one's behavior) is accomplished by tuning the connection weights until some stable behavior is obtained. *Supervised* networks adjust their weights until the output response (for a given input) matches a target response. That target can come from an active teacher, or passively through observing the environment, but it must come from outside the system. *Unsupervised* networks adjust their weights until some internal constraint is satisfied (e.g., maximally different input must have maximally different internal representations). *Backpropagation* (Rumelhart, Hinton, & Williams, 1986) is a popular training algorithm for supervised connectionist networks.

Many connectionist network models are very simple and only contain some 100 units. This does not imply that the part of the brain solving the corresponding task only uses 100 neurons. It is important to understand that these models are not neural models but information processing models of behavior. The models provide examples of how systems with similar computational properties to the brain can give rise to the behaviors observed in infants. As such, they constitute possible explanations of those behaviors in terms of neurally plausible mechanisms. Sometimes, individual units are taken to represent pools of neurons or cell assemblies rather than single neurons. According to this interpretation, the activation level of the units corresponds to the proportion of neurons firing in the pool (e.g., Changeux & Dehaene, 1989).

different methods have yielded sometimes conflicting results on infants' categorization abilities (Mareschal & Quinn, 2001; see also chapters by Rakison & Chicchino and Quinn in this volume), making it difficult to integrate them into an overall picture of category development.

One set of methodologies by which infant categorization has been studied relies on the fact that infants tend to show a preference for novel stimuli (Fantz, 1964). Studies exploiting this novelty preference usually employ a *familiarization* stage in which infants are shown a sequence of images of objects from one category (e.g., cats) on a computer screen. The time that the infants spend looking at each image is measured and is expected to decrease as infants become familiarized with the objects. This stage is followed by a *test* phase in which infants are shown novel stimuli from the familiarized category (e.g., a novel cat) and stimuli from a different category (e.g., a dog). Preference for the object from the different category can then be taken as evidence that the infants have formed a category representation that includes the novel category member (the novel cat) but excludes the object from the other category (the dog). Research based on this paradigm has provided evidence that infants under 6 months of age can form perceptual categories even of complex visual stimuli such as different animals and furniture items (Mareschal & Quinn, 2001; Quinn & Eimas, 1996a; Quinn, Eimas, & Rosenkrantz, 1993). The level (global or basic) at which objects are categorized is dependent on the variability and distribution of information in the environment (Mareschal, French, & Quinn, 2000; French, Mareschal, Memillod, & Quinn, 2004). For example, in one study (Quinn & Eimas, 1996b), 3- to 4-month-olds were familiarized with cats and subsequently were shown to have formed a basic-level category representation of domestic cats that excluded birds, dogs, horses, and tigers. Likewise, when familiarized with chairs, infants formed a basic-level category representation of chairs that excluded couches, beds, and sofas. In a different study (Behl-Chada, 1996), 3- to 4-month-olds were familiarized on different mammals, resulting in their forming of a global-level category representation of mammals that included novel mammals but excluded nonmammals such as birds and fish, as well as furniture. When familiarized with different furniture items, infants formed a global-level category representation of furniture that included novel furniture items but excluded mammals. It therefore seems that infants at 3 to 4 months can show categorization on different levels. However, it has been argued that even younger infants appear to form global distinctions only (Quinn & Johnson, 2000).

Other experimental paradigms are not based on novelty preference and do not involve a familiarization stage. For example, in the generalized imitation paradigm (Mandler & McDonough, 1996), infants are shown a simple action involving toy figures, such as giving a cup of drink to a dog. The infant is then encouraged to imitate this event with different toys, for example, a different dog, a cat, or a car. Category formation is inferred from observing to which novel objects the infants generalize the modeled action. Due to the absence of familiarization, this kind of task is assumed to tap into the background knowledge that infants have acquired during their everyday experiences (Mandler, 2000). In this paradigm, it has been found that global category distinctions (such as animals vs. vehicles) emerge first at around 7 months of age, whereas basic level distinctions (such as cats vs. dogs) do not appear until around 14 months of age (Mandler & McDonough, 1998).

The different experimental paradigms used in infant category formation have also given rise to conflicting theories of the mechanisms underlying early categorization. According to one view (e.g., Quinn, 2004), early category formation is entirely based on the perceptual properties of observed objects. With increasing experience, interacting with objects, and the onset of language, representations gradually become enriched to transcend this purely perceptual information toward more abstract concepts. By contrast, a dual process view of category formation (e.g., Mandler, 2000) assumes two separate mechanisms for perceptual and conceptual categorization, respectively. According to this view, the perceptual mechanism is operational from birth, and a conceptual mechanism develops in the second half of the first year of life. Category formation is then based on integrating the separate representations emerging from both mechanisms.

Whereas the results from preferential looking and generalized imitation studies seem to contradict each other, with infants in preferential looking studies showing categorical differentiation much earlier than in generalized imitation studies, a possible reconciliation can be suggested by highlighting the different task requirements in these paradigms. Preferential looking studies examine within-task on-line category formation and analyze looking behavior to infer category formation. Generalized imitation studies tap into background knowledge and require complex motor responses. Thus, we argue that these different studies can be construed as providing a set of collective insights into the development of a complex neurocognitive system that contains multiple interacting memory systems.

The existence of multiple memory systems is well established in the adult literature (Ashby & Ell, 2001; McClelland, McNaughton, & O'Reilly, 1995). Simply speaking, the idea is that there is a division of labor between a fast learning system in the hippocampus and a slow learning cortically based system. The hippocampus is responsible for the rapid learning of new information, whereas cortical representations develop more gradually and integrate new with previously learned knowledge. Here we suggest that this approach can also account for the unfolding categorization abilities in infants.

Although little is known so far about the development of memory systems in infancy, Nelson (1995) has hypothesized that novelty preference in infants relies on a hippocampal preexplicit memory system that is functional from shortly after birth. According to Nelson, explicit memory becomes functional only after 6 months of age. It is based on the hippocampus as well as on cortical areas such as inferotemporal cortex and entorhinal cortex. For explicit memory to become fully functional, it is thus necessary to develop the entire hippocampus, the relevant cortical areas, as well as connections between hippocampus and cortex. Furthermore, complex tasks such as deferred imitation appear to rely on interactions between the two memory systems, involving the hippocampus as well as occipital, premotor, left inferior prefrontal, and frontal cortices. From this perspective, it is clear that categorization tasks relying on cortical representations will show a later development of categories than those relying on preferential looking.

Previous Connectionist Models of Infant Categorization

Previous connectionist models of infant categorization have often employed autoencoder neural networks (Mareschal, French, & Quinn, 2000; Mareschal & French, 2000; Westermann & Mareschal, 2004). These are simple three-layer backpropagation models in which input and target are the same, that is, the model learns to reproduce its input on the output side (see Figure 11.1). In most autoencoders, the hidden layer is smaller than the input and output layers, forcing the model to extract regularities from the input in order to reproduce it. The rationale behind using these networks for modeling infant categorization is that the network error can be linked to infant looking time. One theory of infant novelty preference is that when infants look at an object, they gradually build up an internal representation of this object, and looking continues until internal representation and object match (Sokolov, 1963). The more unusual an object is, the longer it will take to build this representation, and the longer the object will be fixated. Likewise, in the autoencoder, successive weight adaptations lead to a match between an input (the object) and output (the infant's internal representation of the object). A higher output error requires more adaptation steps and thus can be likened to an infant's longer looking time.

While simple autoencoder models have been successful in accounting for different results from infant looking time studies, they do not take prior knowledge into consideration. Thus, they can only be applied in simulations of within-task category formation that involves familiarization and does not take into account the infant's background knowledge. In the context of Nelson's (1995) framework of memory development, simple autoencoders would implement preexplicit memory only. However, a comprehensive understanding of infant categorization requires that the mechanisms of both within-task and long-term category formation are integrated into a single system. Furthermore, an infant's background knowledge can have an effect even on within-task category formation. For example, one recent study (Pauen & Träuble, 2004) showed that whether infants had cats and dogs at home affected their categorization of cats and dogs in an experimental setting. In another study, Quinn and Eimas (1998) argued that young infants' categorization of humans versus nonhuman animals in a visual preference experiment is affected by differential experience with members from the two classes that occurs prior to the experiment.

Here we describe a model that extends previous categorization models by investigating the unfolding interactions between different memory systems through development. The

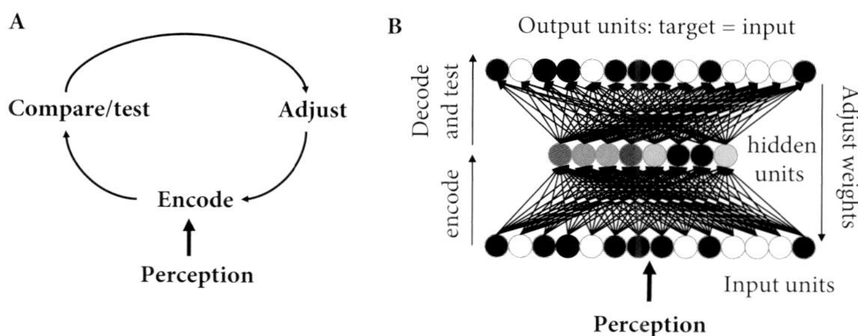

Figure 11.1 Novelty preference as a process of representation construction in (A) infants and (B) connectionist autoencoder networks. (After Mareschal & French, 2000.)

model is loosely linked to the hippocampal/cortical memory systems in the brain. It therefore allows for the investigation of the development of category representations in long-term memory on the basis of experience with the world as opposed to laboratory-based experiments only. By modeling interactions between both memory systems, it is also possible to examine the role of previously acquired knowledge on performance in a laboratory task.

A Dual Memory Model of Categorization in Infancy

The model illustrated in Figure 11.2 consists of two linked autoencoder networks, one of which represents the earliest, preexplicit memory system based on the hippocampus, and the other represents later memory systems that are largely cortically based. In line with theories of adult memory, the "hippocampal" system is characterized by rapid learning (high learning rate) with susceptibility to interference (catastrophic forgetting), and the "cortical" system by slower learning (low learning rate). Unidirectional links between the two components implement interactions between the two memory systems.

Training of the model worked as follows: an input was presented and activation was propagated to the hidden layers. Activation then was cycled back and forth between the hidden layers (which were updating each other's activations)

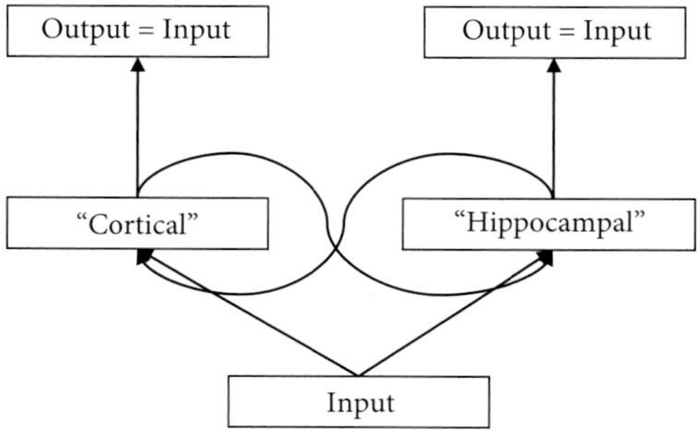

Figure 11.2 The architecture of the dual memory categorization model. (From Westermann & Mareschal, in press.)

until a stable state was reached. Activation was then propagated to the output layers. All weights were adjusted with the backpropagation algorithm at each stimulus presentation.

In the simulations reported here, the network parameters were as follows: learning rate in the hippocampal model, 0.5; learning rate in the cortical model, 0.001; learning rates of the lateral connections between the networks, 0.01; momentum for all weights, 0.4; size of each hidden layer, 15.

The Training Data

Photographs of objects from 19 different basic-level categories previously used to test infants were encoded according to a number of perceptual features. These were maximal height, minimal height, maximal width, minimal width, minimal width of base, number of protrusions, maximal length/width of left, right, lower and upper protrusion, minimal width of lower protrusion, texture, eye separation, face length, and face width. These features comprise both general (geometric) and object specific (facial) characteristics. Feature values were scaled between 0 and 1.

The object categories were chairs, sofas, tables, beds, drawers, horses, giraffes, birds, rabbits, squirrels, elephants, deer, fishes, cars, males, and females. They fell into four global-level categories (furniture, animals, vehicles, humans) all previously used to test infant category formation (Quinn & Eimas, 1996b) and varied in their within-category perceptual similarities. Each category consisted of 10 exemplars (for some categories additional exemplars were created by interpolating the representations of the measured photos). For each category, a prototype was generated by averaging the representations of all members of that category.

The model was trained in two different ways. Familiarization Training was meant to replicate the experience of an infant in a laboratory setting: the model was first familiarized on a set of stimuli until criterion was reached and was then tested on test stimuli. Background Training aimed to capture the experience of an infant with the world by training on random stimuli for random amounts of time before switching to a new random stimulus.

Development of Long-Term Representations

In a first experiment, the hidden representations developed by the cortical component of the model were explored. This was interesting for three reasons: the first was that a neural network that is trained on a sequence of patterns can be subject to catastrophic forgetting (French, 1999) when a new pattern is learned; the representations for previous patterns can be overridden and the learned mapping for these patterns is lost. Here we wanted to investigate if catastrophic forgetting can be avoided through the interactions between the fast and slow components in the model. The second reason for studying the hidden representations of the model was that there was overlap between the perceptual representations of patterns from different categories. This experiment could therefore show how the model clustered exemplars based on perceptual information alone. The third reason was the assumption made in the model that complex responses such as generalized imitation depend on cortical representations. In these tasks, infants show a global-to-basic development of categories and this could be explained by a similar development of cortical category representations.

The model was trained in Background Training mode for 10 epochs, that is, each of the 190 training exemplars were presented to the model in random order, and for random lengths of time (between 1 and 1,000 weight updates), for 10 times. To assess the effect of interactions between the hippocampal and cortical components, the model was trained 10 times with lateral connections between the hidden layers, and 10 times without connections. Results were thus averaged over 10 runs of each model.

Figure 11.3 shows the development of the hidden representations for category prototypes in the cortical component at four points in training, after exposure to 5, 50, 100, and 1,500 stimuli. Over training, the representations become more distinct, with global-level categories (humans, furniture, animals) already well separated after 100 stimuli and basic level subdivisions (e.g., male-female; bed-sofa) visible after 1,500 stimuli.[2] This result provides an explanation for the global-to-basic shift in category development that is found in nonfamiliarization tasks.

The spread of representations was compared for 10 models each trained with and without lateral connections between the cortical (LTM) and hippocampal (STM) components. For the models trained with lateral interactions, the average pairwise distance between cortical hidden representations for all stimuli was 0.74 and for models trained without lateral connections (i.e., with no interaction between memory systems) this distance was 0.38, which was significantly smaller ($F(9) = 34.66, p<.0001$). Thus, hippocampal input to cortex in addition to direct sensory input led to an increased differentiation of cortical category representations, indicating that interactions between memory systems support differentiation of long-term representations and reduce interference between objects.

Effect of Background Knowledge on Familiarization

We investigated the effect of background knowledge of different categories on the time required to reach familiarization criterion in hippocampus-based familiarization tasks. For background knowledge to have an effect, cortical representations must alter hippocampal representations that arise from perceptual experience with objects during a familiarization task.

To investigate this question, a simulation was carried out in which dogs were used as familiarization items, and prior Background Training was on either all items except dogs, or on all items except animals. The prediction was that familiarization times for dogs would reduce more when the Background Training data contained animals than when it did not. In

[2] Because of the relatively limited set of image views used in the training set (e.g., only canonical views of tables), inevitable idiosyncrasies in object representations arose (e.g., the close similarity between dogs and tables in the current simulations). A more representative sample of object views would presumably avoid these spurious similarities.

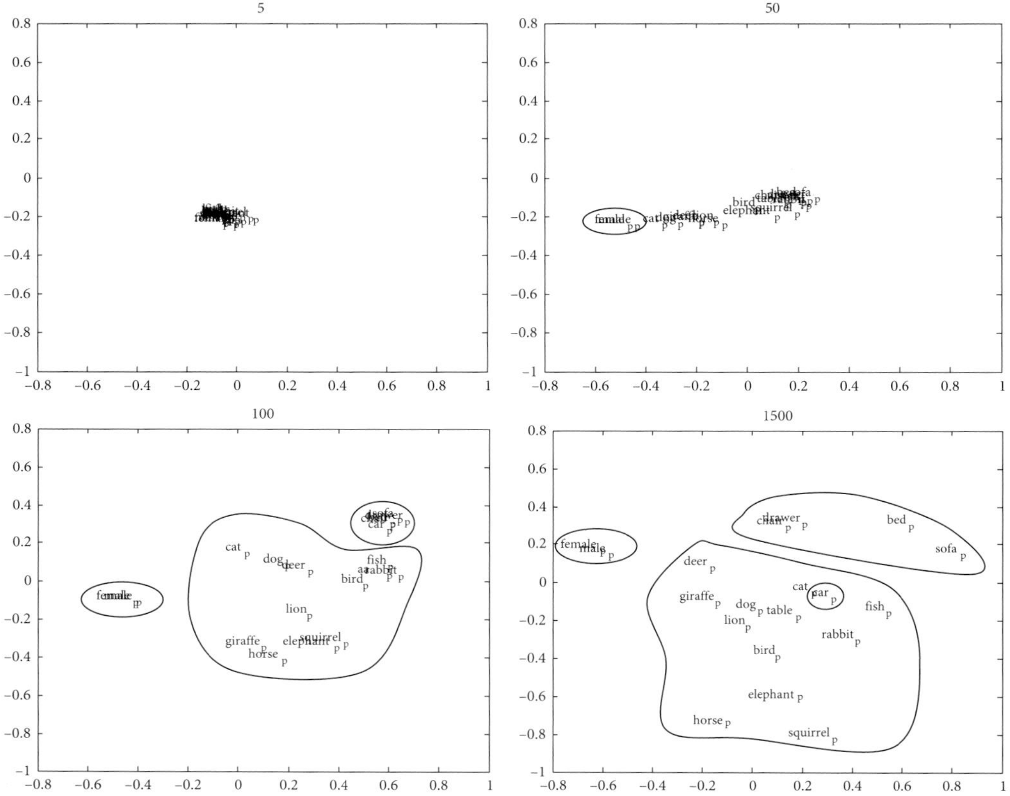

Figure 11.3 Development of the hidden representations of category prototypes (subscript p) in the cortical component of the model. Representations are plotted in terms of their first two principal components. (From Westermann & Mareschal, in press.)

the Animals condition, the model was trained on all stimuli, excluding dogs but including other animals, for 10 epochs (1,800 exemplars). In the No-Animals condition, the model was trained on all stimuli excluding animals for 22 epochs (1,760 exemplars; training was on more epochs than in the Animals condition to ensure an approximately equal number of exemplars).

The results of this simulation are displayed in Figure 11.4A. Background Training (experience with the world) led to a significant decrease in familiarization time. Familiarization time (stimulus presentations necessary to reach error criterion) to dogs was significantly shorter when the model had previous experience with animals than when it had not been trained on background knowledge. However, the specific type of background knowledge also made a difference: models that had prior experience with animals also familiarized significantly faster than those that only had experience with humans, vehicles, and furniture ($F(99) = 3.6967$, $p<.001$). This result indicates that prior learning from experience with the environment can affect an infant's performance in a familiarization experiment in the laboratory.

The effect of prior knowledge on familiarization was further explored for cases in which an infant has experience with members of the specific category that is then tested in the laboratory. For this simulation, one random dog exemplar was removed from the stimulus set. Then, the model was background-trained either on the remaining 9 dogs for 20 epochs (180 exemplars),

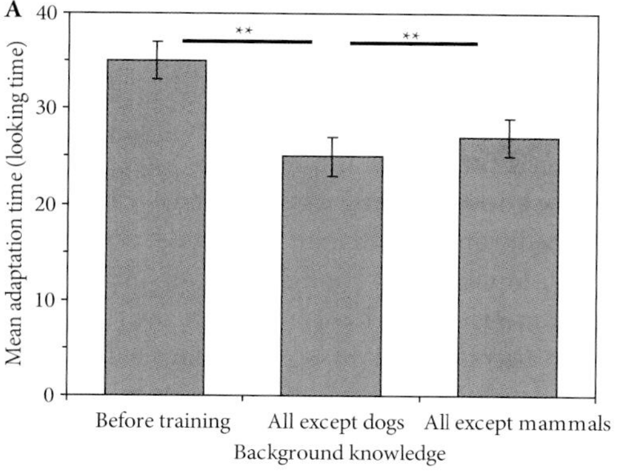

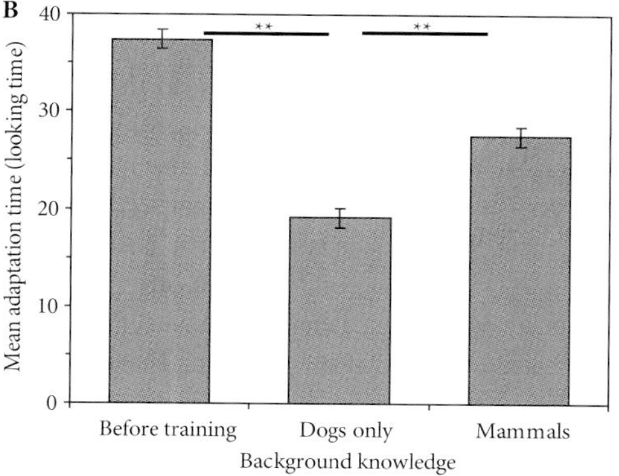

Figure 11.4 (A) Familiarization time to dogs depending on different types of prior knowledge. (B) Familiarization time to dogs depending on whether the model had prior experience with dogs. Results are averaged over 10 runs. (From Westermann & Mareschal, in press.)

or on all mammals except the extracted dog, for 2 epochs. (178 exemplars). The result (Figure 11.4B) showed that the model adapted significantly faster to the dog when it had only been trained on the other dogs than on all mammals ($F(9) = 3.7973$, $p<.01$). This result provides further evidence that adaptation time (looking time) is affected by experience, and that experience with similar objects reduces adaptation time to novel objects. Conversely, this result also shows that familiarization times are fastest when prior experience is maximally similar to the stimuli tested in the familiarization experiment, and that broader experience can slow down familiarization time compared with narrow experience. The mechanism by which previous experience affects current knowledge works through the interactions between the two memory systems: when an input is presented to the model, it activates representations both in the hippocampal and in the cortical network. Through the interconnections between the systems the long-term representations stored in the cortical system feed into the hippocampal system, generating an attractor state in the hippocampal hidden layer that is a blend between the current input and the evoked long-term representations for previously experienced similar stimuli. As a consequence the hippocampal representation becomes more similar to the current input, reducing the novelty of this input.

General Discussion

We began this chapter by reiterating what has been one of the great mysteries of cognitive development research: How does the developing child learn from new experiences while at the same time maintaining a reliable knowledge base? We discussed Bayesian approaches and found that they were promising but failed to address learning and development other than at the computational level of description (Marr, 1982). This, we argued, made them unable to account for developmental transitions and to provide causal explanations that would enable us to explain the errors that atypically developing children make or typically developing children make under cognitive strain. We proposed that it was essential to take the other levels seriously and suggested that connectionist methods provided one tool for doing this. To illustrate this point, we described a well-specified connectionist model of concept learning that explains how prior knowledge interacts with online learning to explain the patterns of concept learning that are observed in early development.

The connectionist simulations reported in this chapter describe preliminary explorations with a multiple memory model of infant category development. However, they raise some important issues about infant studies. Although familiarization/novelty-preference studies examine within-task category formation, the model suggests that presented stimuli in perceptual categorization tasks can activate top-down long-term representations that impact on the formation of representations for the familiarization stimuli. It was not necessary for the models to have background knowledge of the specific basic-level category that was tested in the familiarization task. Instead, experience with other animals and even nonanimal categories was sufficient to speed up familiarization to dogs. These results highlight the need for assessing both the background knowledge of infants and the similarity of experimental stimuli to objects known to the infant in experimental familiarization studies.

The connectionist model also highlighted that it is important to consider which representations are exploited by different experimental paradigms. Cortical representations in the model show a gradual differentiation from global-to-basic level categories, suggesting that tasks based on these representations show the same profile. Thus, the model provides initial evidence that a multiple-memory system perspective provides a useful framework for understanding the development of categorization in infancy. Beyond just explaining the existing typical developmental profiles, this framework can also be used to enable us to explore the effects of damage or atypical development one or another part of the system. Thus, it acts as a tool for bridging between information processing theories of typically and atypically developing children.

Is connectionist modeling incompatible with Bayesian approaches? The answer is a resounding *no*. Because Bayesian models make no commitment to the algorithmic level, they are consistent with any number of computational approaches (see Mitchell, 1997 for an example of this). It is therefore entirely possible that a simple connectionist model could be designed that is consistent with the Bayesian model to explain aspects of child development (see for example, McClelland & Thompson, 2007). In fact, substantial progress has been made in showing the equivalence between some forms of Bayesian learning and existing connectionist learning algorithms (MacKay, 2003; McClelland, 1998).

The advantages of using connectionist models over the principles described by the current Bayesian models are (1) explicit learning mechanisms, (2) access to the knowledge representations (i.e., with an implemented model we can ask question about how knowledge is represented internally and how this affects the way new knowledge and old knowledge can be combined), and (3) change over time. By building a computational model, we can observe how competence gradually changes over time. We can therefore ask how events that occur earlier in development will go on to have effects on events happening later in development.

Finally, the astute reader may have noticed that we opened this chapter by discussing the difficulties of combining prior knowledge with new knowledge and new knowledge with prior knowledge. The Bayesian approach is really all about the first half of this. That is, it examines how prior knowledge is used to modify inferences that an individual child might make on the basis of recent evidence. However, the Bayesian approach remains quiet about how this new knowledge might influence the old knowledge (might change the prior probability distributions). The connectionist model that we described is explicit about both these mechanisms. Indeed, there is a pathway for events in STM to affect representation in LTM while representations in LTM affect events in STM.

In sum, the integration of new and old knowledge during development is at the heart of constructivism. The question of how this is achieved has been grappled with since Piaget's first reflections on this question began almost a century ago. Implemented computational models that are explicit about how knowledge is represented, and how learning occurs provide the tools necessary (we believe) to make substantial progress on this question.

Acknowledgments

This work was supported by EC grants 516542 (NEST) and ESRC grant RES-000-22-3394. Thanks to Paul C. Quinn for providing the images from which the modeling data was derived and for discussions on an early version of this work, and to David Sobel for comments on an earlier draft of this chapter.

References

Anderson, J. R. (1990) *Cognitive psychology and its implications* (4th edition). New York, NY: Freeman and Company.

Ashby, F. G., & Ell, S. W. (2001). The neurobiology of human category learning. *Trends in Cognitive Sciences, 5*, 204–210.

Behl-Chadha, G. (1996). Basic-level and superordinate-like categorical representations in early infancy. *Cognition, 60*, 105–141.

Carey, S. (1985). *Conceptual change in childhood.* Cambridge, MA: MIT Press.

Changeux, J. P., & Dehaene, S. (1989). Neuronal models of cognitive function. *Cognition, 33*, 63–109.

Chater, N., Tenenbaum, J. B., & Yuille, A. (2006). Probabilistic models of cognition: Conceptual foundations. *Trends in Cognitive Sciences, 10*, 292–293.

Elman, J., Bates, E., Johnson, M. H., Karmiloff-Smith, A., Parisi, D., & Plunkett, K. (1996) *Rethinking Innateness: A connectionist perspective on development.* Cambridge, MA: MIT Press.

Fantz, R. L. (1964). Visual experience in infants: Decreased attention to familiar patterns relative to novel ones. *Science, 146*, 668–670.

Fodor, J. A. (1983). *Modularity of mind.* Cambridge, MA: MIT Press.

French, R. M. (1999). Catastrophic forgetting in connectionist networks. *Trends in Cognitive Sciences. 3*, 128–135.

French, R. M., Mareschal, D., Memillod, M., & Quinn P. C. (2004). The role of bottom-up processing in perceptual categorization by 3-to 4-month-old infants: Simulations and data. *Journal of Experimental Psychology—General, 133*, 382–397.

Gelman, S. A. (2003). *The essential child: Origins of essentialism in everyday thought.* New York: Oxford University Press

Gopnik, A., & Tenebaum, J. B. (2007). Bayesian networks, Bayesian Learning and cognitive development. *Developmental Science, 10*, 281–287.

Gopnik, A., Glymour, C., Sobel, D. M., Schulz, L. E., Kushnir, T. & Danks, D. (2004). A theory of causal learning in children: Causal maps and Bayes nets. *Psychological Review, 111*, 1–30.

Heit, E. (1998). A Bayesian analysis of some forms of inductive reasoning. In M. Oaksford & N. Chater (Eds.), *Rational models of cognition* (pp. 248–274). Oxford: Oxford University Press.

Karmiloff-Smith, A. (1998) Development itself is the key to understanding developmental disorders. *Trends in Cognitive Sciences, 2*, 389–398.

Keil, F. C. (1984). Constraints on knowledge and cognitive development. *Psychological Review, 88*, 197–227.

Keil, F. C. (1989). *Concepts, kinds, and cognitive development.* Cambridge, MA: MIT Press.

Kersten, D., Mamassian, P., &Yuille, A. L. (2003). Object Perception as Bayesian Inference *Annual Review of Psychology, 55*, 271–304.

Klahr, D., & Wallace, J. G. (1976). *Cognitive development: An information processing view.* Hillsdale, NJ: Erlbaum.

Lewandowsky, S (1993). The rewards and hazards of computer simulations. *Psychological Science, 4*, 236–243.

MacKay, D. J. C. (2003). *Information theory, inference, and learning algorithms.* Cambridge: Cambridge University Press

Mandler, J. M. (2000). Perceptual and conceptual processes in infancy. *Journal of Cognition and Development, 1*, 3–36.

Mandler, J. M. (2004). *Foundations of mind: Origins of conceptual thought.* New York: Oxford University Press.

Mandler, J. M., & McDonough, L. (1996). Drinking and driving don't mix: Inductive generalization in infancy. *Cognition, 59*, 307–335.

Mandler, J. M., &. McDonough, L. (1998). On developing a knowledge base in infancy. *Developmental Psychology, 34*, 1274–1288.

Marcus, G. F. (2001). *The algebraic mind: Integrating connectionism and cognitive science.* Cambridge, MA: MIT Press.

Mareschal, D., French, R. M., & Quinn, P. (2000). A connectionist account of asymmetric category learning in infancy. *Developmental Psychology, 36*, 635–645.

Mareschal, D., Johnson, M. H., Sirois, S., Spratling, M., Thomas, M., & Westermann, G. (2007a). *Neuroconstructivism Vol. 1: How the brain constructs cognition.* Oxford: Oxford University Press.

Mareschal, D., Sirois, S., Westermann, G., & Johnson, M. H. (Eds.) (2007b). *Neuroconstructivism, Vol. 2: Perspectives and prospects.* Oxford: Oxford University Press.

Mareschal, D., French, R. M., & Quinn P.C. (2000). A connectionist account of asymmetric category learning in early infancy. *Developmental Psychology, 36*, 635–645.

Mareschal, D., & Quinn, P. C. (2001). Categorization in infancy. *Trends in Cognitive Sciences, 4.* 443–450.

Mareschal, D., & Thomas M. S. C. (2007). Computational modeling in developmental psychology. *IEEE Transactions on Evolutionary Computation (Special Issue on Autonomous Mental Development), 11,* 137–150.

Marr, D. (1982). *Vision.* San Francisco: W. Freeman.

McClelland, J. L. (1998). Connectionist models and Bayesian inference. In M. Oaksford & N. Chater (Eds.), *Rational models of cognition* (pp. 21–53). Oxford: Oxford University Press.

McClelland, J.L., McNaughton, B. L., & O'Reilly, R. C. (1995). Why there are complementary learning systems in the hippocampus and neocortex: Insights from the successes and failures of connectionist models of learning and memory. *Psychological Review. 102,* 419–457.

McClelland, J. L., & Thompson, R. M. (2007). Using domain-general principles to explain children's causal reasoning abilities. *Developmental Science, 10,* 333–356.

McLeod, P., Plunkett, K., & Rolls, E. T. (1998). *Introduction to connectionist modeling of cognitive processes.* Oxford: Oxford University Press.

Mitchell, T (1997). *Machine learning.* New York: McGraw Hill.

Nelson, C. A. (1995). The ontogeny of human memory—A cognitive neuroscience perspective. *Developmental Psychology, 31,* 723–738.

Newell, A (1990). *Unified theories of cognition.* Cambridge, MA: Harvard University Press.

Oaksford, M., & Chater, N. (2007) *Bayesian rationality.* Oxford: Oxford University Press.

Pauen, S., & Träuble, B. (2004). *Does experience with real-life animals influence performance in an object examination task?* Paper presented at the Biennial Meeting of the International Conference on Infant Studies, Chicago, IL.

Pearl, J. (2000). *Causality: Models, reasoning and inference.* Cambridge: Cambridge University Press.

Piaget, J. (1952). *The origins of intelligence in the child.* New York: International Universities Press.

Pylyshyn, Z. W. (1984). *Computation and cognition: Towards a foundation for cognitive science.* Cambridge, MA: MIT Press.

Quinn, P. C. (2004). Multiple sources of information and their integration, not dissociation, as an organizing framework for understanding infant concept formation. *Developmental Science, 7.* 511–513.

Quinn, P. C., & Eimas, P. D. (1996a). Perceptual cues that permit categorical differentiation of animal species by infants. *Journal of Experimental Child Psychology, 63,* 189–211.

Quinn, P. C., & Eimas, P. D. (1996b). Perceptual organization and categorization in young infants. In Rovee-Collier & L. C. Lipsitt (Eds.), *Advances in Infancy Research* (pp. 1–36) Norwood, NJ: Ablex.

Quinn, P. C., & Eimas, P. D. (1998). Evidence for a global categorical representation of humans by young infants. *Journal of Experimental Child Psychology, 69,* 151–174.

Quinn, P.C., Eimas, P. D., & Rosenkrantz, S. L. (1993). Evidence for representations of perceptually similar natural categories by 3-month-old and 4-month-old infants. *Perception, 22.* 463–475.

Quinn, P. C., & Johnson, M. H. (2000). Global-before-basic object categorization in connectionist networks and 2-month-old infants. *Infancy, 1,* 31–46.

Rumelhart, D. E., Hinton, G. E., & Williams, R. J. (1986). Learning representations by back-propagating errors. *Nature, 323*(6088), 533–536.

Rumelhart, D. E., & McClelland, J. L. (1986). *Parallel distributed processing: Explorations in the microstructure of cognition.* Volume 1: Foundations (Vol. 1). Cambridge, MA: MIT Press.

Shultz, T. R. (2003). *Computational developmental psychology.* Cambridge, MA: MIT Press.

Shultz, T. R. (2007). The Bayesian revolution approaches psychological development. *Developmental Science, 10,* 357–364.

Shultz, T. R., Schmidt, W. C., Buckingham, D., & Mareschal, D. (1995). Modeling cognitive development with a generative connectionist algorithm. In T. Simon & G. Halford (Eds.), *Developing cognitive competence: New approaches to process modeling* (pp. 347–362). Hillsdale, NJ: Erlbaum.

Simon. T. J., & Halford, G. S., (1995) *Developing cognitive competence: New approaches to process modeling.* Hillsdale, NJ: Erlbaum.

Sokolov, E. N. (1963). *Perception and the conditioned reflex.* Hillsdale, NJ: Erlbaum.

Sternberg, R. J. (1984). *Mechanisms of cognitive development.* San Francisco, CA: Freeman Press.

Thomas, M. S. C. & Karmiloff-Smith, A. (2002). Are developmental disorders like cases of adult brain damage? Implications from connectionist modelling. *Behavioral and Brain Sciences, 25*, 727–788.

Thelen, E. & Smith, L. B. (1994). *A dynamic systems approach to the development of cognition and action*. Cambridge, MA: MIT Press.

Touretzky, D. S., & Pomerleau, D. A. (1994). Reconstructing physical symbol systems. *Cognitive Science*, 18, 345–353.

Westermann, G., & Mareschal, D. (2004). From parts to wholes: Mechanisms of development in infant visual object processing. *Infancy, 5*, 131–151.

Xu, F., & Tenenbaum, J. B. (2007). Word learning as Bayesian inference. *Psychological Review, 114*, 245–272.

Young, R. (1976). *Seriation by children: An artificial intelligence analysis of a Piagetian task*. Basel: Birkhauser.

PART IV

Induction

CHAPTER 12
Development of Inductive Inference in Infancy

David H. Rakison and Jessica B. Cicchino

Imagine, if you will, that you are walking with a friend near a lake and happen upon two bird-like creatures like those depicted below (Figure 12.1). Your friend asks you "If the duck on the left has Mallard blood, does the one on the right also have Mallard blood?" What is your response? On the one hand, you may respond with a "No." After all, although they appear similar in shape and have similar features—for example, eyes, a head, a beak, and webbed feet—at the same time other aspects of their appearance are quite different: one has a brown body and the other a gray body and one has a brown head and the other has a green head. On the other hand, you may respond with a "Yes." Your knowledge of ducks—learned in school or more informally—may allow you to recall that they are the male and female of the same species called *Anas platyrhynchos,* or more commonly, the Mallard duck.

Regardless of your response, the process that you use to make such a decision is called inductive inference. It is the ability to use previous experience to determine how far to generalize a specific observation to a novel instance, or, more formally, the ability to infer that if X_1 has property P then X_2 also has property P. This process is fundamental to human cognition because we can experience only a small portion of the objects, entities, features, and events in the world and must rely on generalization from our previous experience to interpret new objects and events. During a great deal of this experience we form *concepts*—mental representations or depictions—that encapsulate some, but certainly not all, of the properties of the things we have encountered. It is these concepts that we use to generalize during inductive inference as well as during the process of categorization whereby we group similar items together (i.e., if X_1 is a P, then X_2 is also a P). Sometimes we may infer inductively using conceptual knowledge about specific instances—that ducks with certain body and face colorings are Mallards—and at other times we may perform induction by relying on more general knowledge about the statistical regularities in the world (e.g., if an animal is the shape of a duck then it is probably a duck).

Inductive inference is particularly problematic for infants. They have experienced a relatively small fraction of the objects, entities, and events in the environment, and although they undergo perhaps the most rapid period of concept acquisition that occurs during the life span, they possess little in the way of specific or general knowledge about the world. An additional difficulty for the infant is that there is rarely direct feedback during induction; when a novel instance is encountered, the infant must determine how to generalize prior knowledge to it often without the aid of a caretaker. Nonetheless, over the last 10 years, researchers have begun to examine when infants are capable of induction and on what basis they generalize from their previous experience to a novel exemplar.

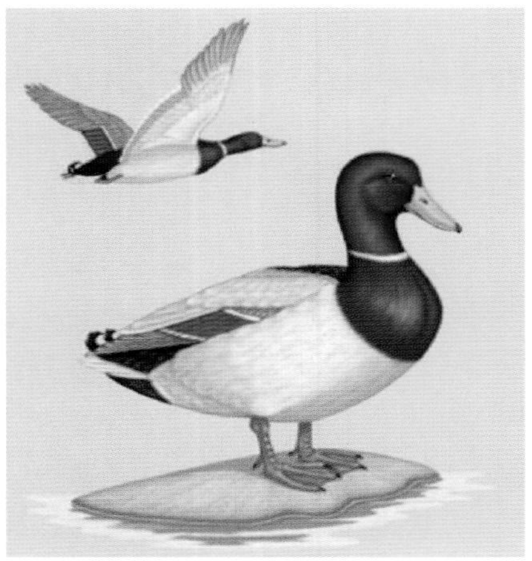

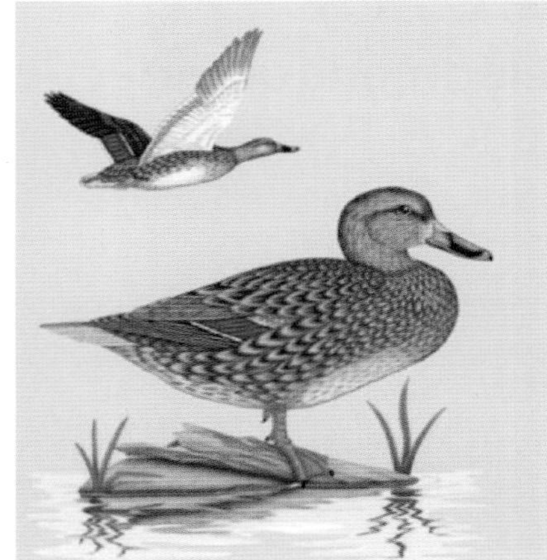

Figure 12.1 Do these ducks have the same blood?

As is common within the infancy literature, there are wildly diverging theoretical views about when inductive inference begins and how it operates. According to one view, as early as 9 months of age, infants' induction primarily is a top-down process that relies on abstract conceptual knowledge about the world (Mandler, 2004; Mandler & McDonough, 1996, 1998; Pauen, 2002; Poulin-Dubois, Frenkiel-Fishman, Nayer, & Johnson, 2006). For instance, it has been suggested that young infants generalize drinking from a dog to a cat not because dogs and cats look alike but because they understand that they are both animals that are capable of similar bodily, sensory, and motion-related actions. Proponents of this perspective theorize that this knowledge develops within the first year of life because infants possess specialized mechanisms that rapidly interpret or recode what is observed into a more conceptual abstract format.

According to an alternative view—the one we present here—induction is initially a bottom-up process that becomes more top-down over time; but crucially, the primary basis for generalization remains the surface features or properties of things (Cicchino & Rakison, 2008; Rakison, 2005). We use the term top-down processes to refer to behaviors that involve accessing prior representations or knowledge, but the term does not (at least in this chapter) imply anything about the content or structure of those representations. We use the term bottom-up processes for those behaviors that rely predominantly on the current, or recent, sensory input. Inherent in our perspective is the notion that general rather than specific mechanisms are the foundation of early learning. From this perspective, infants' extension of an action from dogs to cats or from cars to trucks is not based on knowledge about category membership or an understanding of the characteristics of animals and vehicles. Instead, we propose that infants generalize from one object to another on the basis of the features of those objects—for example, things with legs drink and things with wheels start with keys—and that the specific features that act as the basis for generalization are dependent on the whether or not there is prior knowledge about the observed property or action.

In this chapter, we provide an overview of theoretical arguments and empirical evidence for both the top-down and bottom-up perspectives of infant inductive generalization. The goal of the chapter is to synthesize the research to date in an attempt to provide a coherent view of the development of inductive generalization, the learning mechanisms involved, and to generate ideas for future directions of the area.

The origins of research on inductive inference in infancy

Research on induction in the first years of life did not begin in earnest until the 1990s, perhaps because the visually based paradigms that were used to study infant cognition and perception—notably, habituation and preferential looking—were not considered appropriate to its study. With a growing interest in inductive inference, researchers began to develop experiments that relied not on visual attention but instead on infants' tendency to imitate actions or events that they have observed. These studies laid the groundwork for more recent research by demonstrating that infants as young as 9 to 10 months of age can generalize from one object to another and that there are limits on how far they will extend a given property. For instance, Killen and Uzgiris (1981), who performed one of the first inductive generalization study in which infants were required to perform an action, found that 10- and 16-month-old infants—but not 22-month-olds—are more likely to repeat conventional social actions modeled by an experimenter (e.g., putting a comb to their hair) than counterconventional ones (e.g., putting a comb to a car). Baldwin, Markman, and Melartin (1993) used an exploratory play task to examine inductive inference in 9- and 14-month-olds. Infants were given a brief exposure to the property of a novel toy—for example, a can made a sound when squeezed—and then tested to see if they expected a toy with a similar appearance to have the same property. The results showed that infants in both age groups expected that toys of similar appearance—those that differed only in color or pattern—would have the same property. Finally, Bauer and Dow (1994) found that that 16- and 20-month-olds enacted events they had seen 1 week earlier (e.g., a teddy bear going in a toy crib) with novel, functionally equivalent props (e.g., Big Bird going in a bed).

These studies, although informative about infants' ability to perform inductive generalization more generally shed relatively little light on how and when infants start to use their knowledge about the world to make inferences about the properties of animals, people, vehicles, tools, and so on. There is a large database on such induction in children older than 3 years of age, which suggests that at least by the preschool years, they rely on labels and category knowledge to generalize a novel property (Gelman & Markman, 1986, 1987; cf., Sloutsky & Fisher, 2004). However, it is only since the emergence of novel infant-oriented methodology called the generalized imitation technique (Mandler & McDonough, 1996, 1998; McDonough & Mandler, 1998) that work in this area has progressed at a rapid pace. Because the majority of the work described here used this technique, we describe it here briefly.

The generalized imitation procedure

The generalized imitation, or inductive generalization, procedure uses scale model toys, is simple to implement, and is suitable for infants as young as 9 to 10 months of age and for children as old as 2½ to 3 years. In the prototypical version of the task there is a baseline, a modeling, and a generalization phase. In the baseline phase, infants typically are shown two toys drawn from different categories—for instance, a cat and a truck—as well as a prop that is related to one or perhaps both of them; for instance, a cup. Infants are allowed to interact with the toys and the prop in any way they wish for a brief time without any interaction from the experimenter, after which the toys and prop are withdrawn from view. This phase is included to determine any a priori preference for one of the toys and to discover whether infants perform spontaneously the action they will observe during the next phase of the task. In the modeling phase, the experimenter introduces a novel toy, typically from the same category as one of the first two exemplars and then enacts an action with that toy and the prop. For instance, the experimenter might use a dog to "drink" from the cup while making concurrently an appropriate vocalization such as "sip sip." This action is usually modeled three or four times, after which the novel stimulus is withdrawn.

During the final, generalization phase, infants are presented with the same prop and toys presented in the baseline phase and are encouraged to repeat the action performed by the experimenter. This encouragement can include a hand movement that repeats the motion of the action and a verbal prompt (e.g., Can you show me "sip sip"), but it is the infants' choice to use one or both of the toys to imitate the action they observed in the modeling phase.

Mandler and McDonough's (1996, 1998; McDonough & Mandler, 1998) rationale for this task was as follows. If infants understand that the modeled action is specific to the category of the novel exemplar (e.g., animals drink), they should enact the event with the toy stimulus from the appropriate category and not with the stimulus from the inappropriate category (i.e., they should make the cat drink but not the truck). However, if the two test stimuli are from the same category, and that category is appropriate for the modeling action (e.g., a cat and a rabbit for drinking), then infants should enact the observed event equally often with both stimuli. The dependent variable for the task is typically the object chosen to enact the event, although in variations of the task involving motion-related actions it has also been the way in which the stimuli are moved by infants (Cicchino & Rakison, 2008; Rakison, 2005; Rakison, Cicchino, & Hahn, 2007).

As we shall show, this task has proved a useful tool in gathering data on infants' generalization behavior. At the same time, it is common for researchers to make a number of assumptions in their interpretation of infants' behavior in the task and these assumptions must be re-assessed before strong conclusions can be drawn about the nature of early knowledge. There are also a number of more minor issues with the task—for example, that a human hand moves the toys in the study and that younger infants may not respond in the task due to limited imitation capacities—that will not be discussed here (for discussions, see Cicchino & Rakison, 2008; Rakison, 2005). Below we present research that has been used to support the view that infants' behavior in the task is underpinned by conceptual knowledge about the properties of members of a category (e.g., animals "drink").

The Top-Down Approach to Infant Inductive Generalization

Mandler and McDonough (1996, 1998; McDonough & Mandler, 1998) used the generalized imitation technique to examine whether infants between 9 and 14 months of age understand that animals are capable of certain kinds of actions (e.g., drinking from a cup, going to bed) and that vehicles are capable of different kinds of actions (e.g., starting with a key, giving a ride). The rationale for these studies was to test a top-down view of early induction developed by Mandler (1992; Mandler & McDonough, 1996). According to this view, infants possess a specialized mechanism called perceptual analysis that allows them form perceptual as well as conceptual categories very early in life. The perceptual categories include information about surface appearance and allow infants to identify what an object is; in contrast, the conceptual categories incorporate information about how things move, the actions in which they typically engage, and category relatedness (e.g., "there is a category of animals"). Mandler and McDonough (1996, 1998) argued that infants' induction (and categorization) is driven entirely by their conceptual knowledge about animals, vehicles, furniture, and other superordinate classes. For instance, they claimed that infants' imitations "are based on their conceptual interpretations of what they have observed, not the physical appearance of the items per se" (Mandler & McDonough, 1998, p. 37) and that "conceptual control of inductive generalization begins early in life. There does not seem to be a period in which infants respond only on the basis of physical appearance" (Mandler & McDonough, 1996, pp. 230–231).

What is the evidence in support this view? Mandler and McDonough (1996, 1998) found that infants between 9 and 14 months of age tended to generalize animal properties to novel animals but not vehicles and vehicle properties to novel vehicles but not animals. Thus, infants generalized going to bed to a dog but not a truck and giving a ride to a car but not a dog. They also found that infants generalized these properties for prototypical category members (e.g., a car, a cow) as well nonprototypical category members (e.g., an eagle, a plane). These studies were extended by Mandler and McDonough (1998) who used the same four actions as the modeled properties but in some conditions presented infants with two members of the appropriate category for the action (e.g., after seeing a dog drink from a cup infants were allowed to imitate with a dog and a cat or a dog and a rabbit). The authors predicted that if infants have conceptual knowledge that animals drink or go to bed, then they should enact the action they observe with both of the category appropriate exemplars. This prediction was borne out by the data: infants were just as likely to imitate the animal actions with a cat, a rabbit, and a dog, and they were just as likely to imitate the vehicle actions with a car, a truck, and a motorcycle.

Mandler and McDonough (1998;) presented additional data that they claimed supports the notion infants' inductive inference is based on a conceptual understanding of the behaviors of animals and vehicles. In one series of experiments, Mandler and McDonough (1998) tested infants with domain-general actions—those that are typical of both animals and vehicles such as being washed or going into a building—as well as domain-specific actions that are typical of only one category (e.g., starting with a key or drinking from a cup). Their results indicated that infants at 14 months generalized domain-general actions to animals and vehicles—though it is worth noting that they first imitated with an exemplar from the same category member as the model exemplar—but they generalized the domain-specific actions to the appropriate category members alone. Finally, to examine whether infants' behavior is driven primarily by imitation of what they have seen, Mandler and McDonough (1996) modeled domain-specific events for 14-month-olds with both an appropriate and an inappropriate exemplar; for instance, a dog and a car were put to bed. The results showed that infants were more likely to choose an appropriate exemplar than an inappropriate exemplar for their first action.

More recently, Poulin-Dubois et al. (2006) supported a similar top-down oriented view that infants as young as 14 months of age possess conceptual knowledge about the bodily, sensory, and motion related properties of animate entities. They used the inductive generalization procedure with 14-, 16-, and 20-month-olds to examine whether they would extend properties such as going to bed, looking in a mirror, and jumping over a wall from animals to other animals, from people to animals, and from a monkey to people and animals. The results of the studies showed that 14-month-olds generalized bodily and sensory properties from an animal to another animal rather than a vehicle, and that both 16- and 20-month-olds generalized motion and sensory properties from a person to other mammals rather than to vehicles. They also found that 20-month-olds generalized motion properties from a monkey to people, cats, and tigers but that they generalized sensory properties to people more than to animals.

Reinterpreting the Data: A Bottom-Up Approach to Infant Inductive Generalization

On the surface, the results from these studies with the inductive generalization paradigm indicate that infants are precocious concept formers and that by 14 to 16 months of age, if not earlier, they understand that animals, people, and vehicles engage in distinct bodily (e.g., drinking), sensory (e.g., looking at a sign), and motion-related (e.g., jumping) actions. There are nonetheless a number of reasons to be cautious before jumping to a rich interpretation of infants' performance in the inductive generalization procedure.

First, it remains to be seen to what extent the model exemplar used by the experimenter influences infants' choice during the generalization phase. It could be the case that infants observe which exemplar the experimenter employs to enact the event and then chooses one that is perceptually similar to that exemplar (what has previously been labeled perceptual matching and imitation (Rakison, 2003)). For example, infants may imitate drinking from a cup with a dog rather than a truck after seeing the experimenter use a cat to model the event because the dog is more similar to the cat than the truck. As outlined above, Mandler and McDonough (1996) attempted to address this issue by enacting an event with both an appropriate and inappropriate exemplar; however, although infants were more likely to imitate first with an appropriate exemplar, they were just as likely to use an inappropriate exemplar for their second action (56%) as they were to use an appropriate one for their first action (57%). In other words, infants imitated the actions with both the appropriate and inappropriate exemplars. Mandler and McDonough (1998) claimed that infants' generalization of an action to two animal or two vehicle exemplars is also evidence that they understand in a conceptual sense that both are capable of that action. Yet, this behavior too can be explained by perceptual matching and imitation because both of the test exemplars (e.g., a cat and a rabbit) were perceptually similar to the model exemplar (e.g., a dog). Likewise, in the studies by Poulin-Dubois et al. (2006), infants generalize from a cat to a dog rather than a vehicle, from a person to an animal rather than a vehicle, and from a monkey to a person and an animal. In all of these cases, infants' generalization can be explained by similarity matching to the model exemplar.

One piece of evidence that could be taken as contrary to this explanation is that infants' behavior in the domain-general tasks in which they generalized, for example, going into a building to an animal and a vehicle (Mandler & McDonough, 1998). In other words, if infants use the surface appearance of the model object to generalize to one of the test objects, they should have imitated with only the test animal or the test vehicle—contingent on which was the model—in the domain-specific tasks.

We have two points regarding these data. First, our claim here is not that infants bring no knowledge about the world with them to the laboratory, and it is quite possible that they have learned that a variety of things in the world, including animals and vehicles, go in and out of buildings. As we shall show in the following sections, in our view, infants in the second year of life do have concepts that incorporate how things in the world move around but these concepts do not encapsulate global categories such as animals and vehicles or animates and inanimates as Mandler, Poulin-Dubois, Pauen, and others have suggested. Second, it may nonetheless be the case that infants relied on a matching and imitation strategy during the domain-specific tasks administered by Mandler and McDonough (1998). Careful inspection of their data shows that infants' first imitation tended to be with the exemplar that was from the same category as the model exemplar; when a car was made to move into a building, infants would initially use the novel test vehicle to go into the building and then they would perform a second action with the other test exemplar that belonged to the other category (e.g., an animal moving into the building). Note that this behavior is similar to that found in the task in which both the appropriate and inappropriate exemplar was used to model the events; in our view, it is important to be consistent in evaluating the data such that infants' second action should be not be disregarded in one condition and considered in another.

A second issue concerns the basis for infants' inductive inferences. According to one perspective, early concept learning—and thus categorization and induction—is grounded in specialized learning mechanisms or innate modules (e.g., Gelman, 1990; Mandler, 1992; Premack, 1990; Poulin-Dubois et al., 2006). A corollary of this view is that infants' inductive inferences are based on abstract concepts of animals and vehicles, or even broader notions of animates and inanimates. Thus, when infants generalize a property from a cat to a dog, it is because they understand, in a conceptual sense, that they are both animals and animates and therefore engage in the same kinds of actions.

As stated earlier, we propose that infants may well arrive at the laboratory with experience-based knowledge about the way things move and the actions of which they are capable. We do not subscribe to the idea that this knowledge is embedded in concepts for superordinate domains (e.g., animals) or abstract notions of animacy. The studies by Mandler and McDonough (1996, 1998; McDonough & Mandler, 1998) and Poulin-Dubois et al. (2006) provide no direct evidence whatsoever that infants' concepts contain such information. As an alternative, we have proposed that general, and not specific, mechanisms are the keystone for early learning and that initial representations of the properties of animals, vehicles, and other object involve associative links between those properties and specific surface features (Cicchino & Rakison, 2008; Rakison, 2005; Rakison & Lupyan, 2008). Infants, according to this view, associatively learn the relation between an action—self-propelled motion, looking in a mirror, or drinking from a cup—and the features that are conjointly moving with those features (e.g., legs walking, heads turning, hands grasping). The presence of one of these two associatively learned features is then sufficient to activate the representation of the other; the presence of legs activates the expectation that an object can be self-propelled and goal-directed and the observation that something is self-propelled or goal-directed activates the expectation that an object will have legs. This kind of associative learning means that initially infants may make incorrect generalizations—they may extend a property to any object that possesses the feature associated with an action even if it is from an inappropriate category. However, over time, they make secondary associations to which an action is then extended. For instance, if infants learn the relation between legs and self-propulsion and they then learn that legs and hand are correlated, they will generalize self-propulsion to things with hands as well as legs.

Note that our claim is not that every feature will become associated with the action to which it is connected. It is entirely possible, for example, that young infants will not associate opening mouths with drinking either because mouths often open without drinking or because other aspects of the event may be more salient (e.g., the hand used to reach for the glass or cup). We also acknowledge that at some point in developmental time, infants and young children will generalize on the basis of category membership (e.g., because two objects are both "animals") or even animacy; however, the age at which this occurs is yet to be specified and will vary for different actions and events.

A third, perhaps less problematic, concern is whether infants appreciate that the toy objects used in the task represent real-world objects. This issue is not limited to the inductive generalization procedure and can similarly be levied at other methodologies such as sequential touching (Rakison & Butterworth, 1998) and object examining (Oakes, Madole, & Cohen, 1991) that use scale model objects. According to one perspective, infants understand that the toys in the task are symbolic representations of their real-world equivalents and their performance in the laboratory demonstrates this to be the case (Mandler & McDonough, 1996, 1998). At the same time, there is growing evidence that infants may not have such a deep understanding of the toys that they use to enact the events they observe. Tomasello and collaborators, for example, proposed that children's symbolic understanding of objects is limited until early in the third year of life because those younger than 24 months of age show symbolic skills with gestures but not with objects (Tomasello & Striano, 2001; Tomasello, Striano, & Rochat, 1999). Likewise, using a version of the inductive generalization task, Younger and Johnson (2004) found that children under 2 years of age rarely understand that scale model objects are symbols for their "real" world counterparts.

We are somewhat agnostic on this issue but nonetheless believe that care must be taken in assuming that infants comprehend that the toys in the task are symbolic representations of real-world objects. In our view, scale models serve as appropriate stimuli in the inductive generalization, and object examining tasks because they possess the same features, shape, and structure as the real-world objects they are meant to represent. This means that when infants generalize from one toy object to another—for example, from a model car exemplar to a test truck exemplar—in all likelihood they rely on aspects of the objects that would be used during inductive generalization in the real world. Naturally, the scale model toys are impoverished versions of real-world objects and some features may be minimized or missing entirely; nonetheless, we believe that in general the characteristic features of objects are included in scale model toys and could be used to generalize in the laboratory.

Summary and Predictions of the Model

In our view, it cannot be assumed that infants' behavior in the inductive generalization task is driven by either (a) any knowledge of the properties on which they are tested or (b) abstract conceptual knowledge of the capabilities of animates and inanimates. Figure 12.2 illustrates how infants may respond in any given inductive generalization task contingent on whether or not they come to the task with prior knowledge about the action or event they are shown. Note that regardless of the path one follows, the behavior that would be observed in many of the tasks that have employed the inductive generalization paradigm would be identical. However, this view leads to a number of unique predictions about infants' behavior in the inductive generalization task that would not be generated by a more top-down approach (e.g., Mandler & McDonough, 1996, 1998; Pauen, 2002; Poulin-Dubois et al., 2006).

If infants arrive at the laboratory without any prior knowledge of the actions they are shown, their behavior will be guided by bottom-up processes such that they will most likely imitate with the exemplar most similar to the model exemplar regardless of whether it is appropriate for the action. If infants arrive with some prior knowledge about the event, their behavior is guided more by top-down processes such that they will enact an event with exemplars that possess the appropriate features for the action. The prediction deriving from our theoretical perspective suggests, however, that infants who have some representational content for specific event should generalize actions to objects with the appropriate parts for those actions rather than on the basis of category membership (e.g., being an animal). Finally, at some point in

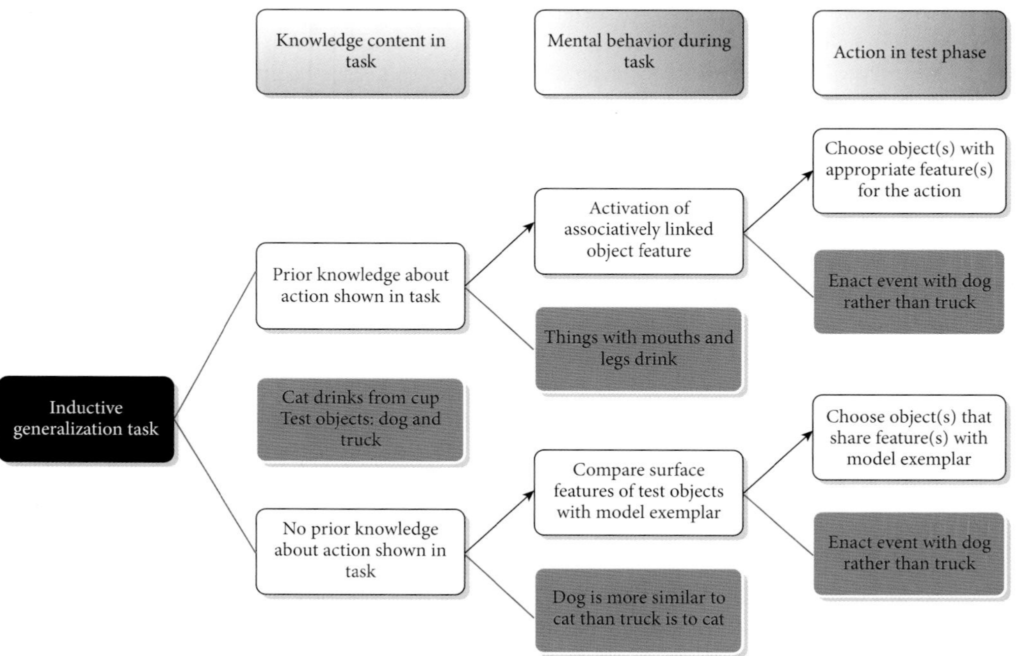

Figure 12.2 Model of infants' behavior in the inductive generalization task contingent on whether they have prior knowledge or no prior knowledge about the action they observe.

developmental time, infants should generalize an action to objects that possess the appropriate parts even if the object that possesses those parts is from an inappropriate category for the action (e.g., a table for walking). In the sections that follow, we outline research using the inductive generalization procedure with infants between 14 and 26 months of age that tested these predictions.

Is Infants' Inductive Inference Based On Prior Knowledge?

Recall that Mandler and McDonough (1996) attempted to address the issue of perceptual matching by modeling bodily actions to 14-month-old infants with both appropriate and inappropriate objects for the actions. Recall also that in their task infants enacted the events they observed with both of the test stimuli. This provides tentative evidence that infants indeed engage in some kind of similarity matching to the model exemplar. However, there are alternative and perhaps better methods to investigate whether infants' behavior in the inductive generalization task is based on perceptual matching. A first step for any bodily, sensory, or motion event that will be studied is to establish whether infants enact it with an appropriate exemplar when modeled with an appropriate exemplar. Assuming this to be the case, there are two potential subsequent approaches. A first method is to model an action only with an inappropriate exemplar. If infants are using a matching strategy, they should enact the action the observed with the inappropriate test exemplar rather than the appropriate test exemplar.

To test whether infants are indeed using a perceptual matching strategy, Rakison (2003, Rakison & Poulin-Dubois, 2000) tested 14-month-old infants with a variety of motion events that were modeled either with an appropriate or inappropriate category exemplar. For each event, a novel appropriate and inappropriate stimulus was presented during the generalization phase. The motion events included motions that were context-specific (e.g., going upstairs for animals, jumping from one ramp to another for vehicles) or context-general (e.g., acting as an agent in a causal event for animals, moving linearly for vehicles). Consistent with the results of other research with the inductive generalization procedure (e.g., Mandler & McDonough, 1996, 1998; Poulin-Dubois et al. 2006), when the events were modeled with a suitable exemplar, infants tended to enact the events with the test stimulus from the appropriate category. For example, when infants observed an experimenter move a cat in a nonlinear walking motion, they enacted the event with a dog rather than a truck. However, when the identical events were modeled with an unsuitable exemplar—for example, a car moving in a walking motion—a separate group of infants of the same age repeated what they had seen with an inappropriate exemplar (e.g., a truck moving in a walking motion). This basic effect held regardless of whether the motions modeled to infants were context specific or context general.

A similar design was employed by Furrer, Younger, and Johnson (2005) to test whether infants relied on perceptual matching and imitation for two of events used by Mandler and McDonough (1996, 1998). Infants at 14 and 16 months of age were tested with one animal action (drinking from a cup) and one vehicle action (starting with a key) and the events were modeled either with a conventional category member or an inappropriate one. In accord with the results of Rakison (2003), infants in both age groups enacted events with the appropriate category exemplar when they observed an experimenter model with a conventional object (e.g., a bus starting with a key) but enacted events with an inappropriate category exemplar when the event was modeled with a counterconventional item (e.g., a dog starting with a key).

Taken together, these results suggest that 14- to 16-month-old infants' behavior in at least some inductive generalization tasks may be based on their ability to compare the similarity of the two test stimuli to the model exemplar. Clearly, this strategy would best be described as bottom-up; infants arrive at the laboratory with little or no knowledge of the events they are shown and must determine during the task—on-line—how perceptually similar are the test stimuli to the one manipulated by the experimenter.

A second method to address the issue of perceptual matching is to use an ambiguous object as the model exemplar. The rationale for this design is that infants are provided no featural cues during the modeling phase and consequently their choice of the appropriate exemplar to enact an event cannot be a result of perceptual matching. Instead, it must be based on prior knowledge about the event and the objects or features of objects that generally engage in that event (Rakison, 2005; Rakison et al., 2007). In one such study to adopt this approach, Rakison et al. (2007) examined infants' inductive generalization of the path that objects take to reach a goal. Seminal work by Gergely, Nádasdy, Csibra, and Biro (1995) suggested that infants as young as 9 to 12 months of age apply a teleological stance—or a naïve theory of rational action—to interpret goal-directed events. In their studies, infants were habituated to a visual event in which a small ball jumped over an obstacle to reach a large ball. In a control condition, infants were habituated to an identical event except that the obstacle was absent. The movement over the block in the experimental condition was rational and goal-directed—it was the only way to reach the larger ball—but the same action in the control condition was goal-directed but not rational. There were two test trials in both conditions in which the obstacle was not present: in one, the smaller ball jumped (the nonrational action), and in the other, the smaller ball moved in a straight line (the rational action) (see Figure 12.3A(i)). Infants in the experimental condition looked longer at the nonrational action than to the rational straight-moving one; in contrast, infants in the control condition looked equally long at the two events. In follow-up experiments, 9- and 12-month-olds behaved similarly when cues to animacy, such as self-propulsion, were absent (Csibra, Gergely, Biro, Koos, & Brockbank, 1999).

To examine when and how infants generalize rational, goal-directed action to animals and not vehicles, Rakison et al. (2007) used the inductive generalization procedure to test 16- and 20-month-olds with a number of similar events to that in Gergely et al. (1995).The four events are presented Figure 12.3. One event (Figure 12.3A(i)) was identical to that used by Gergely et al. (1995). In the other three events, an object moved over a hill (Figure 12.3A(ii)) or travelled across a bridge that was above a valley (Figure 12.3A(iii)) or a sheer drop (Figure 12.3A(iv)). In the test phase, the environment was changed (Figure 12.3B) and the infant was given an animal and a vehicle with which to enact an event. In each case, infants could move the test objects either along a nonrational path similar to that they had observed during the modeling phase or along a rational path (illustrated with a dotted line in Figure 12.3B). The variables of interest were infants' choice of object (either animal or vehicle) and the path that the object was moved as it traveled toward the goal.

In the first experiment with this design, the model exemplar was an animal. The 16-month-old age group in this condition demonstrated more goal-directed motions with the animals than the vehicles; yet, they were just as likely to move the animals along rational as nonrational paths. The 20-month-olds, however, demonstrated goal-directed actions with animals and moved them along a rational path to reach the goal. These results suggest that infants at 20 months of age, but not those at 16 months of age, understand that animals follow rational paths to reach a goal. As with the studies by Mandler and McDonough (1996, 1998), however, these data can be explained by perceptual matching; that is, both the younger and older age groups may have chosen the animal because the model exemplar was an animal.

Consequently, in a follow-up experiment, infants at 16 and 20 months of age were tested with the same design except the model stimuli were ambiguous objects (see Figure 12.4). The stimuli were made from clay and varied in color. This study was also designed to address Csibra et al.'s (1999) claim that animacy cues are neither sufficient nor necessary for a teleological interpretation of an object's behavior. The results of the experiment were somewhat different from those found when the model object was an animal. In contrast to the first experiment, 20-month-olds just as often moved objects along rational and nonrational motion paths and they were just as likely to choose an

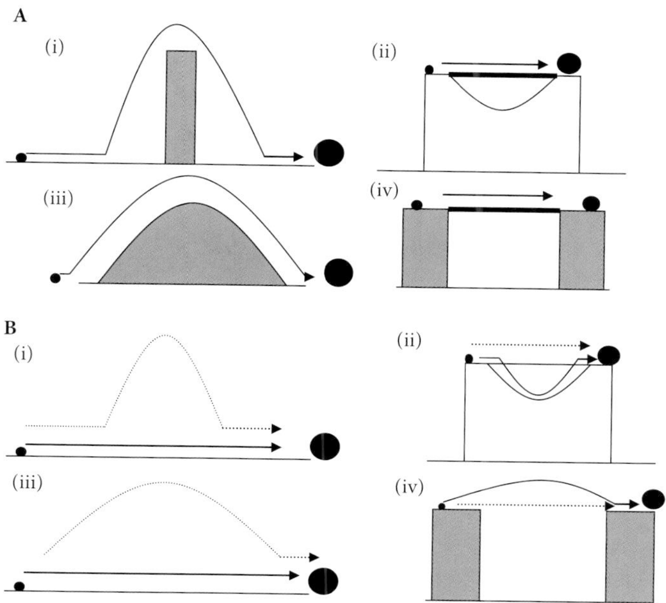

Figure 12.3 (A) Motion events modeled in Rakison et al. (2007). The small circle is the moving object; the large circle represents the goal. The motion paths modeled were (i) jumping over a block, (ii) going across a bridge over a valley, (iii) climbing over a hill, and (iv) going across a bridge over a gap. (B) Motion arenas in generalization phase of Rakison et al. (2007). Rational motion paths are illustrated by the solid line; the nonrational motion paths are illustrated by the dotted line. Note that two of the rational and nonrational paths were linear and two of the rational and non-rational paths were nonlinear.

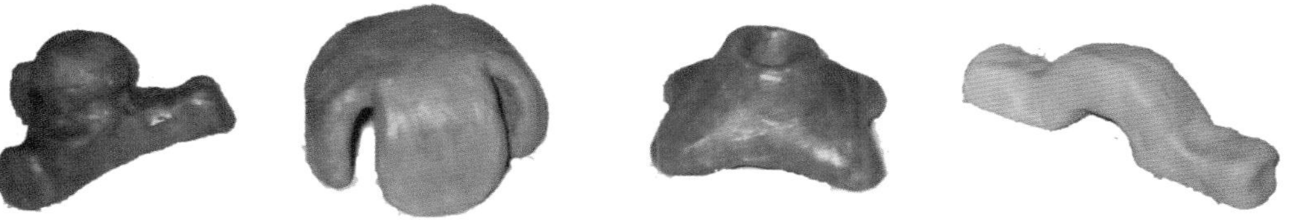

Figure 12.4 Ambiguous blocks used as model exemplars in Experiment 2 of Rakison et al. (2007).

animal as a vehicle to imitate what they had seen. Taken together, these experiments do not support Gergely, Csibra, and colleagues' (Csibra et al., 1999; Gergely et al., 1995) notion that infants apply a teleological stance to the movement of objects as early as 9 months of age. The data suggest that infants as old as 16 months do not understand that objects—specifically, animals—follow a rational path to reach a goal and that infants at 20 months require objects to possess certain surface perceptual cues to interpret their motion toward a goal as rational.

We speculate that infants associate humans, and later animals, with goal-directed actions because these entities invariably move toward goals. What has been labeled a "teleological" interpretation emerges later from experience with the movement of humans and animals, the constraints of the physical world, and the motions typical of those entities. Thus, animates tend to remain in contact with the ground as they move, do not "jump" in the absence of an obstacle, and do "jump" only when there is an obstacle or a gap. Representations that are formed via an associative learning mechanism that is sensitive to such regularities in the world would lead infants to *expect* certain actions—those we label rational—and not others.

Summary

In conjunction, the series of studies described in this section cast doubt about the extent to which infants apply prior knowledge in tasks designed to test their use of this knowledge in inductive inference (see Mandler & McDonough, 1996, 1998; McDonough & Mandler, 1998; Poulin-Dubois et al., 2006). The available data suggest that it cannot be assumed that infants' behavior in the inductive generalization task is guided by abstract knowledge—or indeed any knowledge—about the bodily, sensory, or motion related actions of animals or vehicles. As we outlined earlier, this is not to say that infants in the second year of life have no representations for the various actions of the members of these categories; indeed, as we shall show in the following section, this knowledge is in place by the middle of the second year if not earlier. However, we suggest that caution be taken before interpreting their behavior in the inductive generalization task to mean that they understand—in a conceptual sense—that members of a category engage in specific actions.

The Basis for Induction in Infancy

Clearly, at some point in developmental time, infants do learn about the various bodily, sensory, and motion-related actions of things in the world and will use this knowledge to make inductive inferences, among other things. As we discussed earlier, our view is that the mechanisms that underpin this learning are general rather than specific. Consequently, we do not conform to the view that infants form an abstract concept of animal or vehicle in the first year of life (Gelman, 1990; Leslie, 1995; Mandler, 1992; Premack, 1990). Instead, we have argued that infants' initial representations for actions of entities and objects involve an associative link between those actions and specific, often dynamic, parts (Cicchino & Rakison, 2008; Rakison, 2003, 2005, 2006; Rakison & Lupyan, 2008). For example, an associative learning mechanism that is sensitive to statistical regularities in the world will encode that a cat's legs tend to move only when it self-propels or acts as an agent in a causal event. A prediction that stems from this view is that infants will initially generalize actions or events to objects with the appropriate parts (e.g., legs, hands) rather than objects from the appropriate category that do not possess such parts (e.g., a snake for walking). In a number of recent studies, we have explicitly tested this view by examining the basis for induction in infancy.

In one series of studies to address this issue, Rakison (2005) used a novel version of the inductive generalization procedure to examine infants' knowledge about the path of motion typical of animals and vehicles. In particular, infants at 18 and 22 months of age were tested with two simple motions for animals (walking or hopping and flying) and two simple motions for vehicles (rolling and flying). Contrary to previous experiments with the inductive generalization task, Rakison (2005) presented infants with four test stimuli instead of two during the baseline and testing phases of the experiments. The rationale for this approach was to investigate directly the basis for induction; infants were given stimuli that were either from the appropriate category for the motion, that possessed the appropriate parts for the motion, some combination of the two of these factors, or neither of these factors. For example, if the experimenter modeled nonlinear "walking" with a cat, one test object was a dog (same category, same parts), another was a dolphin (same category, different parts), another was a table (different category, same parts), and another was a car (different category, different parts).

This version of the task gives researchers the tool to examine more closely the basis for early induction; specifically, it allows a test of whether infants generalize bodily, sensory, or motion properties to objects on the basis of category membership or an abstract concept of animacy (Mandler, 2004), or on the basis of specific object parts as we predicted. For the sake of simplicity, we discuss here only the data for the conditions in which land-based motions were modeled (i.e., nonlinear and linear movement in contact with a flat surface).

In the first experiment with this design (Rakison, 2005, Experiment 1), the model exemplars were animals and vehicles with the appropriate parts for the motion in question (i.e., a cat with legs and a car with wheels). In line with the prediction that infants initially associate specific functional parts with specific motion properties, the younger age group enacted the linear and nonlinear motions with objects that possessed the appropriate parts regardless of whether they belonged to the appropriate category for the motion. For instance, having seen an experimenter move a cat in a "walking" motion, infants repeated the action with a dog and a bed. Somewhat surprisingly, however, the older age group enacted the linear and nonlinear motion events only with the test object that was from the appropriate category and possessed the appropriate parts for the motion in question. Note that in a separate study with the same design that tested 14-month-olds' generalization, infants did not choose any particular test object to enact the motions they had observed. This first experiment revealed that 18-month-olds generalize walking to objects with legs and rolling to things with wheels irrespective of category membership. Yet, it remains to be seen whether both age groups' choice of exemplar in the test phase was based on perceptual matching to the model exemplar. It could argued, for example, that the younger age group focused on the legs of the cat and the wheels of the dog and generalized on this basis; the older age group, in contrast, were more constrained in their matching to the model exemplar.

To address this issue, Rakison (2005, Experiments 2 and 3) tested infants at 18 and 22 months of age with the same linear and nonlinear motions and with the same set (Experiment 2) and a different set (Experiment 3) of test exemplars. However, as in the experiments by Rakison et al. (2007), an ambiguous block was the model exemplar for the various land movements (the block was the stimulus on the far right of Figure 12.4). As before, using the ambiguous block as the model exemplar meant that the basis for any generalization of the observed action could only be attributable to prior knowledge brought to the task. The results of the experiment were indeed revealing about the basis for induction and the inductive generalization task. Infants at 18 months of age behaved similarly to those in the first experiment; they enacted the actions they had seen using the exemplars with the appropriate parts for the motion even though they did not necessarily belong to the appropriate category. The 22-month-olds, however, enacted the linear and nonlinear motions with stimuli from the appropriate category regardless of whether they possessed the appropriate parts. In other words, the older age group imitated the nonlinear walking motion with the two animals (e.g., a sheep and a snail) and linear rolling motion with the two vehicles (e.g., a car and a snowmobile).

This latter finding is important for two reasons. First, it suggests that the 22-month-olds in the first experiment were indeed influenced by the model exemplar; why else would infants who are given no information about the identity of the object (as was the case in these later experiments) outperform those who were shown a clearly identifiable category member as a model? Second, although the behavior of the 22-month-olds suggests that they generalized on the basis of category membership (e.g., walking to animals), it remains to be seen whether their choice of the appropriate category without the appropriate parts for the motion was grounded in other, as yet unknown, surface features. For example, it is possible that by 22 months of age infants have learned that things with legs move nonlinearly, that things with legs tend to have eyes, and therefore that things with eyes tend to move nonlinearly. Ongoing research in our laboratory is pursuing this explanation.

The work by Rakison (2005) was a first step in establishing that the initial basis for induction in infancy is not an abstract concept of animal or vehicle but rather is a represented associative link between a dynamic feature (e.g., legs, wheels) and a specific motion. More recently, we have explored the basis for induction for another important characteristic motion of animates, namely, goal-directed action (Cicchino & Rakison, 2008). Goal-directed action can be defined as motion that is aimed at another entity, object, or location and that is governed by an intention (Cicchino & Rakison, 2008; Woodward, Sommerville, & Guajardo, 2001). It has been proposed that infants' earliest appreciation of goal-directed action encompasses the ability to associate actions with the objects at which they are directed (Woodward, 2005) and that in developmental time, this understanding deepens to include the identification of the intentions that motivate these actions (Csibra & Gergely, 1998; Tomasello, Carpenter, Call, Behne, & Moll, 2005). The development of infants' understanding of goal-directed action has received much attention in the literature over the past 10 years, perhaps because the research pertaining to this topic straddles the realms of social cognition and conceptual development.

To examine when and how infants learn that animates but not inanimates are goal-directed, Cicchino and Rakison (2007) used a version of the now classic task developed by Woodward (1998, 1999). In the original tasks, 5- and 9-month-old infants were habituated to an event in which a hand reached for one of two objects on a stage. In the test phase of the study, the locations of the two objects on the stage were switched. Infants viewed a new side test trial in which they saw the hand reach to the same object as that during habituation but to a new location, and a new goal test trial in which they viewed the hand reach toward the same location as that during habituation but toward a different object. It was hypothesized that if infants viewed the hand's action in habituation to be directed at a specific object, they would then look longer at the *new goal* test trial than at the *new side* test trial, because only the new goal test trial violated the relationship between the hand and the object learned during habituation. Infants at both 5 and 9 months of age displayed this pattern of results and looked longer at the new goal test trial than at the new side test trial. However, when infants were presented with a rod, hand-shaped occluder, or mechanical claw that made contact with the object throughout the study instead of a hand, they no longer looked longer at the new goal event than at the new side event.

To examine at what point in developmental time infants generalize goal-directed action to animals and not vehicles, Cicchino and Rakison (2007) tested infants between 14 and 26 months of age with an inductive generalization version of Woodward's (1998) task. Infants saw an experimenter move an object a number of times toward one of two goal objects on a premade environment. Figure 12.5 illustrates the testing environment and the four-goal stimuli (a bed, food, toys, and a ball). After the modeling phase, the locations of the two objects were switched and infants were encouraged to move the same object that the experimenter had moved toward the goal objects. Note that in contrast to the other inductive generalization tasks described in this chapter, in these experiments, infants used the same toy exemplar as the experimenter to enact an event. Unlike the prediction that followed from Woodward's (1998) habituation task, it was hypothesized that if infants attributed goal-directedness to an object, they would move it more often toward the same object as the experimenter had during the modeling phase than toward the same side; if infants did not associate the object with the object it had contacted, performance was expected to be at chance levels.

In a first study designed to address when infants generalize goal-directed action to animals and not vehicles (Cicchino & Rakison, 2008, Experiment 1), 14-, 18-, and 22-month-olds participated in the task with two animals and two vehicles as the test exemplars. When infants were shown an animal moving toward a goal, 14-month-olds did not display a preference for either the location or the path, 18-month-olds moved the toys along the same path as that seen during the modeling phase, and 22-month-olds imitated the action of the experimenter by moving the toys toward the same object as in the modeling phase. In contrast, when infants were shown a vehicle moving toward a goal, infants in all three age groups showed no reliable preference for the either the same object or the same path as that observed in the modeling phase.

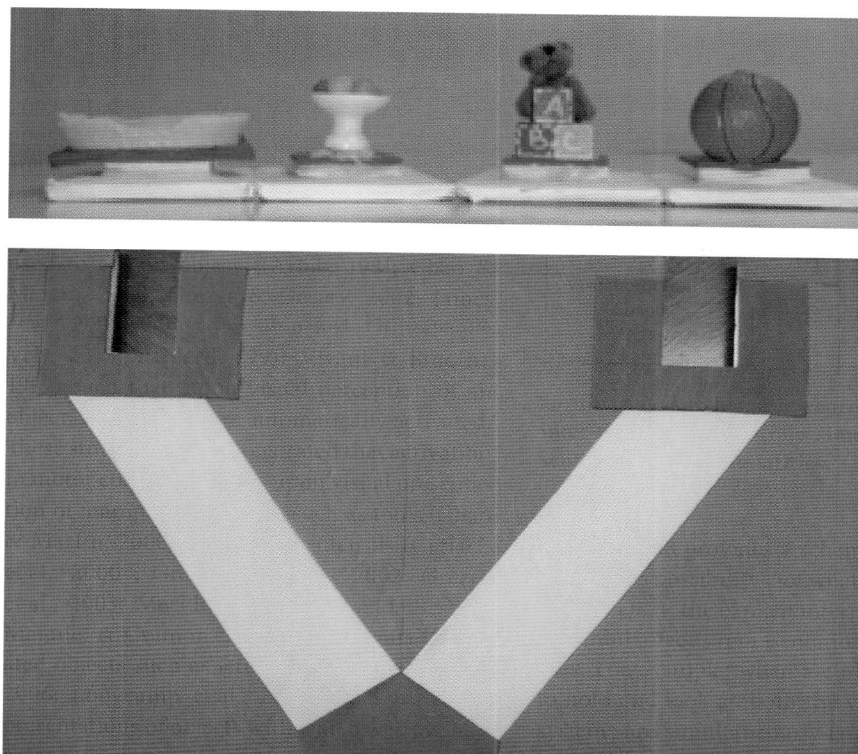

Figure 12.5 **Testing environment and goal stimuli in Cicchino and Rakison (2007).**

This pattern of results suggests that 18-month-old infants associated animals, but not vehicles, with their path of motion but not with their final goal, and that 22-month-olds can selectively associate the actions of nonhuman animals, but not of vehicles, with a goal object.

To address whether the basis for this inductive behavior was an abstract concept of animacy or salient perceptual cues, in a follow-up experiment Cicchino and Rakison (2007, Experiment 3) used the same procedure with 22-month-olds but the test exemplars were an intact scale model cow, a cow missing legs, a cow missing facial features, and a cow missing both facial features and legs. These stimuli are illustrated in Figure 12.6. The rationale for this design was to determine whether infants generalize goal-directed action for animals on the basis of legs, facial features, or a more abstract conceptual representation for animals (in which case they would move only the intact cow toward the same object as that observed during the modeling phase). The results of the experiment showed that 22-month-olds generalized goal-directed action to objects with legs and did so regardless of whether or not they possessed facial features; however, they did not generalize goal-directed action to entities on the basis of facial features alone. This pattern of behavior, which is consistent with that of previous induction and categorization studies (Rakison, 2005; Rakison & Butterworth, 1998), suggests that the presence of legs, but not of facial features, is critical for infants to attribute goal-directedness to animals.

In a final study designed to determine if and when young children generalize goal-directed action to animals more broadly—that is, not

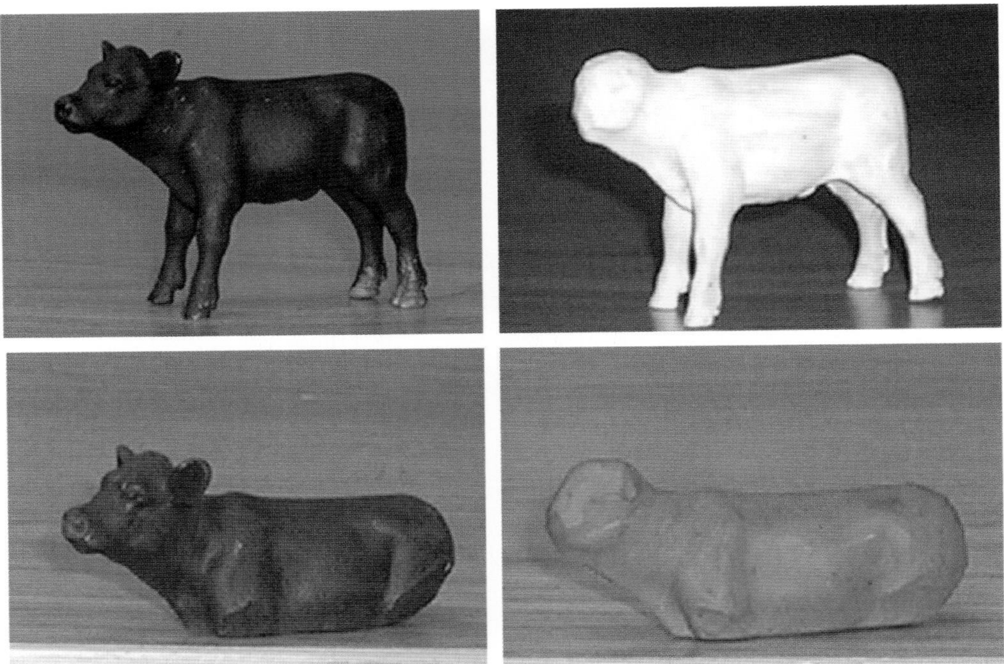

Figure 12.6 **Modified cow stimuli used in Experiment 3 by Cicchino and Rakison (2008).**

on the basis of legs—26-month-olds were tested in the same procedure but the four test stimuli were chosen based on their category membership and whether or not they had legs. The rationale for this choice of stimuli was similar to that in Rakison (2005); one object was an animal with legs (a camel), another was an animal without legs (a snake), one was not an animal but possessed legs (a table), and a final object was not an animal and did not have legs (a car). It was predicted, based on Rakison (2005), that 26-month-olds would generalize goal-directed action to the two animals and not to the objects with legs; however, the results showed that even in the third year of life, children generalize goal-directed action on the basis of parts rather than category membership. In other words, 26-month-olds moved the camel and the table toward the same goal as the experimenter had during the modeling phase, but they did not do so for the snake or the car.

In conjunction, this program of research shows that perceptual features—such as legs—act as the basis for induction for simple motions and goal-directed action for infants and young children (Cicchino & Rakison, 2008; Rakison, 2005). A distinct developmental trend was observed for infants' knowledge of linear and nonlinear land motions; their initial representations involved an associative link between specific features and specific motion paths but later, around 22 months of age, this link was extended to include objects that did not possess those features. In contrast, infants' knowledge of goal-directed action showed a developmental progression in terms of when they started to understand that animals and not vehicles are goal-directed. However, object features remained the basis for induction as late as 26 months of age.

Summary

The studies reported in this section provide strong evidence against the view that infants' inductive inference is based on an abstract conceptual representation for animals, vehicles, and other superordinate categories and that it is not influenced by the surface appearance of objects

(Mandler & McDonough, 1996, 1998; Pauen, 2002; Poulin-Dubois et al., 2006). Clearly, further research on infants' inductive inferences for other motion properties such as self-propulsion or agency is necessary to solidify this claim, and indeed such research is already underway in our laboratory. Nonetheless, the available data cast doubt on the idea that the mechanisms for learning such information are specialized rather than general. Recall that a corollary of such a view is that infants are precocious concept formers, and that they develop rich representations about, for example, animals that incorporate how they move in the world. The experiments discussed here show that such representations are not in place until at least the end of the second year of life, findings that are incompatible with the "top-down" view of Mandler and others.

Concluding comments

In this chapter, we have challenged the predominant "top-down" view of early inductive inference. According to this view, induction and categorization by infants as young as 9 to 11 months of age is based on abstract knowledge about the properties of things that is acquired through specialized mechanisms, modules, or innate principles (Gelman, 1990; Leslie, 1995; Mandler, 1992; Mandler & McDonough, 1996, 1998; Poulin-Dubois et al., 2006). We contested this perspective both on theoretical and empirical grounds.

First, we proposed that infants' concepts for objects and entities are generated via general rather than specific mechanisms. As a corollary of this view, we argued that early knowledge about the properties of things in the world involves an associative links between specific surface features and those properties, and that such representations are not in place until the middle or end of the second year of life (see also Oakes & Madole, 2003; Quinn & Eimas, 1997; Smith, Jones, & Landau, 1996). Second, we argued that care must be taken in interpreting infants' behavior within the inductive generalization procedure. In particular, we claimed that (1) infants' behavior in the task is not always driven by knowledge acquired prior to arriving at the laboratory; and (2) the basis for induction for any property must be studied before conclusions can be drawn about the nature and content of infants' concepts. In support of these views, we provided data from inductive generalization studies with 14- to 26-month-olds that show that infants are influenced by the model exemplar used by the experimenter and that perceptual features—such as legs and wheels—act as the basis for early induction for motion properties.

In light of the fact that research on induction in infancy is a recent development, there is clearly much work to be done. The work to data has focused largely on the bodily, sensory, and motion properties of animals and vehicles but has largely ignored infants' knowledge of other animates—people and insects—and the many categories of inanimate objects (e.g., tools, furniture). Research from our laboratory has started to investigate infants' understanding of the properties of the members of these categories, but important questions remain unanswered. Which surface features are associated with which actions? How are specific feature-property associations generalized to other features? How much experience is required to form such associations? And how do these associations generalized to categories of objects? In time, answers to these, and other, questions will surely be forthcoming. In the meantime, it is the responsibility of researchers to be pragmatic in their interpretation of infants' behavior in the inductive generalization task and to design experiments that will elucidate the nature and content of infants' developmental representations for the objects and entities in the world.

References

Baldwin, D. A., Markman, E. M., & Melartin, E. M. (1993).Infants' ability to draw inferences about nonobvious object properties: Evidence from exploratory play. *Child Development, 64*, 711–728.

Bauer, P. J., & Dow, G. A. (1994). Episodic memory in 16- and 20-month-old children: Specifics are generalized but not forgotten. *Developmental Psychology, 30*, 403–417.

Cicchino, J. B., & Rakison, D. H. (2008). *Infants' attribution of goal-directed action to non-human animals.* Manuscript under review.

Csibra, G., & Gergely, G. (1998). The teleological origins of mentalistic action explanations: A developmental hypothesis. *Developmental Science, 1,* 255–259.

Csibra, G., Gergely, G., Bíró, S., Koós, O., & Brockbank, M. (1999). Goal attribution without agency cues: The perception of 'pure reason' in infancy. *Cognition, 72,* 237–267.

Furrer, S. D., Younger, B .A., & Johnson, K. E. (2005, April) Do planes drink? *Generalized imitation following modeling with an inappropriate exemplar.* Poster presented at the Society for Research in Child Development Biennial Conference, Atlanta, GA.

Gelman, R. (1990). First principles organize attention to and learning about relevant data: Number and the animate–inanimate distinction as examples. *Cognitive Science, 14,* 79–106.

Gelman, S. A., & Markman, E. M. (1986). Categories and induction in young children. *Cognition, 23,* 183–209.

Gelman, S. A., & Markman, E. M. (1987). Young children's inductions from natural kinds: The role of categories and appearances. *Child Development, 58,* 1532–1541.

Gergely, G., Nádasdy, Z., Csibra, G., & Bíró, S. (1995). Taking the intentional stance at 12 months of age. *Cognition, 56,* 165–193.

Killen, M., & Uzgiris, I. C. (1981). Imitation of actions with objects: The role of social meaning. *Journal of Genetic Psychology, 138,* 219–229.

Leslie, A. (1995). A theory of agency. In D. Sperber, D. Premack, & A.J. Premack (Eds.), *Causal cognition* (pp. 121–141). Oxford: Clarendon.

Mandler, J. M. (1992). How to build a baby: II. Conceptual primitives. *Psychological Review, 99,* 587–604.

Mandler, J. M. (2004). *The foundations of mind: Origins of conceptual thought.* New York: Oxford University Press.

Mandler, J. M., & McDonough, L. (1996). Drinking and driving don't mix: Inductive generalization in infancy. *Cognition, 59,* 307–335.

Mandler, J. M., & McDonough, L. (1998). Studies in inductive inference in infancy. *Cognitive Psychology, 37,* 60–96.

McDonough, L., & Mandler, J. M. (1998). Inductive generalization in 9- and 11-month-olds. *Developmental Science. 1,* 227–232.

Oakes, L. M., & Madole, K. L. (2003). Principles of developmental change in infants' category formation. In D.H. Rakison & L.M. Oakes (Eds.), *Early category and concept development: Making sense of the blooming, buzzing confusion* (pp.159–192). New York: Oxford University Press.

Oakes, L. M., Madole, K. L., & Cohen, L. B. (1991). Infant habituation and categorization of real objects. *Cognitive Development, 6,* 377–392.

Pauen, S. (2002). Evidence for knowledge-based category discrimination in infancy. *Child Development, 73,* 1016–1033.

Poulin-Dubois, D., Frenkiel-Fishman, S., Nayer, S., & Johnson, S. (2006). Infants' inductive generalization of bodily, motion, and sensory properties to animals and people. *Journal of Cognition and Development, 7,* 431–453.

Premack, D. (1990). The infants' theory of self-propelled objects. *Cognition, 36,* 1–16.

Quinn, P. C., & Eimas, P. D. (1997). A reexamination of the perceptual-to-conceptual shift in mental representations. *Review of General Psychology, 1,* 171–187.

Rakison, D. H. (2003). Parts, categorization, and the animate–inanimate distinction in infancy. In D. H. Rakison, & L. M. Oakes, (Eds.), *Early category and concept development: Making sense of the blooming buzzing confusion* (pp. 159–192). New York, NY: Oxford University Press.

Rakison, D. H. (2005). Developing knowledge of motion properties in infancy. *Cognition, 96,* 183–214.

Rakison, D. H. (2006). Make the first move: How infants learn about the identity of self-propelled objects. *Developmental Psychology, 42,* 900–912.

Rakison, D. H., & Butterworth, G. (1998). Infants' use of parts in early categorization. *Developmental Psychology, 34,* 49–62.

Rakison, D. H., Cicchino, J. B., & Hahn, E. R. (2007). Infants' knowledge of the identity of rational goal-directed entities. *British Journal of Developmental Psychology, 25,* 461–470.

Rakison, D. H., & Lupyan, G. (2008). Developing object concepts in infancy: An associative learning perspective. *Monographs of the Society for Research in Child Development, 73(1),* 1–110.

Rakison, D. H., & Poulin-Dubois, D. (2000, July). Infants' understanding of animate and inanimate motion events. In D.H. Rakison (Chair),

Components of the animate–inanimate distinction in infancy. Paper presented at the twelfth Biennial International Conference on Infant Studies, Brighton, UK.

Sloutsky, V. M., & Fisher, A. V. (2004). Induction and categorization in young children: A similarity-based model. *Journal of Experimental Psychology: General, 133*, 166–188.

Smith, L. B., Jones, S. S., & Landau, B. (1996). Naming in young children: a dumb attentional mechanism? *Cognition, 60*, 143–171.

Tomasello, M., Carpenter, M., Call, J., Behne, T., & Moll, H. (2005). Understanding and sharing intentions: The origins of cultural cognition. *Behavioral and Brain Sciences, 28*, 675–735.

Tomasello, M., & Striano, T. (2001) Social and object support for early symbolic play. *Developmental Science, 4*, 442–455.

Tomasello, M., Striano, T., & Rochat, P. (1999) Do young children use objects as symbols? *British Journal of Developmental Psychology, 17*, 563–584.

Woodward, A.L. (1998). Infants selectively encode the goal object of an actor's reach. *Cognition, 69*, 1–34.

Woodward, A. L. (1999). Infants' ability to distinguish between purposeful and non-purposeful behaviors. *Infant Behavior and Development, 22*, 145–160.

Woodward, A. L. (2005). The infant origins of intentional understanding. In R. Kail (Ed.), *Advances in child development and behavior* (Vol. 33, pp. 229–262). Oxford: Elsevier.

Woodward, A. L., Sommerville, J. A., & Guajardo, J. J. (2001). How infants make sense of intentional action. In B. Malle, L. Moses & D. Baldwin (Eds.) *Intentions and intentionality: Foundations of social cognition* (pp. 149–169). Cambridge, MA: MIT Press.

Younger, B. A., & Johnson, K. E. (2004). Infants' comprehension of toy replicas as symbols for real objects. *Cognitive Psychology, 48*, 207–242.

CHAPTER 13
The Acquisition of Expertise as a Model for the Growth of Cognitive Structure

Paul C. Quinn

If one is interested in the question of how knowledge is acquired, then the period of infancy becomes an important time window of empirical inquiry. During the first few months of life, infants begin to experience objects from various classes, but at different rates or frequencies of presentation. For example, infants are likely to encounter conspecifics, other humans, more frequently than say, nonhuman animals, even in a family environment that includes a nonhuman animal (cat or dog) as a pet. This feature of infants' early experience allows investigators to ask whether there are differences in the (1) way that infants categorize humans versus nonhuman animals, (2) nature of the category representations formed by infants for humans versus nonhuman animals, (3) perceptual attributes that infants use to categorize humans versus nonhuman animals, and (4) relative amounts of top-down versus bottom-up processing used to categorize humans versus nonhuman animals.

The contrast between how infants respond to humans versus nonhuman animals may represent an expert–novice difference in the early development of perceptual category representations. This interpretation provides the starting point for the broader proposal that the "training and transfer of perceptual expertise" may represent a model for thinking about knowledge acquisition and cognitive development in general. Over the last 10 years, a literature has arisen on how perceptual expertise can emerge in adult participants (Bukach, Gauthier, & Tarr, 2006; Palmeri, Wong, & Gauthier, 2004; Tanaka & Gauthier, 1997). This literature has pointed to two hallmark characteristics of perceptual expertise. One is that objects within an expert domain tend to be recognized at a specific, subordinate, individual-exemplar level, rather than at a generic, basic, category level. For example, a bird expert is likely to identify a sparrow as a "sparrow" rather than as a "bird." This marker of expertise has been referred to as the "downward shift in recognition" (Tanaka, 2001). Notably, the shift corresponds with an effect which has been observed in studies of category learning in adults, namely, that during the time course of learning a category, individuals come to supplement a rule-based or summary structure with a structure that represents the individual exemplars (Gauthier & Tarr, 1997; Johansen & Palmeri, 2002; Smith & Minda, 1998). A second manifestation of expertise is the tendency for objects to be perceived holistically (Gauthier & Tarr, 2002). This mode of perceptual encoding emphasizes that there are performance advantages associated with processing the whole as opposed to processing individual parts (e.g., a whole superiority effect).

Given that the downward shift in recognition and holistic processing effects have been documented as markers of expertise in adults, developmentalists interested in when expertise emerges can ask whether there are any stimulus domains where these effects become evident in infants. In addition, studying how expertise may arise early in development could provide investigators with insights that may not be achieved in studies that *train* expertise in adults. Specifically, adults who acquire expertise in a particular domain have an entire knowledge base that can be recruited as the expertise is acquired. By contrast, young infants who may develop expertise are doing so without an extensive knowledge base, and thus one may be better able to determine how the expertise affects the representation of generic nonexpert object information that is being acquired in the same developmental time window as the expertise. That is, by studying how expertise emerges in young infants, one may be in a stronger position to assess how that expertise structures the acquisition of nonexpert information, thereby providing a more informed sense of how information can accrue to existing representations and form a domain of knowledge. On this basis, investigations of the effects of expertise development in infants may inform studies examining how the training of expertise may bring about cognitive change in adults.

The chapter will begin by asking whether infants can form category representations for nonhuman animals, via what stimulus attributes such representations might be formed, and whether infants are forming these category representations on the basis of stimulus images presented in the laboratory. The chapter will proceed to a discussion of whether infants categorize humans, and whether the category structure that infants use to represent humans differs from the structure infants use to represent nonhuman animals. Also considered will be the stimulus information infants use to represent humans as well as whether infants respond to human images presented in the laboratory on the basis of knowledge about humans acquired prior to arrival at the laboratory. The chapter will conclude with the thesis that what infants know about nonhuman animals can be likened to what novices know about generic object categories, whereas what infants know about humans can be likened to what experts know about their domain of expertise.

Categorization of Nonhuman Animals by Young Infants

Looking Time Studies

A familiarization/novelty-preference procedure has been used to study how infants categorize nonhuman animals such as cats and horses (Mareschal & Quinn, 2001). Infants are presented with multiple instances from a common category during familiarization and then with a preference test pairing a novel instance from the familiar category and a novel instance from a novel category. Categorization is inferred if infants generalize their familiarization to the novel instance from the familiar category and display a preference for the novel instance from the novel category. The preference is measured in looking time, and it is important to demonstrate in control procedures that the preference cannot be attributed to (1) an a priori preference for instances of the novel category over instances of the familiar category or (2) the inability to discriminate among instances of the familiar category. Concluding that categorization has occurred based on this pattern of performance accords well with the traditional way categorization has been defined in the adult concept literature, namely, as equivalent responding to discriminably different instances from a common class based on some internalized representation of the class (Bruner, Goodnow, & Austin, 1956).

With the familiarization/novelty-preference procedure, 3- to 4-month-old infants familiarized with a dozen visual images of cats have generalized their familiarization to novel cats and displayed novel category preferences for exemplars of birds, dogs, and horses (Oakes & Ribar, 2005; Quinn, Eimas, & Rosenkrantz, 1993; Younger & Fearing, 1999). Likewise, same-aged infants familiarized with photographic instances of horses have generalized their familiarization to novel horses and shown novel category preferences for exemplars of cats, giraffes, and zebras (Eimas & Quinn, 1994). These novel category preferences are not attributable to a priori preference, nor can they be explained by an inability to discriminate among the familiar category instances. The results indicate that infants can form individuated category representations for cats and horses, each of which excludes instances of the other as well as exemplars of other basic-level nonhuman animal categories.

Examples of the cats can be seen in seen in Figure 13.1, where it can be observed that the images presented to the infants are realistic and depict different breeds of cats in a variety of colors and stances. The variation amongst the exemplars decreases the likelihood that the infants could represent one or more spurious stimulus attributes that are common to a small set of stimulus images but not necessarily diagnostic of "catness" as it exists in the natural world. It should also be mentioned that each category was represented by 18 different instances. Having this many stimuli included in each category allowed each individual infant to be presented with a randomly selected set of 12 exemplars during familiarization, and with randomly selected pairings of novel stimuli from the familiar and novel categories during the preference test. This feature of the experimental design increases the ecological validity of the study given that no two infants are likely to experience the same set of cats in the same order during early development. Finally, Figure 13.1 makes clear that the stimuli from within a category are highly discriminable and this underscores again that the preferences cannot be attributed merely to processes of perceptual discrimination between categories (cf., Bauer, Dow, & Hertsgaard, 1995; Dueker & Needham, 2005; Pauen, 2002; Xu, 1997). The infants can discriminate between the different instances of the cats just as readily as they can discriminate between a cat and a dog, yet they are also able to look through this variation so as to group together the various cat images into a common representation that excludes the dog images.

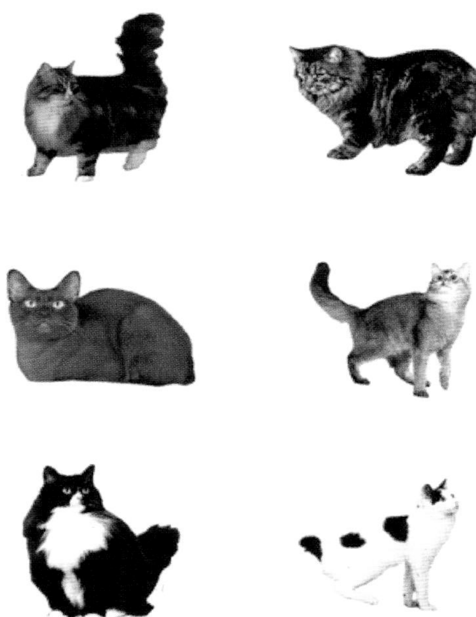

Figure 13.1 Examples of the cat images presented in the studies investigating infants' categorization of nonhuman animals.

Neural Correlates

As a complement to the behavioral looking-time studies demonstrating category formation for the various nonhuman animal species by infants, Quinn, Westerlund, and Nelson (2006) recently investigated whether neural correlates of category learning by infants might be measurable. They did so by developing an event-related potential (ERP) analog of the behavioral looking-time procedure. This involved placing a 64-channel Geodesic Sensor Net on the head of the participating infants to record their brain wave activity (Tucker, 1993). Attempting to make the ERP recording procedure equivalent to the behavioral looking-time procedure can be challenging given that ERPs are measured for short, discrete, half-second presentations of visual stimuli, whereas in the behavioral looking-time studies, the images are continuously available for 10 to 15 s at a time. In an effort to provide the infants in the ERP procedure with an amount of category structure at least somewhat comparable to that presented in the looking-time studies, Quinn et al. compensated for the shorter-duration stimuli by presenting more of them, while at the same time remaining cognizant of the limited attention span of infants and the total number of stimulus presentations the infants would tolerate. These considerations led to an experimental design in which infants were presented with 36 cat images followed by 20 novel cat images interspersed with 20 dog images.

It should also be acknowledged that the participants in the ERP studies were 6-month-olds, approximately 2.5 months older than the 3- to 4-month-old participants in the behavioral studies. The age change was necessitated because pilot testing revealed a substantially higher attrition rate of the younger infants participating in the ERP procedure. The higher attrition rate could be attributed to a greater likelihood for the younger age group to engage in head movements during stimulus presentations, thereby creating artifacts in the resulting neural activity that make it difficult to determine what portions of the neural response were due to the head movement and what portions were due to the stimulus presentation. Fortunately, 6-month-olds, like their younger counterparts, have been shown to form category representations for nonhuman animal species in behavioral looking-time procedures (Eimas & Quinn, 1994), thereby facilitating comparison with outcomes obtained from ERP procedures. A 6-month-old wearing the geodesic sensor net is depicted in Figure 13.2.

The analytical plan involved partitioning the results (i.e., the neural activations observed in different parts of the scalp up to a second and a half after stimulus presentation) into four different conditions: cats 1–18, cats 19–36, novel cats, and novel dogs. The rationale is that if there is a neural signal that corresponds with category learning, then the responses to cats 1–18 and the novel dogs (reflecting initial experience with exemplars of a category) are equivalent. The responses to cats 19–36 and the novel cats (reflecting a learned category of cats) should also be equivalent, but different from the responses to cats 1–18 and the novel dogs.

With regard to expectations for how the amplitude and latency of the brain wave components of infants might be affected in a category learning procedure, the only guide was the brain wave responsiveness of infants observed in studies of simple recognition memory (e.g., Nelson, 1994; Reynolds & Richards, 2005). Of interest is a late-slow wave component observed in the time window between 1,000 and 1,500 ms after stimulus presentation. The amplitude of the slow wave has been associated with the differentiation of familiar and novel stimuli. In

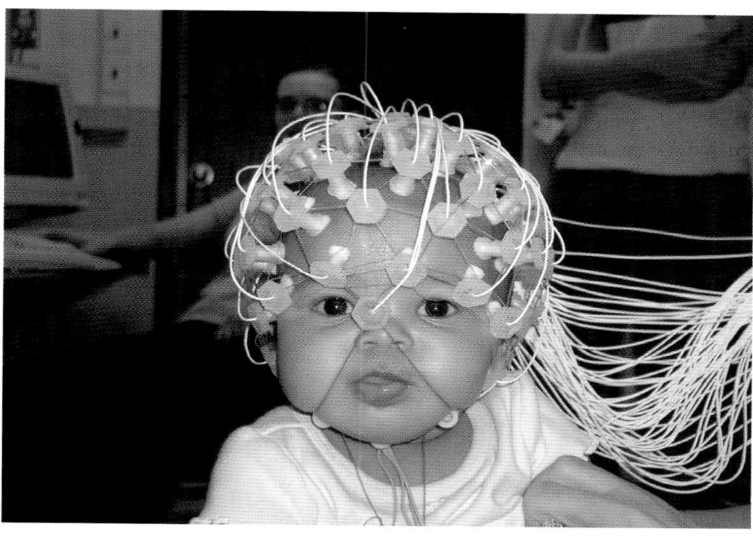

Figure 13.2 A 6-month-old infant wearing the Geodesic sensor net (Courtesy of Alissa Westerlund).

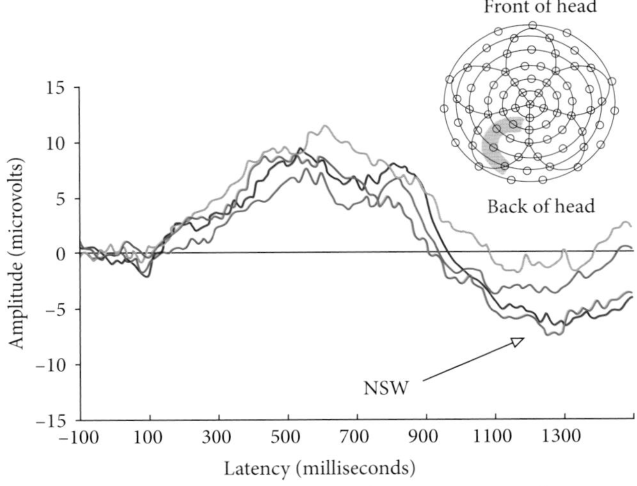

Figure 13.3 Grand average infant ERPs reflecting the negative slow wave (NSW) response to the first set of familiar cats (blue), second set of familiar cats (red), novel cats (orange), and novel dogs (green) for a group (average) of left occipital-parietal electrodes.

particular, a slow wave that returns to baseline has been associated with the recognition of familiarity, whereas a slow wave that deflects away from baseline in either the positive or negative direction is associated with the detection of novelty. As is depicted in Figure 13.3, greater negative amplitude was recorded over left occipital parietal scalp in the time window between 1,000 and 1,500 ms after stimulus onset in response to cats 1–18 and novel dogs than in response to cats 19–36 and novel cats. This analysis reveals that the infant's brain responded to novel cats with activity equivalent to that displayed for cats 19–36. More generally, it points to the neural instantiation of a key behavioral indicant of categorization: responding to the novel as if it is familiar. That there is distinct brain activity corresponding to the formation of a category representation for the exemplars presented during familiarization (e.g., the cats) provides convergent evidence with the looking-time studies and indicates a neural preparedness at 6 months to represent category information on the basis of perceptual experience.

Perceptual Processes Supporting Category Formation by Infants: What is the Significance?

With infant category learning of nonhuman animal species evident in both brain and behavior, one can ask what the larger significance of these findings is for the conceptual development literature. As described by Rogers and McClelland (2004), "...these studies are viewed as being important for conceptual development, because they demonstrate that in many cases, the visual similarities apparent from photographs of real objects can be sufficient to allow the discrimination of semantic categories" (p. 124). To expand on the observation of Rogers and McClelland, the studies of infant learning of nonhuman animal categories suggest that young infants possess abilities to divide the world of objects into perceptual clusters that approximate a basic level of exclusivity. These perceptual cluster representations later come to have conceptual significance for adults. As such, the conceptual representations found later in development can be viewed as informational enrichments of the category representations that infants form on the basis of perceptual experience.

To provide a concrete example of the aforementioned ideas, consider infants who are presented with exemplars of cats and horses. The looking time and ERP studies suggest that the exemplars are not experienced as an undifferentiated bunch of grapes, but rather as separate groups that fall into distinct representations. These representations could then serve as placeholders for the acquisition of the more abstract and nonobvious information that occurs beyond infancy, through language and more formal learning of semantic categories. Thus, over time, the perceptual placeholder representation for horses will come to include the information that horses eat hay, carry heavy loads, give birth to foals, have horse DNA, and are labeled as "horses," whereas the perceptual placeholder representation for cats will come to include the information that cats eat tuna, hunt mice, give birth to kittens, have cat DNA, and are labeled as "cats." The acquisition of this additional information serves to enrich the original perceptually based category representations to the point that they attain the richness and boundedness of the more mature conceptual representations of children and adults.

It is important to acknowledge that this view does not deny that in some instances, the more abstract information can supplant the more perceptual information when the two sources of information are placed in competition as determinants of category identity (Keil, 1989). This type of evidence has been used to support an "essentialist" view of concept development (Gelman, 2003), a perspective that argues that the organization of perceptual experience is not sufficient to explain the full course of category development. While "essentialist" arguments are persuasive, the claims have been challenged on the grounds that at least some of the evidence in which nonobvious features win over perceptual features as indicators of category identity was obtained because of salience differences between the individual features presented in the comparisons (Jones & Smith, 1993). Moreover, Hampton, Estes, and Simmons (2007; see also Hampton, 1995) have actually presented cases in which a majority of research participants weight characteristic perceptual features more heavily than defining essentialist features in decisions about category identity.

Arguments about the relative force of perceptual and nonobvious features aside, the major claim here is that it is difficult to envision how a child could go from experiencing cats and horses as an undifferentiated bunch of grapes to representing cats as having cat DNA and horses as having horse DNA without the perceptual placeholder representations that organize the individual cats and horses into distinct representations serving as facilitating intermediaries. In other words, it is hard to imagine how a child could even acquire the more abstract attributes and map them onto their correct object referents without having category representations available from perceptual experience to serve as support structures. Mapping attributes onto objects on a case by case would arguably be a much slower and labor-intensive process. The perceptual category representations of infants may thus form an important linkage mechanism for conjoining concrete object classes with their nonobvious attributes in an efficient manner.

It is also important to acknowledge that the emphasis in interpreting the category learning abilities is on the demonstration of perceptual parsing skills. There is no evidence, for example, that infants who are familiarized with cats or horses in the laboratory are leaving the laboratory with long-term memory representations for these classes. The claim is that infants are demonstrating perceptual grouping or clustering abilities in the laboratory that are presumably engaged when infants encounter cats and horses in the course of experience in the world outside the laboratory (or images of them as depicted in videos and picture books). The latter representations are those believed to be the ones that serve as the supports for the acquisition of the nonobvious attributes that occurs beyond the infancy period.

What Perceptual Information Do Young Infants Use to Categorize Nonhuman Animals?

Although the chapter has thus far centered on the learning of category representations formed on the basis of perceptual experience, what has not yet been considered is the question of what perceptual attributes infants are using to construct the category representations. One can ask whether it is the whole of the stimulus images that infants are using or whether it is a particular part or the pattern of correlation across multiple parts. The answer to this question is not obvious, given that the animal category representations sorted by infants include cats, dogs, and horses, where the exemplars of each category possess attributes in common such as a head, torso, legs, and a tail.

Quinn and Eimas (1996) examined the abilities of 3- to 4-month-olds to categorize cats versus dogs when provided with the whole stimuli, just the heads (with the body occluded), or just the bodies (with the head occluded) during both the familiarization and preference test portions of the experiment. The results were that the infants categorized when presented with the whole stimuli (this outcome should not be surprising given that it constitutes a replication of results already described) and also when presented with just the heads, although not with just the bodies. The findings indicate that the head provided a sufficient basis for the infants to categorize cats versus dogs.

The conclusion of Quinn and Eimas (1996) is supported by an additional study in which infants were familiarized with whole cat or dog images and then preference tested with hybrid stimuli, i.e., cat head on dog body versus dog head on cat body (Spencer, Quinn, Johnson, & Karmiloff-Smith, 1997). Examples of the stimuli are presented in Figure 13.4. Infant preference followed the direction of the novel category head. That the head region provided infants with the information to separate cats and dogs into different category groupings is consistent with the broader idea that young infants' category representations for nonhuman animal species are structured by perceptual part or attribute information that can be detected from the surfaces of the exemplars. In other words, young infants may represent nonhuman animal categories on a featural basis. Interestingly, adults also seem to emphasize the head when representing nonhuman animal species (Reed, McGoldrick, Schackelford, & Fidopiastis, 2004).

Head Preference: Attentional Bias or Diagnostic Feature?

A question of recent interest has been why infants use the heads to categorize the cats as separate from the dogs. Use of the head could arise from a biasing mechanism that orients infant attention to attend to head information that is present in a visual scene (Johnson & Morton, 1991). Such a biasing mechanism would be adaptive in

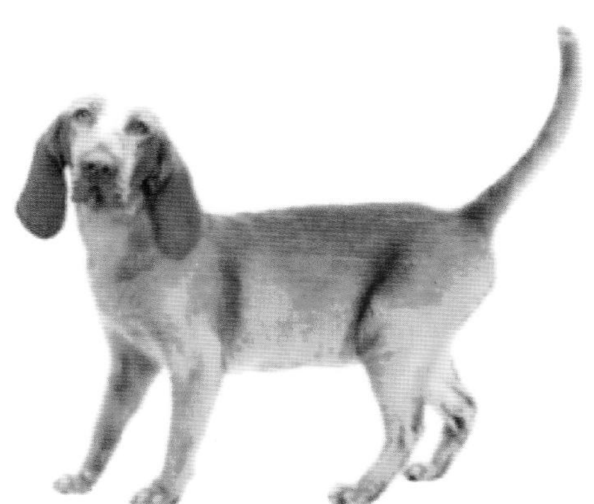

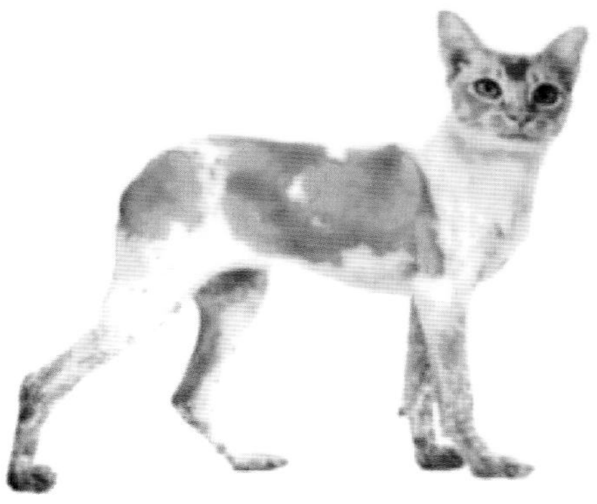

Figure 13.4 Examples of the cat–dog hybrid stimuli presented to the infants in Spencer et al. (1997).

terms of insuring that infants will attend to and eventually recognize faces. It is also possible that the infants simply learn that the head is the most diagnostic part of the stimulus and that the head feature is flexibly created as the basis for the category representation during the course of experience with the exemplars (Quinn, Schyns, & Goldstone, 2006). This possibility seems reasonable to suggest given that the head may have fewer degrees of freedom relative to the body in terms of the various stances presented to the infants (Reed, Stone, & McGoldrick, 2005). As such, it might be more easily extracted as an invariant feature.

To tease apart whether use of the heads was due to top-down or bottom-up influences, Mermillod, French, Smeets, and Spencer (2005) employed an empirical strategy based on computational modeling. In particular, Mermillod et al. followed the lead of Mareschal and French (1997) who proposed that the learning that occurs in infant looking time experiments is analogous to the learning that occurs in simple connectionist networks. In particular, the extent to which an infant continues to look at a stimulus reflects the difference between the actual stimulus and the mental representation of the stimulus in the same way that error in an autoassociative network reflects the extent to which output does not match with input. Mermillod et al. simulated the Spencer et al. (1997) experiments with the hybrid stimuli by training an autoencoder on cat or dog images, with each image expressed as an input vector with 7 features from the head and 7 from the body. When the network was tested on the hybrid images presented in accord with the same input scheme, the head preference observed in the experiment with the infants was not reproduced. Error was equivalent for both kinds of the hybrid images, instead of there being greater error for the images with the novel category head. This finding is consistent with the idea that the head preference does not arise from bottom-up processes deriving the head as a diagnostic feature from the statistics of the input.

Another approach taken to address the question of why infants rely on the head rather than the body to partition cats and dogs into separate categories has relied on eye tracking to measure the eye movements that infants use to scan the visual images that they are presented with in the category learning task. This in turn allows one to conduct the same behavioral experiments that have used looking time as a measure of categorization performance and learn where on the stimulus images the infants are fixating. On the assumption that stimulus regions used for categorization will be preferentially fixated over those not used, Quinn, Doran, Reiss, and Hoffman (2009) reasoned that if the head preference results from a biasing mechanism, then infants should fixate more on the heads than the bodies of the exemplars throughout the course of the familiarization portion of a category learning procedure. Alternatively, if the infants are learning that the head is the most diagnostic region of the stimuli, then the head preference should emerge during the course of the familiarization trials.

Quinn et al. (2009) tested 6-month-old infants on the eye-tracking version of the categorization familiarization task. The findings were that 46% of the fixation time that was on the stimulus was on the head and 54% on the body, percentages that remained constant throughout familiarization. The percentages take on additional meaning when one considers that the head area represented only 17.5% of the whole stimulus area of the cat and dog images; the body took up the remaining 82.5%. This means that on a per unit area basis, equating for the size difference between the head and the body, when the infants are fixating the stimulus, they are actually spending 80% of their fixation time per unit area of the head and 20% of their fixation time per unit area of the body.

The results are consistent with the idea that the reliance on the head for the categorical parsing of cats and dogs arises from a biasing mechanism. However, one could still argue that infants are simply orienting to the head because it contains high contrast internal features and infants are attracted to the most visible portion of the stimulus (Banks & Salapatek, 1981). To address this possibility, a control study was undertaken that repeated the eye-tracking version of the category familiarization procedure, but with stimulus images that were inverted (Quinn et al., 2009). If the head preference resulted from infants' simply orienting to the most visible portion of the stimulus, then it should still be observed with inversion. However, if the infants orient to the head because of a bias that is in place to facilitate face recognition, then one would not expect it to be present with stimulus inversion, given that inversion changes the normal configuration of facial features, and faces are believed to be recognized on a configural basis by infants in the age range investigated (Cohen & Cashon, 2001).

The results of the control study revealed that in the inversion condition only 11% of the fixation time on the stimulus was on the head, whereas 89% was on the body. This outcome suggests that when the images are inverted, the relative distribution of fixations to the head and body regions are proportional to the relative areas of these regions. The control results indicate that the bias to fixate on the head over the body in the initial experiment is not because the head contains high-contrast features. When the images were inverted, the fixation time to the head was substantially reduced despite the same sensory power emanating from the head region across the two experiments. This finding provides evidence that infants use the head to categorize upright cat and dog images because of a preexisting biasing mechanism that responds to face information.

As proposed by Johnson and Morton (1991), a bias to attend to face information present in a visual display may play a facilitative role in terms of allowing infants to attend to and recognize members of their own species and also specific persons such as the primary caregiver. The present studies suggest that the bias could more broadly assist conceptual development by allowing infants to differentiate categories that have faces (e.g., animals) and those that do not (e.g., furniture), as well as partition classes marked by distinctive facial make-ups (e.g., cats vs. dogs). The bias may also aid infants in selecting from among various features that are potentially available in the input (i.e., head or body), and in this way "set the system on the trajectory of learning" (Thelen & Smith, 1994, p. 315). Such biases may be especially important in determining the course of concept acquisition in a system that is otherwise characterized by flexibility.

On-Line Learning or Preexisting Representations?

One question not yet considered is whether the representations that human infants form for nonhuman animals are learned as the infants are presented with images of the categories during the course of the familiarization trials or whether the experiments are tapping into representations that were formed on the basis of experiences that occurred prior to arrival at the laboratory. A way of addressing this issue is to ask if infant experience with a home pet affects categorization performance. That is, if a group of infants is reared with a pet at home that belongs to the same category as that experienced during the familiarization trials of a category learning experiment, one can ask if this group performs differently than another group of infants reared in a household without a pet. Because a number of our studies have involved the category contrast of cats versus dogs, the most common family pets, we have had the opportunity to compare the performance of 3- to 4-month-old infants without a pet at home with those who had a cat or dog as a pet a home that was a match with the cat or dog category presented during familiarization of a category learning task. This analysis has not yielded a reliable difference. The lack of an effect of a home pet on infant performance on categorization tasks involving nonhuman animals is consistent with the idea that the infants are processing the stimuli based on the information presented in the laboratory tasks rather than on the basis of representations that existed prior to arrival at the laboratory.

Another clue to whether infant categorization of nonhuman animals is based on within-task learning or preexisting representations comes from an asymmetry that is observed when one compares the performance of infants familiarized with cats or dogs and tested with novel cats versus novel dogs (Quinn et al., 1993). In particular, when infants are familiarized with cats, they prefer dogs over novel cats; however, when infants are familiarized with dogs, attention is divided evenly between cats and novel dogs. This asymmetry is surprising given that on an a priori basis, one might predict that infants presented with a category contrast in a completely balanced experimental design would show evidence of categorization in both directions (cat to dog or dog to cat) or in neither direction. The asymmetrical pattern of preference is actually consistent with the possibility that there could be a spontaneous preference for dogs that would interfere with a novel category preference for cats after familiarization with dogs and work in concert with a novel category preference for dogs after familiarization with cats. However, when infants were presented with a category preference test involving cat–dog pairings, no spontaneous preference was observed; the infants attended equally to the cat and dog images.

Another explanation for the asymmetry arose because visual inspection of the stimuli suggested that the dog images were more variable than those of the cats. As noted earlier, an attempt had been made to gather cat and dog images for presentation to the infants that were representative of the categories as they existed in nature. Nevertheless, the differences between the Calico, Siamese, Tabby, and Birman breeds, for example, seemed not to match the variation among the French Poodles, Bulldogs, Collies, and Terriers.

To develop a more quantitative account of the category variability explanation for the performance asymmetry, a number of the surface attributes of the cat and dog images were measured. The attributes included those from the head and face (given the importance of this region for the category distinction) along with those corresponding with the basic skeletal dimensions of stimuli. The measurements allowed each stimulus to be expressed as a vector of values that could be presented as input to a connectionist autoencoder (Mareschal, French, & Quinn, 2000). When the autoencoder was trained on either cat or dog images and then tested with novel cat versus dog images, it reproduced in the form of network error what had been observed in infant looking time. In particular, when trained on cat images, the network produced a high level of error for dog images and little error for novel cat images. In contrast, when trained on dog images, the network produced equivalent amounts of error for cat and novel dog images.

Because the network had only the measurements of the stimuli to learn from, and was able to simulate the behavior of the infants, the indication is that the key to explaining the performance asymmetry lies in the statistics of the input presented to the infants. This suggestion is confirmed through detailed examination of the distribution of values measured for the individual attributes of the cat and dog images. Consider the attribute of nose width. What can be seen in Figure 13.5 is that the distribution of values of the nose width attribute corresponding to the dog images is broader than that of the cat images, thereby creating an inclusion relation in which the cat values are subsumed by the dog values. This inclusion relation was observed for a majority of the attributes.

The outcome of the analysis of the individual attributes provides an explanation for the original category learning performance asymmetry of the infants: Following familiarization with cats, there is a good likelihood that a dog image will follow outside of the familiarized range of values and be detected as novel; however, after familiarization with dogs, there is a strong probability that a cat image will fall within the familiarized range of values, and not

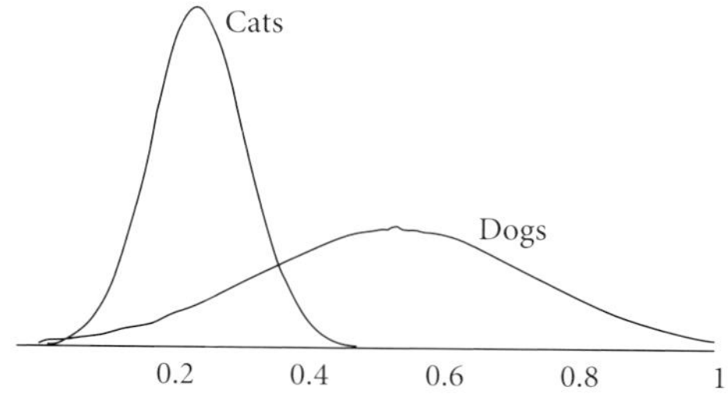

Figure 13.5 Gaussian probability distributions generated from the means and standard deviations of the normalized nose width feature of cats and dogs.

be viewed as novel. In other words, infants form a category representation for cats that excludes dogs, and a category representation for dogs that includes cats, and these representations are predictable from the on-line learning of the statistical structure of the images. The computational account of the cat–dog categorization asymmetry is thus consistent with the null effect of the home pet assessment in suggesting that infants are learning their category representation for nonhuman animals based on within-task learning (i.e., the information presented during laboratory familiarization procedures).

A representation for humans

An Inclusive Category

Given that infants in the studies just reviewed showed evidence of categorizing classes of nonhuman animals, the issue arose as to how infants would categorize humans. The general question of how humans are conceptualized among other animals has met with different answers in the cognitive literature. For example, Carey (1985) has proposed that humans are the prototype for other animals, whereas Medin and Waxman (2007) have argued that humans are represented as having a dual status inclusive of a general representation in which humans are represented as being like other animals and a more specific representation in which humans are represented as being distinct from other animals. In addition, there has been discussion of whether infants represent humans as intentional agents that are not constrained by physical principles (Kuhlmeier, Bloom, & Wynn, 2004), or as solid, material objects (Saxe, Tzelnic, & Carey, 2005). There has also been the suggestion that infants represent the configuration of parts that make up the human body (Gliga & Dehaene-Lambertz, 2005), although with debate regarding when during early development this configural representation emerges (Slaughter & Heron, 2004).

What the infant studies thus far described have not addressed is the question of whether infants categorize humans as similar to or different from categories of nonhuman animals. Given the perceptual differences between humans and nonhuman animals (i.e., humans wear clothes, stand upright, and have arms) and given the abilities of young infants to separate various nonhuman animal species into different categories, the expectation was that infants would represent humans as distinct from categories of nonhuman animals. To determine whether this was the case, 3- to 4-month-olds were presented with a dozen photographic images of clothed humans (males and females) in standing, walking, and running poses, and then preference tested with a novel human paired with a horse or cat image (Quinn & Eimas, 1998). Counter to expectation, the infants generalized their familiarization to the novel humans, cats, and horses; they did not exhibit novel category preferences for the cats or horses. In addition, a control experiment assessing a priori preference showed that infants did not have a spontaneous preference for looking at humans over cats or horses. This latter outcome means that the null results in the categorization experiment could not be explained by a spontaneous preference for humans interfering with novel category preferences for cats or horses. In addition, adult observers did not judge the exemplars of the human category to be more variable than the exemplars of the horse or cat categories, thereby weakening potential explanations based on inclusion relations.

The next step was to investigate further how infants represent humans by familiarizing with human stimuli and preference testing with additional contrast categories. This further testing was necessary because the null results of the initial investigation (i.e., the generalization to cat and horse exemplars) left open the question of whether infants were categorizing humans at all or whether they were forming a broad category representation that was inclusive of nonhuman animals. The additional contrast categories consisted of exemplars of fish and cars. The fish allow one to determine how infants would respond to a nonmammalian animal category and the cars enable one to learn how infants would react to a nonanimal category with no obvious overlap with humans in terms of perceptual attributes.

The findings were that infants familiarized with humans generalized their familiarization to the fish, but preferred the cars. The overall pattern of outcomes indicates that infants were in fact forming a category representation for humans, one that was sufficiently broad so as to include novel humans, cats, horses, and even fish, but not cars.

An Asymmetry and an Exemplar-based Representation

The next question became why there was a difference in exclusivity in how infants represented the categories of nonhuman animals and humans. That is, the infants were forming a category of humans that included nonhuman animals, but they were also forming category representations for nonhuman animal species that excluded exemplars from contrasting nonhuman animal species. What lies behind the asymmetry? One possibility for the "overshoot" in the human representation is because infants have greater experience with humans including parents, siblings, and caregivers than they have with nonhuman animal species. Differential experience and knowledge have been used to account for why young children use humans as the prototype for their projections about other animals in children's inductive reasoning tasks (Inagaki & Hatano, 1999). Supporting this experiential account of the asymmetry is the finding that children who have experience raising goldfish use goldfish as well as humans as a base for inductive generalization (Inagaki, 1990).

If differential experience with humans versus nonhuman animals affects infants' categorization for these classes, then one might expect that the nature of the representation that infants have for humans and nonhuman animals will be different. In particular, following from the studies that have investigated the time course of category learning in adults (Gauthier & Tarr, 1997; Johansen & Palmeri, 2002; Smith & Minda, 1998) and the downward shift in recognition associated with enhanced experience (Tanaka, 2001), one might expect infants to represent the less experienced categories (i.e., nonhuman animals) in terms of summary structures (i.e., prototypes), whereas the representation for the more frequently experienced category would be supplemented by information about the individual exemplars. To investigate this possibility, a group of 3- to 4-month-olds was presented either with a dozen images of humans or cats. The infants were then administered two preference tests: one was the standard test of categorization pairing a novel exemplar from the novel category with a novel exemplar from the familiar category (i.e., novel cat versus novel human), the other was a test probing the nature of the representation (i.e., novel exemplar from the familiar category versus familiar exemplar from the familiar category). This latter test is based on the following rationale: if infants are representing the category solely as a summary structure, then there should be a null preference; however, if infants are also representing the category in terms of individual exemplars, then they should prefer the novel exemplar.

The results were that infants familiarized with cats preferred a novel human over a novel cat in the test of categorization, but did not prefer a novel over a familiar cat in the test of exemplar memory. In contrast, infants familiarized with humans did not prefer a novel cat over a novel human, but did prefer a novel over a familiar human. The findings indicate first that the exclusivity difference in the way that infants represent humans versus nonhuman animals is actually a full-blown asymmetry. That is, infants form a category of humans that includes cats, whereas they form a category representation for cats that excludes humans. Second, there are differences in the nature of the representation such that infants represent nonhuman animals as a summary structure, possibly a prototype that encompasses an averaging of the familiar exemplars, whereas the human representation is supplemented by information about the individual exemplars. Of interest is that category-level recognition of other species and individual recognition of conspecifics have also been demonstrated in monkeys (Humphreys, 1974) and have been attributed to differential experience (Sugita, 2008) indicating that the effects are not human-specific.

An Attractor Account Based on Differential Experience

How does one tie together the notions of differential experience, the inclusivity–exclusivity difference, and the exemplar–prototype distinction into a coherent account of how infants categorize and represent humans versus nonhuman animals? The account proposed here maintains that infants who are presented with images of humans and nonhuman animals in the laboratory bring different knowledge bases about humans and nonhuman animals into the laboratory prior to their participation in the categorization task and then come to represent different information during on-line learning while being familiarized with the stimulus images. As depicted in Figure 13.6A, infants may bring to the task of learning about humans a summary representation for humans along with representations of individual humans (i.e., parents, siblings, caregivers) into the experiment. They then learn about the individual exemplar humans presented during familiarization. By contrast, in Figure 13.6B, infants may *not* bring preexisting representations of nonhuman animals to the task of learning about nonhuman animals and form only a summary representation of the nonhuman animals during the course of familiarization with them. As a consequence of these differences in prior knowledge base and within-task learning, infants end up with an expansive representation for humans, which is broadly accepting of stimuli that have attributes in common with humans (e.g., a head attached to a torso with skeletal appendages). In this way, the human representation comes to act as an attractor or perceptual magnet for nonhuman animals. By contrast, the individual representations for nonhuman animal species are tightly constructed around prototype structures, do not have attractor properties, and thus come to exclude humans.

Evidence from computational simulations is consistent with the account of the human–nonhuman animal categorization asymmetry that is based on prior knowledge about humans (Mermillod, French, Quinn, & Mareschal, 2004). The same connectionist autoencoder that was shown capable of reproducing the cat–dog asymmetry was not able to simulate the human–nonhuman animal asymmetry. In particular, when the network was trained on either horses or humans, and then tested on novel horses and novel humans, the network produced consistently more error for the images from the novel categories, irrespective of the trained category. However, when a long-term memory component that received prior training on humans was added and coupled with the short-term memory

A After familiarization with humans

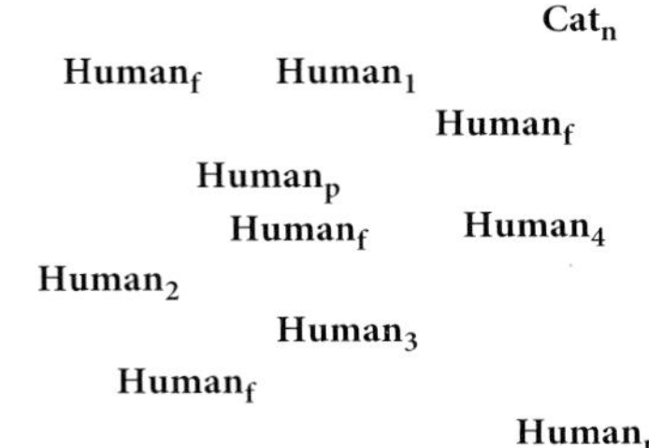

B After familiarization with cats

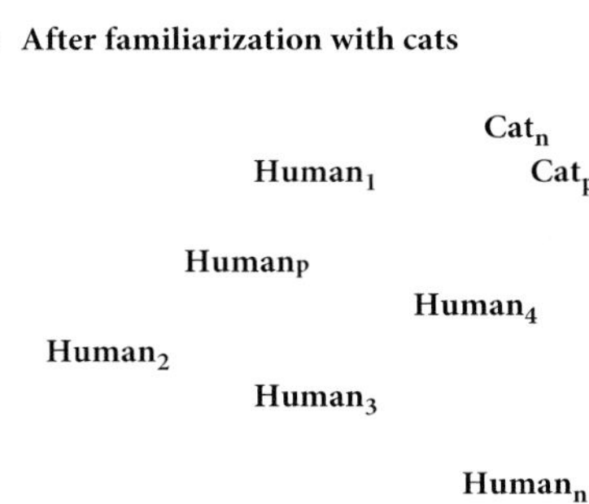

Figure 13.6 **A schematic depiction of the mental space used to represent humans and cats after familiarization with humans (A) or cats (B). The numbers correspond to individual exemplars of humans represented before the familiarization trials. The letter p corresponds with a summary (prototype) representation formed either during familiarization (in the case of cats) or before familiarization (in the case of humans). The letter f corresponds with individual exemplars represented during the familiarization trials, and the letter n corresponds with novel individual exemplars presented during the preference test trials.**

component for learning about the images presented during familiarization, the human–nonhuman animal asymmetry was reproduced. That is, the "dual network" architecture, when trained on humans, produced equivalent error for novel humans and novel horses; however, when trained on horses, the network produced small error for novel horses and large error for novel humans. The network simulations provide additional evidence that the human–nonhuman animal asymmetry reflects the different knowledge base that infants have for humans versus nonhuman animals.

The finding that infants include nonhuman animals in their representation for humans is consistent with work of Pauen (2000) who reported that 5-month-old infants included different mammals in their representation for humans in a habituation–dishabituation categorization task. The human–nonhuman animal asymmetry in infant categorization also appears to foreshadow the human–nonhuman animal asymmetry in child induction that was reported by Carey (1985) and subsequently investigated by others (Atran et al., 2001). The asymmetry was initially interpreted by Carey in terms of young children's failure to distinguish naive psychology from naive biology, although other investigators have more recently suggested an important role for differential exposure and expertise (Inagaki, 1990; Ross, Medin, Coley, & Atran, 2003), which is in keeping with the framework proposed here. As described by Inagaki and Hatano (2006), "young children draw analogically on their knowledge about humans when attributing properties to less familiar living entities... Young children do this because they possess fairly rich knowledge about humans compared with their knowledge about other animals..." (pp. 177–181). The results reported here suggest that the seeds of the human-based inference or person analogy system of reasoning observed in children may be planted very early in development. Here then may be an example of how differential perceptual experience that infants have with humans versus nonhuman animals leads infants to become more expert in representing humans with the eventual consequence that such expertise comes to structure how children come to conceptualize the biological world.

What Perceptual Information Do Young Infants Use to Categorize Humans?

While differential experience may be necessary to account for the human–nonhuman animal categorization asymmetry, it may not be sufficient. This is because the human representation included nonhuman animals, but excluded cars, even though neither contrast category was likely to be experienced much by infants in the first 3 to 4 months of life. This aspect of the results points to a role for perceptual information shared by humans and nonhuman animals, but not by cars, without specifying what that perceptual information is.

On the one hand, the evidence described earlier indicated that infants represent nonhuman animals on a featural basis (Quinn & Eimas, 1996; Spencer et al., 1997). On the other hand, the expertise hypothesis predicts that infants would represent humans on a holistic basis (Gauthier & Tarr, 2002). To evaluate the stimulus information that was the basis for the human–nonhuman animal categorization asymmetry, 3- to 4-month-olds were presented with the category contrast of cats versus humans in experimental conditions in which the whole stimulus, just the head (with body information occluded) or just the body (with head information occluded), was available for processing from each image during both familiarization and preference test (Quinn, 2004). The major finding was that a category representation for humans that included cats and a category representation for cats that excluded humans was observed only in the whole stimulus condition. This result indicates that the human–nonhuman animal asymmetry is based on holistic processing of the overall structure of the stimulus. That holistic information shared by humans and nonhuman animals is likely to consist of the head, a body torso, and skeletal appendages.

A recent study has shown further that a representation for humans that includes nonhuman animals is observed only when the human images presented during familiarization are in an upright orientation (Quinn, Lee,

Pascalis, & Slater, 2007). When these data are considered in conjunction with the Quinn (2004) findings and the observation that inversion disrupts configural processing (Freire, Lee, & Symons, 2000), the suggestion is that the holistic information that is the basis for the incorporation of nonhuman animals into the human representation has a configural aspect. That is, the head, body, and skeletal appendages may need to be in a particular arrangement in order for the attractor effect to occur. Although the precise nature of the configural arrangement of head, body, and skeletal appendages is difficult to specify based on a single set of inversion results, it may be the case that skeletal appendages attached to the head rather than the body would violate the arrangement (Slaughter & Heron, 2004), although further studies using a "feature scrambling" methodology would be needed to confirm this suggestion.

The idea that the human versus nonhuman animal categorization asymmetry in infants is rooted in both the frequency and similarity structure of one's experience with various object classes may have a parallel with an occurrence observed in the word learning literature. In particular, increased experience with a particular class of objects leads to a tendency observed in child word learners to extend the label associated with that class to less familiar, similar classes of objects, although not to less familiar, dissimilar classes of objects (Clark, 1973). Moreover, in a connectionist simulation designed to capture this behavior, a model that was trained with dog patterns appearing more frequently than other mammals, extended the label dog to goats and even robins, but not to oak trees (Rogers & McClelland, 2004). The correspondence between behavior and computational simulation observed in both infant categorization and child lexical acquisition suggests that a common learning process operating on the regularities of a structured environment may underlie both phenomena.

On-Line Learning or Preexisting Representations?

Earlier in the chapter, it was argued that infants categorize nonhuman animals based on learning taking place during the familiarization trials of a laboratory categorization task. Behavioral and computational analyses supported this assertion. It was also argued that infants categorize humans based at least in part on information that infants had acquired about humans prior to their arrival at the laboratory. In the present section, evidence is offered to buttress this latter claim. The evidence comes from how infants process particular attributes of humans, namely, the gender and race of their faces. In the initial study, 3- to 4-month-olds were presented with photographic images of eight male or female faces and then preference tested with a novel male face and a novel female face (Quinn, Yahr, Kuhn, Slater, & Pascalis, 2002). The results were asymmetrical: infants familiarized with male faces preferred novel female faces, however, infants familiarized with female faces did not prefer novel male faces over novel female faces. Notably, the same asymmetry was previously reported by Leinbach and Fagot (1993) who used a serial habituation–dishabituation procedure and a different set of face stimuli with 5- to 12-month-olds. That the asymmetry was observed in two different labs with different stimuli and under different procedural variants suggests that the phenomenon is robust (see also Strauss, Newell, & Best, 2003, for an additional report of female face preference in 5- to 8-month-olds).

The question now became how to interpret the asymmetry. The form of the asymmetry is suggestive of an a priori preference. That is, if infants prefer female over male faces, then such a preference would have facilitated a novel category preference for female faces after familiarization with male faces, but interfered with a novel category preference for male faces after familiarization with female faces. To investigate the possibility of an a priori preference for female over male faces, 3- to 4-month-olds were administered a spontaneous preference test that consisted of male–female face pairings presented without a familiarization period. The infants looked more at the female faces.

It now became important to determine what perceptual or cognitive factors might contribute to the heightened visual attention to the female faces on the part of the infants. One possibility is that the female faces were marked by longer hair than the male faces; however, when the spontaneous preference test was repeated with hair cues removed, the preference for the female faces was unaffected. Another possibility is that the female faces were marked by higher-contrast internal features possibly related to greater cosmetic use. Arguing against this account is the result that the female face preference dropped to chance when the spontaneous preference test was repeated with inverted heads without hair. If the female preference was driven by more sensory power in the female faces, then it should have been preserved with the inversion manipulation, given that the individual face features are presented in both upright and inverted orientations. The inversion finding indicates that the female preference depends on the perception of faces in the upright orientation that depicts the canonical arrangement of internal features.

With lower-level perceptual factors failing to provide an account of the female face preference, one can ask whether a higher-level cognitive factor might be determining performance. All of the infants discussed thus far from the Quinn et al. (2002) study had a female primary caregiver. Given that familiarity is known to play a role in face processing by young infants (e.g., Bartrip, Morton, & DeSchonen, 2001), it seemed reasonable to suggest that infants with female primary caregivers might look more toward female faces than male faces because the female faces bore a greater resemblance to the face of the caregiver. If this was the case, then it should be possible to reverse the spontaneous preference in a sample of infants raised by male primary caregivers. Eight such infants were presented with the upright faces without hair, and 7 of the 8 displayed a preference for the male faces (see also Quinn et al., 2003). The findings indicate that how infants respond to faces in a laboratory task is influenced by what they know about faces prior to arrival at the laboratory. More generally, how infants respond to human images is affected by what previously acquired knowledge they possess about humans.

The idea that previously acquired knowledge is a determinant of how infants respond to information about humans in laboratory experiments receives additional support from studies examining how infants respond to race information in faces. When newborn Caucasian infants, just 2 to 3 days old on average, are presented with Caucasian faces paired with African, Asian, or Middle-Eastern faces, examples of which are shown in Figure 13.7, no consistent preferences for one or another race were observed (Kelly et al., 2005). However, when 3-month-old Caucasian infants reared by Caucasian caregivers and exposed to predominantly Caucasian faces were tested with the same face pairings as the newborns, the 3-month-olds displayed a reliable preference for the Caucasian (own-race) faces. In addition, when 3-month-old Chinese infants reared with Chinese caregivers and with little or no exposure to other-race faces were presented with the face pairings, they manifested a reliable preference for the Chinese (own-race) faces (Kelly, Liu et al., 2007). The preference for own-race faces was also observed in a contrast of 3-month-old Israeli infants who preferred Caucasian faces and Ethiopian infants who preferred African faces (Bar-Haim, Ziv, Lamy, & Hodes, 2006).

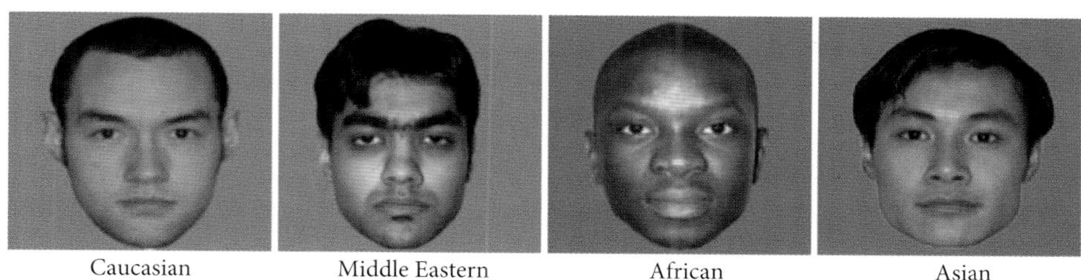

Figure 13.7 Examples of the stimuli used in Kelly et al. (2005, 2007a).

Bar-Haim et al. demonstrated further that Israeli-born infants of Ethiopian parentage who had extensive exposure to both Caucasian and African faces did not prefer either group of faces. The results indicate that differential exposure to faces from different racial groups during the first 3 months of postnatal experience is sufficient to produce a visual preference for same-race faces. The findings provide another demonstration that knowledge acquired about humans outside the laboratory can affect how infants visually attend to human visual images presented inside the laboratory.

In addition to the spontaneous visual attention preferences that have been observed for faces matching the gender of the primary caregiver and same-race faces at 3 to 4 months, there also appears to be superior recognition memory. Specifically, 3- to 4-month-olds reared by female primary caregivers presented with a series of female faces, preferred a novel over familiar female face; however, when presented with a series of male faces, there was no differential preference for a novel over familiar male face (Quinn et al., 2002). In addition, although 3-month-old Caucasian infants exposed predominantly to Caucasian faces and 3-month-old Chinese infants exposed predominantly to Chinese faces performed as well on a recognition memory task involving either own- or other-race faces, 6- and 9-month-old infants demonstrated superior recognition memory for own-race faces (Kelly, Quinn, et al., 2007b; Kelly et al., in press). These findings indicate that differential experience within the category of humans occurring outside the laboratory can produce processing differences on laboratory tasks that measure abilities which go beyond spontaneous preference (i.e., exemplar memory).

Categorization of Humans Versus Nonhuman Animals by Infants: An Expert–Novice Distinction

The findings reviewed in the previous sections of the chapter have compared how young infants categorize humans versus nonhuman animals. The data suggest that infants categorize nonhuman animals at a basic level of exclusivity, on the basis of part information, via a summary representation, and because of learning taking place within the experimental task. In contrast, infants categorize humans at a global-level of exclusivity with magnet-like properties, on the basis of holistic information, with an exemplar representation, and via recruitment from a preexisting knowledge base.

The various differences between how infants categorize humans versus nonhuman animals can be interpreted with different theoretical accounts. For example, as Carey (1985) has argued about child induction, perhaps it is the case that infants have not yet separated the psychological domain of humans from the biological domain of nonhuman animals. Another way to think about the differences is that they reflect an expert–novice distinction. In support of this conjecture, two of the differences in how infants respond to nonhuman animals versus humans are consistent with behavioral markers of expertise that have been reported for adults. First, consistent with the findings that novices identify objects at the basic level (Murphy & Smith, 1982; Rosch, Mervis, Gray, Johnson, & Boyes-Braem, 1976), infants categorized nonhuman animals at the basic level. In addition, in accord with the results that expertise training in adults shifts the entry level at which recognition occurs to the subordinate level (Tanaka, 2001; Tanaka, Curran, & Sheinberg, 2005; Tanaka & Taylor, 1991), infants represented humans at the level of individual exemplars. Second, in concert with the data showing that experts tend to encode information about a stimulus across a wide spatial extent inclusive of the entire stimulus and are less able to attend selectively to individual parts (Gauthier & Tarr, 2002), infants represented humans based on information about their configural structure, but represented nonhuman animals based on part information.

An additional characteristic that has been associated with the acquisition of expertise in adults also appears to manifest itself in terms of how infants process information about humans. Specifically, even within domains of expertise, experience can affect how exemplars are processed (Bukach et al., 2006). Within the domain of faces, for example, adults have been shown to remember faces from their own race better than faces from other races (Malpass & Kravitz, 1969). Likewise, within the category of humans, infants reared by female caregivers have demonstrated superior recognition memory for female relative to male faces, and infants exposed predominantly to individuals from a particular race have displayed superior recognition memory for same-race faces.

The present results showing that infants respond to humans versus nonhuman animals at different levels of specificity is also consistent with evidence from the anthropology literature showing that different cultures differ in the level of specificity at which they recognize objects depending on the amount of experience they have with those objects (Malt, 1995). For example, Dougherty (1978) reported that Tzetlal Mayan children reared in a nonindustrialized culture were more likely to name plants at a subordinate category level, whereas American children reared in Berkeley, California were more likely to name the plants at a basic category level. Just as expertise effects can arise within a culture based on differential experience with different classes, it can also arise as a consequence of cultural differences in experience with various categories.

There is yet another parallel that may be drawn between what is observed with infants' representation of humans versus nonhuman animals and what has been reported in the adult expertise literature. Concurrently with recognizing humans at a more specific level (as individual exemplars) than nonhuman animals (as members of a basic-level category), infants were also able to represent humans at a global level that included nonhuman animals. As described earlier, these two effects that take infants' representation in two different directions, toward increased specificity *and* generality, may be related. Specifically, the addition of individual exemplars to a summary structure that comes with increased experience is what serves to expand the range of variation of the attributes that are represented for the category, thereby giving rise to the increased inclusivity of the category and its attractor properties. Moreover, this trend toward increased distinctiveness *and* commonality observed in the infant representation for humans has also been observed in studies of acquired expertise in adults. For example, Murphy and Wright (1984), in a comparison of novices and experts on child psychopathology, found that experts were more likely than novices to list both distinctive and common features of disorders. Thus, not only are experts able to recognize instances from their domain at more specific levels than novices, they are also better able to recognize commonalities across a domain. Notably, the dual trends toward both differentiation and generalization that occur with increased experience have also been reported in the trajectory of learning observed in connectionist networks operating on input where one class is presented more frequently than others (Rogers & McClelland, 2004). An important facet of the simulation work is that it links together the differentiation and generalization behavior in a common framework in which the representational space devoted to the more experienced class becomes larger than that allocated to less experienced classes.

The generalization aspect of expertise may be especially relevant for cognitive development and the structuring of domains of knowledge. For example, for children to develop a domain of biological knowledge, they will need to represent a broad category of animals that includes both humans and nonhuman animals. Despite the perceptual differences between humans and nonhuman animals, infants display an ability to generalize from humans to nonhuman animals based on their underlying commonalities. Thus, in perhaps the same sense in which physics experts look past superficial similarities and group physics problems based on nonobvious resemblances (Chi, Feltovich, & Glaser, 1981), infants may develop a category representation for animals that includes both humans and nonhuman animals based on abstract structural information about overall biological form (e.g., a head attached to a body with skeletal appendages). By this account, the generalization from humans to nonhuman animals may represent an important component in the construction of a broad concept of animal. And in this way, the acquisition of expertise may represent an important vehicle for the growth of category structure during early cognitive development.

Acknowledgments

Preparation of this chapter was supported by Grants HD-42451 and HD-46526 from the National Institute of Child Health and Human Development. The author thanks Scott P. Johnson for inviting the contribution, and the participants in the NYU-BUG workshop for comments that helped to structure the major themes of the chapter.

References

Atran, S., Medin, D. L., Lynch, E., Vapnarsky, V., Ucan Ek', E., & Sousa, P. (2001). Folkbiology doesn't come from folkpsychology: Evidence from Yukatec Maya in cross-cultural perspective. *Journal of Cognition and Culture, 1,* 4–42.

Banks, M. S., & Salapatek, P. (1981). Infant pattern vision: A new approach based on the contrast sensitivity function. *Journal of Experimental Child Psychology, 31,* 1–45.

Bar-Haim, Y., Ziv, T., Lamy, D., & Hodes, R. M. (2006). Nature and nurture in own-race face processing. *Psychological Science, 17,* 159–163.

Bartrip, J., Morton, J., & De Schonen, S. (2001). Responses to mother's face in 3-week to 5-month old infants. *British Journal of Developmental Psychology, 19,* 219–232.

Bauer, P. J., Dow, G. A., & Hertsgaard, L. A. (1995). Effects of prototypicality on categorization in 1- to 2-year-olds: Getting down to basic. *Cognitive Development, 10,* 43–68.

Bruner, J. S., Goodnow, J. J., & Austin, G. A. (1956). *A study of thinking.* New York: Wiley.

Bukach, C. M., Gauthier, I., & Tarr, M. J. (2006). Beyond faces and modularity: The power of an expertise framework. *Trends in Cognitive Sciences, 10,* 159–166.

Carey, S. (1985). *Conceptual change in childhood.* Cambridge, MA: MIT Press.

Chi, M. T., Feltovich, P. J., & Glaser, R. (1981). Categorization and representation of physics problems by experts and novices. *Cognitive Science, 5,* 121–152.

Clark, E. V. (1973) What's in a word? On the child's acquisition of semantics in his first language. In T. E. Moore (Ed.), *Cognitive development and the acquisition of language* (pp. 65–110). New York: Academic Press.

Cohen, L. B. & Cashon, C. H. (2001). Do 7-month-old infants process independent features or facial configurations? *Infant and Child Development, 10,* 83–92.

Dougherty, J. W. D. (1978). Salience and relativity in classification. *American Ethnologist, 5,* 66–80.

Dueker, G., & Needham, A. (2005). Infants' object category formation and use: Real world context effects on category use in object processing. *Visual Cognition, 12,* 1177–1198.

Eimas, P. D., & Quinn, P. C. (1994). Studies on the formation of perceptually based basic-level categories in young infants. *Child Development, 65,* 903–917.

Freire, A., Lee, K., & Symons, L. A. (2000). The face-inversion effect as a deficit in the encoding of configural information: Direct evidence. *Perception, 29,* 159–170.

Gauthier, I., & Tarr, M. J. (1997). Becoming a "Greeble" expert: Exploring mechanisms for face recognition. *Vision Research, 37,* 1673–1682.

Gauthier, I., & Tarr, M. J. (2002). Unraveling mechanisms for expert object recognition: Bridging brain activity and behavior. *Journal of Experimental Psychology: Human Perception and Performance, 28,* 431–446.

Gelman, S. A. (2003). *The essential child: Origins of essentialism in everyday thought.* Oxford: Oxford University Press.

Gliga, T., & Dehaene-Lambertz, G. (2005). Structural encoding of body and face in human infants and adults. *Journal of Cognitive Neuroscience, 17,* 1328–1340.

Hampton, J. A. (1995). Testing the prototype theory of concepts. *Journal of Memory and Language, 34,* 686–708.

Hampton, J. A., Estes, Z., & Simmons, S. (2007). Metamorphosis: Essence, appearance, and behavior in the categorization of natural kinds. *Memory & Cognition, 35,* 1785–1800.

Humphreys, N. K. (1974). Species and individuals in the perceptual world of monkeys. *Perception, 3,* 105–114.

Inagaki, K. (1990). The effects of raising animals on biological knowledge. *British Journal of Developmental Psychology, 8,* 119–129.

Inagaki, K., & Hatano, G. (1999). Chidren's understanding of mind–body relationships.

In M. Siegal & C. Peterson (Eds.), *Children's understanding of biology and health* (pp. 23–44). Cambridge, UK: Cambridge University Press.

Inagaki, K., & Hatano, G. (2006). Young children's conception of the biological world. *Current Directions in Psychological Science, 15,* 177–181.

Johnson, M. H., & Morton, J. (1991) *Biology and cognitive development: The case of face recognition.* Oxford, UK: Blackwell.

Johansen, M. K., & Palmeri, T. J. (2002). Are there representational shifts during category learning? *Cognitive Psychology, 45,* 482–553.

Jones, S. S., & Smith, L. B. (1993). The place of perception in children's concepts. *Cognitive Development, 8,* 113–139.

Keil, F. C. (1989). *Concepts, kinds, and cognitive development.* Cambridge, MA: MIT Press.

Kelly, D. J., Liu, S., Ge, L., Quinn, P. C., Slater, A. M., Lee, K., et al. (2007). Cross-race preferences for same-race faces extend beyond the African versus Caucasian contrast in 3-month-old infants. *Infancy, 11,* 87–95.

Kelly, D. J., Liu, S., Lee, K., Quinn, P. C., Pascalis, O., Slater, A. M., et al. (in press). Development of the other-race effect in infancy: Evidence towards universality? *Journal of Experimental Child Psychology.*

Kelly, D. J., Quinn, P. C., Slater, A., Lee, K., Ge, L., & Pascalis, O. (2007b). The other-race effect develops during infancy: Evidence of perceptual narrowing. *Psychological Science, 18,* 1084–1089.

Kelly, D. J., Quinn, P. C., Slater, A. M., Lee, K., Gibson, A., Smith, M., et al. (2005). Three-month-olds, but not newborns, prefer own-race faces. *Developmental Science, 8,* F31–F36.

Kuhlmeier, V. A., Bloom, P., & Wynn, K. (2004). Do 5-month-old infants see humans as material objects? *Cognition, 94,* 95–103.

Leinbach, M. D., & Fagot, B. I. (1993). Categorical habituation to male and female faces: Gender schematic processing in infancy. *Infant Behavior & Development, 16,* 317–332.

Malpass, R. S., & Kravitz, J. (1969). Recognition for faces of own and other race. *Journal of Personality and Social Psychology, 13,* 330–334.

Malt, B. (1995). Category coherence in cross cultural perspective. *Cognitive Psychology, 29,* 85–148.

Mareschal, D., & French, R. M. (1997). A connectionist account of interference effects in early infant memory and categorization. In M. G. Shafto & P. Langley (Eds.), *Proceedings of 19th Annual Conference of the Cognitive Science Society* (pp. 484–489). Mahwah, NJ: Erlbaum.

Mareschal, D., French, R. M., & Quinn, P. C. (2000). A connectionist account of asymmetric category learning in early infancy. *Developmental Psychology, 36,* 635–645.

Mareschal, D., & Quinn, P. C. (2001). Categorization in infancy. *Trends in Cognitive Sciences, 5,* 443–450.

Medin, D. L. & Waxman, S. R. (2007). Interpreting asymmetries of projection in children's inductive reasoning. In A. Feeney & E. Heit (Eds.), *Inductive reasoning* (pp. 55–80). New York: Cambridge University Press.

Mermillod, M., French, R. M., Quinn, P. C., & Mareschal, D. (2004). The importance of long-term memory in infant perceptual categorization. In R. Alterman & D. Kirsh (Eds.), *Proceedings of the 25th Annual Conference of the Cognitive Science Society* (pp. 804–809). Mahwah, NJ: Erlbaum.

Mermillod, M., French R. M., Smeets, H., & Spencer, J. (2005). A neural network investigation of the head preference: problems explaining empirical results by bottom-up processes alone. In A. Cangelosi, G. Bugmann, & R. Borisyuk (Eds.), *Modeling Language, Cognition & Action: Proceedings of the Ninth Neural Computation and Psychology Workshop* (Vol. 16, pp. 361–366). Singapore: World Scientific.

Murphy, G. L., & Smith, E. E. (1982). Basic level superiority in picture categorization. *Journal of Verbal Learning and Verbal Behavior, 21,* 1–20.

Murphy, G. L., & Wright, J. C. (1984). Changes in conceptual structure with expertise: Differences between real-world experts and novices. *Journal of Experimental Psychology: Learning, Memory, and Cognition, 10,* 144–155.

Nelson, C. A. (1994). Neural correlates of recognition memory in the first postnatal year of life. In G. Dawson & K. Fischer (Eds.), *Human behavior and the developing brain* (pp. 269–313). New York: Guilford Press.

Oakes, L. M., & Ribar, R. J. (2005). A comparison of infants' categorization in paired and successive familiarization tasks. *Infancy, 7,* 85–98.

Palmeri, T. J.,Wong, A., & Gauthier, I. (2004). Computational approaches to the development of perceptual expertise. *Trends in Cognitive Sciences, 8,* 378–386.

Pauen, S. (2000). Early differentiation within the animate domain: Are humans something special? *Journal of Experimental Child Psychology, 75,* 134–151.

Pauen, S. (2002). Evidence for knowledge-based category discrimination in infancy. *Child Development, 73,* 1016–1033.

Quinn, P. C. (2004). Is the asymmetry in young infants' categorization of humans versus non-human animals based on head, body, or global Gestalt Information? *Psychonomic Bulletin & Review, 11,* 92–97.

Quinn, P. C., Doran, M. M., Reiss, J. E., & Hoffman, J. E. (2009). Time course of visual attention in infant categorization of cats versus dogs: Evidence for a head bias as revealed through eye tracking. *Child Development, 80,* 151–161.

Quinn, P. C., & Eimas, P. D. (1996). Perceptual cues that permit categorical differentiation of animal species by infants. *Journal of Experimental Child Psychology, 63,* 189–211.

Quinn, P. C., & Eimas, P. D. (1998). Evidence for a global categorical representation of humans by young infants. *Journal of Experimental Child Psychology, 69,* 151–174.

Quinn, P. C., Eimas, P. D., & Rosenkrantz, S. L. (1993). Evidence for representations of perceptually similar natural categories by 3- and 4-month-old infants. *Perception, 22,* 463–475.

Quinn, P. C., Lee, K., Pascalis, O., & Slater, A. M. (2007). In support of an expert–novice difference in the representation of humans versus non-human animals by infants: Generalization from persons to cats occurs only with upright whole images. *Cognition, Brain, & Behavior* (Special Issue on the Development of Categorization), *11,* 679–694.

Quinn, P. C., Schyns, P. G., & Goldstone, R. L. (2006). The interplay between perceptual organization and categorization in the representation of complex visual patterns by young infants. *Journal of Experimental Child Psychology, 95,* 117–127.

Quinn, P. C., Westerlund, A., & Nelson, C. A. (2006). Neural markers of categorization in 6-month-old infants. *Psychological Science, 17,* 59–66.

Quinn, P. C., Yahr, J., Kuhn, A., Slater, A. M., & Pascalis, O. (2002). Representation of the gender of human faces by infants: A preference for female. *Perception, 31,* 1109–1121.

Reed, C. L., McGoldrick, J. E., Shackelford, R., & Fidopiastis, C. (2004). Are human bodies represented differently from other animate and inanimate objects? *Visual Cognition, 11,* 523–550.

Reed, C. L., Stone, V. E., & McGoldrick, J. E. (2005). Not just posturing: Configural processing of the human body. In W. Prinz, M. Shiffrar, I. Thornton, G. Knoblich, & M. Grosjean (eds.), *The human body: From the inside out* (pp. 229–258). Oxford, UK: Oxford University Press.

Reynolds, G. D., & Richards, J. E. (2005). Familiarization, attention, and recognition memory in infancy: An ERP and cortical source localization study. *Developmental Psychology, 41,* 598–615.

Rogers, T. T., & McClelland, J. L. (2004). *Semantic cognition: A parallel distributed processing approach.* Cambridge, MA: MIT Press.

Ross, N., Medin, D. L., Coley, J. D., & Atran, S. (2003). Cultural and experiential differences in the development of folkbiological induction. *Cognitive Development, 18,* 25–47.

Rosch, E., Mervis, C. B., Gray, W., Johnson, D., & Boyes-Braem, P. (1976). Basic objects in natural categories. *Cognitive Psychology, 8,* 382–439.

Saxe, R., Tzelnic, T., & Carey, S. (2006). Five-month-old infants know that humans are solid, like inanimate objects. *Cognition, 101,* B1–B8.

Slaughter, V., & Heron, M. (2004). Origins and early development of human body knowledge. *Monographs of the Society for Research in Child Development, 69,* Serial number 276.

Smith, J. D., & Minda, J. P. (1998). Prototypes in the mist: The early epochs of category learning. *Journal of Experimental Psychology: Learning, Memory, and Cognition, 24,* 1411–1436.

Spencer, J., Quinn, P. C., Johnson, M. H., & Karmiloff-Smith, A. (1997). Heads you win, tails you lose: Evidence for young infants categorizing mammals by head and facial attributes (Special Issue: Perceptual Development). *Early Development and Parenting, 6,* 113–126.

Strauss, M. S., Newell, L. C., & Best, C. A. (April, 2003). The perception and recognition of faces by infants, preschoolers, and individuals with autism. In C. A. Nelson (Organizer), *The development of facial expertise.* Symposium conducted at the meeting of the Society for Research in Child Development, Tampa, FL.

Sugita, Y. (2008). Face perception in monkeys reared with no exposure to faces. *Proceedings of the National Academy of Sciences, 105,* 394–398.

Tanaka, J. W. (2001). The entry point of face recognition: Evidence for face expertise. *Journal of Experimental Psychology: General, 130,* 534–543.

Tanaka, J. W., Curran, T., & Sheinberg, D. L. (2005). The training and transfer of real-world perceptual expertise. *Psychological Science, 16,* 145–151.

Tanaka, J. W., & Gauthier, I. (1997). Expertise in object and face recognition. In R. L. Goldstone, P. G. Schyns, & D. L. Medin (Eds.), *The psychology of learning and motivation* (Vol. 36, pp. 83–125). San Diego: Academic Press.

Tanaka, J. W., & Taylor, M. (1991). Object categories and expertise: Is the basic level in the eye of the beholder? *Cognitive Psychology, 23,* 457–482.

Thelen, E., & Smith, L. B. (1994). *A dynamic systems approach to the development of cognition and action.* Cambridge, MA: MIT Press.

Tucker, D. M. (1993). Spatial sampling of head electrical fields: The geodesic sensor net. *Electroencephalography and Clinical Neurophysiology, 87,* 154–163.

Xu, F. (1997). From Lot's wife to a pillar of salt: Evidence that physical object is a sortal concept. *Mind & Language, 12,* 365–392.

Younger, B. A., & Fearing, D. D. (1999). Parsing items into separate categories: Developmental change in infant categorization. *Child Development, 70,* 291–303.

CHAPTER 14
Similarity, Induction, Naming, and Categorization: A Bottom-up Approach

Vladimir M. Sloutsky

People are remarkably smart: they know language, possess complex skills, and function in a complex dynamic environment. However, they do not exhibit evidence of this knowledge at birth and one of the central and most interesting issues in the study of human cognition is the question of how people acquire this knowledge in the course of development. One possibility is that sensory and cognitive systems have the capacity to extract regularities from structured input. However, this possibility has been frequently criticized as an untenable candidate for a complete story. In particular, it has been often argued that input data are severely underdetermined: the same data are compatible with multiple possibilities. Consider a visual occlusion phenomenon presented in Figure 14.1: the same event presented in Figure 14.1A is compatible with events presented in Figures 14.1B, C, D, and E, or an infinite number of other possibilities, and there is not enough information in the input to decide among these possibilities. However, under many conditions, even very early in development, people are more likely to expect the situation presented in Figure 14.1B than situations presented in Figure 14.1C and 14.1D (Kellman & Spelke, 1983; Spelke, 1990, but see Johnson, 2003).

Similarly, when adults label objects for young children (e.g., "Look, look, a dax!"), a mere co-occurrence of an object and a word is not sufficient for determining that the word refers to the object. In fact, the word could refer to a variety of things, including, any part of the object, its color, texture, manner of motion, or the speaker's attitude toward the situation. Again, despite the fact that the referential situation appears to be severely under constrained, even very young children somehow manage to determine that the word (at least if it is a noun) refers to the object (see Woodward & Markman, 1998, for a review).

It has been argued that these examples indicate that infants and young children perform these tasks with some expectations about the language and the world (e.g., they may expect words to refer to objects). This hypothesis raises a number of important questions. Where does this knowledge come from? How is this knowledge represented? And how do infants and young children deploy this knowledge? If the input is under constrained, then the "cognitive" constraints imposed on the input cannot be acquired from the input, and hence these constraints have to be a priori. Therefore, according to this position, some aspects of structured knowledge (e.g., knowledge of syntax, semantics, or visual organization) are a priori and the task of learning is to recognize these structures in the input. To reflect the fact that the constraints are a precondition rather than a consequence of learning, I will refer to this position as a "top-down approach." "Top-down" here refers to the origins of knowledge and many constraints that emerge in the bottom-up manner (in the course of learning) do not have "top-down" origins.

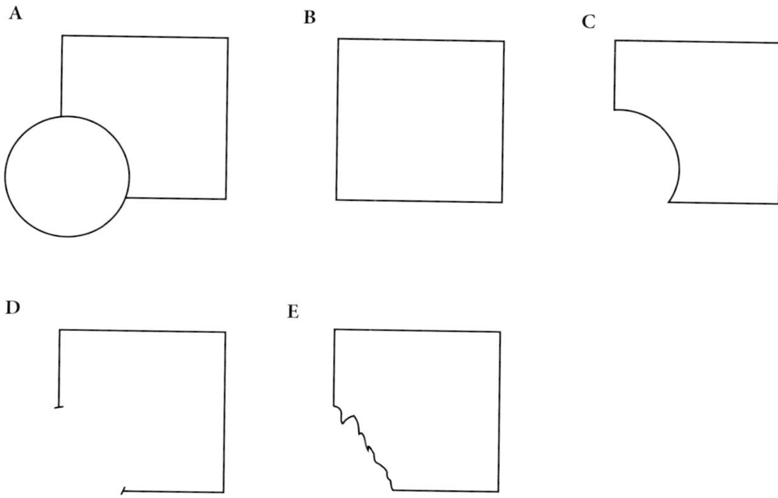

Figure 14.1 An example of visual occlusion, B–E. Possible states of the world compatible with A.

However, there is a growing body of evidence indicating that input is substantially richer than the above examples imply and that human learning is powerful enough to extract regularities from structured, albeit somewhat noisy, input. Of course, if this is the case, then people may not need a priori constraints. To reflect the fact that regularities are extracted from data (rather than imposed on the data), I will refer to this position as a "bottom-up" approach. The primary focus of this chapter is whether learning and cognitive development are constrained by a priori knowledge (and are thus top-down processes) or by the nature of the input and by learning mechanisms (and are thus bottom-up processes).

Top-down versus bottom-up learning

We say that a process is *top-down* when an outcome of a process is determined by a higher-order structure. For example, the number of light bulbs produced in North Korea in a given year (as well as their price) is completely determined by a government plan. The plan is not influenced by market conditions, but is designed to affect these conditions. Therefore, the plan, rather than the market conditions, prescribes the manufacturers' output, and radically different market conditions may result in a similar or identical output. Similarly, if cognitive development is a top-down process, then acquisition of syntax, the development of perception, and the development of generalization (such as word leaning or categorization) are constrained by knowledge, beliefs, or biases that are independent of input. As a result, radically different input conditions should result in similar linguistic and perceptual development outcomes.

Alternatively, we say that the process is *bottom-up* when an outcome of the process stems from an interaction of simpler processes, none of which alone can determine the outcome. In this case, the regularity in the outcome emerges from regularities in the input. For example, although it cannot be known in advance how many light bulbs will be produced in the United States in a given year, the production (as well as the price) is a function of market conditions (e.g., the cost of energy, the amount of construction activity, etc.), and it is likely that similar market conditions will result in somewhat similar production outcomes. Similarly, acquisition of syntax, the development of perception, and the development of generalization is a joint function of the regular input and the ability of the organism to extract and exploit these regularities.

The distinction between top-down and bottom-up approaches to learning has been recurring under different names. For example, in the domain of language learning, there has been a distinction between inductive and deductive approaches to language learning (e.g., Wexler & Culicover, 1980; Xu & Tenenbaum, 2007). According to the former view, learners extract regularities from linguistic input. In contrast, according to the latter view, learners entertain a fixed set of a priori hypotheses, and the role of input is to eliminate the inappropriate hypotheses, thus enabling the learner to settle on the correct hypothesis.

In this chapter, I focus on a different domain—the ability to extend knowledge from known to novel. People deploy this ability every time they (1) extend a known word to a novel entity (i.e., in naming or label extension), (2) treat a novel entity as a member of a familiar class (i.e., categorization), and (3) extend a property from a familiar entity to a novel entity (i.e., projective induction).

This ability to extend knowledge from known to novel, or inductive generalization, and the development of this ability are interesting and controversial issues in human cognition. Some researchers propose a top-down approach to generalization, arguing that even early in development, conceptual knowledge is a critical component of inductive generalization (Gelman, 2003; Gelman & Wellman, 1991; Keil, Smith, Simons, & Levin, 1998). This position is commonly known as knowledge-based (or naïve theory) approach. Others suggest that inductive generalization may develop in a bottom-up manner, with similarity playing a critical role in early induction (Colunga & Smith, 2005; French, Mareschal, Mermillod, & Quinn, 2004; Rogers & McClelland, 2004; Sloutsky, 2003; Sloutsky & Fisher, 2004a). While both positions agree that bottom-up processes, such as similarity computation, play a role (e.g., Keil et al.,1998; Keil, 2003), there is less agreement about the role and origins of top-down knowledge. For example, there no agreement on whether these top-down constraints are necessary for inductive generalization, when these constraints come online, and where they come from.

Top-down approaches to generalization

According to this position, even at the outset of development, infants and young children have a repertoire of "smart" conceptual assumptions about the language and the world (R. Gelman, 1990; Gelman & Markman, 1987; Gelman & Wellman, 1991; Keil, 1989; Mandler, 1997, 2004; Soja, Carey, & Spelke, 1991; Wellman & Gelman, 1992). Although conceptual knowledge plays a prominent role in top-down approaches, it is hard to pin down what exactly the top-down theorists mean by "conceptual knowledge" is. One possibility is that conceptual knowledge is knowledge that cannot be observed directly, but has to be inferred. Therefore, knowledge that birds have wings is perceptual, whereas knowledge that birds and fish share many biological properties is conceptual. Another issue that remains unclear is the origin of conceptual knowledge. Does conceptual knowledge emerge as generalization over data? Or does it exist independently of data? And if the latter is the case, where does it come from? Although these questions remain unanswered, conceptual knowledge plays a prominent role in top-down theories of generalization.

According to some accounts (see Massey & R. Gelman, 1988; Spelke, 1994) conceptual knowledge constrains (or even overrides) perceptual input, while remaining impervious to perceptual input. Conceptual effects in an inductive generalization task have been described as follows. When "trying to determine whether to draw an inference from object A to object B, a child would not simply calculate the similarity between the two objects. Rather the child would determine whether A and B belong to members of the same natural kind category that encompasses both A and B" (Gelman & Coley, 1991, p. 185). Therefore, according to this account of generalization, abstract (and not directly perceptible) category information is of greater importance than appearance information. Furthermore, identification of an abstract category is a necessary step in inductive generalization, and therefore induction in young children is category-based (e.g., Gelman, 1988).

Overall, among the putative conceptual assumptions, two are especially important for inductive generalization. The category assumption is the belief that individual entities are members of more general categories and that members of the same category share many unobserved properties. The linguistic assumption is the belief that words (especially count nouns) denote categories rather than individuals. When performing induction, people rely on these assumptions to conclude that entities sharing a label belong to the same kind, and therefore share many unobservable properties. For instance, when shown a picture of a yellow fish and told that this fish needs branchia to breathe, children are more likely to generalize this property to a red fish than to a turtle or a couch (Gelman, 1988). Presumably, children apply the two assumptions to infer that since the entities have a matching label (i.e., both are referred to as "a fish"), these entities belong to the same kind, and therefore they share many important properties.

Supporting Evidence

There are several lines of research supporting the idea of the linguistic and category assumptions in infants and children. For example, in support of the linguistic assumption, Markman and Hutchinson (1984) demonstrated that in an absence of a label, children may group things thematically (e.g., a police car and a policeman), whereas when the police car was named "a dax" and children were asked to select another "dax," they selected the passenger car, thus grouping the cars together. More recently, Gelman and Heyman (1999) demonstrated that young children were more willing to generalize properties from one person to another when both persons were referred to by a noun (i.e., "carrot-eaters") than when both were referred to by a descriptive sentence (e.g., "both like to eat carrots"). Furthermore, infants and children may also expect words to refer to categories, although, younger infants may hold this expectation not only for count nouns, but also for other speech sounds (e.g., Balaban & Waxman, 1997; Booth & Waxman, 2002).

There is also evidence supporting the idea that young children expect things to belong to categories and they expect members of the same category to share important properties. This evidence stems primarily from the study of inductive generalization. For example, Gelman and Markman (1986) presented young children with a Target item and two Test items, with one Test item looking more like the Target and another Test item sharing the label with the Target. Participants were also told that one Test item had a hidden property (e.g., "This one has hollow bones"), whereas another Test item had a different hidden property (e.g., "This one has solid bones"), and asked to induce a hidden property to the Target. Results indicated that young children tended to induce properties from the identically labeled, but not from the similarly looking item. Similar findings were reported with infants. Specifically, when objects were not labeled, infants generalized nonobvious properties based on appearance similarity, whereas when objects were labeled participants were using labeling information (Welder & Graham, 2001).

Challenges to the Top-Down Approach

There are several challenges to the idea that early generalization is driven by top-down conceptual assumptions. Some of these challenges stem from findings indicating that conceptual knowledge is not an a priori constraint, but is rather a product of learning and development. Other challenges stem from findings questioning the very existence of particular conceptual assumptions early in development.

Most importantly, empirical evidence does not lend unequivocal support to the idea that children's inductive generalization is driven by a priori assumptions, such as the linguistic and the category assumptions. In particular, several lines of research on categorization, word learning, and projective induction cast doubt on the existence of a priori assumptions in infants and young children (Colunga & Smith, 2005; French et al.,2004; Oakes & Madole, 2003, Rakison, 2003, Smith, Jones, & Landau, 1996; Yoshida & Smith, 2005). For example, it has been demonstrated that category learning in early infancy can be readily accounted for by the distribution of feature values within a category and across categories (French et al.,2004). It has been also found that when categorizing objects or inducing properties, the type of property infants focus on changes in the course of development (e.g., Madole, Oakes, & Cohen, 1993; Rakison, 2003). Similarly, "biases" that drive word learning have been found to come on-line in the course of learning rather than being a priori. For example, Smith, and colleagues (e.g., Smith, Jones, Landau, Gershkoff-Stowe, & Samuelson, 2002) examined the developmental course of the "shape bias"—the tendency of toddlers to extend a novel word to items that have the same shape as the originally labeled item. These researchers hypothesized that the shape bias is not a prerequisite, but a consequence of word leaning. The underlying idea is that in the course of language acquisition, babies first detect that a particular shape co-occurs with a particular label (e.g., "cup-shaped" objects are called "cups," while "ball-shaped" objects are called "balls"). As the corpus of evidence grows, they detect a more abstract regularity: similar-shaped entities have the same name, and this more abstract regularity, in turn, makes shape an important predictor of category membership. If this hypothesis is correct, then the shape bias is a function of word learning experience and it should emerge as children accumulate their vocabularies. This is exactly what Smith and colleagues found, thus presenting evidence that the "shape bias" in naming is not an a priori assumption, but is a product of learning.

Additional challenges to the top-down approach come from studies with preschoolers (i.e., 3- to 5-year-old children). For example, there are recent findings indicating that effects of labels on categorization and induction may be driven by attentional factors and do not have to stem from the linguistic assumption (Napolitano & Sloutsky, 2004; Sloutsky & Napolitano 2003). In particular, Amanda Napolitano and I demonstrated that under many conditions, auditory input (including linguistic input) automatically captures young children's attention, thus overshadowing (or attenuating processing of) corresponding visual input. Therefore, it is possible that (due to overshadowing effects) shared labels contribute to the overall similarity of compared entities (Sloutsky & Fisher, 2004a; Sloutsky & Lo, 1999), and thus to both categorization and induction.

Furthermore, there are reasons to be skeptical whether some of the findings, which are being used as evidence for linguistic and category assumptions, do in fact constitute such evidence. For example, Anna Fisher and I (Sloutsky & Fisher, 2004a) reexamined young children's performance on Gelman and Markman (1986) task. Similar to the original task, we presented 4- to 5-year-olds with triads of items, with each triad consisting of a target and two test items (these are presented in Figure 14.2B). Also, as

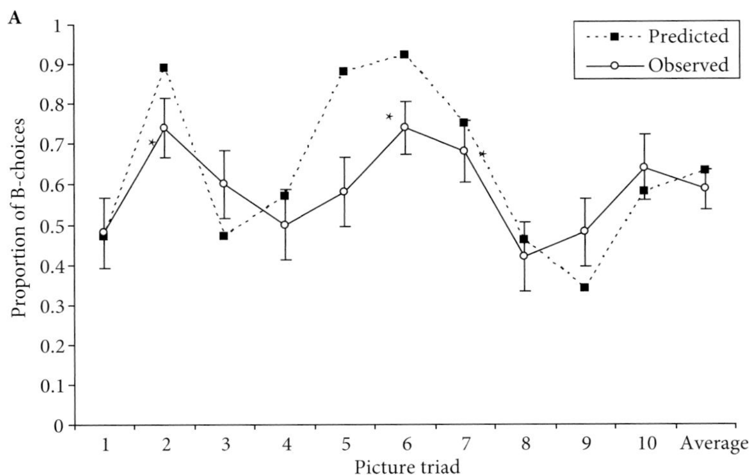

Figure 14.2 (Originally presented in Sloutsky & Fisher, 2004a). (A) Predicted and observed proportions of B-choices by stimuli triads in induction task. Error bars represent standard errors of the mean. (B) Stimuli used in Gelman and Markman (1986). ***Note*****: *Above chance; $p < .05$. Triad 1: Bird-Bat-Bird. Triad 2: Coral-Plant-Coral. Triad 3: Flower-Sea Anemone-Flower. Triad 4: Snake-Worm-Snake. Triad 5: Bug-Leaf-Bug. Triad 6: Starfish-Pinecone-Starfish. Triad 7: Squirrel-Rabbit-Squirrel. Triad 8: Dinosaur-Rhinoceros-Dinosaur. Triad 9: Lizard-Snake-Lizard. Triad 10: Fish-Dolphin-Fish.**

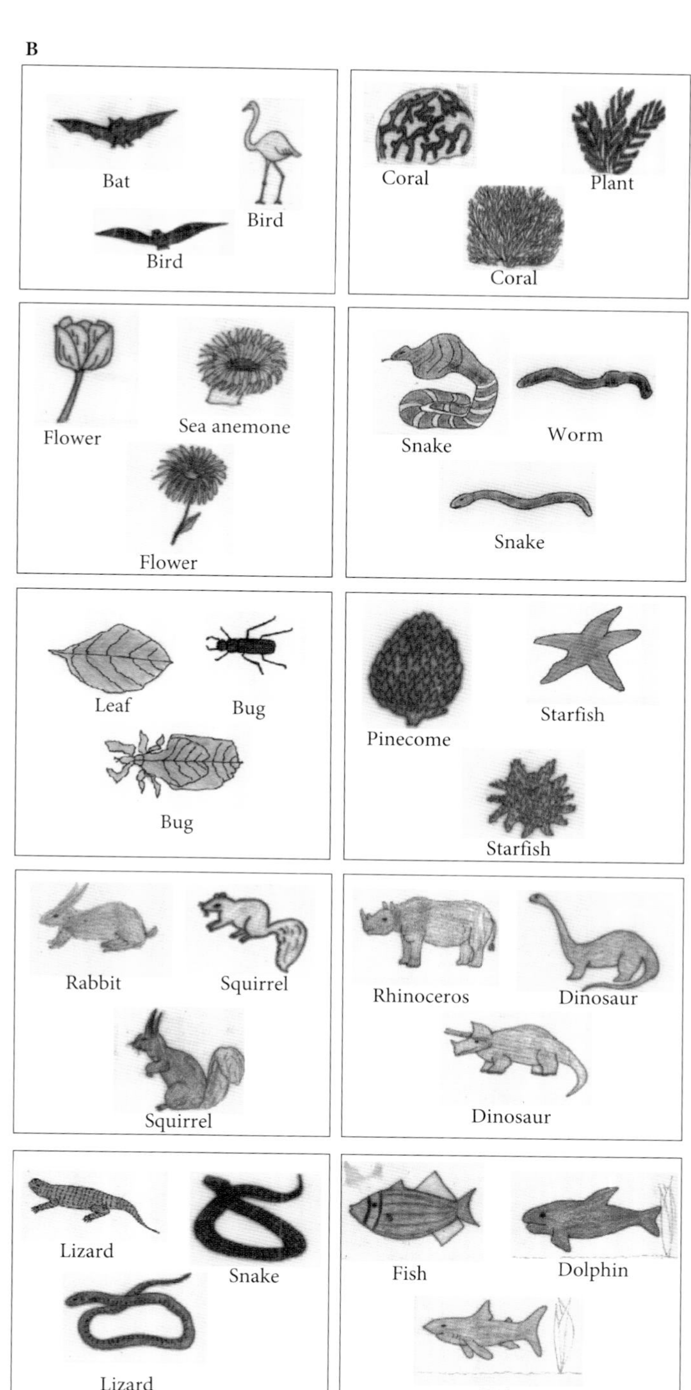

Figure 14.2 (Continued)

in the original task, we named items, such that one test item shared the label with the target, whereas the other appeared more similar to the target. Finally, as in the original task, we told participants that each of the test items had a particular nonobvious property and asked them to guess the property of the target. The entire procedure, including pictures, labels, and properties were identical to the original study. In addition, prior to the experiment proper, we conducted a separate experiment estimating for each triad the similarity of the test items to the target.

While replicating the overall mean reported by Gelman and Markman, we demonstrated that (a) children's performance varied drastically across picture triads (which should not be the case if induction was driven by a set of assumptions), (b) appearance similarity made a sizable contribution to induction, and (c) a simple model of similarity (the model is presented below) very accurately predicted how children perform on individual triads (see Figure 14.2A for a comparison of predicted and observed means). Therefore, a detailed analysis of children's performance does not support the conclusion that in the presence of shared labels, children ignore appearance information.

Another serious challenge to the idea that early generalization is constrained by a priori conceptual knowledge is that it is unclear how this knowledge (even if it existed) could be implemented and deployed in real-life situations. For example, in order for infants and young children to ignore salient (yet surface-level) perceptual information in favor of nonobservable and thus less salient conceptual information, they should have a substantial level of control over their attention. However, there is little evidence indicating that young children have sufficient control of attention, enabling them to focus on less salient (yet deep) information, while ignoring more salient (yet surface) information.

Bottom-up approaches to generalization

According to this view, young children generalize on the basis of multiple commonalities, or similarities, among presented entities. Because members of the same category often happen to be more perceptually similar to each other than they are to nonmembers (i.e., a yellow fish is more similar to a red fish than it is to a turtle or a couch), children are more likely to generalize properties to members of a category than to nonmembers. Furthermore, common labels could be features directly contributing to perceptual similarity rather than denoting a common category (Sloutsky & Fisher, 2004a; Sloutsky & Lo, 1999). Proponents of this view challenge the position that young children hold conceptual assumptions, and they argue that induction with both familiar and novel categories is similarity-based. In the remainder of this section, I will consider a recently proposed model of generalization (SINC standing for Similarity, Induction, Naming, and Categorization) that considers categorization, induction, and naming as variants of similarity-based generalization (see Sloutsky & Fisher, 2004a).

SINC Model

Overview

SINC assumes that young children consider linguistic labels as attributes of objects that contribute to similarity among compared entities. This assumption has been supported empirically (Sloutsky & Lo, 1999; Sloutsky, Lo, & Fisher, 2001). Qualitatively, SINC suggests that linguistic labels contribute to similarity of compared entities and that similarity drives induction and categorization in young children. The model is based on the product-rule model of similarity (Estes, 1994; Medin, 1975) that specifies similarity among nonlabeled feature patterns. In the product-rule model, similarity is computed using the following equation:

$$\mathrm{Sim}(i, j) = S^{N-k} \qquad (14.1)$$

where N denotes the total number of relevant attributes, k denotes the number of matches, and S ($0 \le S \le 1$) denotes values (weights) of a mismatch. For example, suppose that one is presented with two visual patterns (e.g., schematic faces A and B). Further suppose that these patterns consist of four distinct features (i.e., the shape of the face, eyes, and nose, and the size of ears) that the patterns share two of these features (i.e., the shape of the face and eyes) and differ on the other two. Assuming that $S = 0.5$ [the value frequently derived empirically (Estes, 1994)], similarity between A and B would be equal to 0.25 (i.e., 0.5^2). Note that similarity between entities decreases very rapidly with a decrease in the number of mismatches, approximating the exponential decay function discussed elsewhere (Nosofsky, 1984). For example, if the faces shared only one of the four features, their similarity would be equal to 0.125 (i.e., 0.5^3). On the other hand, if the faces shared all four features, they would be identical, and their similarity would be equal to 1 (i.e., 0.5^0).

According to SINC, similarity of labeled feature patterns could be calculated using the following equation:

$$\mathrm{Sim}(i,j) = W_{\mathrm{Label}}^{1-L} S_{Vis.attr}^{N-k} \left\{ \begin{array}{l} L = 1, \text{if } L_i = L_j \\ L = 1, \text{ otherwise} \end{array} \right\} \qquad (14.2)$$

Again, N denotes the total number of visual attributes, k denotes the number of matches, $S_{\mathrm{vis.attr.}}$ denotes values (attentional weights) of a mismatch on a visual attribute, W_{Label} denotes values of label mismatches, and L denotes a label match.

When there is a label match, $L = 1$ and $W_{\mathrm{Label}} = 1$; when there is a label mismatch, $L = 0$ and $W_{\mathrm{Label}} < 1$. Note that S and W (their values vary between 0 and 1) denote attentional weights of mismatches and the contribution of S and W is large when these parameters are close to 0 and is small they are close to 1. This is because the closer the value of these parameters to 1, the smaller the contribution of a mismatch to the detection of difference, while the closer the value to 0, the greater the contribution to the detection of difference. When two entities are identical on all dimensions (i.e., there are no mismatches), their similarity should be equal to 1; otherwise, it is smaller than 1.

Note that, according to the model, when neither entity is labeled (i.e., $W_{\mathrm{Label}} = 1$), similarity between the entities is determined by the number of overlapping visual attributes, thus conforming to Equation 14.1. Labels are presented as a separate term in the equation because they are expected to have larger attentional weight than most visual attributes (Sloutsky & Lo, 1999). In the case that the weight of a label does not differ from that of other attributes, the label will become one of the attributes in the computation of similarity, and Equation 14.2 becomes Equation 14.1.

Why would labels contribute to similarity? And what might be a mechanism underlying the greater weight of labels at earlier age demonstrated in previous research (e.g., Sloutsky & Lo, 1999)? One possibility is that labels have larger weights because they are presented auditorily, and auditory processing dominates the visual processing in infancy and early childhood, but this dominance decreases with age (Lewkowicz, 1988a, 1988b; Sloutsky & Napolitano, 2003). Alternatively, it is possible that larger weights of labels are grounded in a special status of sounds of human speech (Balaban & Waxman, 1997; Waxman & Markow, 1995). We discuss both possibilities in the "Why Do Labels Contribute to Similarity" section.

Finally, SINC suggests that if the child is presented with a Target feature pattern (T) and Test feature patterns (A and B) and asked which of the Test patterns is more similar to the Target, the child's choice for one of the Test items (e.g., Test B) could be predicted using a variant of the Luce's choice rule presented in the following equation:

$$P(B) = \frac{\mathrm{Sim}(T,B)}{\mathrm{Sim}(T,B) + \mathrm{Sim}(T,A)} \qquad (14.3)$$

We argue that if induction and categorization in young children are indeed similarity-based, then this model that predicts similarity judgment in young children (e.g., Sloutsky & Lo, 1999) should be able to predict their induction.

However, for the majority of naturalistic visual stimuli patterns, it is impossible to individuate features and calculate feature overlap (e.g., think about photographs of two animals and the multiplicity of perceptual features that they have). At the same time, perceptually rich naturalistic stimuli constitute the most interesting and informative test of the proposed model.

Because neither N nor k presented in Equation 14.1 are determinable a priori for perceptually rich naturalistic stimuli, we made several additional steps to apply the model to naturalistic stimuli. Denoting similarity of Test stimuli A and B to the Target as S^x and S^y, respectively, and performing simple derivations from Equation 14.3 allow us to get equations predicting categorization and induction performance. First, consider the case when entities are not labeled. Substituting Sim(T,B) and Sim(T,A) by S^x and S^y, we get the following equation:

$$P(B)=\frac{S^x}{S^x+S^y}=\frac{S^x}{S^x\left(1+S^{y-x}\right)}=\frac{1}{1+\frac{S^y}{S^x}} \qquad (14.4)$$

For the labeled entities, derivations remain essentially the same, except for the W_{Label} parameter. The parameter equals to 1, if there is a label match, otherwise it varies from 0 to 1, and the smaller the value of W, the greater the contribution of label mismatch. Therefore, in the case of labeled entities, the probability of selecting the item that shares the same label (say item B if it shares the label with the Target) could be derived as follows:

$$P(B)=\frac{S^x}{S^x+WS^y}=\frac{S^x}{S^x\left(1+WS^{y-x}\right)}=\frac{1}{1+\frac{WS^y}{S^x}} \qquad (14.5)$$

In short, Equations 14.4 and 14.5 should predict participants' induction responses in label and no-label conditions, respectively. In other words, their willingness to induce from Test B to the Target should be a function of the ratio of S^y/S^x (i.e., of similarity of A and B to the Target) when no labels are provided, and it should be a joint function of S^y/S^x and W (i.e., the attentional weight of label) when labels are provided. Note that Equation 14.5 reflects a situation when the Target and Test B have the same labels, whereas Test A has a different label. For the purpose of expository convenience, in the description of data and in figures, I will refer to the Test stimulus sharing the label with the Target as "Test B." Note that both W and S^y/S^x can be estimated from data, and therefore Equations 14.4 and 14.5 can be used for predicting specific probabilities of induction and categorization.

One important (and testable) consequence of this proposal is that because linguistic labels contribute to similarity in a quantitative manner rather than in a qualitative "all-or-nothing" manner, they should also make a quantitative contribution to induction as well. Therefore, the top-down approach and SINC make different predictions about the effect of linguistic labels on induction. If inductive generalization is made solely on the basis of linguistic label (as predicted by the linguistic assumption), then induction should be independent of appearance similarity. Alternatively, SINC predicts that labels make a quantitative contribution to similarity and thus to induction.

Empirical Findings Generated by SINC

SINC is a model implementing a theory of inductive generalization, which can predict a wide range of phenomena across a variety of tasks. These phenomena include: (1) effects of labels on similarity early in development; (2) effects of phonological similarity of labels on induction; (3) low-level attentional mechanisms underlying effects of labels on similarity and induction; (4) flexible (yet nondeliberate) adjustment of attentional weights of different sources of information; (5) differential effects of induction on recognition memory at different points of development; (6) dissociation between label and category information; (7) integration of labeling and appearance information in the course of similarity judgment and induction; and (8) interrelationships among induction, categorization, naming, and similarity.

First, it has been demonstrated that early in development, labels contribute to similarity of compared entities (Sloutsky & Fisher, 2004a; Sloutsky & Lo, 1999). In particular, when two entities share a label, young children tend to consider these entities as looking more alike than when the same entities are presented without labels, and, as we explain below, these effects stem from attentional factors, such as auditory information overshadowing (or attenuating processing) of corresponding visual information

(Napolitano & Sloutsky, 2004; Robinson & Sloutsky, 2004; Sloutsky & Napolitano, 2003).

Second, if labels are features contributing to the overall similarity, then it is possible that labels are perceived as subjectively continuous variables, in which case, not only the identity, but also phonological similarity of labels would contribute to the overall similarity and to induction. Therefore, the theory underlying SINC suggests that phonological similarity of labels may contribute to induction. There is recent evidence supporting this prediction (Fisher & Sloutsky, 2004): Young children were more likely to generalize a property from a test item to a target item if the test and target items had a phonologically similar label (e.g., *Guma* and *Gama*) than if it had a phonologically different label (*Guma* and *Fika*). Furthermore, young children tended to extend phonologically similar words to visually similar entities.

Third, according to SINC, effects of words on similarity and thus on induction stem from low-level attentional mechanisms rather than from an understanding of the conceptual importance of labels. Based on this idea, it was predicted that words, as well as other auditory stimuli, may affect processing of corresponding visual information. This prediction was confirmed empirically: For infants and young children, auditory information overshadows corresponding visual information (Napolitano & Sloutsky, 2004; Robinson & Sloutsky, 2004; Sloutsky & Napolitano, 2003). In particular, when discriminable visual and auditory stimuli (including human speech) were presented together, discrimination of visual (but not of auditory) stimuli decreased compared to a unimodal baseline.

Fourth, because effects of words and visual information on induction stem from attentional mechanisms rather than from understanding of the conceptual importance of labels or appearances, SINC predicts that contribution of labels or appearance to induction can be changed by changing attentional weights of labels or appearance through associative training. This prediction was supported in a set of experiments (Fisher & Sloutsky, 2006; Sloutsky & Spino, 2004). In one set of experiments (Sloutsky & Spino, 2004), attention to labels or to appearances was manipulated by varying their predictive values (when a cue is consistently nonpredictive, attention to this cue decreases, see Hall, 1991, for a review). After training, participants were presented with an induction task, which was repeated again 3.5 months after training. It was found that as a result of training, young children exhibited (depending on the training condition) either appearance-based or label-based induction, with either pattern being different from pretraining induction. Furthermore, 3.5 months after training, young children retained these effects of training.

Fifth, SINC enabled a novel prediction regarding effects of induction on recognition memory. Recall that according to SINC, early induction is driven by similarity, whereas according to the knowledge-based approach, even early in development induction is category-based and is driven by more abstract category information. To address this issue, Anna Fisher and I developed the Induction-then-Recognition (ITR) paradigm, allowing the distinction between these two possibilities (see Sloutsky & Fisher, 2004a, 2004b).

The ability of ITR to distinguish between these possibilities is based on the following reasoning. Research on false-memory phenomena showed that deep semantic processing of studied items (including grouping of items into categories) often increases memory intrusions—false recognition and recall of nonpresented "critical lures" or items semantically associated with studied items (e.g., Koutstall & Schacter, 1997; Thapar & McDermott, 2001). Thus "deeper" processing can lead to lower recognition accuracy when critical lures are semantically similar to studied items. In contrast to deep processing, focusing on perceptual details of pictorially presented information results in accurate recognition (Marks, 1991). Therefore, a memory test administered after an induction task may reveal information about how items were processed during the induction task. If participants processed the items relatively abstractly as members of a category (i.e., they performed category-based induction), then they would likely have difficulty discriminating studied targets from conceptually similar critical lures. If, on the other hand, they processed items more concretely, focusing on perceptual details (i.e., they performed similarity-based induction), then they should discriminate relatively well. This is exactly what we found: After performing induction with pictures of members of familiar categories (e.g., cats), young children exhibited greater recognition accuracy than did adults, with recognition gradually decreasing with increasing age (Fisher & Sloutsky, 2005a; Sloutsky & Fisher, 2004a, 2005). Their accuracy, however, dropped to the level of adults when they were trained to perform induction in a category-based manner—by deciding whether the test and the target items belong to the same kind.

Unlike some top-down approaches that consider linguistic labels as category proxies, SINC clearly differentiates between labeling information and category information: According to SINC, linguistic labels contribute to induction by contributing to similarity rather than by denoting categories. Initial evidence for this distinction comes from the fact that young children's induction is not category-based (Fisher & Sloutsky, 2005a; Sloutsky & Fisher, 2004a, 2004b), yet labels contribute to early induction by affecting similarity (Sloutsky & Fisher, 2004a; Sloutsky et al.,2001).

More direct evidence for the distinction comes from a set of recent studies using the ITR paradigm (Fisher & Sloutsky, 2005b). Note that in the recognition studies using the ITR paradigm discussed above (Fisher & Sloutsky, 2005a; Sloutsky & Fisher, 2004a, 2004b), pictures were not accompanied by labels. If label and category information are the same for young children, then when presented entities are labeled, children should exhibit effects of semantic processing—low-recognition accuracy stemming from high hits and elevated false alarms. Furthermore, effects of category labels (i.e., the words *Cat* referring to each individual cat) should differ from those of individual labels (i.e., a different count noun referring to each member of a category). In particular, only the former, but not the latter should promote category-based induction. However, because SINC does not consider category labels to be category markers, the prediction is different. In particular, because labels may overshadow corresponding visual information, introduction of labels may disrupt encoding of visual information, thus resulting in a decreased proportion of hits. Furthermore, category labels and individual labels should have comparable effects on recognition memory. This is exactly what was found—individual label and category labels exerted similar effects on recognition memory (Fisher & Sloutsky, 2005b). However, when young children were trained to perform category-based induction (Fisher & Sloutsky, 2005b), not only did their induction performance increase, but participants also exhibited patterns of recognition accuracy that were similar to those of adults (i.e., high hits and elevated false alarms).

We also found that labels and visual similarity jointly contribute to induction early in development, and SINC can quantify these contributions: For example, as mentioned above, SINC accurately predicted young children's performance on individual triads with Gelman and Markman (1986) stimuli and, as predicted, children's induction was driven by the overall similarity rather than by reliance on labels. Also, as shown in Figure 14.3, SINC accurately predicts young children's performance on a similarity judgment task (Figure 14.3A) and on induction and categorizations tasks (Figure 14.3B). Finally, SINC assumes the interrelatedness of similarity, induction, and categorization, and results support this assumption, pointing to high intercorrelations among similarity, induction, and categorization (Sloutsky & Fisher, 2004a).

However, it could be argued that reliance on similarity does not constitute unequivocal evidence against the idea that conceptual assumptions constrain generalization. For example, it has been argued that categorization and induction "reflect an interaction of perceptual knowledge, language, and conceptual knowledge" (Gelman & Medin, 1993, p. 159). Therefore, it is important to know whether or not young children's generalization is driven by the category and linguistic assumptions.

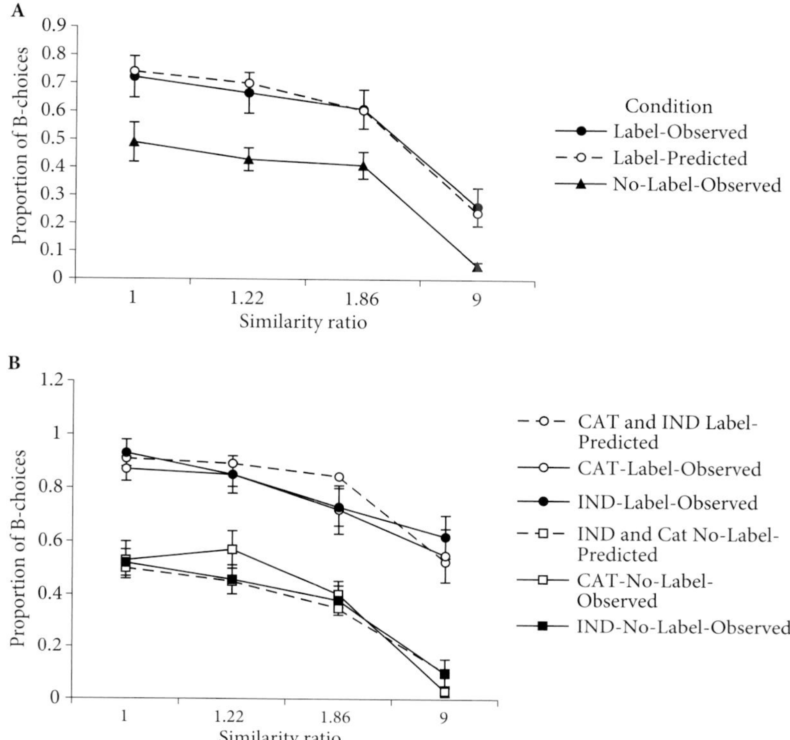

Figure 14.3 (Originally presented in Sloutsky & Fisher, 2004a). (A) Predicted and observed probabilities of B-choices as a function of similarity ratio and labeling in the similarity judgment task. (B) Predicted and observed probabilities of B-choices as a function of similarity ratio and labeling in induction and categorization tasks. Error bars represent standard errors of the mean.

In an attempt to answer this question, we conducted a study, in which 4- to 5-year-olds learned a novel category and then performed an induction task (Sloutsky, Kloos, & Fisher, 2007). The category was bound by a relational inclusion rule rather than by similarity (see Figure 14.4 for examples). After successfully learning the category, participants were presented with a triad induction task, such that one test item shared category membership with the target and another was similar to the target (while being a member of a different category). Despite the fact that young children ably learned the categories and readily categorized items throughout the experiment, they did not use this knowledge when making inductions, relying instead on appearance similarity. Therefore, there is little evidence that top-down conceptual information is an important factor in early generalization, even when this information is directly given to young children.

WHY DO LABELS CONTRIBUTE TO SIMILARITY?

As mentioned above, linguistic labels play an important role in the early generalization: if two items are accompanied by the same label, young children are more likely to generalize properties from one item to another than when labels are different or no labels are introduced. In an attempt to explain these effects, two classes of explanations have been proposed. According to the language-specific explanation, young children assume that (a) entities are members of categories and (b) count nouns

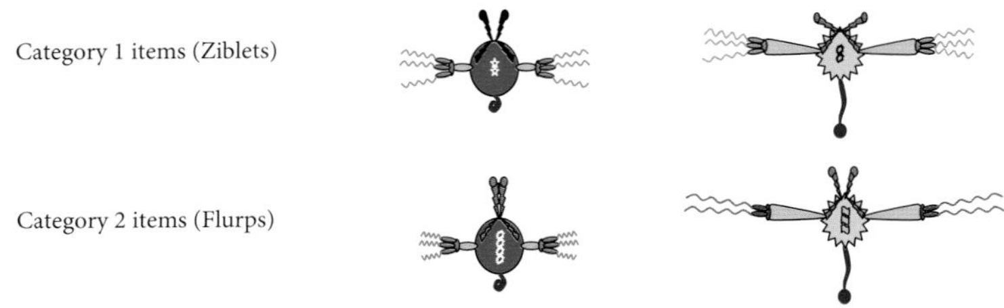

Figure 14.4 Examples of stimuli used by Sloutsky, Kloos, and Fisher (2007).

convey category membership (Gelman & Coley, 1991). Furthermore, for 9-month-old infants, even speech sounds devoid of morphosyntactic information may communicate category membership (Balaban & Waxman, 1997). These assumptions lead young children and infants to infer that entities that are denoted by the same count noun belong to the same category (Gelman & Markman, 1986; Markman, 1989; see also Waxman & Markow, 1995 for a discussion). Therefore, according to the language-specific explanation, if entities share a label presented as a count noun, then this shared count noun suggests that entities belong to the same category (thus supporting categorization), and further, belonging to the same category indicates that the members of the category share nonobvious properties (thus supporting inductive inference about these properties).

However, it is also possible that effects of labels stem from attentional factors, such as auditory information overshadowing (or attenuating processing) of corresponding visual information (Napolitano & Sloutsky, 2004; Robinson & Sloutsky, 2004; Sloutsky & Napolitano, 2003). As a result of overshadowing, young children may consider entities that share the label as looking more similar (Sloutsky & Fisher, 2004a; Sloutsky & Lo, 1999), with similarity affecting inductive generalization.

Initial evidence for overshadowing was presented in the Sloutsky and Napolitano (2003) study, in which 4-year-olds and adults were presented with an auditory-visual target item (AUD_TVIS_T), where the visual and the auditory components were presented in synchrony. The Target was followed by one of the four test items. Some test items were identical to the target items (i.e., AUD_TVIS_T). Other test items had either the auditory component changed ($AUD_{new}VIS_T$), the visual component changed (AUD_TVIS_{new}), or both components changed ($AUD_{new}VIS_{new}$). Participants had to respond *same* if the two compound stimuli had the same auditory and visual components, and to respond *different* if either the auditory or visual component differed between the target and test items. The auditory components consisted of unfamiliar nonlinguistic sounds and the visual components consisted of unfamiliar images (e.g., geometric shapes). If participants encode both auditory and visual stimuli, then they should accept target items as the *same* and reject items that had either new visual or new auditory components.

It was found that 4-year-olds failed to report that the visual components changed when stimuli were cross-modal, whereas they had no difficulty noticing when the same visual components changed in the unimodal condition (see Figure 14.5 for overshadowing effects in 4- and 6-year-olds). As shown in Figure 14.5, processing of visual stimuli was not difficult per se: in the absence of auditory stimuli, young children ably encoded the visual stimuli, whereas when both visual and auditory stimuli were presented simultaneously, encoding of visual (but not of auditory) stimuli decreased compared to a unimodal baseline (Napolitano & Sloutsky, 2004; Robinson & Sloutsky, 2004; Sloutsky & Napolitano, 2003). The results presented in Figure 14.5 also indicate that there was a decrease in overshadowing effects between 4 and 6 years of age. Furthermore, we found no evidence of overshadowing in adults: adults ably processed both auditory and visual stimuli.

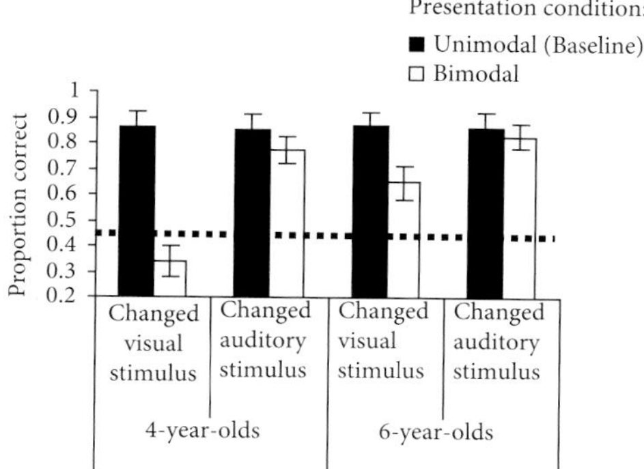

Figure 14.5 Recognition accuracy by modality, presentation condition and age. Error bars represent standard errors of the mean.

Finding overshadowing effects in young children and the decrease of these effects in the course of development enabled us to make predictions about infants' ability to encode cross-modal stimuli. If overshadowing effects decrease with age, then infants should exhibit even stronger overshadowing effects than young children. These predictions were confirmed empirically (Robinson & Sloutsky, 2004). In a set of experiments, Chris Robinson and I (Robinson & Sloutsky, 2004) presented the same auditory and visual compounds to infants, children, and adults. In the infant task, 8-, 12-, and 16-month-olds were familiarized to an auditory-visual compound ($AUD_T VIS_T$). At test, infants were presented with four test trials where either the auditory component changed ($AUD_{new} VIS_T$), the visual component changed ($AUD_T VIS_{new}$), both components changed ($AUD_{new} VIS_{new}$), or neither component changed ($AUD_T VIS_T$). If infants encode the auditory component during familiarization, then they should increase looking when the auditory component changes at test (i.e., $AUD_{new} VIS_T - AUD_T VIS_T > 0$), and if infants encode the visual stimulus, then they should increase looking when the visual component changes at test. Even though infants ably encoded the visual stimuli when presented unimodally, they often failed to encode visual stimuli when paired with an auditory stimulus (auditory overshadowing). Furthermore, infants exhibited auditory overshadowing under a wider range of stimulus conditions than children and adults.

Although these auditory overshadowing effects should hinder forming word-object associations, it is well known that 14- and 15-month-olds can form such associations (e.g., Schafer & Plunkett, 1998; Werker, Cohen, Lloyd, Casasola, & Stager, 1998). To examine whether words also overshadow corresponding visual input, we paired the same visual stimuli that were used in Robinson and Sloutsky (2004) with nonsense words (Sloutsky & Robinson, 2008). Results presented in Figure 14.6A indicate that 8- and 12-month-olds only encoded the word, whereas 16-month-olds encoded both the word and visual stimulus. Thus, at 8 and 12 months of age, both unfamiliar words and unfamiliar sounds overshadowed visual input, whereas, at 16 months, words did not overshadow corresponding visual input. Therefore, when cross-modal stimuli are presented for a protracted period of time (such as in familiarization or habituation paradigms), by 16 months of age, words stop interfering with visual processing, whereas nonlinguistic sounds continue to interfere.

Why is there a difference between encoding visual stimuli accompanied by words and by sounds at 16 months of age? First, it is possible that human speech is a special class of stimuli for humans, with infants and young children having broad assumptions that words refer to categories (e.g., Waxman & Booth, 2003). Thus, according to this "language-specific hypothesis," labels play a special role in processing of visual information by directing children's attention to visual input (e.g., Balaban & Waxman, 1997; Baldwin & Markman, 1989; Xu, 2002). Alternatively, it is possible that the decreased interference of words in visual processing at 16 months of age stems from familiarity effects: by that age, human speech may become more familiar than many other sounds (e.g., Jusczyk, 1998; Napolitano & Sloutsky, 2004), and, under repeated presentation conditions, more familiar stimuli may be processed faster and may be less likely to interfere with processing of visual stimuli. If familiarity can account for the increased processing of visual input, then prefamiliarizing infants to the nonlinguistic sounds

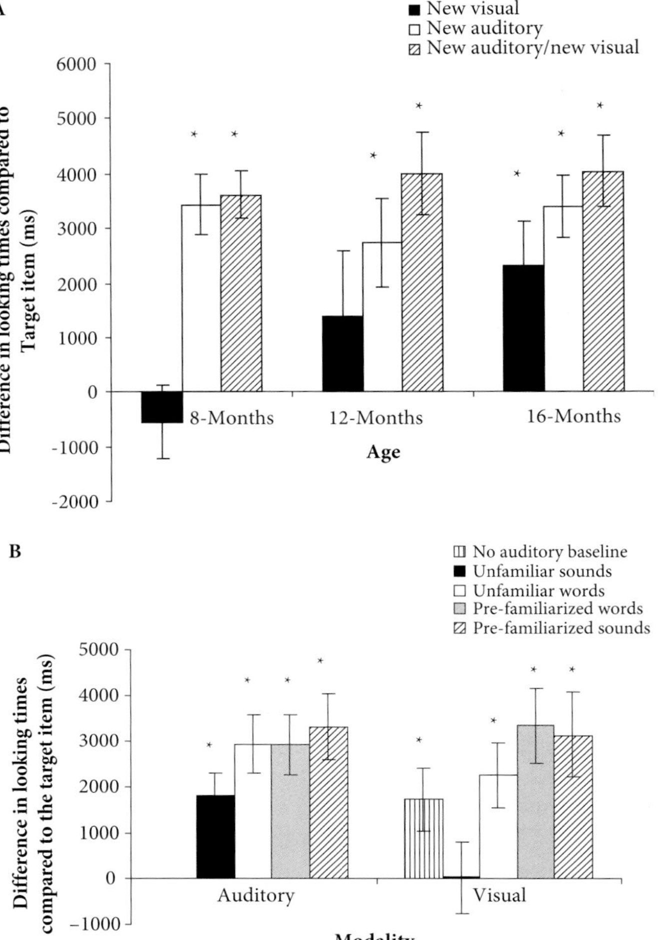

Figure 14.6 (A) Encoding of auditory and visual stimuli at 8-, 12-, and 16-months of age. (B) 16-month-olds' encoding of auditory and visual components across different auditory conditions.

prior to the experiment proper should attenuate overshadowing effects.

To determine whether the effects of words at 16 months were language-specific or stemmed from familiarity, we conducted another experiment, in which 16-month-olds were presented with the same visual patterns accompanied by the same auditory input (i.e., either linguistic or non-linguistic). However, prior to the experiment proper, participants were prefamiliarized to the auditory input. Note that the presence of prefamiliarization was the only difference between this and the previous experiment. As can be seen in Figure 14.6B, across the different auditory conditions, infants ably encoded auditory input. In contrast, encoding of visual input was affected by the familiarity of the auditory input. When the auditory input was unfamiliar, the sounds overshadowed corresponding visual input and the words did not interfere with processing of visual input (compared to the unimodal baseline). However, when infants were first prefamiliarized to the auditory component (either sound or word), prefamiliarized sounds and words facilitated processing of corresponding visual input—in these conditions, infants were more likely to encode the visual stimuli than in a unimodal baseline. Therefore, under these conditions, familiar auditory stimuli tuned attention to corresponding visual input.

Taken together, these findings present evidence that early in development, auditory input may affect attention allocated to visual input and in the course of development, visual processing becomes more independent from auditory processing. If this is the case, then effects of words may stem from the dynamics of cross-modal processing rather than from conceptual assumptions. As processing of visual input becomes more independent of processing of auditory input and as children learn that under many conditions, words are reliable cues, effects of words may become more "conceptual" in nature. This account may elucidate mechanisms underlying effects of words on early generalization: many of these effects may stem from auditory input affecting processing of visual input. In addition, this account suggests that the importance of words is not "given," but is acquired in the course of learning and development.

Unresolved issues

In sum, SINC—a bottom-up model reviewed in this chapter—can account well for early generalization. First, the model accurately predicts children's performance on similarity judgment, induction, and categorization tasks. I presented evidence from induction, categorization, and recognition memory tasks, indicating that early generalization is driven by similarity rather than by abstract conceptual information. Second, the model quantifies effects of labels on similarity and generalization early in development, and the theory underlying SINC suggests the mechanism driving the effects of labels. I presented evidence indicating that labels affect similarity (and thus generalization) by attenuating visual processing. The reviewed findings indicate that many effects of labels may stem from dynamics of cross-modal processing rather than from conceptual assumptions about the language and the world. These ideas also explain why phonologically similar labels may affect early generalization in a manner similar to that of identical labels. Finally, the model suggests that the contribution of various predictors (e.g., labels, appearances, etc.) to early generalization is determined by attention allocated to these predictors. The fact that attention allocated to predictors (i.e., attentional weights of the predictors) is not fixed, but can be flexibly (yet nondeliberately) adjusted in a course of learning suggests how generalization can change in the course of learning and development. At the same time, there are several issues that remain unresolved. Most importantly, SINC cannot account for many aspects of mature generalization, such as some of the sophisticated strategies exhibited by adults, or for the transition from the early to mature generalization. These are interesting challenges that have to be addressed in the future.

Conclusions

In this chapter, I considered two broad theoretical approaches to cognitive development. One approach advocates the importance of a priori constraints in cognitive development (i.e., the top-down approach). Evidence for these constraints comes from a variety of studies with infants and young children, indicating that even early in development, infants and children treat some aspects of input as more "important" or central than others. Another approach argues that people have powerful learning mechanisms enabling them to extract regularities from the input (i.e., the bottom-up approach). Proponents of the latter approach argue that conceptual knowledge is not a priori, but it emerges in the course of learning and development. Therefore, whenever children treat some aspects of input as more "important," these "important" stimuli have to be natural "attention grabbers"; otherwise the importance of these stimuli has to be learned. In the course of learning, children may realize that some stimuli are regular and reliable predictors of other important events and they may start treating the reliable predictors differently from the less reliable ones.

I then reviewed a recently proposed bottom-up model of inductive generalization and several phenomena predicted by the model; some of these phenomena present challenges to the top-down approach. I specifically focused on the role of label and appearance information in induction and presented evidence that labels affect induction by contributing to the overall similarity of compared items. I also considered a mechanism that may underlie the effects of labels on generalization: I suggested that labels (and other sounds) contribute to similarity by overshadowing (or attenuating processing of) corresponding visual input and presented supporting evidence from studies with infants and young children. Finally, I discussed how effects of words may change in the course of development as a function of increasing familiarity of human speech.

I also tried to make it clear throughout the chapter that much of the developmental story remains a mystery. Despite the significant advances in the study of inductive generalization in the past 20 years, the most interesting developmental question has not been answered: How do people become so smart, acquiring extraordinary complex knowledge that shapes their striking intellectual abilities? A detailed answer to this question would likely to constitute the most significant contribution to the study of cognitive development.

Acknowledgments

This research was supported by grants from the NSF (BCS-0720135) and from the Institute of Education Sciences, U.S. Department of Education (R305H050125) to VM.S. The opinions expressed are those of the authors and do not represent views of the awarding organizations. I thank Anna Fisher and Chris Robinson for helpful comments.

References

Balaban, M. T., & Waxman, S. R. (1997). Do words facilitate object categorization in 9-month-old infants? *Journal of Experimental Child Psychology, 64*, 3–26.

Baldwin, D. A., & Markman, E. M. (1989). Establishing word–object relations: A first step. *Child Development, 60*, 381–398.

Booth, A. E., & Waxman, S. R. (2002). Word learning is 'smart': Evidence that conceptual information affects preschoolers' extension of novel words. *Cognition, 84*, 11–22.

Colunga, E. & Smith, L. B. (2005). From the lexicon to expectations about kinds: A role for associative learning. *Psychological Review, 112*, 347–382.

Estes, W. K. (1994). *Classification and cognition.* New York: Oxford University Press.

Fisher, A. V., & Sloutsky, V. M. (2004). When mats meow: Phonological similarity of labels and induction in young children. In K. Forbus, D. Gentner, & T. Regier (Eds.), *Proceedings of the XXVI Annual Conference of the Cognitive Science Society.* Mahwah, NJ: Erlbaum.

Fisher, A. V., & Sloutsky, V. M. (2005a). When induction meets memory: Evidence for gradual transition from similarity-based to category-based induction. *Child Development, 76*, 583–597.

Fisher, A. V., & Sloutsky, V. M. (2005b). Effects of category labels on induction and visual processing: Support or interference? In B. G.Bara, L. Barsalou, & M. Bucciarelli (Eds.), *Proceedings of the XXVII Annual Conference of the Cognitive Science Society.* Mahwah, NJ: Erlbaum.

Fisher, A. F., & Sloutsky, V. M. (2006). Flexible attention to labels and appearances in early induction. In R. Sun and N. Miyake (Eds.). *Proceedings of the XXVIII Annual Conference of the Cognitive Science Society* (pp. 220–225). Mahwah, NJ: Erlbaum.

French, R. M., Mareschal, D., Mermillod, M., & Quinn, P. C. (2004). The role of bottom-up processing in perceptual categorization by 3- to 4-month-old infants: Simulations and data. *Journal of Experimental Psychology: General, 133*, 382–397.

Gelman, R. (1990). First principles organize attention to and learning about relevant data: Number and the animate–inanimate distinction as examples. *Cognitive Science, 14*, 79–106.

Gelman, S. A. (1988). The development of induction within natural kind and artifact categories. *Cognitive Psychology, 20*, 65–95.

Gelman, S. A. (2003). *The essential child: Origins of essentialism in everyday thought.* London: Oxford University Press.

Gelman, S. A., & Coley, J. (1991). Language and categorization: The acquisition of natural kind terms. In S. A. Gelman, S. & J. P. Byrnes (Eds.), *Perspectives on language and thought: Interrelations in development* (pp. 146–196). New York: Cambridge University Press.

Gelman, S. A., & Heyman, G. D. (1999). Carrot-eaters and creature-believers: The effects of lexicalization on children's inferences about social categories. *Psychological Science, 10*, 489–493.

Gelman, S. A., & Markman, E. (1986). Categories and induction in young children. *Cognition, 23*, 183–209.

Gelman, S. A., & Markman, E. M. (1987). Young children's inductions from natural kinds: The role of categories and appearances. *Child Development, 58*, 1532–1541.

Gelman, S. A., & Medin, D. L. (1993). What's so essential about essentialism? A different perspective on the interaction of perception, language, and concrete knowledge. *Cognitive Development, 8*, 157–167.

Gelman, S. A., & Wellman, H. M. (1991). Insides and essences: Early understanding of the obvious. *Cognition, 38*, 213–244.

Hall, G. (1991). *Perceptual and associative learning.* New York: Oxford University Press.

Johnson, S. P. (2003). Development of fragmented versus holistic object perception. In G. Schwarzer & H. Leder, Helmut (Eds.), *The development of face processing* (pp. 3–17). Ashland, OH: Hogrefe & Huber Publishers.

Jusczyk, P. W. (1998). *The discovery of spoken language.* Cambridge, MA: MIT Press.

Keil, F. C. (2003). Categories, cognitive development and cognitive science. In D. H. Rakison & L. M. Oakes (Eds.), *Early category and concept development: Making sense of the blooming buzzing confusion* (pp. vi–xi). New York: Oxford University Press.

Keil, F. C. (1989). *Concepts, kinds, and cognitive development.* Cambridge, MA: MIT Press.

Keil, F. C., Smith, W. C., Simons, D. J., & Levin, D. T. (1998). Two dogmas of conceptual empiricism: Implications for hybrid models of the structure of knowledge. *Cognition, 65*, 103–135.

Kellman, P. J., & Spelke, E. S. (1983). Perception of partly occluded objects in infancy. *Cognitive Psychology, 15*, 483–524.

Koustall, W., & Schacter, D. L. (1997). Gist-based false recognition of pictures in older and younger adults. *Journal of Memory & Language, 37*, 555–583.

Lewkowicz, D. J. (1988a). Sensory dominance in infants: 1. Six-month-old infants' response to auditory-visual compounds. *Developmental Psychology, 24*, 155–171.

Lewkowicz, D. J. (1988b). Sensory dominance in infants: 2. Ten-month-old infants' response to auditory-visual compounds. *Developmental Psychology, 24*, 172–182.

Mandler, J. M. (1997). Development of categorisation: Perceptual and conceptual categories. In G. Bremner, A. Slater & G. Butterworth (Eds.), *Infant development: Recent advances* (pp. 163–189). Hove, England: Psychology Press.

Mandler, J. (2004). *The foundations of mind: Origins of conceptual thought.* New York, NY: Oxford University Press.

Madole, K. L., Oakes, L. M., & Cohen, L. B. (1993). Developmental changes in infants' attention to function and form–function correlations. *Cognitive Development, 8*, 189–209

Markman, E. (1989). *Categorization and naming in children.* Cambridge, MA: MIT Press.

Markman, E. M., and Hutchinson, J. E. (1984). Children's sensitivity to constraints on word meaning: Taxonomic versus thematic relations. *Cognitive Psychology, 16*, 1–27.

Marks, W. (1991). Effects of encoding the perceptual features of pictures on memory. *Journal of Experimental Psychology: Learning, Memory, and Cognition, 17*, 566–577.

Massey, C. M., & Gelman, R. (1988). Preschooler's ability to decide whether a photographed unfamiliar object can move itself. *Developmental Psychology, 24*, 307–317.

Medin, D. (1975). A theory of context in discrimination learning. In G. Bower (Ed.), *The psychology of learning and motivation* (Vol. 9, pp. 263–314). New York: Academic Press.

Napolitano, A. C., & Sloutsky, V. M. (2004). Is a picture worth a thousand words? The flexible nature of modality dominance in young children. *Child Development, 75*, 1850–1870.

Nosofsky, R. M. (1984). Choice, similarity, and the context theory of classification. *Journal of Experimental Psychology: Learning, Memory, & Cognition*, 10, 104–114.

Oakes, L. M., & Madole, K. L. (2003). Principles of developmental changes in infants' category formation. In D. H. Rakison & L. M. Oakes (Eds.), *Early category and concept development: Making sense of the blooming, buzzing confusion* (pp. 132–158). New York: Oxford University Press.

Rakison, D. H. (2003). Parts, motion, and the development of the animate–inanimate distinction in infancy. In Rakison & L. M. Oakes (Eds.), *Early category and concept development: Making sense of the blooming, buzzing confusion* (pp. 159–192). New York, NY: Oxford University Press.

Robinson, C.W., & Sloutsky, V.M. (2004). Auditory dominance and its change in the course of development. *Child Development, 75*, 1387–1401.

Rogers, T. T. and McClelland, J. L. (2004). *Semantic cognition: A parallel distributed processing approach*. Cambridge, MA: MIT Press.

Schafer, G., & Plunkett, K. (1998). Rapid word learning by fifteen-month-olds under tightly controlled conditions. *Child Development, 69*, 309–320.

Sloutsky, V. M. (2003). The role of similarity in the development of categorization. *Trends in Cognitive Sciences, 7*, 246–251.

Sloutsky, V. M. & Fisher, A. V. (2004a). Induction and categorization in young children: A similarity-based model. *Journal of Experimental Psychology: General, 133*, 166–188.

Sloutsky, V. M., & Fisher, A. V. (2004b). When development and learning decrease memory: Evidence against category-based induction in children. *Psychological Science, 15*, 553–558.

Sloutsky, V. M. & Fisher, A. V. (2005). Similarity, Induction, Naming, and Categorization (SINC): Generalization or Inductive Reasoning? Response to Heit and Hayes. *Journal of Experimental Psychology: General, 134*, 606–611.

Sloutsky, V. M., Kloos. H., & Fisher, A. V. (2007). What's beyond looks? Reply to Gelman and Waxman. *Psychological Science, 18*, 556–557.

Sloutsky, V. M., & Napolitano, A.C. (2003). Is a picture worth a thousand words? Preference for auditory modality in young children. *Child Development, 74*, 822–833.

Sloutsky, V. M., & Lo, Y.-F. (1999). How much does a shared name make things similar? Part 1: Linguistic labels and the development of similarity judgment. *Developmental Psychology, 35*, 1478–1492.

Sloutsky, V. M., Lo, Y.-F., & Fisher, A. (2001). How much does a shared name make things similar? Linguistic labels, similarity and the development of inductive inference. *Child Development, 72*, 1695–1709.

Sloutsky, V. M., & Spino, M. A. (2004). Naive theory and transfer of learning: When less is more and more is less. *Psychonomic Bulletin and Review, 11*, 528–535.

Sloutsky, V. M., & Robinson, C. W. (2008). The role of words and sounds in visual processing: From overshadowing to attentional tuning. *Cognitive Science, 32*, 354–377.

Smith, L. B., Jones, S. S., & Landau, B. (1996). Naming in young children: A dumb attentional mechanism? *Cognition, 60*, 143–171.

Smith, L. B., Jones, S. S., Landau, B., Gershkoff-Stowe, L., & Samuelson, L. (2002). Object name learning provides on-the-job training for attention. *Psychological Science, 13*, 13–19.

Soja, N. N., Carey, S., & Spelke, E. S. (1991). Ontological categories guide young children's inductions of word meaning Object terms and substance terms. *Cognition, 38*, 179–211.

Spelke, E. S. (1990). Principles of object perception. *Cognitive Science, 14*, 29–56.

Spelke, E. S. (1994). Initial knowledge: Six suggestions. *Cognition, 50*, 431–445.

Thapar, A., & McDermott, K. B. (2001). False recall and false recognition induced by presentation of associated words: Effects of retention interval and level of processing. *Memory & Cognition, 29*, 424–432.

Werker, J. F., Cohen, L. B., Lloyd, V. L., Casasola, M., & Stager, C. L. (1998). Acquisition of word–object associations by 14-month-old infants. *Developmental Psychology, 34*, 1289–1309.

Waxman, S. R., & Booth, A. E. (2003). The origins and evolution of links between word learning and conceptual organization: New evidence from 11-month-olds. *Developmental Science, 6*, 130–137.

Waxman, S. R., & Markow, D. B. (1995). Words as invitations to form categories: Evidence from 12- to 13-month-old infants. *Cognitive Psychology, 29*, 557–302.

Welder, A.N., & Graham, S.A. (2001). The influences of shape similarity and shared labels on infants' inductive inferences about nonobvious object properties. *Child Development, 72*, 1653–1673.

Wellman, H. M., & Gelman, S. A. (1992). Cognitive development: Foundational theories of core domains. *Annual Review of Psychology, 43*, 337–375.

Wexler, K., & Culicover, P. W. (1980). *Formal principles of language acquisition*. Cambridge MA: MIT Press.

Woodward, A. L., & Markman, E. M. (1998). Early word learning. In W. Damon, D. Kuhn & R. Siegler (Eds.), *Handbook of child psychology, Volume 2: Cognition, perception and language* (pp. 371–420). New York: John Wiley and Sons.

Xu, F. (2002). The role of language in acquiring object kind concepts in infancy. *Cognition, 85*, 223–250.

Xu, F., & Tenenbaum, J. B. (2007). Word learning as Bayesian inference. *Psychological Review, 114*, 245–272.

Yoshida, H., & Smith, L. B. (2005) Linguistic cues enhance the learning of perceptual cues. *Psychological Science, 16*, 90–95.

PART V

Foundations of Social Cognition

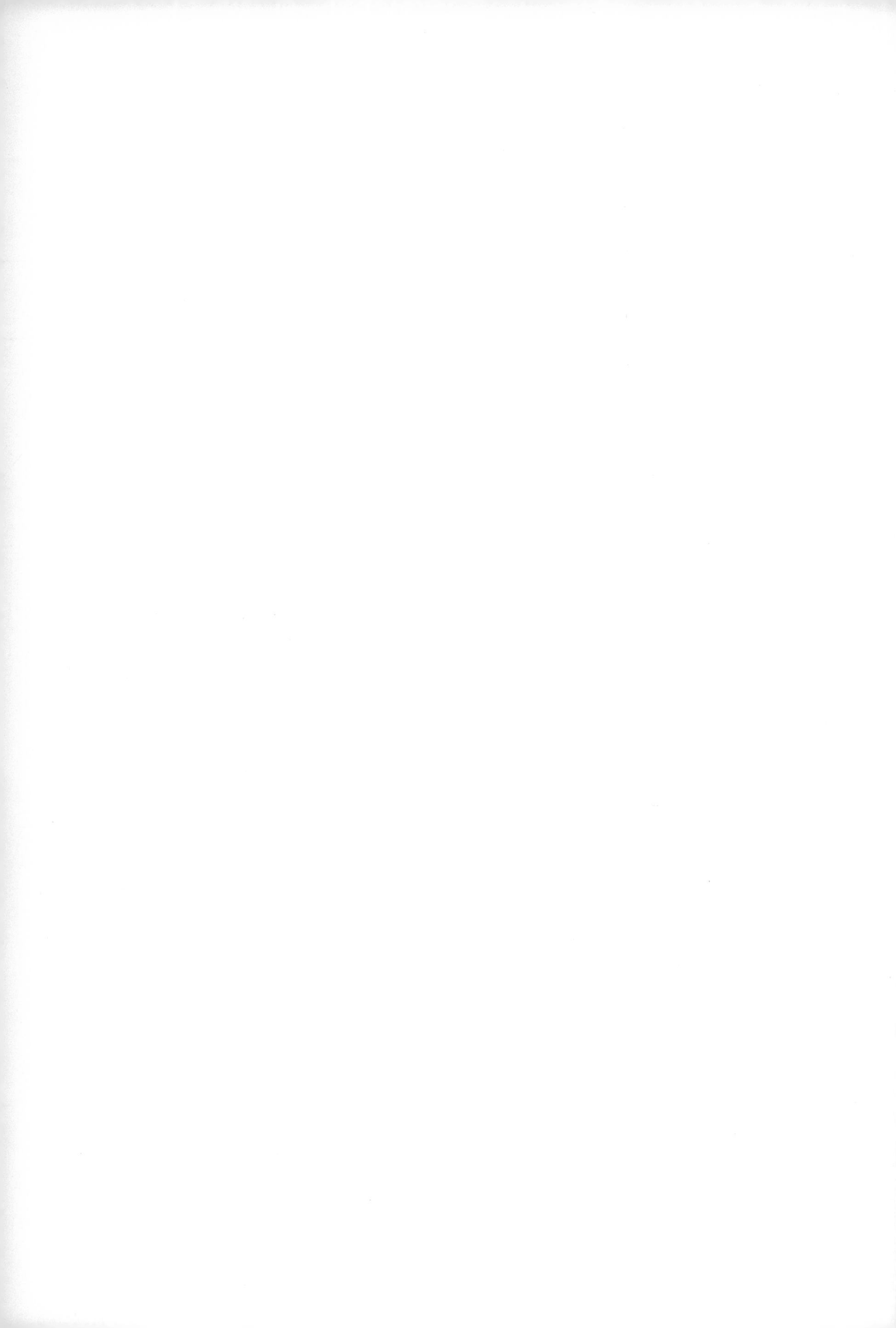

CHAPTER 15
Building Intentional Action Knowledge with One's Hands

Sarah Gerson and Amanda Woodward

Understanding others' actions as intentional is fundamental to everyday social life. Adults view even the simplest and most concrete actions not as sheer movements, but rather as actions organized by intentions. To illustrate, observing a group of children and a ball traversing a soccer field, we perceive the motions of the former, but not the latter, as structured with respect to a goal, in this case the goal of driving the ball across the field to score. This foundational aspect of social perception is a critical ingredient in social, cognitive, and linguistic development. In the first years of life, children acquire a great deal of knowledge from other people. By 12 to 18 months of age, if not earlier, this learning is mediated by an analysis of others' intentions (Baldwin & Moses, 2001; Meltzoff, 1995; Tomasello, 1999). Deficiencies in this ability have devastating developmental effects, as seen in individuals with autism. In this chapter, we will consider the potential origins of the ability to discern others' intentions in acting.

Recent findings have shown that by the middle of the first year, infants represent certain actions in terms of their intentional structure (Gergely & Csibra, 2003; Kuhlmeier, Wynn, & Bloom, 2003; Luo & Baillargeon, 2007; Woodward, 1998; Woodward & Guajardo, 2002). For example, in a series of studies from our laboratory (Guajardo & Woodward, 2004; Woodward, 1998, 1999, 2003), infants 6 months of age and older viewed events in which a person reached toward and grasped one of two toys. The question of interest was whether infants, like adults, would represent this event as goal-directed, that is, in terms of the relation between the agent and her goal. Following habituation, the positions of the two toys were switched. Then the experimenter reached for either a new toy in the same place (new-object trials) or the same toy in a new place (new-side trials). Infants looked longer to the new-object trials than the new-side trials, indicating that they represented the event in terms of the relation between agent and goal, rather than strictly in terms of physical properties such as the movement and position of the actor's arm.

Critically, several subsequent findings confirmed that infants' responses in this paradigm indicate more than an association between the hand and the object it grasps. Rather, infants encoded the reaching events in terms of the relational structure of the action. This conclusion is supported by the outcomes of comparison events in which one object moves toward another, but, unlike the hand, the moving object is not readily construed as an agent. For example, in one control condition, infants saw a mechanical claw move toward and grasp a toy (Woodward, 1998). If infants only encoded the association between two "objects" (the hand and toy or the claw and toy), their responses in these two situations would be equivalent. However, infants in the mechanical claw condition looked equally long at the new-object and new-side test events.

Additional evidence that infants attend to relations between agents and goals comes from recent work by Luo and Baillargeon (2007): 12-month-old infants did not show selective attention to goal change events if the agent could only see one of two objects during habituation (the other object was visible to the infant but hidden from the experimenter's view). In this paradigm, the association between the hand and the goal-object was identical to Woodward's (1998) paradigm but the actor's knowledge of the potential goals differed. Therefore, it can be concluded that infants considered the agent's intentional relations to the objects, rather than simply the association of the hand with the object it grasped. These findings also indicate that infants understand that an agent's goals are limited by perception.

Infants' sensitivity to the goal structure of others' actions is also evident in other paradigms, including those that assess imitative responses (Hamlin, Hallinan, & Woodward, in press; Meltzoff, 1995) and other overt spontaneous social behaviors in experimental contexts (Behne, Carpenter, Call, & Tomasello, 2005). For example, like older infants and children, 7-month-old infants selectively reproduce the goals of observed actions, thereby revealing, with their hands, the same goal analysis that has been shown in looking time studies (Hamlin et al., in press; Mahajan & Woodward, 2007).

Toward the end of the first year of life, infants become increasingly able to discern the goal structure of more complex actions. By 9 to 12 months, for example, infants represent others' gaze as indicating relations between the looker and the object at which her eyes are pointed. Evidence for this ability comes from looking time studies (Johnson, Ok, & Luo, 2007; Phillips, Wellman, & Spelke, 2002; Sodian & Thoermer, 2004; Woodward, 2003) and studies assessing infants' overt social responses (Moll & Tomasello, 2004; Tomasello & Haberl, 2003). Further, by this same age, infants represent goals that span individual actions. For example, they can represent the relation between actions on a tool or intermediary and the attainment of an ultimate goal (Gergely & Csibra, 2003; Sommerville, Hildebrand, & Crane, in press; Sommerville & Woodward, 2005; Woodward & Sommerville, 2000).

Origins of Intentional Understanding

While this evidence makes clear that the ability to recover intentional structure from observed actions exists early in life, the ontogenetic origins of this ability are still in question. How do the beginnings of these understandings appear? How do changes in understanding come about? As is the case in other domains of infant cognition, current positions on these questions range from the strongly nativist (e.g., Biro & Leslie, 2006; Gergely & Csibra, 2003; Kiraly, Jovanovic, Prinz, Aschersleben, & Gergely, 2003) to strongly emphasizing the role of experience (e.g., Meltzoff, 1995; Tomasello, 1999; Woodward, 2005). At this point, there is little direct evidence available to distinguish among these views because most studies have not investigated developmental change and its possible causes. Instead, studies have typically taken a "snapshots" approach, seeking evidence for focal abilities at a particular point in time but not considering how these abilities may change as a function of other events in development.

In this chapter, we will attempt to begin to fill this void by considering a category of experience that has long been hypothesized to contribute to intentional understanding, namely first-person agentive experience. The idea that action production and action understanding are linked in development has been around for over a century (Baldwin, 1897; Piaget, 1953). A number of current proposals have at their core the idea that one's own actions provide unique insight into the structure of others' actions (Barresi & Moore, 1996; Meltzoff, 1995; Tomasello, 1999).

Theoretically, it seems reasonable that one's own experience as an agent could provide useful information for understanding other agents. A true test of this general hypothesis requires (1) measuring infants' analysis of observed action structure and (2) relating this measure to variations in infants' own actions. We turn first to recent studies that have done just this, and in so doing provided initial evidence that this general proposal is on the right track. We will then turn to the much harder question of *why* self-produced experience might have an effect on the development of action understanding. This question will lead us to consider recent work on mirror systems, the limits of mirror systems, and the role of analogy in conceptual development.

Evidence for Links Between Action Production and Action Understanding

As researchers began to document infants' emerging sensitivity to the goal structure of action, a coincidence became apparent. Infants and children are generally able to produce particular actions around the same age at which they are also able to understand these actions in others. Around 4 to 5 months of age, infants begin to make intentional grasps themselves (Bertenthal & Clifton, 1998; Rochat, 1989) and also begin to understand grasp as goal-directed (Woodward, 1998). Around 9 to 12 months of age, infants begin to engage in shared attention and triadic interactions (Adamson & McArthur, 1995; Carpenter, Nagell, & Tomasello, 1998) and also begin to understand gaze and pointing as implying a relation between the agent and the target of her attention (Brune & Woodward, 2007; Woodward, 2003; Woodward & Guajardo, 2002). Also, as infants are first able to produce goal-directed action sequences (around 9 to 12 months of age; Bates, Carlson-Luden, & Bretherton, 1980; Piaget, 1953), they begin to understand the ultimate goal of a means–end sequence that another person performs (Sommerville & Woodward, 2005; Woodward & Sommerville, 2000).

Two approaches have been taken to follow up on these coincidences to determine whether, in fact, they reflect developmental relations between acting and understanding actions. The first is to assess, within the same infants, correlations between action production and action perception. The second is to intervene to change infants' self-produced experience and then assess the effects of this intervention on infants' action perception.

Correlational Evidence

During times of developmental change, a great deal of individual variation can be seen in children at a given age, and therefore, links between motor capabilities and understanding of these actions can be examined keeping age constant. For example, between 10 and 12 months of age, a great deal of variability exists in infants' ability to produce planful actions such as pulling a cloth to get a toy. There is also individual variation in the ability to understand goal structure in these kinds of means–end sequences. In a paradigm assessing the understanding of these means–end actions, Sommerville and Woodward (2005) habituated infants to sequences in which an actor pulled a cloth in order to get a toy on its far edge. The question was whether infants represented the actor's action on the cloth as directed at the ultimate goal (the toy) or at the cloth itself. To address this question, after habituation, infants were shown test events in which the toys' positions were reversed and the actor only produced the first action in the sequence, grasping a cloth. Thus, infants viewed new-cloth trials, on which the actor grasped the other cloth, which now supported the previous goal toy, or new-toy trials, on which the actor grasped the same cloth as before, which now held a different toy. Twelve-month-olds looked longer on new-toy trials than new-cloth trials, showing that they represented the action on the cloth as directed at the toy. Ten-month-olds, in contrast, were variable in their responses, showing no reliable group preference. At this age, there was a correlation between infants' own cloth-pulling abilities and their looking time responses (see Figure 15.1). Infants who were well organized in their own ability to pull a cloth to get a toy looked longer on new-toy trials, whereas infants who were unable to produce an organized and planful cloth-pulling action looked longer on new-cloth trials. Importantly, this finding demonstrated that infants who were unable to perform this means–end action were not completely disorganized concerning their understanding of the intention behind this action when observing another. Instead, these infants understood this

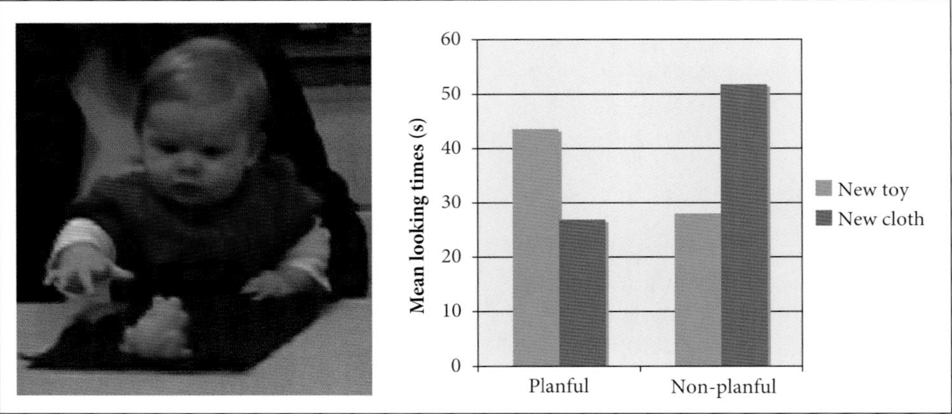

Figure 15.1 Infants who were able to produce planful cloth-pulling actions themselves were sensitive to the means–end structure of an observed sequence of actions. From Sommerville and Woodward (2005).

action on a simpler level, wherein the end-goal of the action was the cloth, as if it were a simple grasp.

Other studies have found additional correlations between infants' own abilities to act and their responses to others' actions. For example, between 9 and 12 months of age, a great deal of individual variation exists in infants' production of point and engagement in shared attention; there is also individual variation in the ability to understand point and gaze. Woodward and Guajardo (2002) found a relation between infants' ability to produce object-directed points and their understanding of point in a habituation paradigm. In addition, a study by Brune and Woodward (2007) supported the correlation between production and understanding of pointing and also found a correlation between infants' engagement in shared attention and understanding of gaze as object-directed at 10 months of age.

This correlational evidence is important in that it demonstrates a specific link between production and understanding of particular actions. In addition, these results demonstrate that data from looking time studies is clearly related to developments in infants' overt actions. Most importantly for the current arguments, this evidence provides an initial view of the link between action production and action understanding and how this link may lead to developmental change. It demonstrates that the developmental concordance in time reviewed above is more than mere coincidence. Importantly, however, correlational evidence does not shed light on the causal contributors to this relation. Next, we will discuss evidence that goes beyond correlations in an attempt to examine causality.

Intervention Evidence

In intervention studies, infants at the cusp of performing a particular skill are trained or supported in a new self-produced action and then the effect of the training on their understanding of that action is assessed. This approach provides clearer evidence about the effects of acting on action understanding. For example, 3-month-olds are generally not yet skilled in producing goal-directed grasps and they do not typically understand the relation between another's grasp and his or her goal. In a study by Sommerville, Woodward, and Needham (2005), infants received training in which they were able to manipulate the movement of toys using Velcro mittens. Infants' object-directed touching (as indicated by simultaneous looking and touching of the toys) increased with the use of the mittens. After training, infants responded to observed mittened reaching actions as goal-

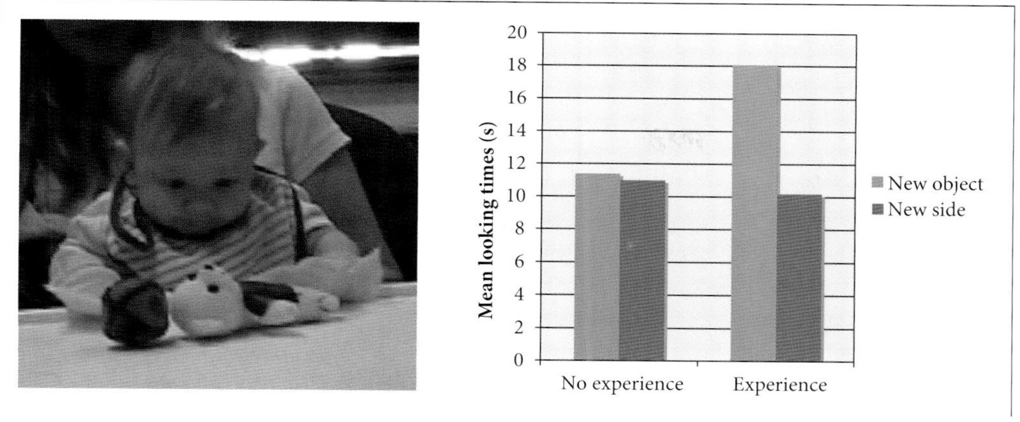

Figure 15.2 Infants given experience producing object-directed actions with Velcro mittens were sensitive to the goal structure of an observed mittened reach. From Sommerville et al. (2005).

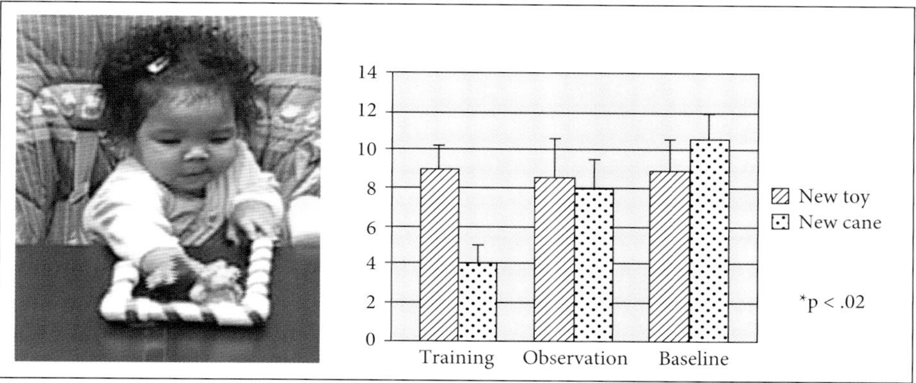

Figure 15.3 Infants given training producing cane-pulling actions were sensitive to the means–end structure of an observed sequence of actions. From Sommerville et al. (in press).

directed in the habituation paradigm described earlier (see Figure 15.2). That is, infants who had undergone training showed a strong novelty response on new-object trials but not on new-side trials. In contrast, infants who had not undergone training looked equally on the two kinds of test trials. Moreover, in the training group, there was a strong correlation between the extent to which infants had engaged in object-directed actions with the mittens and the degree of their novelty response on new-object trials. Thus, engaging in object-directed action seemed to drive infants' subsequent responses to observed reaching events. These results support the conclusion that infants' own actions provide structure for the perception of others' actions.

Similar intervention effects have also been found with means–ends actions such as cane-pulling (Sommerville et al., in press). In this study, 10-month-old infants trained to use a cane to reach for a toy were able to understand the ultimate goal of a cane-pulling sequence in a habituation paradigm (they looked longer to a reach for the old cane to get a new toy than a reach for a new cane to get the old toy; see Figure 15.3). Moreover, as in Sommerville et al.'s (2005) study, infants' success in cane-pulling during training was correlated with their response to the habituation events. Infants who were more successful at cane-pulling during training showed stronger attention to the goal structure of the habituation events. Critically, first-person experience had unique effects on infants' analysis of the observed actions. Infants who received observational, rather than active, training recovered attention to both test events, indicating that they detected the changes in the test events, but did not respond differentially to the new-toy versus the new-cane events.

Work by Meltzoff and Brooks provides further evidence that self-produced experience can inform infants' analysis of others' actions. In a previous study, Brooks and Meltzoff (2002) used infants' propensity to follow gaze as a measure of their understanding of attentional relations. They found that, 14 and 18, but not 12-month-old, infants understood that an adult wearing a blindfold was not attending to an object in the direction of her head turn. Specifically, 14- and 18-month-old infants were less likely to follow the direction of the adults' gaze when the adult was wearing a blindfold, but 12-month-olds continued to follow the adults' "gaze" under these conditions. However, in an intervention study (Meltzoff & Brooks, in press), after 12-month-old infants were given experience wearing a blindfold, they inhibited the tendency to follow gaze when the adult was wearing the blindfold. Thus, self-produced experience with the blindfold seemed to give them insight into the perceptual experience of others in the same situation.

These three examples demonstrating the effects of intervention suggest that being an agent provides infants with information about others' actions. There are a number of issues that require further investigation. For one, the relative impacts of self-produced and matched observational experience require further study. Sommerville et al. (in press) findings indicate that self-produced experience has unique effects on infants' action perception, but whether this is always the case is not yet known. Even so, evidence from these studies is strongly suggestive of a causal link between action production and understanding. Ongoing work in our laboratory seeks to replicate and extend these findings.

Theoretical Links Between Action Production and Action Understanding

Natural concordance in time, correlational data, and intervention data all support the conclusion that a link exists between action production and understanding. But why? One possibility is that by acting, infants produce for themselves examples for observational analysis. There is evidence that infants analyze the structure of observed actions in several ways that could support the extraction of goal information. First, infants attend to the outcomes of actions, and, in some cases, use these to infer the function, and perhaps goal, behind the action. For example, in a study by Hauf, Elsner, and Aschersleben (2004), 12- and 18-month-old infants were more likely to imitate an action that produced a sound than an action that did not produce any effect. Further, in some cases, action effects (such as moving an object to a new location) may help infants to interpret the goals of ambiguous actions (Biro & Leslie, 2006; Kiraly et al., 2003; but see Heineman-Pieper & Woodward, 2003).

In addition, infants are sensitive to statistical regularities in temporally extended events (Kirkham, Slemmer, & Johnson, 2003; Saffran, Aslin & Newport, 1996; see also Gomez, Kirkham, and Saffran chapters in this volume), and may therefore be able to extract recurring patterns in actions. Baldwin, Baird, Saylor, & Clark (2001) found that 10- and 11-month-old infants were sensitive to units in naturalistic action that corresponded to those defined by goal completions to adult observers. This finding may, in part, reflect infants' statistical analysis of action elements that typically co-occur as units (Baird & Baldwin, 2001).

Clearly, self-produced actions would provide data for these kinds of statistical learning mechanisms to exploit. However, here we explore the further possibility that self-produced actions also provide unique information for the perception of goal-directed action. In support of this possibility, consider what infants seem not to learn by watching alone. Infants are constant witnesses to goal-directed actions like grasping, looking, and tool use, but knowledge about the goal structure of these actions is not evident from the start. Rather, as described earlier, infants' sensitivity to the goal structure of these actions emerges, at different points, during the first year of life.

Self-Produced Actions as Unique Sources of Information

Unlike observed actions, which can only provide information "at the surface" (e.g., the sequelae of actions), the regular patterns in self-produced actions could also provide unique information about the underlying goal structure of action. Agency requires representing the goals of one's actions at some level. To coordinate complex actions in service of a goal, or to acquire a new goal-directed skill, like reaching by gradually gaining control over the relevant effectors, individuals must continue to represent the goals that structure their actions and adjust their actions as needed to attain the goal. This information could potentially be recruited to then interpret the perceived actions of others.

This general idea has been broadly proposed in the developmental literature (Barresi & Moore, 1996; Meltzoff, 2005; Sommerville & Woodward, in press; Tomasello, 1999). Accounts differ, however, on two important dimensions: the nature of the information carried from self to other and the means by which information about the self is related to the actions of another person. On the first dimension, some have proposed that infants or young children derive mental state information from first-person experience, which they then use to infer similar states in others (e.g. Meltzoff, 2005). In contrast, it is possible that the information available to infants from first-person experience is in terms of action level descriptions, rather than mental states. On the second dimension, some have hypothesized that children extend information from self to others via a process of analogical mapping (e.g., Barresi & Moore, 1996). In contrast, others have suggested a direct link between self and other, in the form of shared representations for one's own and others' actions (Hauf, Aschersleben, & Prinz, 2007; Meltzoff, 2005; Sommerville et al., 2005). Although current evidence suggests that there is some truth to the general proposal that self-produced actions provide unique information for perceiving others' actions, it does not indicate which of these more specific accounts is correct. Indeed, more than one of them could provide an accurate depiction of different aspects of action knowledge development.

In one current proposal, Meltzoff (2005) proposes a developmental framework, nicknamed the "like me" account, in which information about self and other is directly connected because both are instantiated in a common supramodal representation and grounded in a common body schema. This direct connection provides infants with a means for apprehending the inner states that correlate with others' observed actions, and it also supports imitation. By imitating an observed action, Meltzoff proposes, infants gain information, via their own experience, about the inner states of the other person. Meltzoff further proposes that infants do not begin with full-fledged conceptions of mental states like intention or perception, but rather they construct these concepts in the course of back and forth information sharing about their own and others' actions. In this way, action understanding is direct and linked with internal states from the onset and infants' understanding of their own and others' mental lives becomes more abstract with development.

A somewhat different view has been elaborated by Barresi and Moore (1996). In this account, as in Meltzoff's, information derived from first-person experience is critical for understanding the mental lives of others. Their perspective, however, views the connection between self and other as indirect and emerging through analogical mapping. According to their perspective, triadic interactions, in which individuals jointly attend to an object or event, are a key element in understanding the relation between self and others. Through joint engagement with an adult, the infant can directly align the actions of himself or herself with the actions of another individual. This physical alignment of actions provides the basis for the building of an intentional schema through analogy.

Below, we propose an alternative account, similar in some respects to each of these perspectives, but also differing in several respects. Our proposal is informed by recent findings concerning the mirror system and recent debates concerning the nature of information this system provides the perceiver. To foreshadow, we propose that direct and indirect, mental and action-level information sharing occur at different points during development. Initially, the information provided by self-produced actions provides a direct, action-level description of goal-directedness. This beginning point sets up the conditions for subsequent analogical mappings, which lead to more abstract levels of analysis. Before elaborating our proposal, we first review relevant research on the mirror system.

Role of mirror representations in action perception

Findings from the past decade provide evidence for a direct link between neurocognitive systems that subserve action production and action perception. The first evidence for this link came from primate research that identified neurons in motor regions that discharge both during the performance and the observation of goal-directed actions (Rizzolatti & Arbib, 1998; Rizzolatti & Fadiga, 1998). Subsequent research in humans has similarly indicated shared neural (Buccino et al, 2001; Grafton, Arbib, Fadiga, & Rizzolatti, 1996; Grezes & Decety, 2001; Iacoboni et al., 1999) and cognitive (Hommel, Musseler, Aschersleben, & Prinz, 2001) representations for perceiving and producing actions. Evidence in humans does not isolate individual neurons. Instead, researchers ask whether common brain regions support the production and perception of action. Our focus is not on the exact nature of the neural representations, but rather the functions that mirror representations may support in development. Specifically, three important functional characteristics of mirror representations have been revealed across a number of studies: (1) they provide a direct link between action and perception, (2) they are selectively sensitive to goal-directed action, and (3) they are shaped by motor experience. Below, we will review evidence for each of these features. We will then discuss the status of infancy research in this area.

Rizzolatti and colleagues (Rizzolatti & Arbib, 1998; Rizzolatti & Fadiga, 1998) found that neurons fire during both performance and observation of actions in monkeys, thus providing neural evidence for the link between action production and perception. In research with humans, transcranial magnetic stimulation (TMS) studies have found a selective increase in motor-evoked potentials during observation of actions that are specific to those muscles used in the action (Fadiga, Fogassi, Pavesi, & Rizzolatti, 1995; Gangitano, Mottaghy, & Pascual-Leone, 2001). In addition, evidence of corresponding areas of activation in the premotor cortex during action observation and execution has been found in functional magnetic resonance imaging (MRI) and positron emission tomography (PET) studies (Buccino et al, 2001; Grafton et al., 1996; Grezes & Decety, 2001; Iacoboni et al., 1999). More recently, electroencephalography (EEG) studies have found a suppression of mu rhythm in both the production and the observation of actions (Altschuler, Vankov, Wang, Ramachandran, & Pineda, 1997; Cochin, Barthelemy, Roux, & Martineau, 1999). The mu rhythm is evident over motor areas, and is suppressed by movement, intended movement, or observation of movement (Muthukumaraswamy, Johnson, & McNair, 2004; Pineda, Allison, & Vankov, 2000). Together, these diverse findings point to the existence of shared neural representations for the production and perception of action.

Rizzolatti, Fogassi, & Gallese (2001) also found that mirror neurons in monkeys only discharged to an agent grasping an object, not to either the agent or object alone, suggesting that these neurons are selectively responsive to goal-directed actions (Gallese, Fadiga, Fogassi, & Rizzolatti, 1996). Similar findings have been obtained in humans. For example, Muthukumaraswamy and colleagues (2004) found mu rhythm suppression occurred when adults viewed a grasping action of an object but not when this same action was produced without an object present. In humans, mirror representations seem to be sensitive to goals at more abstract levels as well, responding to events beyond the simple attainment of objects to include such actions as a dance movement or the use of chopsticks (Calvo-Merino, Glaser, Grezes, Passingham, & Haggard, 2005; Calvo-Merino, Grezes, Glaser, Passingham, & Haggard, 2006; Järveläinen, Schürmann, & Hari, 2004).

Work by Calvo-Merino and colleagues (2005, 2006) highlights the expertise-driven nature of mirror representations. In one study, male dancers showed motor activation during the observation of dance movements they regularly produced but not during observation of movements regularly performed by female dancers, with which the males were extremely familiar but had no firsthand experience producing. Additionally, simple effects of gender were accounted for in that males watching females perform an action common to both genders did show activation of the mirror system. These findings demonstrate that action experience can lead to activation of the system and that mirror system activity is dependent on possessing a motor representation for an action rather than simply having visual knowledge of the action. Additional evidence that action experience influences the mirror system is provided by Catmur, Walsh, & Heyes (2007). In this study, training in producing an action opposite to the one being observed reversed mirror effects, demonstrating that the mirror system is reliant on sensorimotor learning.

Mirror Systems in Infancy

Due to limitations in techniques for brain imaging with infants, the majority of work concerning the mirror system in humans has been done with adults. Currently, brain-based evidence of mirror systems in infants is extremely limited, but behavioral studies have provided indirect support for the idea that the mirror system may be functioning in human infants (see Lepage & Theoret, 2007). For example, neonatal imitation, in which newborn infants are able to imitate tongue protrusions without the ability to see the action they make themselves suggests a correspondence between representations of self and other in infancy (Meltzoff & Moore, 1989). In addition, the evidence from looking time studies with older infants that is discussed above, in which infants' understanding of goal-directed actions is correlated with their actions, is consistent with the notion that mirror system activity exists in infancy.

A study by Falck-Ytter, Gredeback, and von Hofsten (2006) provides additional indirect support for the existence of mirror representations in infancy. Previous research has shown that adults produce systematic, proactive eye movements during the production of goal-directed actions. That is, adults make predictive eye movements in order to control and coordinate their actions. The same kind of predictive eye movements are made when an adult is watching others produce similar goal-directed actions (Flanagan & Johansson, 2003). This finding is consistent with the possibility that a common system drives both attention to one's own actions and attention to others' actions. Following on this finding, Falck-Ytter and colleagues asked whether infants anticipate the goals of observed actions. They showed infants sequences in which a person placed each of a set of balls into a container. Like adults, 12-month-old infants anticipated the goal of this sequence, looking to the bucket reliably before the ball's arrival. In contrast, infants who viewed the same ball movements, this time without a human mover, followed the balls, but did not anticipate their arrival at the bucket. Based on these results, these researchers speculate that the mirror system is active in infancy and drives infants' predictive attention to observed actions.

A recent study provides the only brain-based evidence for the presence of a mirror system in human infants. Shimada and Hiraki (2006) conducted a study that examined brain activity during action observation in 7- and 8-month-old infants. In this study, the sensorimotor area was identified during a motor task in which adult participants were prompted to engage in repetitive hand movements and infant participants engaged in structured free-play. Then, the activity of motor areas was measured using near-infrared spectroscopy during action observation (in one condition, infants watched an experimenter manipulate a toy) in both adults and infants. The sensorimotor area was selectively activated during live action observation in both adults and infants. This area was not activated when observing a live object-motion condition in which the object moved on its own. Additionally, coding of the infants' arm movements during free-play indicated that the observed motion was part of the motor repertoire of most infants, supporting the claim that the mirror system is sensitive to motions within an individual's motor repertoire, even in infancy.

Mirror representations: mental state or action level descriptions?

Mirror representations provide a direct path between actions of self and others that may be in place from infancy. They respond selectively to goal-directed actions and are shaped by agentive experience. A critical open question, however, is the extent to which mirror representations make contact with mental state concepts. Debates in the literature on the functions of mature mirror systems have highlighted this issue.

Some theorists have taken up the mirror system findings as evidence in favor of simulation theory. The simulationist account posits that individuals can gain an understanding of others' mental states by mentally simulating those actions themselves (Goldman, 1989; Gordon, 1986; Harris, 1989; Heal, 1998). This theory proposes a direct link between first-person mental states and the comprehension of others' mental states. In this way, individuals can "mirror" the actions of another and come to understand another's actions based on their own past experience (without analyzing or building a theory). To illustrate, Gallese and Goldman (1998) proposed that mirror systems allow an individual to detect mental states in others because mirroring creates a match between mental activity of the observer and the actor, and, thus, the observer is able to use his or her own mental processes to understand and predict the mental goals of others. Blakemore and Decety (2001) also proposed that mental states can be inferred directly from biological motion through a process of simulation.

Other researchers have countered this view with the argument that the mirror system may be useful in determining motor intentions but that it is not sufficient for understanding prior intentions and mental states more generally. Representing prior intentions entails an understanding of intentions as mental states that exist independent of the particular actions used to achieve the intended goal. Motor intentions, in contrast, are specified at the level of the goal at which a particular action is directed. Jacob and Jeannerod (2005) argue that perceiving an action will lead to an understanding of motor intention but cannot lead to the understanding of an agent's prior intention. They state, for example, that infants' understanding of a basic grasp in a habituation paradigm may be due to motor simulation, but that this simulation is only possible for basic actions and intentions. Prior intentions, however, wherein the goal is not inherent in the action itself (i.e., opening a drawer in order to retrieve a pen from inside), cannot be represented by mirror systems alone.

In its strongest form, the claim that the mirror system can only be used on the most basic level has been disputed by subsequent evidence that mirror neurons in primates and mirror systems in humans can represent not only the goals of simple actions, but also overarching goals that structure action sequences (Fogassi et al., 2005; Iacoboni et al., 2005). For example, Fogassi and colleagues (2005) found mirror neurons in macaque monkeys that fired differentially to grasping actions that preceded eating versus placing of the grasped object when there were contextual cues to support one of these two analyses of the grasp. Thus, these neurons reflected processing, not of the basic action itself (grasping), but rather the ultimate goal at which the grasp was apparently directed (eating versus placing). Further, Ferrari, Rozzi, and Fogassi (2005) report the existence of "grasping" mirror neurons that fired for grasping done by varied effectors (e.g., the hand, the mouth or even a tool), thus indicating that mirror systems can reflect goal representations that are relatively abstract, at the level of action plans.

Even so, mirror representations alone seem unlikely to account for the full range of mental state knowledge humans eventually acquire. To illustrate, Saxe (2005) argues that if belief attribution derived from direct simulation, then the pervasive belief attribution errors seen in children (and even in adults) would be difficult to explain. Rather, these errors indicate that people's judgments about others' epistemic states are the product of an interpretive system (theory of mind) that can, in some cases, generate incorrect analyses.

This debate concerning more mature mirror systems sheds light on the probable limitations of developing mirror systems in infants. Mirror systems, on their own, seem unlikely to directly yield higher order mental state descriptions. At the very least, however, they would provide action level or even plan level descriptions of actions as structured in relation to a goal. Descriptions at this level, whether or not they make contact with mental state concepts, could account for many of the infant findings reviewed in this chapter. For example, when an infant responds selectively to the change in the goal of a grasp in a habituation paradigm, this response, at a minimum, reflects an understanding of the relational goal structure of grasping actions (see also Gergely & Csibra, 2003). It may also reflect the attribution of a mental state, such as wanting the object or liking the object, but as of yet there is not strong evidence for this in infants under 12 months of age (see Biro & Leslie, 2006; Gergely & Csibra, 2003; Onishi & Baillargeon, 2005; and Woodward, 2005 for different perspectives on this issue).

Thus, we assume at this point that, at a minimum, infants in the first year have action level and plan level representations of goal-directed action, leaving open the possibility that they may also represent information about the inner states that drive action. In addition to accounting for the data from younger infants, the structural level of description could provide an initial representational kernel for the subsequent development of intentional action knowledge. We turn next to this possibility.

Relational Action Representations and Structure Mapping: A Proposal

We propose that early in the first year, as infants begin to organize their own actions with respect to external goal objects, they acquire relational action representations that enable the perception of others' actions as structured by goals. Thus, as infants acquire new ways of acting (i.e., reaching, using a tool to acquire an object, pointing), they also attain new action level representations of each of these actions. These representations may reflect the activity of a mirror system that, as reviewed above, reflects representations accessible to both action production and action perception, is tuned to actions that are goal-directed, and is shaped by motor experience. This proposal is motivated by the findings, reviewed above, that (1) young infants encode others' actions as goal-directed and they express this action analysis in their overt actions as well as their looking time responses; (2) infants' goal encoding is correlated with developments in their own actions; (3) interventions that shape infants' own actions also affect their responses to others' actions; and (4) initial evidence suggesting that self-produced actions exert unique, or especially potent, effects on infants' action perception.

On our proposal, the action representations infants initially glean from agentive experience may be limited in two ways: They may be specific to particular actions and they may describe action in structural rather than rich mentalistic terms. Despite these limitations, they reflect a critical aspect of action structure, namely, that actions are structured by the relation between the agent and his or her goal. We propose that this relational core provides a basis for generalizing initial knowledge so as to create broader classes of goal-directed actions and to move toward more abstract representations of goals.

The literature on conceptual generalization in older children and adults provides a model of how this process could occur in infancy. In particular, Gentner and her colleagues have described a general cognitive mechanism that can extract increasingly abstract levels of relational similarity across instances (Gentner,

1988; Gentner & Medina, 1998). Because it yields abstract relational representations, this structure mapping engine (SME) seems especially well suited to the case of goal-directed action. The structure mapping engine is essentially an analogy maker. Instances are aligned based on similar features and this alignment promotes attention to other shared dimensions. Alignment and comparison supports the detection of abstract, relational similarities that may not be initially obvious to the observer.

To illustrate, in one set of studies, Loewenstein and Gentner (2001) showed 3-year-old children a toy bone hidden in relation to an object in a model room (e.g., under the bed). Then, children were shown another model room that had different-looking exemplars of each piece of furniture, similarly arranged to the first room. They were told there was a bone in the same place in this room. Children were generally unsuccessful in finding the second bone, suggesting they found it difficult to apply the relational information (the bone is under the bed) to the new, dissimilar room. To facilitate children's ability to see the common relational structure between the two rooms, Loewenstein and Gentner showed a second group of children two nearly identical model rooms with bones hidden in the same location. Then, children saw the dissimilar test room and were asked to find the bone hidden in the "same place." In this condition, children generally succeeded in finding the bone. Thus, alignment of perceptually similar instances supported children's ability to extract the common relational structure among even dissimilar instances. These effects were strongest when children could directly compare the first two models at the same time. However, even comparison across sequentially presented models helped.

Further, alignment of perceptually similar instances also supports children's extraction of higher-order relations. For example, Loewenstein and Gentner (2001) found that the opportunity to compare similar rooms also facilitated the extraction of embedded relational similarities. Specifically, on some trials, the bone was hidden under one of two identical chairs. To find the hidden bone, children had to represent not only the relation between the bone and the hiding place (i.e., *under the chair*) but also the relation between the chair and other objects in the room (i.e., *under the chair that is next to the bed*). The older children in the study were able to use comparisons of this embedded relational structure to find the hidden bone. Furthermore, Kotovsky and Gentner (1996) found that aligning items based on relatively concrete relations facilitated 4-year-old children's subsequent ability to discern higher-order relational structure. For example, if children were trained with perceptually similar examples of the relation small-big-small, they were then better able to detect the higher-order relational similarity between small-big-small patterns and A-B-A patterns in other dimensions (e.g., dark-light-dark). These examples show that beginning with relatively concrete comparisons can support the extraction of higher-order relational structure.

If infants, like older children, engage in structure mapping, then this mechanism could explain how initial, self-generated action representations become more general and abstract. For one, it would provide a mechanism for moving beyond particular actions, e.g., grasping with the hand, to categories of actions that subsume a broader range of instances, e.g. obtaining objects with varied hand postures or other affectors. As in Loewenstein and Gentner's (2001) studies, infants may begin by detecting relational similarities among similar-looking actions (e.g., grasping with the hands), and by so doing become more sensitive to the relational similarity among more disparate actions.

Recent findings show that infants sometimes detect goal relations for events in which objects are moved or obtained by unusual hand postures or inanimate agents (Biro & Leslie, 2006; Hauf et al., 2004; Kiraly et al., 2003). These results are generally taken as evidence that infants possess abstract concepts of intention that arise independent of experience (see Biro & Leslie, 2006; Kiraly et al., 2003). However, many of these findings would also be expected if infants generalized familiar action representations via structure mapping. Specifically, these extensions seem to occur most readily when (1) infants have a well-established relational action representation and (2) the situation promotes alignment between the infants' action representation and the novel event. First, the propensity to view unusual events as goal-directed is more often seen in older than younger infants, and those experiments that include infants at multiple ages find age differences (Biro & Leslie, 2006; Gergely, Nadasdy, Csibra, & Biro, 1995; Hauf et al., 2004). It could be assumed that age is a reasonable proxy for the robustness of infants' self-produced action representations. Second, infants more readily construe unusual events as goal-directed when they involve unusual hand postures than when they involve inanimate agents (Biro & Leslie, 2006; Hauf et al., 2004; Woodward, 1998). This effect may be due to the presence of hands supporting alignment with familiar hand actions.

Structure mapping may also facilitate extracting and generalizing the relational structure of embedded actions, such as using a tool to draw an object near before grasping it. Tool use presents a challenge for the perceiver because the action on the tool does not make direct contact with the goal object. Sommerville and colleagues' (in press) work suggests that self-produced means–end action provides insight into the embedded relational structure of others' actions. Once this is in place, structure mapping would allow infants to generalize this structure across diverse tool use events. For example, an infant who had experienced and observed multiple cloth-pulling events might then be able to discern means–end structure in a novel tool use event, just as children in Kotovsky and Gentner's (1996) study were able to detect higher-order relational similarities among patterns after aligning multiple instances of the relation.

Structure mapping can extract relational similarities starting at the level of pure object similarity, with no initial relational content. However, as detailed above, we hypothesize that infants begin one step ahead in this process in that they bring with them relational representations of some actions. This differs from Barresi and Moore's (1996) view of the role of analogy in extracting intentional relations. In their view, infants do not begin with relational representations, but rather derive them from the physical alignment of their own actions with the actions of others. For this reason, they hypothesize that triadic interactions are especially important for the process. On our proposal, infants may represent intentional relations before they reliably engage in triadic interactions.

Beginning with a relational kernel would have several advantages. Real world actions are not as neatly packaged as are habituation events or stimuli in analogical mapping experiments. Hand trajectories and shapes differ as different objects are grasped. People seldom grasp the same object again and again. Furthermore, except in some specific contexts, like triadic interactions, it is relatively rare for infants' actions to be directed at the same objects as others' actions at the same time. Thus, infants must be able to extract common goal structure across exemplars that are varied and distributed in time. Therefore, the conditions that have been shown to support the extraction of relational structure from initial object similarity may rarely occur in the domain of action, especially early in infancy. Beginning with a few self-generated relational action representations would support infants' ability to identify others' goal-directed actions in the face of the challenges posed by variability and temporal dispersion. As work with older children has shown, once children have established relational representations, they are less dependent on surface similarity and physical alignment of instances in extending this relational information to new instances.

Furthermore, hands move in many ways, not all of them object-directed. If infants began only with the ability to map events in terms of similarities in the objects involved, they might note that events with hands that grasp, gesture, snap, tap, scratch, etc. are all similar in that they involve hands. However, they would miss the critical underlying similarity that unites disparate goal-directed actions (e.g., lifting a box with two hands and picking up a cheerio with a pincer grip) and makes them different from other "hand events." Relational action representations would highlight for infants the common relational structure of goal-directed actions, thus distinguishing them from other hand movements or motion events.

In summary, we propose that infants begin with self-generated, relational action representations that guide their perception of others' actions. Structure mapping provides one means for going beyond these initial representations, allowing infants to discern common relational structure across diverse actions. In this way, infants may take the first step in separating goals from the particular actions that pursue them.

This independence from particular actions is one critical piece of what it means to understand a goal or plan as a mental state. Thus, it is possible that structure mapping plays a role in the development of folk concepts of mental states. We assume that this is only part of the story. Mature mental state concepts are embedded in and defined by theory-like systems of knowledge (Wellman, 1990). The acquisition of such knowledge systems involves the interplay of cognitive learning mechanisms in the child and information from the environment, including linguistic information. Indeed, Gentner (2003) has highlighted the role of language in supporting the acquisition of abstract relational concepts. Gentner and Medina (1998) have proposed a similar account for the role of structure mapping in the acquisition of folk theoretical knowledge in other domains, for example the concept of essences in folk biology.

Mental state knowledge becomes increasingly rich during the preschool years (Wellman, 1990). Even as early as 18 to 24 months of age, children verbally express knowledge about mental states, such as states of attention, emotions, and intentions (Bartch & Wellman, 1995). Further, recent experiments suggest that by these same ages children may understand belief states (Csibra & Southgate, 2006; Onishi & Baillargeon, 2005; Southgate, Senju, & Csibra, 2007; Surian, Caldi, & Sperber, 2007). This interpretation of the findings is debated, but at the very least, these studies demonstrate relatively rich understanding of others' states of attention. It is beyond the scope of this chapter to resolve this debate. Nevertheless, by these ages, we think it is possible that joint contributions of action analysis and linguistic input could contribute to initial mental state concepts.

Conclusion

In this chapter, we have presented a constructivist hypothesis regarding the development of action and intention understanding. We propose that emerging abilities to act, mirror representations, and analogy each play an important role in this constructive process. The development of intention understanding occurs through the progression from an initial structural understanding of goal-directed actions provided by mirror systems to a more abstract understanding through application of general purpose analogical mapping processes. Mirror systems may get the process started, but further ontogenetic processes are needed to produce the abstract action knowledge children eventually attain.

Our account is similar to Meltzoff's (2005) "like me" hypothesis in many important ways. We concur that action understanding is grounded in shared representation of self and other, and that action knowledge develops from relatively concrete to abstract forms during infancy and early childhood. Our account differs in two respects. For one, we propose that the extension of self-generated action representations to others can take place without the infant or child needing to engage in motor imitation. On Meltzoff's account, engagement in imitation is critical for infants' interpretation of others' intentions in acting. On our view, action representations acquired from first-person experience can then function "off-line" to provide structure for perceiving other's actions.

Further, we suggest that these action representations can undergo change as a function of observational extension. An infant with well-structured means-end action representations may extend them to observed actions with a novel tool, and by so doing, enrich the action knowledge they can bring to bear in future events. That is, once it is engaged, structure mapping can operate on observational as well as self-produced examples. This proposal is consistent with the finding that by the second year of life, infants engage in observational learning, imitating new actions with artifacts or tools. Even so, because they bring with them relational content, self-produced actions may continue to render especially powerful effects on children's emerging action knowledge.

A second difference between our proposal and Meltzoff's is that we are more conservative in our estimation of whether and when infants conceive of others' actions as being caused by mental states. In Meltzoff's account (2005), inner or mental states are part of what is extended from self to other from the start. As we have described, we think it is also possible to account for young infants' action knowledge in structural terms, and we further hypothesize that structural representations of goal-directed action may provide a foundation for later emerging mental state concepts. On the other hand, our account does not make a clear prediction of when in this chain of events the first "mental" concepts will arise. In fact, we think the question of when an action representation counts as "mental" is complex and difficult to address given evidence from infancy research (see Woodward, 2005).

Our proposal, though consistent with much of what is currently known, raises a number of questions to motivate future research. To start, we propose that infants' own actions yield relational action representations that observation alone cannot provide. If we are right, then laboratory manipulations of infants' own actions should change their perceptual responses in ways that observational training does not. Recent findings from Sommerville's group (Sommerville et al., in press) are consistent with this hypothesis, but more work is needed to test the limits of this hypothesis. Further, we hypothesize that structure mapping processes play a role in the generalization of infants' action knowledge. If we are right, then the same kinds of laboratory manipulations that have been shown to influence older children's generalization of relational information should influence infants' responses to action structure. Work currently underway in our laboratory is investigating each of these hypotheses.

Finally, our account predicts that the action representations derived in infancy contribute to the eventual emergence of folk concepts of mental states. Evidence in favor of this final prediction comes from several recent longitudinal studies documenting that infants' action analysis predicts their responses, some years later, on verbal theory of mind measures (Aschersleben & Hohenberger, 2007; Kuhlmeier & Yamaguchi, 2007; Poulin-Dubois & Olineck, 2007; Wellman, Phillips, Dunphy-Lelii, & Lalonde, 2004). Infants who respond more systematically to the intentional structure of others' actions go on to become preschoolers who respond more systematically on classic theory of mind assessments, like the false-belief task. Thus, the initial steps we have begun to uncover during infancy seem to begin a long journey in the construction of folk psychology.

Acknowledgments

The writing of this chapter was supported, in part, by NIH grant HD35707 to A.W. We thank Annette Henderson and Scott Johnson for their insightful comments on earlier versions of this manuscript.

References

Adamson, L. B., & McArthur, D. (1995) Joint attention, affect, and culture. In C. Moore, & P. J. Dunham (Eds.), *Joint attention: Its origins and role in development* (pp. 205–222). Hillsdale, NJ: Lawrence Erlbaum Associates, Inc.

Altschuler, E. L., Vankov, A., Wang, V., Ramachandran, V. S., Pineda, J. A. (1997). Person see, person do: human cortical electrophysiological correlates of monkey see monkey do cells [Abstract]. *Society for Neuroscience, 719.*

Aschersleben, G., & Hohenberger, A. (2007). *Does infant action interpretation predict later theory of mind abilities?* Paper presented at the Meetings of the Jean Piaget Society, Amsterdam, The Netherlands.

Baird, J., & Baldwin, D. A. (2001). Making sense of human behavior: Action parsing and intentional inference. In B. F. Malle, L. J. Moses, & D. A. Baldwin (Eds.), *Intention and intentionality: Foundations of social cognition.* Cambridge, MA: MIT Press.

Baldwin, J. M. (1897). *Social and ethical interpretations in mental development: A study in social psychology.* New York: Macmillan.

Baldwin, D. A., Baird, J. A., Saylor, M. M., & Clark, M. A. (2001). Infants parse dynamic action. *Child Development, 72,* 708–717.

Baldwin, D. A., & Moses, L. J. (2001). Links between social understanding and early word learning: Challenges to current accounts. *Social Development, 10,* 309–329.

Barresi, J., & Moore, C. (1996) Intentional relations and social understanding. *Behavioral and Brain Sciences, 19,* 107–129.

Bartch, K., & Wellman, H. M. (1995). *Children talk about the mind.* New York: Oxford Press.

Bates, E., Carlson-Luden, V., & Bretherton, I. (1980). Perceptual aspects of tool using ininfancy. *Infant Behavior and Development, 3,* 127–140.

Behne, T., Carpenter, M., Call, J., & Tomasello, M. (2005) Unwilling versus unable: Infants' understanding of intentional action. *Developmental Psychology, 41,* 328–337.

Bertenthal, B., & Clifton, R. K. (1998). Perception and action. In W. Damon, D. Kuhn, & R. Siegler (Eds.), *Handbook of child psychology: Cognition, perception and language* (pp. 51–102). New York: Wiley.

Biro, S., & Leslie, A. M. (2006). Infants' perception of goal-directed actions: development through cue-based bootstrapping. *Developmental Science, 10,* 379–398.

Blakemore, S. J., & Decety, J. (2001). From the perception of action to the understanding of intention. *Nature Reviews Neuroscience, 2,* 561–567.

Brooks, R., & Meltzoff, A. N. (2002). The importance of eyes: How infants interpret adult looking behavior. *Developmental Psychology, 38,* 958–966.

Brune, C., & Woodward, A. L. (2007). Social cognition and social responsiveness in 10-month-old infants. *Journal of Cognition and Development, 8,*133–158.

Buccino, G., Binkofski, F., Fink, G. R., Fadiga, L., Fogassi, L. et al. (2001). Action observation activates premotor and parietal areas in a somatotopic manner: an fMRI study. *European Journal of Neuroscience, 13,* 400–404.

Calvo-Merino, B., Glaser, D. E., Grezes, J., Passingham, R. E., & Haggard, P. (2005). Action observation and acquired motor skills: An fMRI study with expert dancers. *Cerebral Cortex, 15,* 1243–1249.

Calvo-Merino, B., Grezes, J., Glaser, D. E., Passingham, R. E., & Haggard, P. (2006). Seeing or doing? Influence of visual and motor familiarity in action observation. *Current Biology, 16,* 1905–1910.

Carpenter, M., Nagell, K., & Tomasello, M. (1998). Social cognition, joint attention, and communicative competence from 9 to 15 months of age. *Monographs of the Society for Research in Child Development, 63,* serial no. 255.

Catmur, C., Walsh. V, & Heyes, C. (2007). Sensorimotor learning configures the human mirror system. *Current Biology, 17,* 1527–1531.

Cochin, S., Barthelemy, C., Roux, S., & Martineau, J. (1999). Observation and execution of movement: Similarities demonstrated by quantified electroencephalography. *European Journal of Neuroscience, 11,* 1839–1842.

Csibra, G., & Southgate, V. (2006). Evidence for infants' understanding of false beliefs should not be dismissed. *Trends in Cognitive Science, 10,* 4–5.

Fadiga, L., Fogassi, L. Pavesi, G., & Rizzolatti, G. (1995). Motor facilitation during action observation: A magnetic stimulation study. *Journal of Neurophysiology, 73,* 2608–2611.

Falck-Ytter, T., Gredeback, G., & von Hofsten, C. (2006). Infants predict other people's action goals. *Nature Neuroscience, 9,* 878–879.

Ferrari, P. F., Rozzi, S., & Fogassi, L. (2005). Mirror neurons responding to observation of actions made with tools in monkey ventral premotor cortex. *Journal of Cognitive Neuroscience, 17,* 212–226.

Flanagan, J.R. & Johansson, R.S. (2003). Action plans used in action observation. *Nature, 424,* 769–771.

Fogassi, L., Ferrari, P. F., Gesierich, B., Rozzi, S., Chersi, F., & Rizzolatti, G. (2005). Parietal lobe: From action organization to intention understanding. *Science, 308,* 662–667.

Gallese, V., Fadiga, L., Fogassi, L., & Rizzolatti, G. (1996). Action recognition in the premotor cortex. *Brain, 119,* 593–609.

Gallese, V., & Goldman, A. (1998). Mirror neurons and the simulation theory of mind reading. *Trends in Cognitive Science, 12,* 493–501.

Gangitano, M., Mottaghy, F. M., & Pascual-Leone, A. (2001). Phase-specific modulation of cortical motor output during movement observation. *NeuroReport, 12,* 1489–1492.

Gentner, D. (1988). Metaphor as structure mapping: the relational shift. *Child Development, 59,* 47–59.

Gentner, D. (2003). Why we're so smart. In D. Gentner & S. Goldin-Meadow (Eds.),

Language in mind (pp. 195–236). Cambridge, MA: MIT Press.

Gentner, D., & Medina, J. (1998). Similarity and the development of rules. *Cognition, 65,* 263–297.

Gergely, G., & Csibra, G. (2003). Teleological reasoning in infancy: The one-year-olds' naive theory of rational action. *Trends in Cognitive Sciences, 7,* 287–292.

Gergely, G., Nadasdy, Z., Csibra, G., & Biro, S. (1995). Taking the intentional stance at 12 months of age. *Cognition, 56,* 165–193.

Goldman, A. (1989). Interpretation psychologized. *Mind and Language 4,* 161–185.

Gordon, R. M. (1986). Folk psychology as simulation. *Mind and Language, 1,* 158–171.

Grafton, S. T., Arbib, M. A., Fadiga, L., & Rizzolatti, G. (1996). Localization of grasp representations in humans by PET: 2. Observation compared with imagination. *Experimental Brain Research, 112,* 102–111.

Grezes, J., & Decety, J. (2001). Functional anatomy of execution, mental simulation, observation and verb generation of action: A meta-analysis. *Human Brain Mapping, 12,* 1–19.

Guajardo, J. J., & Woodward, A. L. (2004). Is agency skin-deep? Surface attributes influence infants' sensitivity to goal-directed action. *Infancy , 6,* 361–384.

Hamlin, J. K., Hallinan, E. V., & Woodward, A. L. (2008). Do as I do: 7-month-old infants selectively reproduce others' goals. *Developmental Science, 11,* 487–494.

Harris, P. (1989). *Children and emotion.* Oxford: Blackwell Publishers.

Hauf, P., Aschersleben, G., & Prinz, W. (2007). Baby do-baby see! How action production influences action perception in infants. *Cognitive Development, 22,* 16–32.

Hauf, P., Elsner, B., & Aschersleben, G. (2004). The role of action effects in infant's action control. *Psychological Research, 68,* 115–125.

Heal, J. (1998). Co-cognition and off-line simulation: Two ways of understanding the simulation approach. *Mind and Language, 13,* 477–498.

Heineman-Pieper, J., & Woodward, A. (2003). Understanding infants' understanding of intentions: Two problems of interpretation (A reply to Kiraly et al., 2003). *Consciousness and Cognition, 12,* 770–772.

Hommel, B., Musseler, J., Aschersleben, G., & Prinz, W. (2001). The theory of event coding (TEC): A framework for perception and action planning. *Behavioral and Brain Sciences, 24,* 849–937.

Iacoboni, M., Molnar-Szakacs, I., Gallese, V., Buccino, G., Mazziotta, J. C., & Rizzolatti, G. (2005). Grasping the intentions of others with one's own mirror neuron system. *PLoS Biology, 3,* 529–535.

Iacobani, M., Woods, R. P., Brass, M., Bekkering, H., Mazziotta, J. C., & Rizzolatti, G. (1999). Cortical mechanisms of human imitation. *Science, 286,* 2526–2528.

Jacob, P., & Jeannerod, M. (2005). The motor theory of social cognition: A critique. *Trends in Cognitive Science, 9,* 21–25.

Järveläinen, J., Schürmann, M., & Hari, R. (2004). Activation of the human primary motor cortex during observation of tool use. *NeuroImage, 23,* 187–192.

Johnson, S. C., Ok, S., & Luo, Y. (2007). The attribution of attention: Nine-month-olds' interpretation of gaze as goal-directed action. *Developmental Science, 10,* 530–537.

Kiraly, I., Jovanovic, B., Prinz, W., Aschersleben, G., & Gergely, G. (2003). The early origins of goal attribution in infancy. *Consciousness & Cognition, 12,* 752–769.

Kirkham, N., Slemmer, J., & Johnson, S. (2002). Visual statistical learning in infancy: Evidence for a domain general learning mechanism. *Cognition, 83,* B35–B42.

Kotovsky, L., & Gentner, D. (1996). Comparison and categorization in the development of relational similarity. *Child Development, 67,* 2797–2822.

Kuhlmeier, V., Wynn, K., & Bloom, P. (2003). Attribution of dispositional states by 12-month-olds. *Psychological Science, 14,* 402–408.

Kuhlmeier, V., & Yamaguchi, M. (2007). *How does infants' performance on goal-attribution tasks relate to other social-cognitive skills?* Paper Presented at the Meetings of the Jean Piaget Society, Amsterdam, The Netherlands.

Lepage, J., & Theoret, H. (2007). The mirror neuron system: grasping others' actions from birth? *Developmental Science, 10,* 513–529.

Loewenstein, J., & Gentner, D. (2001). Spatial mapping in preschoolers: Close comparisons facilitate far mappings. *Journal of Cognition and Development, 2,* 189–219.

Luo, Y., & Baillargeon, R. (2007). Do 12.5-month-old infants consider what objects other see when interpreting their actions? *Cognition, 105,* 489–512.

Mahajan, N., & Woodward, A. L. (2007). *Imitation of animate versus inanimate agents in seven-month-old infants.* Poster presentation at the biennial meetings of the Cognitive Development Society, Santa Fe, NM.

Meltzoff, A. N. (1995). Understanding the intentions of others: Re-enactment of intended acts by 18-month-old children. *Developmental Psychology, 31*, 1–16.

Meltzoff, A. N. (2005). Imitation and other minds: The "like me" hypothesis. In S. Hurley & N. Chater (Eds.), *Perspectives on imitation: From neuroscience to social science* (pp. 55–77). Cambridge, MA: MIT Press.

Meltzoff, A. M. & Brooks, R. (2008). Self-experience as a mechanism for learning about others: A training study in social cognition. *Developmental Psychology, 44,* 1257–1265.

Meltzoff, A. N., & Moore, M. K. (1989). Imitation in newborn infants: Exploring the range of gestures imitated and the underlying mechanisms. *Developmental Psychology, 25,* 954–962.

Moll, H., & Tomasello, M. (2004). 12- and 18-month-old infants follow gaze to space behind barriers. *Developmental Science, 7,* F1–F9.

Muthukumaraswamy, S. D., Johnson, B. W., & McNair, N. A. (2004). Mu rhythm modulation during observation of an object-directed grasp. *Cognitive Brain Research, 19,* 195–201.

Onishi, K. H., & Baillargeon, R. (2005). Do 15-month-old infants understand false beliefs? *Science, 308,* 255–258.

Phillips, A. T., Wellman, H. M., & Spelke, E. S. (2002). Infants' ability to connect gaze and emotional expression to intentional action. *Cognition, 85,* 53–78.

Pineda, J. A., Allison, B. Z., & Vankov, A. (2000). The effects of self-movement, observation, and imagination on mu rhythms and readiness potentials (RP's): toward a brain-computer interface (BCI). *IEEE Transactions on Rehabilitation Engineering, 8,* 219–222.

Poulin-Dubois, D., & Olineck, K. M. (2007). *From intention-in-action to intention-in the mind: Infants' goal detection and intentional imitation predict later theory of mind.* Presentation Presented at the Meetings of the Jean Piaget Society, Amsterdam, The Netherlands.

Piaget, J. (1953). *The origins of intelligence in the child.* London: Routledge & Kegan Paul.

Rizzolatti, G., & Arbib, M. A. (1998). Language within our grasp. *Trends in Neuroscience, 21,* 188–194.

Rizzolatti, G., & Fadiga, L. (1998). Grasping objects and grasping action meanings: the dual role of the monkey rostroventral premotor cortex (area F5). *Novartis Foundation Symposium, 218,* 81–95.

Rizzolatti, G., Fogassi, L., & Gallese, V. (2001). Neurophysiological mechanisms underlying the understanding and imitation of action. *Nature Reviews Neuroscience, 2,* 661–670.

Rochat, P. (1989). Object manipulation and exploration in 2- to 5-month-olds. *Developmental Psychology, 25,* 871–884.

Saffran, J. R., Aslin, R. N., & Newport, E. L. (1996). Statistical learning by 8-month-old infants. *Science, 274,* 1926–1928.

Saxe, R. (2005). Against simulation: The argument from error. *Trends in Cognitive Science, 9,* 174–179.

Shimada, S., & Hiraki, K. (2006). Infant's brain responses to live and televised action. *Neuroimage, 32,* 930–939.

Sodian, B., & Thoermer, C. (2004). Infants' understanding of looking, pointing, and reaching as cues to goal-directed action. *Journal of Cognition & Development, 5,* 289–316.

Sommerville, J. A., Hildebrand, E. A., & Crane, C. C. (2008). Experience matters: The impact of doing versus watching on infants' subsequent perception of tool use events. *Developmental Psychology, 44,* 1249–1256.

Sommerville, J. A., & Woodward, A. L. (2005). Pulling out the intentional structure of action: The relation between action processing and action production in infancy. *Cognition, 95,* 1– 30.

Sommerville, J. A., & Woodward, A. L. (in press). The link between action production and action processing in infancy. In F. Grammont, D. Legrand, & P. Livet (Eds.), *Naturalizing intention in action.*

Sommerville, J. A., Woodward, A. L., & Needham, A. (2005). Action experience alters 3-month-old infants' perception of others' actions. *Cognition, 96,* B1–B11.

Southgate, V., Senju, A., & Csibra, G. (2007). Action anticipation through attribution of false belief by 2-year-olds. *Psychological Science, 18,* 587–192.

Surian, L., Caldi, S., & Sperber, D. (2007). Attribution of beliefs by 13-month-old infants. *Psychological Science, 18,* 580–586.

Tomasello, M. (1999). *The cultural origins of human cognition.* Cambridge, MA: Harvard University Press.

Tomasello, M., & Haberl, K. (2003). Understanding attention: 12- and 18-month-olds understand what is new for other persons. *Developmental Psychology, 39,* 906–912.

Wellman, H. M. (1990). *The child's theory of mind.* Cambridge, MA: MIT Press.

Wellman, H. M., Phillips, A. T., Dunphy-Lelii, S., & Lalonde, N. (2004). Infant understanding of persons predicts preschool social cognition. *Developmental Science, 7,* 283– 288.

Woodward, A. L. (1998). Infants selectively encode the goal object of an actor's reach. *Cognition, 69,* 1–34.

Woodward, A. L. (1999). Infants' ability to distinguish between purposeful and non-purposeful behaviors. *Infant Behavior and Development, 22,* 145–160.

Woodward, A. L. (2003). Infants' developing understanding of the link between looker and object. *Developmental Science, 6,* 297–311.

Woodward, A. L. (2005). The infant origins of intentional understanding. In R. V. Kail (Ed.), *Advances in child development and behavior* (Vol. 33, pp. 229–262). Oxford: Elsevier.

Woodward, A. L., & Guajardo, J. J. (2002). Infants' understanding of the point gesture as an object-directed action. *Cognitive Development, 17,* 1061–1084.

Woodward, A. L., & Sommerville, J. A. (2000). Twelve-month-old infants interpret action in context. *Psychological Science, 11,* 73–76.

CHAPTER 16
A Neoconstructivistic Approach to the Emergence of a Face Processing System

Francesca Simion and Irene Leo

Introduction to the Neoconstructivistic Approach

Developmental theories have been dominated by two different views both on the origin of knowledge and on the initial mechanisms that form the basis for cognitive development. On one view, knowledge emerges on the basis of domain-general mechanisms of learning that are sufficient to explain how children learn about specific domains of knowledge such as language, number, space, or faces. Although Piagetian, behaviorist, and more recently connectionist theories fall within this view, Piaget's position, known as "epigenetic constructivism," differs because cognitive development is considered as the outcome of a self-organizing system that is structured and shaped by its interaction with the environment.

On the competing view, the early appearance of abilities hitherto unsuspected has supported the notion that knowledge begins early in life and constitutes parts of humans' innate endowment. Some authors maintain that human cognition is built on domain-specific system of knowledge and that natural selection may have favored the evolution of mechanisms that give rise to this knowledge (e.g., Kellman, 1993). More specifically, the human mind is considered to be a collection of special purpose mechanisms, each shaped, through adaptation to the environment during the course of evolution, to perform a particular function. This nativistic view asserts that humans are born either with the innate capacity to develop information processing systems or "cognitive modules" that allow them to make sense of the world, or that learning is guided by innately specified and content-specific principles that determine the entities on which subsequent learning takes place (e.g., Gelman, 1990; Spelke, 1991).

In this perspective, deeply influenced by Chomskyan linguistics (1988) and by Fodor's modularity theory (1983), the infant comes into the world well prepared to process different domains of knowledge. For example, the infant comes preprepared for processing faces, language, space, and number, each in very different ways. Accordingly, cognition would be specialized from the outset in processing content-specific inputs able to mediate complex cognitive functions (e.g., Spelke, 1991; Wynn, 1995). This approach seems to preclude the "epigenetic constructivist principle" to development because biological forms are not considered as a product of any dynamic interactions between the genes and the environment.

The dichotomy between general and specific innate mechanisms as determinants of cognitive development has been overcome by the neoconstructivistic approach to cognition that combines these two different explanations and states that nativism and epigenetic principles are not incompatible because it can be assumed the existence of some innate specified predispositions that would give the epigenetic process a head start in each domain of knowledge. Such predispositions are supposed not to be knowledge-impregnated and content-specific but instead are presumed to be less detailed specifications that some nativists presuppose. Indeed, in the neoconstructivism approach, the cognitive activity is seen as emerging gradually as a product of the interaction between innate constraints and the structure of the input provided by the species-typical environment (de Schonen, 2002; Elman et al., 1996; Johnson, 1993; Michel & Moore, 1995; Nelson & Luciana, 2001). More specifically, this theoretical perspective suggests that the specific cognitive systems are the product of a "process of modularization"; that is to say, the modular architecture is the result of a gradual development rather than being innately specified. The modules are not hardwired nor of fixed neural architecture; they are the outcome of a continuous process that emerges through the dynamic of a probabilistic epigenesis that progressively leads to an increasing functional specialization of neural circuits (Bates & Elman, 1993; Johnson, 1997; Karmiloff-Smith, 1992).

Consequently, brain specialization, domain specificity, and cognitive modules rather than being assumed as genetically prespecified are considered to emerge epigenetically and developmentally through the interaction with postnatal environment. Evolution have prespecified many innate biological constraints on development that are domain-general mechanisms becoming "domain-specific" with the process of development. During this process, the same general mechanisms have been used repeatedly to process a certain class of stimuli and in so doing they become specific. Some apparent constraints contribute to the development of new structures and new modes of functioning, which will be advantageous at later stages of development (Karmiloff-Smith, 1992) and provide starting points that channel the subsequent perceptual and cognitive development (e.g., Turkewitz & Kenny, 1982). For instance, it has been proposed that the constraints imposed by the development of the sensory systems may actually facilitate subsequent perceptual development by reducing the range of stimuli that the infant has to deal with.

Within this theoretical framework, the notion of innate constraints are described as architectural, computational, and temporal biases that shape information processing, limiting the types of input to be selected and constraining the computations on the input. Consequently, the word "constraints" does not carry on any negative connotation, but rather, it possesses a positive connotation. In fact, constraints are defined as biases in the information processing due to the properties of the brain architecture or of the perceptual systems in a given period of development. Benefits from these biases consist in selectively focusing the cognitive system toward certain aspects of the surrounding environment or facilitating processing of certain kinds of inputs, thus strengthening learning of some categories of stimuli rather than others, and, consequently, tuning the system to become specialized.

To summarize, in contrast to the classic nativist/modular thesis that considers the infant brain as provided with built-in specific representational contents, the neoconstructivistic approach stresses the role of a number of innately specified constraints or biases in the emergence of representations and thus in the origins of knowledge. There is the idea that specific cognitive structures may arise from primary, general innate constraints shaped by the nature of the experience the organism is exposed to (Karmiloff-Smith, 1992).

Brain development is viewed in terms of an increasing restriction of the fate of component elements, such as neurons and neural circuits. In other words, as development proceeds, neurons and cortical circuitry become increasingly specialized, dedicated to particular functions and less capable of change. The cerebral cortex does not appear to contain intrinsic prespecified representations to support functions such as face recognition or linguistic processing. Rather, the appropriate representations emerge through the constraints of the complex cortical and subcortical networks and through the interaction between the infant and the statistical regularities latent in its environment. Endogenous constraints select the successive aspect of the environment to which paying attention and, interacting with the structure of the input typical of the infant's environment, guide and shape the gradual emerging of specialized processing (Werker & Vouloumanos, 2001). Domain-specific cognitive activity is, therefore, strictly linked to the exposure to certain experiences, i.e., activity-dependent (Greenough & Black, 1992). Experience appears to play a prominent role in recruiting the cortical areas potentially suited to be activated by certain stimuli. The activation of these cortical and functional networks leads as a consequence to a process of a progressive specialization that emerges on condition that the critical type of input is provided within the sensitive time window and, in this sense, is activity-expectant (Nelson 2001, 2003). For instance, it has been demonstrated that deprivation of early visual input due to bilateral congenital cataract in the first months of life impairs face processing, even years after surgery (e.g., Le Grand, Mondloch, Maurer, & Brent, 2003). This suggests that the normal visual experience is a necessary condition to develop an expert face processing system (e.g., Geldart, Mondloch, Maurer, de Schonen, & Brent, 2002; Le Grand et al., 2003).

The fact that some perceptual and/or attentional biases toward certain characteristics of sensory information enhance learning processes weakens the classical contraposition between nature and nurture, because innate predispositions are not stable and unchangeable and are not distinct and separated from learned behaviors. On the contrary, innate predispositions represent the necessary conditions to constrain and to determine learning itself (Elman et al., 1996).

In light of this theoretical framework, since development cannot be explained in terms of innate, built-in representational contents, it becomes relevant for developmental researchers to investigate what types of general perceptual constrains and attentional biases are present in the first months of life and how they contribute to the specialization of the cognitive system.

The general goal of this chapter is to examine (1) whether some constraints or prewired attentional biases are present at birth; (2) if these constraints are general or specific, and (3) how they contribute to guide and shape cognitive activity.

In order to address these issues, a peculiar class of visual stimuli, namely faces, will be taken into consideration because faces form a special class of visual objects elaborated in adults by a specific face system. The first part of the chapter focuses on the mechanisms underlying infants' visual preference for faces and on the visuoperceptual constraints that induce newborns to prefer faces.

The second part of the chapter will review the studies on the nature of the information newborns actually process and encode when they look at faces as compared to nonface stimuli, more specifically, whether the recognition of faces at birth requires the same nonspecific generalized perceptual abilities that are involved in processing all types of visual stimuli.

Mechanisms Underlying Face Preference at Birth

Evidence from behavioral, brain lesion, and neuroimaging studies suggests that in adults face processing involves distinct, domain-specific perceptual processing (Maurer, Le Grand, & Mondloch, 2002; Schwaninger, Carbon, & Leder, 2003) carried out by dedicated brain areas (e.g., Farah, Rabinowitz, Quinn, & Liu, 2000; Kanwisher, 2000). The functional and neural specialization present in the adult face processing system renders faces an ideal class of stimuli in order to investigate the time course and the factors affecting such specialization. Some authors claim the existence of a specialized system for face processing already at birth (experience-independent; e.g., Farah et al., 2000), while others raise the possibility that such specialization is a product of experience (experience-dependent; e.g., Gauthier & Logothetis, 2000; Gauthier & Tarr, 1997, 2002), so developmental studies carried out with newborns become critical to disentangle this issue. The preference discovered in the first days of life to orient to and attend at faces has been interpreted as supporting the existence of an innate, content-specific mechanism for face processing in the human system. When presented with face-like and nonface-like patterns, newborns spontaneously look longer at and orient more frequently toward the configuration that represents a face (e.g., Johnson & Morton, 1991; Valenza, Simion, Macchi Cassia, & Umiltà, 1996). Face preference at birth has been demonstrated with both static and moving stimuli (Easterbrook, Kisilevsky, Muir, & Laplante, 1999; Goren, Sarty, & Wu, 1975; Kleiner, 1987; Macchi Cassia, Simion, & Umiltà, 2001), and with both schematic and veridical images of faces (Johnson & Morton, 1991; Macchi Cassia, Turati, & Simion, 2004; Valenza et al., 1996).

However, a matter of dispute concerns the mechanisms underlying face preference at birth because the presence of such a preference could be due to either the existence of general biases or a content-specific mechanism.

Three different hypotheses have been proposed to explain newborns' preference for faces. The first, named the "sensory hypothesis," maintains that faces are not different from other visual stimuli and that certain classes of stimuli are preferred by newborns as a result of the general properties of the early stages of visual processing.

This hypothesis is based on the predictions of the linear system model (LSM) (e.g., Banks & Salapatek, 1981; Kleiner, 1987; Kleiner & Banks, 1987). Any two-dimensional, achromatic pattern can be described on the basis of the spatial frequencies, amplitude (contrast), orientation, and phase of its constituent sine wave gratings. For any pattern, two functions may be derived: the amplitude spectrum, comprising the amplitude and orientation of the component spatial frequencies; and the phase spectrum, comprising the phase and orientation of the components. The LSM holds that the attractiveness of a pattern is determined solely by the amount of effective energy of that pattern. The amplitude spectrum of the pattern is filtered through the contrast sensitivity function (CSF) of the subject. Each age has an appropriate CSF, so in newborns CSF removes all information at frequencies greater than 2 cycles per degree (c/d). In a choice situation, newborns' visual preferences are for those stimuli that provide spatial frequency and contrast information that fit the visual window—the CSF—better than the pattern with which it is paired. Basically, the LSM claims that newborns' preferences for visual patterns are determined solely by their visibility. Faces would not be different from other visual stimuli that are preferred simply because they possess more appropriate sensory properties.

This hypothesis succeeded in explaining preferences for a variety of visual configurations but failed to entirely account for newborns' preference for face-like patterns (Valenza et al., 1996). In fact, empirical evidence demonstrated that newborns still prefer a face-like pattern even when it is contrasted to a stimulus of equal (Johnson, Dziurawiec, Ellis, & Morton, 1991; Kleiner, 1987) or greater (Valenza et al., 1996) visibility.

The second hypothesis, named the "structural hypothesis" (Johnson & Morton, 1991; Morton & Johnson, 1991), maintains that faces are special for the newborn because human infants possess a device (i.e., *Conspec*), which contains structural information concerning the visual characteristics of conspecifics. In particular, this information would be concerned with the relative spatial location of elements within the pattern, like three high-contrast blobs in the correct relative locations for the eyes and mouth on a stimulus of about the right size. Recently, this model of the development of face processing has been revised and updated. Johnson (2005) maintains that newborns' face preference is due to the existence of a "low-spatial-frequencies face-configuration detector" supported by a fast subcortical route. The existence of a content-specific template, i.e., "a face detector," allows the human visual system to detect faces and explains the specific bias toward faces present at birth (Johnson, 2005). The face detector (Conspec in the original Morten & Johnson model) is responsible only for face detection and triggers attention toward faces, because it is a very specialized orienting mechanism. At around 2 months of age, a second cortical mechanism, *Conlearn*, that benefits from experience with faces, replaces Conspec, whose function is essentially to "set" Conlearn.

An alternative account of face preference in newborns proposed that the visual preference for faces at birth reflects a preference for a collection of general structural properties, including both the low-level components such as the contrast and the spatial frequencies content and the higher level components such as the structural properties of a stimulus described by the phase spectrum according to a Fourier analysis (e.g., Macchi Cassia et al., 2004; Simion, Macchi Cassia, Turati, & Valenza, 2001, 2003; Simion, Valenza, Macchi Cassia, Turati, & Umiltà, 2002).

This hypothesis maintains that the human visual system possesses some general predispositions toward certain general properties embodied in a face and that the preference for faces present since birth is in fact a preference for a collection of general properties. Each single property present in a face such as symmetry along the vertical axis, the presence of more elements in the upper part, the congruent distributions of the inner elements according to the shape of the contour, could trigger newborns' attention and in so doing determine face preference.

To summarize this third hypothesis is in line with the neoconstructivistic approach to cognition and is consistent with both the existence of a more domain-general system responsive to general properties of the stimuli and with the presence of a limited number of innately specified domain-general predispositions that only with time and experience would activate specific circuits and specific computations in response to domain-specific inputs. The presence of general, nonspecific constraints on visual processing might be sufficient to produce the emergence of the functional specialization for faces observed later in development through the process of modularization. The evidence that supports the idea that faces may be perceived at birth by general mechanisms that can also operate on nonface stimuli is mainly grounded in evidence suggesting that faces are not the only class of stimuli that can trigger newborns' attention and induce a preference. For example, when horizontal gratings were paired with vertical gratings, newborns preferred the horizontal ones (Farroni, Valenza, Simion, & Umiltà, 2000; Slater, Earle, Morison, & Rose, 1985; Slater & Sykes, 1977). These data suggest that the structural configuration of a pattern is a crucial factor in determining newborns' preference for geometrical stimuli as well as for faces.

To test whether face preference could be explained either on the basis of some general structural properties that other stimuli may share with faces or by specific mechanisms, two series of experiments were carried out in our laboratory. In the first series of experiments, we tested the presence of general, noncontent-specific attentional biases toward some structural properties as determinants of face preferences. In the second series of experiments, we contrasted the hypothesis supporting the existence of a specific mechanism with the hypothesis supporting the existence of general mechanisms.

The rationale of the first series of experiments was that if we were able to demonstrate that some nonspecific structural properties can engage attention with stimuli other than faces and that these structural properties are the same as those present in a face, then it may be concluded that these structural properties could explain face preference at birth.

Two general structural properties present in a face were tested in our laboratory: congruency and the top-down asymmetry in the disposition of the elements in the upper part.

Congruency was defined by the presence of a congruent or corresponding relationship between the shape and orientation of the bounded area, delimiting the pattern and the spatial disposition of the included features. Faces can be described as a congruent stimulus in that they typically display a greater number of features (the eyes), in the widest, upper portion of the face outline and only one feature (the mouth) in the narrowest bottom part. By the use of geometrical stimulus (both triangles and trapezoids), it has been shown that when a congruent and a noncongruent disposition of the elements within a pattern were compared, newborns show a significant tendency to prefer the configuration that displays a congruent spatial disposition of the elements (Figure 16.1). Evidence revealed that when embedded in geometric nonface-like stimuli, the congruency

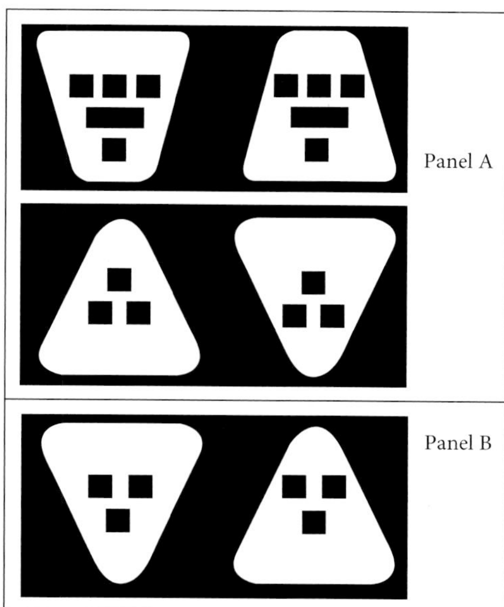

Figure 16.1 The geometric patterns used in Macchi Cassia et al. (2008). Panel A: The congruent and noncongruent nonface-like patterns. Panel B: The congruent and noncongruent face-like patterns.

property is capable of inducing a preferential response, which was not overcome by the preference for the face-like arrangement of the inner elements (Macchi Cassia, Valenza, Simion, & Leo, 2008).

The second property, tested with geometrical stimuli in a visual preference task, was the presence of more elements in the upper part, i.e. the up-down asymmetry in the distribution of the elements (Simion et al., 2002; Turati, Simion, Milani, & Umiltà, 2002). Three groups of newborns were presented with three different pairs of stimuli, each composed of an upright geometrical configuration, with a greater number of high-contrast areas in the upper part, and an upside-down configuration with more elements in the lower part (Simion et al., 2002; Turati et al., 2002). Results were clear in showing that at birth there is a preference for up-down asymmetrical patterns with more elements in the upper part because newborns both orient more frequently to and look longer at the upright configurations (Simion et al., 2002).

The same results were replicated with face-like stimuli and with real faces in which we disrupted the geometry of the face. The upright stimuli with two blobs randomly located in the upper part of the configuration were always preferred over the upside-down stimuli (e.g., Simion et al., 2003; Turati et al., 2002). The evidence in all of these experiments was in favor of the existence of an attentional bias toward up-down asymmetrical patterns, because in all the experiments, a pattern was always preferred when its more salient part was the upper one (Figure 16.2). Given that faces are up-down asymmetrical stimuli, we hypothesized that the preference for faces at birth could be due to the presence of such a general property in the stimulus.

After this first step, a second series of experiments was carried out to contrast the two models that explain face preference as due to general or specific mechanisms. The model supporting the existence of a specific built-in mechanism, i.e., Conspec in Johnson's terminology (Johnson & Morton, 1991) predicts that newborns are sensitive to face geometry, that is to the correct disposition of the elements within a face or, according to the up to date model, to the correct disposition of the eyes (Johnson, 2005). In contrast, our model supporting the existence of general biases toward up-down asymmetrical patterns predicts that the number of elements in the upper part is crucial in determining face preference (Simion et al., 2001, 2003). To test the opposite predictions of these two models, we disrupted the geometry of the face by manipulating the location of the three elements and this stimulus was contrasted with a face-like stimulus with a natural disposition of the internal elements. Results showed that when a face-like stimulus or real face were contrasted with a nonface stimulus, paired for the number of elements in the upper part, no preference for the stimuli with a natural disposition of the inner elements was obtained, either for the face-like stimulus or for the real face (Figure 16.3). Even more interesting were the results showing that when either a face-like or a real face were contrasted with a stimulus with more elements in the upper part, newborns prefer the pattern

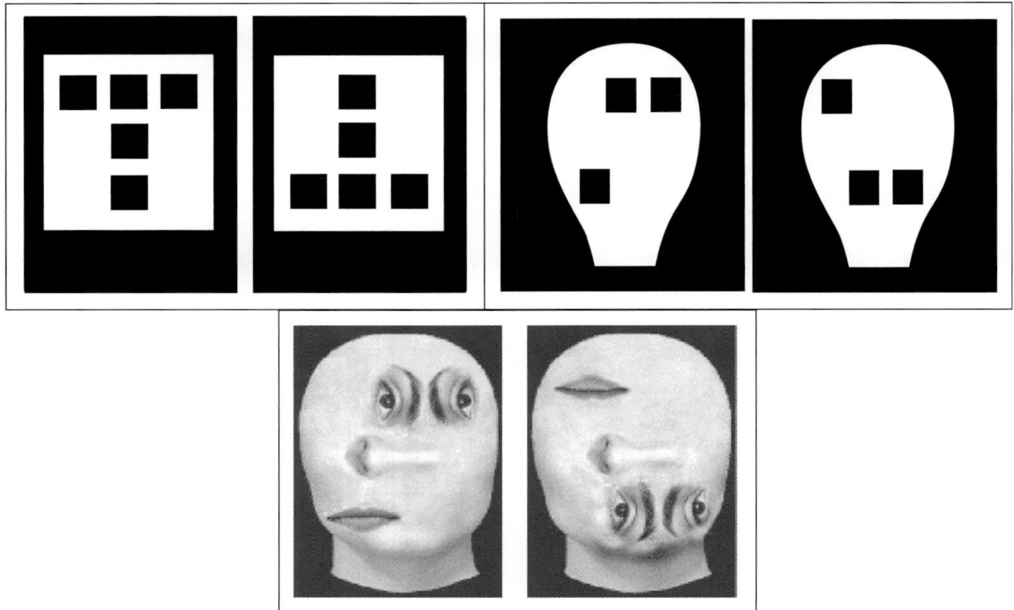

Figure 16.2 Stimuli used to test the preference for up-down asymmetrical patterns (Macchi Cassia et al., 2004; Simion et al., 2002; Turati et al., 2002).

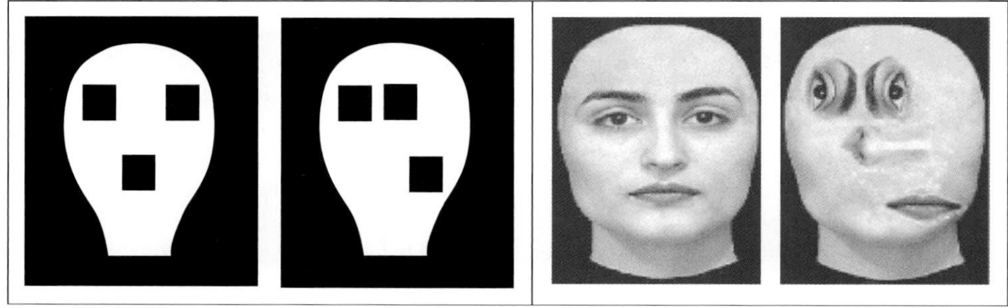

Figure 16.3 Schematic head shaped configurations and real faces used to test the role of a specific mechanism versus the existence of general attentional biases (Macchi Cassia et al., 2004; Turati et al., 2002).

with more elements in the upper part (e.g., Simion et al., 2003; Turati et al., 2002).

Overall, since newborns' visual behavior was affected by the up-down arrangement of the inner features and by congruency independently of whether such arrangement was or not face-like, these findings strongly support the hypothesis on the existence of general attentional biases toward structural properties of the stimuli. Preference for faces at birth may be explained by the result of the cumulative effect of this set of noncontent-specific biases toward some psychophysical properties of the stimuli that best match the characteristics of the human visuoperceptual system rather than by the existence of a specific face detector.

The effect of the up-down asymmetry on newborns' preference, for instance, might be derived from endogenous constraints that characterize their visual system. Specifically, we have proposed that newborns may find top-heavy patterns more easily detectable than other stimuli because of the existence at birth of an upper-visual-field advantage in visual sensitivity (e.g., Simion et al., 2002; Turati et al., 2002). Indeed, in several species, a major role in visual exploration of the upper visual field is played by the superior colliculus (Sprague, Berlucchi, & Rizzolati, 1973), which is supposed to affect considerably newborns' visual behavior (Atkinson, Hood, Wattam-Bell, & Braddick, 1992; Braddick et al., 1992; Bronson, 1982; Johnson, 1995). Some computational models support a similar interpretation based on the constraints on the newborns' visual system and on the properties of the neurons in area V1 (e.g., Acerra, Burnod, & de Schonen, 2002).

Overall, the results obtained in our laboratory support the idea that faces at birth are perceived by domain-general mechanisms that can also operate on nonface stimuli such as geometrical figures. Face preference is in fact a preference for some general bottom-level properties and higher-level configurational properties that faces share with other visual stimuli.

In other words, we maintain that the visuoperceptual system allows newborns to perceive not only the psychophysical low-level information embedded in a stimulus (i.e., spatial frequency and contrast that determines its visibility), but also the higher-level structural and configural properties. Newborns are sensitive to some general configural/structural properties of the stimuli so the preference for faces is in fact a preference for such general properties.

To conclude, the evidence presented in this first part is in line with a neoconstructivist view that maintains that the adult-specific face system arises from innate general predispositions that tune the system toward certain aspects of the external environment, and through experience, neural and functional specialized processes develop. We argue that the face processing system to develop in its adult-like expert form might not require a highly specific template (i.e., a face-detector) but rather, a number of general biases that work together to provide the minimal information that would be sufficient to bootstrap the system.

In this same vein, Nelson (2001) suggests that the development of face processing is an experience-expectant process that, with increasing exposure to faces, produces a "perceptual narrowing" to this class of stimuli, with a consequent increase in the selectivity of infants' behavioral responses to human faces (e.g., Pascalis, de Haan, & Nelson, 2002). Some of the strongest evidence supporting this account comes from behavioral studies that showed a perceptual narrowing to the stimuli most consistently present in the individual-specific environment, as speech sound and faces (e.g., Cheour et al., 1998; Kelly et al., 2005; Kuhl et al., 1992; Pascalis et al., 2002).

From General to Specific Constraints

The presence at birth of general perceptual biases on visual processing seems sufficient to cause the human face to be a frequent focus of newborns' visual attention, allowing, through experience, the gradual development of a face processing system. Based on the evidence provided by the studies with newborns reviewed above, we investigate whether and how infants' preferential response to faces becomes specific for this stimulus category during the first months of life.

Behavioral studies suggest that in 3-month-old infants, preferential responses to faces become more specific to the face category (e.g., Bar-Haim, Ziv, Lamy, & Hodes, 2006; Kelly et al., 2007; Kelly et al., 2005). Neuropsychological studies either with scalp-recorded brain electric potentials (event-related potential, ERP) (Halit, deHaan, & Johnson, 2003) or performed with positron emission topography (PET) (Tzourio-Mazoyer et al., 2002) support the conclusion that the first signs of cortical specialization for faces can be observed in infants of 2–3 months of age.

The question driving our behavioral studies was to verify whether the same general biases that induce face preference at birth still operate and explain face preference 3 months later. More specifically, we tested whether the general structural property such as up-down asymmetry that induces face preference at birth still operates at 3 months of age when a certain degree of cortical specialization for faces begins to emerge (e.g., Halit et al., 2003; Tzourio-Mazoyer et al., 2002).

The results from a first experiment showed that when contrasting photographs of real faces in the canonical upright orientation with the upside-down version, 3-month-old infants show a visual preference for the upright face (Turati, Valenza, Leo & Simion, 2005).

After having observed a face preference in 3-month-old infants, we investigated whether the same bias present at birth toward up-down asymmetrical nonface patterns was still present 3 months later (Turati et al., 2005). To test this hypothesis, the same experiments with geometrical figures carried out with newborns (Simion et al., 2002) were replicated with 3-month-old infants. Results indicated that the responses of 3-month-olds varied as a function of the two different types of up-down asymmetrical stimuli that were presented.

When infants were shown elements organized into a T, their visual behavior appeared to be radically different from that exhibited by newborns (Simion et al., 2002), in that the visual preference for the top-heavy upright T disappeared when contrasted with an inverted T. However, when the other type of stimuli, with four elements in the upper or lower half of the configuration, was considered, a different pattern of results emerged: that is, 3-month-olds' behavior paralleled that shown by newborns with the top-heavy configuration being preferred over the bottom-heavy configuration. These results suggest that, in 3-month-old infants, the determinants of preference for nonface top-heavy patterns are still active but are less powerful than in newborns. This weak preference for up-down asymmetrical patterns suggests that the bias toward up-down asymmetry might still be present but cannot be the sole factor in determining 3-month-olds' preference for faces (Turati et al., 2005). To test this possibility, we directly compared a natural face and a top heavy scrambled face with more elements in the upper part. Results showed that 3-month-old infants always prefer the real face, demonstrating that at this age up-down asymmetry in the distribution of the inner features can not longer be considered as a crucial factor able to induce infants' preference for a face (Simion, Turati, Valenza, & Leo, 2006).

These findings suggest that the bias toward up-down asymmetric stimuli at birth acts as an early facilitating factor that leads to an increased specialization for faces later in development and contradicts the hypothesis that similar general constraints mediate face preference during infancy (Simion et al., 2006).

Recent evidence from an adult fMRI study supports this conclusion by showing enhanced activation in cortical regions involved in face processing (the right fusiform face area, rFFA) in response to nonface-like top-heavy stimuli (Caldara et al., 2006). In line with this claim, adult ERPs revealed that manipulation of the up-down arrangement of the features within scrambled faces modulated the response properties of the N170 (Macchi Cassia, Kuefner, Westerlund, & Nelson, 2006). Together these findings demonstrated that the adult face processing system still shows sensitivity to the up-down asymmetry and that this property seems to play a crucial role in the development of the face system.

Overall the developmental data support the notion that different mechanisms underlie face preference at birth and in 3-month-old infants. Face preference in newborns can be explained by general attentional biases toward sensory and structural properties of these stimuli. On the contrary, the same general mechanisms still active cannot explain face preference 3 months later.

Consistent with the neoconstructivist approach to cognition, our results demonstrate that, likely by virtue of the prolonged exposure to human faces, the mechanisms responsible for infant's face preference shift from being broadly tuned to a wide range of visual stimuli to being increasingly tuned to the human face (Nelson, 2001).

Face recognition

The current developmental models on face processing diverge as for either the nature of the mechanisms that attract newborns toward faces or the existence of special processes to discriminate and recognize individual faces at birth and during the course of development.

In adults, the behavioral signatures of face-specific processing derive from three specific effects present with faces unlike with other objects: the inversion effect (e.g., Yin, 1969), the part-whole effect (e.g., Tanaka & Farah, 1993), and the composite effect (e.g., Young, Hellawell, & Hay, 1987).

The "inversion effect" is a decrement in performance that occurs when stimuli are inverted (i.e., turned upside-down) and is greater for faces as compared with other classes of familiar and complex objects, such as houses, airplanes, etc. (e.g., Valentine, 1988; Yin, 1969). When faces are inverted, adults continue to be able to use featural information (such as the eyes, mouth, nose or ears) nearly as well, but are impaired in their ability to use configural information (such as the spatial interrelationship of facial features) (e.g., Bartlett & Searcy, 1993; Leder & Bruce, 2000).

The second behavioral marker is the "part-whole effect" in which adults are more accurate in recognizing the identity of a feature (e.g., nose) when it is presented in the context of the whole face rather than as an isolated features (e.g., Tanaka & Farah, 1993). Houses, scrambled faces, and inverted faces did not produce this whole/part advantage, suggesting that these types of stimuli are instead recognized on the basis of featural information.

In the "composite effect," subjects are slower to identify one half of the chimeric face if it is aligned with consistent other-face than if the two half-faces are misaligned (e.g., Young et al., 1987). This phenomenon demonstrates that when upright faces are processed, the facial features are so strongly integrated that it becomes difficult to parse the face into isolated features (e.g., Hole, 1994).

Taken together, these effects suggest that upright faces are processed in a distinctive configural manner than processing each of the parts of the face independently.

According to Maurer et al., (2002), configural processing can be divided into three types: (1) sensitivity to first-order relations, that is to the basic arrangement of its features with two eyes above a nose, which is above a mouth; (2) holistic processing, integrating facial features into a whole, thus rendering individual features less accessible; (3) sensitivity to second-order relations, encoding of the spacing among facial features. Previous research has shown that adults process all of these three types of configural information (e.g., Tanaka & Farah, 1993; Searcy & Bartlett, 1996) and that they are able to identify faces using both featural and configural information (e.g., Carey & Diamond, 1977; Freire & Lee, 2001; Maurer et al., 2002). These behavioral data were explained either on the basis of the existence of special-purpose, domain-specific mechanism selectively activated by faces (i.e., the face specific hypothesis) (e.g., Farah et al., 2000), or on the basis of domain-general mechanisms involved in processing not only faces but all the stimuli that require a high level of expertise and task-specific processes (i.e., a process specific hypothesis) (e.g., Gauthier, William, Tarr, & Tanaka, 1998).

This latter hypothesis seems to be consistent with a neoconstructivistic approach to cognition because it maintains that by virtue of the prolonged experience with faces and due to the fine-grained discrimination necessary to process faces, the neural networks should become specialized not only for faces but for all the stimuli that share the same perceptual level of expertise (expertise hypothesis; e.g., Gauthier, Tarr, Anderson, Skudlarski, & Gore, 1999).

The following section of the present chapter focuses on newborns' ability to recognize individual faces and on the information newborns actually process and encode when they discriminate, learn, and recognize individual faces. More specifically, our focus is to investigate the nature of the operations that are utilized to process faces and whether such operations are exclusively involved in face processing at birth.

WHAT KIND OF VISUAL INFORMATION NEWBORNS PROCESS AND ENCODE WHEN THEY RECOGNIZE A FACE?

The literature is consistent in showing that newborns can recognize individual faces despite limited visual abilities. There is considerable evidence of an ability to discriminate among faces and recognize an individual face within a very short time after birth (e.g., Bushnell, 2001; Pascalis, de Schonen, Morton, Deruelle & Fabre-Grenet, 1995; Walton, Bower & Bower, 1992). The mother's face is recognized and preferred over a female stranger's face within hours from birth (Bushnell, 2001; Bushnell, Sai, & Mullin, 1989; Pascalis et al., 1995). The ability to discriminate the mother from a stranger is present also when the task requires memory processes. Using a visual preference technique, Bushnell (2001) demonstrated that newborns still recognize and prefer their mother's face after a separation of 15 min. This study suggests that memory for the mother's face is established in a long-term store within a few days from birth.

Newborns' ability to recognize their mother's face seems to be the product of a more general capacity to discriminate and recognize individual human faces. Pascalis and de Schonen (1994) demonstrated that, after habituation with a photograph of a stranger's face, 4-day-old infants looked longer at a new face than at the familiar one. This evidence demonstrates that newborns are able to learn about a specific individual face to which they are repeatedly exposed within a short time after birth.

Despite convergent evidence on newborns' ability to learn and discriminate individual faces, little is known about the kind of visual information newborns' face recognition relies on. Some studies seem to suggest that there is an inability of newborns to respond to the internal features of the face. In a study by Pascalis et al. (1995), in which the mother's face was preferred over that of a female stranger, newborns' preference for the face disappeared when only the inner features of the two faces were visible (i.e., when both women wore scarves around their heads) and the outer contour of the head and hairline were masked. Based on these findings, the authors concluded that, in order to recognize and prefer the mother, newborns used the outer features of the face rather than the configuration of the internal features.

Nevertheless, some studies conducted in our laboratory demonstrated that this conclusion cannot be considered definitive. We have shown, in three different sets of experiments, that newborns are able to process the internal information contained on both face and nonface stimuli. To be specific, the first set of experiments was carried out to investigate newborns' ability to discriminate, recognize, and learn inner visual information embedded in the face-like and nonface-like configurations that differ in the shape of the inner elements (Simion, Farroni, Macchi Cassia, Turati, & Dalla Barba, 2002).

The results demonstrate that newborns discriminated between two schematic face-like and nonface-like configurations that differed exclusively in the shape of the internal local elements. Hence, learning processes with well-contrasted nonface-like patterns do not appear different from those of face-like patterns.

Further support to these conclusions comes from previous studies carried out to test whether newborns can discriminate between arrays that are identical with respect to the global characteristics (i.e., columns of filled or unfilled elements), but different with respect to the shape of the filled elements contained within the two filled columns (i.e., square elements vs. diamond elements; Farroni et al., 2000) (Figure 16.4, Panel A).

Results showed that newborns are able to discriminate the individual filled elements of the array of a stimulus and can organize such elements into a holistic percept (Farroni et al., 2000). Moreover, even more interesting are the results showing that newborns are able to discriminate the individual elements of the array even when they are embedded in an identical areas and external contour (Figure 16.4, Panel B) (Farroni et al., 2000).

Put together, the findings obtained with face-like and geometric stimuli converge to suggest that the operations involved in face processing are the same that occur to process any visual stimuli (e.g., de Schonen & Mancini, 1995; de Schonen, Mancini, & Liegeois, 1998; Johnson, 1993, 1997).

However, this evidence cannot be extended by default to the case of real faces because faces are far more complex stimuli than schematic

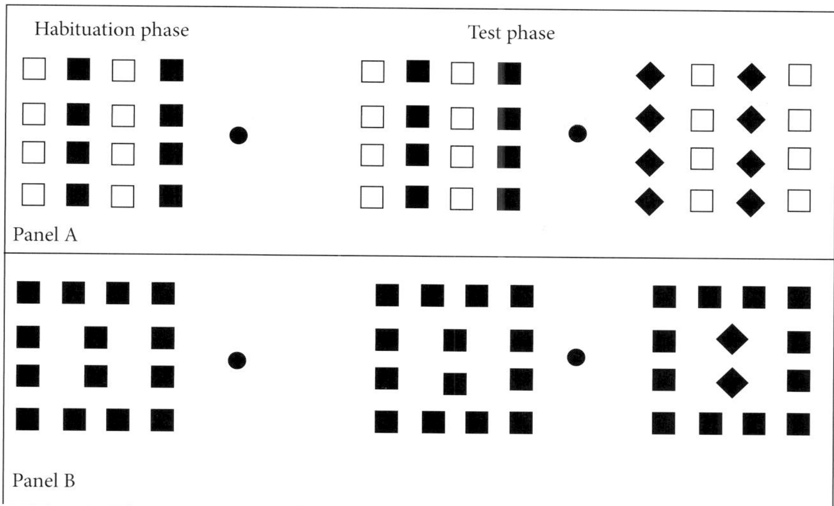

Figure 16.4 Examples of the stimuli used in Farroni et al. (2000) in the habituation and test phases. Panel A: The familiar stimulus was alternating columns of black (filled) and white (unfilled) squares. In one of the two stimuli of the preference test phase the internal elements varied. Panel B: The familiar stimulus was a square frame in which two filled black squares were arranged vertically. The two stimuli of the preference test phase had identical areas and different internal elements.

face-like configurations, which usually display inner elements all with an identical shape. As a result, it is possible that the visibility of the features within a real face is lower than the visibility of the elements that characterizes schematic black and white face-like patterns. Therefore, it is possible that, within a few days from birth, infants are constrained by their limited visual capacities to discriminate and recognize faces relying on their most salient characteristics, that is the shape of the hair and the outer contour (Pascalis et al., 1995).

This hypothesis appears unlikely as demonstrated by our third set of studies. The results show that newborns were able to discriminate and recognize experimentally familiarized images of real faces in three different conditions: when the faces were fully visible, when only the inner features were visible, and when the outer features alone were visible (Turati, Macchi Cassia, Simion, & Leo, 2006). The evidence supports the conclusion that newborns are able to recognize upright faces both when faces were fully visible, and when only the inner or outer features are present. The presence of only the inner or the outer parts of the face is sufficient to produce effective recognition at birth (Turati et al., 2006). These findings are in line with the previous results demonstrating that newborns can discriminate geometrical stimuli when the external contour is identical (Farroni et al., 2000). The limited resolution capacities of the visual system at birth do not prevent few-day-old infants to discriminate the information embedded in the inner portion of stimuli (e.g., Farroni et al., 2000; Simion et al., 2002; Turati et al., 2006).

Overall, the results discussed so far support the view that recognition of face-like, geometric, and real faces is mediated by a general pattern-learning mechanism dedicated to acquiring information about any visual pattern independent of whether they are face or nonface stimuli (de Schonen, 2002; de Schonen & Mancini, 1995; Johnson, 1993; Johnson & de Haan, 2001; Pascalis & de Schonen, 1994).

Although it has been demonstrated that at birth, the inner facial features alone convey sufficient information in order to recognize a face, the data leave open the question whether newborns relied on the local or configural information. Indeed, these types of information are not independent of each other, because every change in the local information implies a change in the configuration.

What is the Nature of the Operations that Occur on Face Recognition at Birth?

In order to investigate whether, early in life, face recognition relies upon the encoding of the local facial features (local information) or configural information (e.g., Maurer et al., 2002; Rhodes, Brake, & Atkinson, 1993), we investigated whether newborns' ability to recognize individual faces is affected by orientation (Turati et al., 2006). In the available literature (e.g., Valentine, 1988; Yin, 1969), the inversion effect has been taken as diagnostic of configural processing. An analogue of the "inversion effect," similar to the one observed with adults (e.g., Leder & Bruce, 2000; Yin, 1969), has been documented in 4-month-old infants, who have been shown to be impaired in a recognition task with inverted faces as compared to upright faces (Turati, Sangrigoli, Ruel, & de Schonen, 2004). Moreover, it has been shown that stimulus inversion disrupts newborns' preference for attractive over unattractive face ("attractiveness effect"; Slater et al., 2000).

In this vein, we examined whether newborns' ability to recognize a full face or a face in which only the outer or the inner features were visible is preserved when the face is presented inverted, that is rotated 180°. Results showed that the inversion of the face differentially affected newborns' recognition in the three examined conditions. Newborns were still able to recognize a face as familiar only in the two conditions in which the external features were present (i.e., full face and external features only). In contrast, recognition was disrupted when only the inner portion of the inverted face was present. Overall, the lack of recognition for upside down faces in the inner features condition suggests that, early in life, faces are processed on the basis of configural information.

The presence of an inversion effect at birth might be interpreted as due either to face-specific processes or to the early experience that newborns accumulate in the first days of life with a monooriented stimulus such as a face. However, a third possible explanation could be put forward in terms of a general superiority effect of the global level in individual discrimination (Kimki, 1992). In both adults and infants, visual processing is dominated by configural-holistic properties, defined as properties that depend on the interrelations among the stimulus components. Line segments are discriminated better when presented in a contextual frame than when presented in isolation (i.e., pattern-line effect; Pomerantz & Pristach, 1989). These effects demonstrated that the global level that involves the use of relational information is extracted at early stages of the perceptual processing and interferes with the processing of the local features. The best example comes from a replication of the global–local paradigm (Navon, 1977) with newborns. The study utilized compounded hierarchical patterns in which larger figures (i.e., cross or rhombus) are constructed from the same set of smaller figures. In the global–local paradigm, the primacy of the holistic properties is inferred from the perceptual advantage of the global level of the stimulus over the local level (Figure 16.5).

Our results demonstrated that newborns are able to discriminate both the local and the global levels (see New-Local and New-Global conditions on Panel A, Figure 16.5). In contrast, recognition of the local features was impaired in the condition when conflicting information at the global level interfered with identification of the local features (i.e., there was an asymmetric global-to-local interference, see Panel B, Figure 16.5) (Macchi Cassia, Simion, Milani, Umiltà, 2002). The presence of an asymmetrical interference between the two levels of information, which is consistent with a global advantage effect already documented with stimuli other than faces in newborns (Macchi et al., 2002) as well as in 3-month-old infants (Ghim & Eimas, 1988), might be responsible of the inversion effect obtained in the inner features condition with faces in our study.

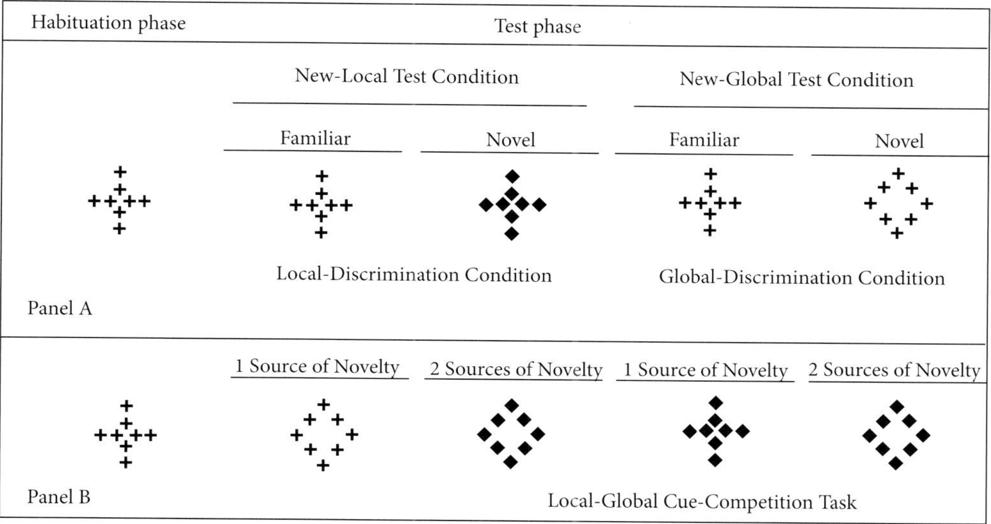

Figure 16.5 Examples of stimulus arrangements used during the habituation and test phase in Macchi Cassia et al. (2002).

When the face is in the upright orientation, newborns encode both the levels (i.e. the local and the global levels) with a superiority of the global/configural one that allows recognition of the face. In contrast, when the face is turned upside down newborns are impaired in using the global/configural information and due to the limited capacities of their visual system cannot rely upon the only use of the featural information.

Collectively, these results suggest that the visuoperceptual system at birth constrains newborns to process those coarse visual cues of a face or nonface stimuli strictly dependent on low spatial frequencies that convey configural information.

Recent evidence supports this conclusion by demonstrating that the visual information newborns use to process and recognize a face is based on low rather than high spatial frequencies bands (de Heering et al., 2008). According to some authors, young infants' poor visual acuity and contrast sensitivity limit encoding to information carried by lower spatial frequencies. The cortical neural networks begin to form stable networks on the basis of this input and will eventually become specialized for configural processing of any visual pattern–included faces (e.g., de Shonen & Mathivet, 1989). In line with this reasoning, research on infant hemispheric specialization showed that discrimination of face as well as non face stimuli in 4-month-old infants are based on configural differences carried out more effectively by the right hemisphere as compared to the left (e.g., Deruelle & de Schonen, 1991, 1998; de Schonen, Dereulle, Mancini & Pascalis, 1993). This is probably because the right hemisphere matures at a faster rate than the left hemisphere during this period of early infancy when visual input is limited to lower spatial frequencies (e.g., de Schonen & Mathivet, 1990). As result, young infants should be sensitive to configural information.

General conclusions

Evidence reviewed in this chapter is relevant to explain the factors affecting the emergence of a specialized system to process faces during the initial steps of development. The first section focuses on the mechanisms underlying infants' visual preference for faces and the results are clear in indicating that some general biases allow newborns to orient toward certain structural properties that faces share with other stimuli. More intriguing for the topic of a progressive specialization of the system to process faces are the results showing that the same general biases cannot explain face preferences at birth and 3 months later. The replication of the same experiments at these two different age levels reveals a modification in the determinants of 3-month-old infants' face preference, in that, contrary to what happens at birth, face preferences cannot be explained by general attentional biases.

At 3 months of age, face preference appears to be the product of more specific mechanisms that respond more selectively to the perceptual characteristics that distinguish faces from other stimulus categories. As already suggested by some computational models (Acerra et al., 2002; Bednar, 2003), this change in the mechanisms underlying face preference in the first months of life might be viewed as the gradual and progressive emergence of an increasingly complex system for face processing rather than the appearance of a novel and independent cortical mechanism such as Conlearn, allowing finer face encoding and thus better recognition (Gliga & Csibra, 2007). Consistent with the neocostructivistic approach, it can be suggested that as a function of experience, the nonspecific neural and functional networks become progressively specialized for processing the category of visual stimuli to which infants are most extensively exposed—that is, faces.

The same general conclusion can be extended to the processing underlying face recognition. Evidence suggests that at birth, the system seems not to be specialized to process faces because the perceptual processes carried out to recognize different categories of stimuli did not differ. The visuoperceptual system at birth permits newborns to process and to discriminate the information embedded in any visual pattern independent of whether they are face or nonface stimuli. Evidence supports the claim that the visual system at birth constraints newborns to process those coarse visual cues either of a face or nonface stimuli that convey configural information.

Overall, the pattern of results is in agreement with a neoconstructivism perspective that explains the early emergence of face processing as a result of the interaction between innate constraints and the structure of the input provided by the species-typical environment (e.g., Elman et al., 1996). Evidence from our laboratory suggests that face specificity is not prewired, but rather arises from general perceptual processes that, during development, become progressively tuned to the human face, as a result of extensive experience with this stimulus category. Consequently, face at birth would simply represent a particular exemplar of a broader category of stimuli that share common structural and configural properties. As it is suggested by recent event-related potential (e.g., de Haan & Nelson, 1999; de Haan, Pascalis, & Johnson, 2002) and behavioral studies (e.g., Pascalis et al., 2002), with increasing exposure to faces during the first months of life, the category of faces shows an increasing degree of segregation: neural and behavioral responses to this class of stimuli become more and more specific, as a result of the narrowing of the infants' perceptual window. The data presented in this chapter are in line with an experience-expectant perspective (Nelson, 2003) that emphasizes the relevance of both general constraints of the human visuoperceptual system and exposure to certain experiences shortly after birth to drive the system to become functionally specialized to process faces in the first months of life.

Acknowledgments

The studies reported in the chapter were supported by grants from the Ministero dell'Università e della Ricerca Scientifica e Tecnologica (No. 2003112997_004 and No. 2005119101_003). The authors are deeply indebted to Dr. Beatrice Dalla Barba and the nursing staff at the Pediatric Clinic of the University of Padova for their collaboration. We thank the parents and infants who participated in these studies. We thank also Sandro Bettella for writing the software.

References

Acerra, F., Burnod, I., & de Schonen, S. (2002). Modeling aspects of face processing in early infancy. *Developmental Science, 5*, 98–117.

Atkinson, J., Hood, B., Wattam-Bell, J., & Braddick, O. (1992). Changes in infants' ability to switch visual attention in the first three months of life. *Perception, 21*, 643–653.

Banks, M. S., & Salapatek, P. (1981). Infant pattern vision: A new approach based on the contrast sensitivity function. *Journal of Experimental Child Psychology, 31*, 1–45.

Barr-Haim, Y., Ziv, T., Lamy, D., & Hodes, R. M. (2006). Nature and narture in own-race face processing. *Psychological Science, 17*, 159–163.

Bartlett, J.C., & Searcy, J. (1993). Inversion and configuration of faces. *Cognitive Psychology, 25*, 281–316.

Bates, E. A., & Elman, J. L., (1993). Connectionism and the study of change. In M. Johnson (Ed.), *Brain development and cognition: A reader* (pp. 420–440). Oxford: Blackwell Publishers.

Bednar, J. A. (2003). The role of internally generated neural activity in newborn and infant face preferences. In O. Pascalis, & A. Slater (Eds.), *The development of face processing in infancy and early childhood: Current perspectives* (pp. 133–142). New York: Nova Science Publishers.

Braddick, O., Atkinson, J., Hood, B., Harkness, W., Jackson, G., & Vargha-Cadem, F. (1992). Possible blindsight in infants lacking one cerebral hemisphere. *Nature, 360*, 461–463.

Bronson, G. W. (1982). Structure, status and characteristics of the nervous system at birth. In P. Stratton (Ed.), *Psychobiology of the human newborn* (pp. 99–118). New York: Wiley.

Bushnell, I. W. R. (2001). Mother's face recognition in newborn infants: Learning and memory. *Infant and Child Development, 10*, 67–74.

Bushnell, I. W. R., Sai, F., & Mullin, J. T. (1989). Neonatal recognition of the mother's face. *British Journal of Developmental Psychology, 7*, 3–15.

Caldara, R., Seghier, M. L., Rossion, B., Lazeyras, F., Michel, C., & Hauert, C. A. (2006). The fusiform face area is tuned for curvilinear patterns with more high-contrasted elements in the upper part. *NeuroImage, 31*, 313–319.

Carey, S., & Diamond, R. (1977). From piecemeal to configurational representation of faces. *Science, 195*, 312–314.

Cheour, M., Ceponiene, R., Lehtokoski, A., Luuk, A., Allik, J., Alho, K., et al. (1998). Development of language-specific phoneme representations in the infant brain. *Nature Neuroscience, 1*, 351–353.

Chomsky, N. (1988). *Language and the problems of knowledge: The Managua lectures*. Cambridge, MA: MIT Press.

de Haan, M., & Nelson, C. A. (1999). Brain activity differentiates face and object processing by 6-month-old infants. *Developmental Psychology, 34*, 1114–1121.

de Haan, M., Pascalis, O., & Johnson, M. (2002). Specialization of neural mechanisms underlying face recognition in human infants. *Journal of Cognitive Neuroscience, 14*, 199–209.

de Heering, A., Turati, C., Rossion, B., Bulf, H., Goffaux, & Simion, F. (2008). Newborns' face recognition is based on spatial frequencies below 0.5 cycles per degree. *Cognition, 106*, 444–454.

Deruelle, C., & de Schonen, S. (1991). Hemispheric asymmetries in visual pattern processing in infancy. *Brain and Cognition, 16*, 151–179.

Deruelle, C., & de Schonen, S. (1998). Do the right and left hemispheres attend to the same visuospatial information within a face in infancy? *Developmental Neuropsychology, 14*, 535–554.

de Schonen, S. (2002). Epigenesis of the cognitive brain: a task for the 21st Century. In L. Backman & C. von Hofsten (Eds.), *Psychology at the turn of the millenium* (pp. 55–88). Hove, UK: Psychology Press.

de Schonen, S., Dereulle, C., Mancini, J., & Pascalis, O. (1993). Hemispheric differences in face processing and brain maturation. In B. de Boysson-Bardies, S. de Schonen, P. W. Jusczyk, P. McNeilage, & J. Morton (Eds.), *Developmental neurocognition: Speech and face processing in the first year of life* (pp. 149–163). Dordrecht, Netherlands: Kluwer.

de Schonen, S., Mancini, J., & Liegeois, F. (1998). About functional cortical specialization: The development of face recognition. In F. Simion & G. Butterworth (Eds.), *The development of sensory, motor, and cognitive capacities in early infancy* (pp. 103–116). Hove, UK: Psychology Press.

de Schonen, S., & Mathivet, E. (1989). First come, first served: A scenario about the development of hemispheric specialization in face recognition during infancy. *European Bulletin of Cognitive Psychology, 9*, 3–44.

de Schonen, S., & Mathivet, E. (1990). Hemispheric asymmetry in a face discrimination task in infants. *Child Development, 61*, 1192–1205.

Easterbrook, M. A., Kisilevsky, B. S., Muir, D. W., & Laplante, D. P. (1999). Newborns discriminate schematic faces from scrambled faces. *Canadian Journal of Experimental Psychology, 53*, 231–241.

Elman, J. L., Bates, E. A., Johnson, M. H., Karmiloff-Smith, A., Parisi, D., & Plunkett, K. (1996). *Rethinking innateness. A connectionist perspective on development.* Cambridge, MA: The MIT Press.

Farah, M. J., Rabinowitz, C., Quinn, G. E., & Liu, G. T. (2000). Early commitment of neural substrates for face recognition. *Cognitive Neuropsychology, 17*, 117–123.

Farroni, T., Valenza, E., Simion, F., & Umiltà, C. (2000). Configural processing at birth: Evidence for perceptual organization. *Perception, 29*, 355–372.

Fodor, J. (1983). *The modularity of mind. An essay on faculty psychology.* Cambridge, MA: The MIT Press.

Freire, A., & Lee, K. (2001). Face recognition in 4- to 7-year-old: processing of configural, featural, and paraphernalia information. *Journal of Experimental Child Psychology, 80*, 347–371.

Gauthier, I., & Logothetis, N. K. (2000). Is face recognition not so unique after all? *Cognitive Neuropsychology, 17*, 125–142.

Gauthier, I., & Tarr, M. J. (1997). Becoming a "greeble" expert: Exploring mechanisms for face recognition. *Vision Research, 37*, 1673–1682.

Gauthier, I., & Tarr, M. J. (2002). Unraveling mechanisms for expert object recognition: Bridging brain activity and behavior. *Journal of Experimental Psychology: Human Perception and Performance, 28*, 431–446.

Gauthier, I., Tarr, M. J., Anderson, A. W., Skudlarski, P., & Gore, J. C. (1999). Activation of the middle fusiform "face area" increases with expertise in recognizing novel objects. *Nature Neuroscience, 2*, 568–573.

Gauthier, I., Williams, P., Tarr, M. J., & Tanaka, J. (1998). Training "greeble" experts: A framework for studying expert object recognition processes. *Vision Research, 38*, 2401–2428.

Geldart, S., Mondloch, C. J., Maurer, D., de Schonen, S., & Brent, H. P. (2002). The effect of early visual deprivation on the development of face processing. *Developmental Science, 5*, 490–501.

Gelman, R. (1990). First principles organize attention to and learning about relevant data: number and the animate–inanimate distiction as examples. *Cognitive Science, 1*, 79–106.

Ghim, H. R., & Eimas, P. D. (1988). Global and local processing by 3- and 4-month-old infants. *Perception & Psychophysics, 43*, 165–171.

Gliga, T., & Csibra, G. (2007). Seeing the face through the eyes: A developmental perspective on face expertise. *Progress in Brain Research, 164*, 323–339.

Goren, C., Sarty, M., & Wu, P. (1975). Visual following and pattern discrimination of face-like stimuli by newborn infants. *Pediatrics, 56*, 544–549.

Greenough, W. T., & Black, J. E. (1992). Induction of brain structure by experience: Substrates for cognitive development. In M. Gunnar & C. A. Nelson (Eds.), *Behavioral developmental neuroscience. Vol. 24. Minnesota symposia on child psychology* (pp. 35–52). Hillsdale, NJ: Erlbaum.

Halit, H., de Haan, M., & Johnson, M. H. (2003). Cortical specialization for face processing: Face sensitive event-related potential components in 3- and 12-month-old infants. *Neuroimage, 19*, 1180–1193.

Hole, G. J. (1994). Configurational factors in the perception of unfamiliar faces. *Perception, 23*, 65–74.

Johnson, M. H. (1993). Constraints on cortical plasticity. In M. J. Johnson (Eds.), *Brain development and cognition. A reader* (pp. 703–721). Cambridge, MA: Blackwell.

Johnson, M. H. (1995). The development of visual attention: A cognitive neuroscience perspective. In M. S. Gazzaniga (Ed.), *The cognitive neurosciences* (pp. 735–747). Cambridge, MA: MIT Press.

Johnson, M. H. (1997). *Developmental Cognitive Neuroscience: An Introduction.* Oxford: Blackwell.

Johnson, M. H. (2005). Subcortical face processing. *Nature Reviews Neuroscience*, 6, pp. 766–774.

Johnson, M. H., & de Haan, M. (2001). Developing cortical specialization for visual-cognitive function: The case of face recognition. In J. L. McClelland & R. S. Seigler (Eds.), *Mechanisms of cognitive development: Behavioral and neural perspectives* (pp. 253–270). Mahwah, NJ: Erlbaum.

Johnson, M. H., Dziurawiec, S., Ellis, H., & Morton, J. (1991). Newborns' preferential tracking of face-like stimuli and its subsequent decline. *Cognition, 40*, 1–19.

Johnson, M. H., & Morton, J. (1991). *Biology and cognitive development. The case of face recognition.* Oxford, England: Basil Blackwell.

Kanwisher, N. (2000). Domain specificity in face perception. *Nature Neuroscience, 3*, 759–763.

Karmiloff-Smith, A. (1992). *Beyond modularity.* Cambridge, MA: MIT Press.

Kellman, P. J. (1993). Kinematic foundations of infant visual perception. In C. Granrud,

Visual perception and cognition in infancy (pp. 121–173). Hillsdale, NJ: Erlbaum.

Kelly, D. J., Liu, S., Ge, L., Quinn, P. C., Slater, A. M., Lee, K., et al. (2007). Cross-race preferences for Same-race faces extend beyond the Afreican versus Caucasian contrast in 3-month-old infants. *Infancy, 11*, 87–95.

Kelly, D. J., Quinn, P. C., Slater, A. M., Lee, K., Gibson, A., Smith, M., et al. (2005). Three-month-olds, but not newborns, prefer own-race faces. *Developmental Science, 8*, F31–F36.

Kimki, R. (1992). Primacy of wholistic processing and global/local paradigm: A critical review. *Psychological Bulletin, 112*, 24–38.

Kleiner, K.A. (1987). Amplitude and phase spectra as indices of infants' pattern preferences. *Infant Behavior & Development, 10*, 49–59.

Kleiner, K. A., & Banks, M. S. (1987). Stimulus energy does not account for 2-month-old infants' face preference. *Journal of Experimental Psychology: Human, Perception and Performance, 13*, 594–600.

Kuhl, P. K., Williams, K. A., Lacerda, F., Stevens, K. N., & Lindblom, B. (1992). Linguistic experience alters phonetic perception in infants by 6 months of age. *Science, 255*, 606–608.

Leder, H., & Bruce, V. (2000). When inverted faces are recognized: The role of configural information in face recognition. *The Quartely Journal of Experimental Psychology A, 53*, 513–536.

Le Grand, R., Mondloch, C. J., Maurer, D., & Brent, H. P. (2003). Expert face processing requires visual input to the right hemisphere during infancy. *Nature Neuroscience, 6*, 1108–1112.

Macchi Cassia, V., Kuefner, D., Westerlund, A., & Nelson, C. A. (2006). Modulation of face-sensitive event-related potentials by canonical and distorted human faces: The role of vertical symmetry and up-down featural arrangement. *Journal of Cognitive Neuroscience, 18*, 1343–1358.

Macchi Cassia, V., Simion, F., Milani, I., & Umiltà, C. (2002). Dominance of global visual properties at birth. *Journal of Experiment Psychology: General, 131*, 398–411.

Macchi Cassia, V., Simion, F., & Umiltà, C. (2001). Face preference at birth: The role of an orienting mechanism. *Developmental Science, 4*, 101–108.

Macchi Cassia V., Turati C., & Simion, F. (2004). Can a non specific bias toward top-heavy patterns explain newborns' face preference? *Psychological Science, 15*, 379–383.

Macchi Cassia, V., Valenza, E., Simion, F., & Leo, I. (2008). Congruency as a non-specific perceptual property contributing to newborns' face preference. *Child Development, 79*, 807–820.

Maurer, D., Le Grand, R., & Mondloch, C. J. (2002). The many faces of configural processing. *Trends in Cognitive Sciences, 6*, 255–260.

Michel, G. F., & Moore, C. L. (1995). *Developmental psychobiology: An integrative science.* Cambridge, MA: MIT Press.

Morton, J., & Johnson, M. H. (1991). CONSPEC and CONLEARN: A two-process theory of infant face recognition. *Psychological Review, 98*, 164–181.

Navon, D. (1977). Forest before trees: The precedence of global features in visual perception. *Cognitive Psychology, 9*, 353–383.

Nelson, C. A. (2001). The development and neural bases of face recognition. *Infant and Child Development, 10*, 3–18.

Nelson, C. A. (2003). The development of face recognition reflects an experience-expectant and activity-dependent process. In O. Pascalis & A. Slater (Eds.), *The development of face processing in infancy and early childhood: Current perspectives* (pp. 79–97). New York: Nova Science Publishers.

Nelson, C. A., & Luciana, M. (Eds.). (2001) *Handbook of developmental cognitive neuroscience.* Cambridge, MA: MIT Press.

Pascalis, O., de Haan, M., & Nelson, C. A. (2002). Is face processing species-specific during the first year of life? *Science, 296*, 1321–1323.

Pascalis, O., & de Schonen, S. (1994). Recognition memory in 3- to 4-day-old human neonates. *Neuroreport, 5*, 1721–1724.

Pascalis, O., de Schonen, S., Morton, J., Deruelle, C., & Fabre-Grenet, M. (1995). Mother's face recognition by neonates: A replication and an extension. *Infant Behavior & Development, 18*, 79–85.

Pomerantz, J. R., & Pristach, E. A. (1989). Emergent features, attention, and perceptual glue in visual form perception. *Journal of Experimental Psychology: Human Perception and Performance, 15*, 635–649.

Rhodes, G., Brake, S., Atkinson, A. P. (1993) What's lost in inverted faces? *Cognition, 47*, 25–57.

Schwaninger, A., Carbon, C. C., & Leder, H. (2003). Expert face processing: Specialization and constraints. In G. Schwarzer & H. Leder (Eds.), *Development of face processing* (pp. 81–97). Gottingen: Hogrefe.

Searcy, J. H., & Bartlett, J. C. (1996). Inversion and processing of component and spatial-relational information in faces. *Journal of Experimental Psychology: Human Perception and Performance, 22,* 904–915.

Simion, F., Farroni, T., Macchi Cassia, V., Turati, C., & Dalla Barba, B. (2002). Newborns' local processing in schematic face-like configurations. *British Journal of Developmental Psychology, 20,* 465–478.

Simion, F., Macchi Cassia, V., Turati, C., & Valenza, E. (2001). The origins of face perception: Specific vs. non-specific mechanisms. *Infant and Child Development, 10,* 59–65.

Simion, F., Macchi Cassia, V., Turati, C., & Valenza, E. (2003). Non-specific perceptual biases at the origins of face processing. In O. Pascalis & A. Slater (Eds.), *The development of face processing in infancy and early childhood: Current perspectives.* (pp. 13–25). New York: Nova Science Publishers.

Simion, F., Turati, C., Valenza, E., & Leo, I. (2006). The emergence of cognitive specialization in infancy: The case of face preference. In M. Johnson & M. Munakata (Eds.), *Processes of Change in Brain Development: Attention and Performance XXI* (pp. 189–208). Oxford: University Press.

Simion, F., Valenza, E., Macchi Cassia, V., Turati, C., & Umiltà, C. (2002). Newborns' preference for up-down asymmetrical configurations. *Developmental Science, 5,* 427–434.

Slater, A., Bremner, G., Johnson, S.P., Sherwood, P., Hayes, R., & Brown, E. (2000). Newborn infants' preference for attractive faces: The role of internal and external facial features. *Infancy, 1,* 265–274.

Slater, A., Earle, D.C., Morison, V., & Rose, D. (1985). Pattern preferences at birth and their interaction with habituation induced novelty preferences. *Journal of Experimental Child Psychology, 39,* 37–54.

Slater, A., & Sykes, M. (1977). Newborn infants' responses to square-wave gratings. *Child Development, 48,* 545–553.

Spelke, E.S. (1991). Physical knowledge in infancy: Reflections on Piaget's theory. In S. Carey & R. Gelman (Eds.) *The epigenesis of mind: Essays on biology and cognition* (pp. 133–169). Hilsdale, NJ: Erlbaum.

Sprague, J.M., Berlucchi, G., & Rizzolatti, G. (1973). The role of the superior colliculus and pretectum in vision and visually guided behavior. In R. Jung (Ed.), *Handbook of sensory physiology* (Vol. 7, pp. 27–101). Berlin: Springer-Verlag.

Tanaka, J.W., & Farah, T. (1993). Parts and wholes in face recognition. *The Quarterly Journal of Experimental Psychology A, 46,* 225–245.

Turati, C., Macchi Cassia, V., Simion F., & Leo, I. (2006). Newborns' face recognition: The role of inner and outer facial features. *Child Development, 77,* 297–311.

Turati, C., Sangrigoli, S., Ruel, J., & de Schonen, S. (2004). Evidence of the face-inversion effect in 4-month-old infants. *Infancy, 6,* 275–297.

Turati, C., Simion, F., Milani, I., & Umiltà, C. (2002). Newborns preference for faces: What is crucial? *Developmental Psychology, 38,* 875–882.

Turati, C., Valenza, E., Leo, I., & Simion, F. (2005). Three-month-old visual preference for faces and its underlying visual processing mechanisms. *Journal of Experimental Child Psychology, 90,* 255–273.

Turkewitz, G., & Kenny, P. A. (1982). Limitations on input as a basis for neural organization and perceptual development: a preliminary theroretical statement. *Developmental Psychobiology, 15,* 357–368.

Tzourio-Mazoyer, N., de Schonen, S., Crivello, F., Reutter, B., Aujard, Y., & Mazoyer, B. (2002). Neural correlates of woman face processing by 2-month-old infants. *Neuroimage, 15,* 454–461.

Valentine, T. (1988). Upside-down faces: A review of the effect of inversion upon face recognition. *British Journal of Psychology, 79,* 471–491.

Valenza, E., Simion, F., Macchi Cassia, V., & Umiltà, C. (1996). Face preference at birth. *Journal of Experimental Psychology: Human Perception and Performance, 22,* 892–903.

Walton, G. E., Bower, N. J. A., & Bower, T. G. R. (1992). Recognition of familiar faces by newborns. *Infant Behavior & Development, 15,* 265–269.

Werker, J. F., & Vouloumanos, A. (2001). Speech and language processing in infancy: A neurocognitive approach. In C.A. Nelson & M. Luciana (Eds.), *Handbook of Developmental Cognitive Neuroscience* (pp. 269–280). Cambridge, Mass: MIT Press.

Wynn, K. (1995). Origins of numerical knowledge. *Mathematical Cognition, 1,* 35–60.

Yin, R. K. (1969). Looking at upside-down faces. *Journal of Experimental Child Psychology, 81,* 141–145.

Young, A. W., Hellawell, D., & Hay, D. C., (1987). Configural information in face perception. *Perception, 16,* 747–759.

PART VI

The Big Picture

CHAPTER 17
A Bottom-up Approach to Infant Perception and Cognition: A Summary of Evidence and Discussion of Issues

Leslie B. Cohen

As the author of the final chapter in this book, I have been given the impossible task of summarizing and evaluating the evidence reported by all the previous speakers at this conference. We were all also given instructions to emphasize general methodological and theoretical issues, the "big picture" so to speak, rather than the details of specific studies. Although I cannot possibly do the former, I will try to do the latter and in so doing will at least raise some of the issues mentioned by other speakers.

The evolution of research on infant perception and cognition over the past 50 years has been truly astounding. In the 1950s and 1960s, infants were blasted with bright lights and loud noises while their reflexive responses were being measured. In the late 1960s and 1970s, it was discovered that infants preferred to look longer at something novel than at something familiar and this preference was exploited to study infant memory. From the mid-1970s through the 1980s, it became clear that one could not understand how well an infant remembered until one knew what the infant remembered. That realization, in turn, led to the use of habituation and related memory paradigms as tools to investigate infant visual and auditory information processing. An explosion of studies appeared on basic visual, auditory, speech, and intermodal perception. In the 1980s and 1990s, the types of information processing attributed to infants became more relational, more abstract, i.e., more cognitive. Infants' ability to categorize, their understanding of causal relations, and their knowledge of objects, events, and even simple rules were just some of the topics being investigated. Finally, as we enter the new century, infant cognition and information processing is becoming more integrated with infant language acquisition. Sensitivity to correlated information and statistical regularities are being shown to be critically important to language segmentation, the formation of syntactic regularities, and categorical structure.

As great as these advances have been, most research on these topics has tended to suffer from one glaring weakness, a lack of emphasis on development and the mechanisms underlying developmental change. To be sure, a reasonable percentage of published studies have tested infants at different ages. Some of them have even reported interesting age differences, i.e., differences other than younger infants cannot do what older ones can do. But rarely, have they taken the next step and attempted to describe or explain the principles or mechanisms by which these changes occur. A couple of real exceptions have been the books by Karmiloff-Smith (1992) who explained how a modular organization of some cognitive ability can develop gradually

This chapter is based upon a paper presented at NSF Sponsored Workshop: A Neoconstructivist Approach to Early Cognitive Development. New York, October, 2006.

through experience, and the book by Elman et al. (1996) that showed how connectionist models do, in fact, make explicit assumptions about mechanisms of developmental change.

Constructivist Principles of Developmental Change

Over the years, our laboratory has investigated many different aspects of infant perception and cognition. Most of these investigations have looked specifically at developmental changes in infants' information processing abilities. From these studies, as well as from those reported by many other investigators, we have found some striking similarities. Infants often seem to progress in a bottom-up fashion. That is, infants initially appear to process simple isolated units, and then move to the relationship or integration of those simple units into higher-order units. Furthermore, this appears to be a domain-general progression. This progression has been reported on many topics from simple form and object perception, to complex face identification, to an understanding of moving objects in causal events, and even to an infant's ability to learn word–object associations. We have summarized much of this evidence previously (e.g., Cohen & Cashon, 2003, 2006), and that evidence has led us to formulate the following set of constructivist principles to describe these developmental changes:

1. *Infants are endowed with a hierarchical information processing system.* This statement simply affirms that infants can process information at multiple levels of abstraction.

2. *Infants form higher units from relationships among lower units.* These relationships may be correlational, conditional, or even causal. By far, most research to date has examined relations that based upon correlations or statistical associations.

3. *Higher units serve as components for still-higher units.* This proposition simply asserts the bottom-up or constructivist nature of this hierarchy. For example, Object A may come to be associated with one type of movement, M1, and become Moving Object A. Similarly, Object B and its movement, M2, may become associated as Moving Object B. Then, when Moving Object A repeatedly precedes and makes contact with Object B, leading to Moving Object B, the entire sequence can be organized as a conditional or even a causal event (Cohen, Amsel, Redford, & Casasola, 1998).

4. *There is a bias to process information using the highest-formed units available.* This is really a simplifying assumption. Given that someone can process information at multiple levels, it usually will be more efficient to begin at the highest, most inclusive or abstract level available. When an infant is looking at her mother, it certainly would be more appropriate and adaptive for her to process the mother's face and her actions as a whole, rather than trying to process the eye, the eyebrow, the relationship between the eye and the hairline, the configuration of those parts with the rest of the face, the mouth and its movement, etc. all separately either in series or in parallel.

5. *If higher units do not respond, lower units are utilized.* This is really a fallback provision. There are occasions when attempting to process information at the highest level available fails for some reason. On those occasions, people (including infants) do not automatically give up. Instead, they often will drop down to a lower level and attempt to process information at that level. Assimilating information at that level eventually may lead them back to a higher level. One could consider this provision an instance of top-down processing rather than bottom-up processing.

This fallback tends to occur when the system is overloaded. In our research, we have found examples of infants falling to a lower level when

(a) the complexity of the task is increased,
(b) the infant has to process a category rather than a single instance,
(c) uncertainty or noise is added to the task, and
(d) some additional meaning is added to the task

Several examples of this fallback provision with infants will be described later in this chapter.

6. *These principles apply throughout development and across domains.* These principles can be seen to apply to many different tasks at many different ages. No particular level or unit being processed is tied to one particular age. It is not the case that 4-month-olds always process information in an elementary form and 6-month-olds always process it in an integrated form. The unit of processing at any one age is more a function of the level of expertise on a particular task. In fact, these principles may be more appropriately considered principles of learning rather than principles of development. As one learns a new task, whether it is to ride a bicycle, play Monopoly, or use Excel, one begins by acquiring some basic elements such as how to pedal, move a piece, or enter a number. However, once a person becomes relatively proficient at that level, he/she operates at an entirely different level, going to the store, owning a whole row, or analyzing a set of data. The same may be true for an infant. But the tasks are more basic and immediate, recognizing a face, getting fed, predicting an object's movement. This point will be raised again toward the end of the chapter. Perhaps infant perceptual-cognitive development and learning (i.e., the development of expertise in some domain) are not that different. It is just that infants gradually are becoming experts about the immediate physical and social worlds around them.

Evidence for Constructivist Principles

Evidence for these principles has been reported many times in the past. A detailed account of much of this evidence has been presented most recently in Cohen and Cashon (2006). I will not attempt to duplicate that account here. Instead I will summarize briefly several examples of developmental changes occurring across a variety of different topics within infant perception and cognition. It should be obvious from this account that similar types of changes occur repeatedly but that the ages involved depend upon the particular topic or skill. Almost all of these studies used some version of a habituation or familiarization paradigm in which infants were familiarized with one or more habituation stimuli and then tested with novel and familiar stimuli to determine if infants responded differently to the two.

1. *Angle perception studies.* One of the earliest set of studies we conducted on this topic examined developmental changes in infants' perception of a simple angle (Cohen & Younger, 1984). In these studies, 6- and 12-week-old infants were habituated to an acute 45° angle made with thick black lines. The infants were then shown four test angles, in counterbalanced order. One angle was identical to the one presented during habituation. It, *AfOf*, was the familiar angle with lines in familiar orientations. A second angle, *AfOn*, was the familiar angle rotated so that the lines were in novel orientations. The third, *AnOf*, was a novel 135° angle, but the line orientations were familiar. They were the same as in the 45° angle used in habituation. Finally, the fourth, *AnOn*, was a novel angle with novel line orientations. The results were clear-cut. Six-week-olds looked longer only when the orientation of the lines changed (i.e., at *AfOn* and *AnOn*). In contrast, the 12-week-olds looked longer only when the angle changed (i.e., at *AnOf* and *AnOn*). These results indicated that 6-week-olds were processing one or more individual line segments, while 12-week-olds were integrating those line segments into complete angles.

Alan Slater (Slater, 1995; Slater, Mattock, Brown, & Bremner, 1991) replicated this study with 1-month-old infants and found they too responded to a change in line segment orientation. He then turned the study into a category task by habituating infants to the same angle, but on each trial in a different rotation. Now he claimed they were responding to the angle since in the test they looked longer at a novel angle than at the familiar angle. However, he admits that there may be a simpler possibility. They may be responding to the "size of the blob" at the apex of the angle. An acute angle has a larger low spatial frequency "blob" at its apex than does an obtuse angle. This "blob theory" is supported by another study reported by Slater and Morrison (reported in Slater, 1995) that showed infants had to be 3 months of age before they responded categorically to a simple geometric shape. Thus, it was unlikely that 1-month-old infants in Slater et al. (1991) were responding categorically. If, on the contrary, infants were responding to the size of the blob, then one could claim both that infants progress from processing individual line segments to entire angles and that turning the task into a category problem made it more difficult, and as a consequence, infants fell back to yet a simpler way of processing the angle (i.e., in terms of the size of the blob). Both claims, of course, would be consistent with the constructivist principles stated earlier.

2. *Object unity studies.* In a classic set of studies reported by Kellman and Spelke (1983), 4-month-old infants were habituated to a rod moving left and right (i.e., translating) behind an occluder. Only the top and bottom portions of the rod were visible. In the test phase of the experiment, the occluder was absent and infants saw either the pieces of the rod they had seen before or the entire rod. Infants looked longer at the separated pieces. The authors concluded that the common motion of the upper and lower pieces produced the perception, or inference, of an entire rod. Many subsequent studies examined the limits of this perception of object unity (see Johnson, 2000 for one review) but for my purposes among the most interesting are those by Slater, Johnson, Kellman, and Spelke (1994) and by Slater, Johnson, Brown, and Badenoch (1996) that showed newborns do exactly the opposite. They look longer at the solid rod than at the separated pieces. If one wishes to argue that infants at 4 months are integrating the pieces into a solid rod, then by the same logic, one should argue that newborns are perceiving the separate pieces, a view consistent with our constructivist principles.

Furthermore, additional evidence by Eizenman and Bertenthal (1998) indicates another developmental change between 4 and 6 months of age. If the partially hidden rod is seen rotating (like a propeller) rather than translating from left to right, 4-month-olds fall back and respond to the separate pieces as familiar. They have to be 6 months of age before they respond to the entire rod as familiar. If one assumes that a rotating rod is more complex than a translating rod by virtue of the continuing changing rod/occluder angle, then research on object unity provides additional evidence for the fallback provision.

3. *Face perception studies.* Infant face perception has been and continues to be a very popular area of investigation. One topic within that area is how infants perceive and organize the features of a face. We have both examined and written extensively about this topic (e.g., Cashon & Cohen, 2003, 2004; Cohen & Cashon, 2001) and our conclusions have been that developmental changes between 3 and 7 months of age tend to follow our constructivist principles. The procedure we used is an instance of the "switch design" in which infants are habituated to two separate pictures of female faces and then are tested with a familiar face, a new face, and most critically, a composite constructed by combining the external features of one face with the internal features of the other, familiar face. The question is whether infants respond to the composite face as old or new. If they treat it as new, it must be because they are relating the external with the internal features. We tested infants with both upright and inverted faces. What we found was an interesting series of developmental changes. At 3 months of age, infants treated the composite face, both upright and inverted, as old suggesting they were processing independent features. By 4 months of age, they responded to both upright and inverted composites as new, suggesting they were now processing the relationship among internal and external features. This pattern of results, of course, fits with our constructivist view. At 6 months of age, they reverted back to responding to the composites as old. However at 7 to 10 months of age, they differentiated between inverted and upright faces. Inverted composite faces were still processed as old but upright composite faces were new once again. Our interpretation was that infants had indeed advanced from processing independent features at 3 months to processing the relationship among features at 4 months. Faces, of course, were very interesting, moving stimuli with both visual and auditory components. However, by

6 months of age, faces were far more. They were social, personal, interactive, perhaps, even more than that. During their waking hours, infants spent much of their time in a sitting position and faces were becoming more meaningful when seen upright than when seen inverted. This additional meaningful component tended to overload their processing system temporarily and the infants reverted to a simpler way of processing. By 7 months of age, that meaningful component was incorporated (assimilated) into their understanding of a face and now they processed upright and inverted faces differentially.

4. *Causal perception studies.* Of all topics available within infant perception and cognition, our laboratory has made the most extensive study of infant causal perception and its development. Research on infant causal perception was originally inspired by Michotte (1963) who showed that when adults see one spot move laterally, hit a second spot that then begins to move, they perceive the event as the first spot causing or initiating the second spot's movement. In groundbreaking work with infants, Leslie (Leslie, 1982, 1986; Leslie & Keeble, 1987) found a similar phenomenon with 6-month-old infants. He made a movie of an event in which one block moved across a screen, hit, and directly launched a second block. He also made a slight variation of the event in which a delay occurred between the first block's contact and movement of the second block, and a variation in which a spatial gap remained between the first and second blocks. By habituating infants to one event and then testing on these other events, Leslie found that 6-month-olds treated the direct launching (i.e., causal) differently from the others and concluded that infants perceive the causal relation in the direct launching event.

We began by replicating Leslie's results with 6-month-olds. We (Cohen & Amsel, 1998) then tested younger infants and found that 4-month-olds responded to the continuous movement and 5.5-month-olds responded to both spatial and temporal differences between events, but not to the causality. Thus, a constructivist developmental progression appeared once again. However, that was just one part of the story. When we made the task more complex by using pictures of realistic toys rather than squares or circles 6 month olds could no longer do it (Cohen & Oakes, 1993). They had to be 10 months of age before they could perceive the causality. Furthermore, when we made that task more complex by using different toys on each trial, thereby turning it into a category problem, even the 10-month-old infants could not do it and reverted back to processing the spatial and temporal differences between events, but not the causality. Thus, we found evidence for the fallback as well.

Finally, we made the event more complex by embedding the simple direct launching event in a longer sequence (Cohen, Rundell, Spellman, & Cashon, 1999). We called these events "causal chains." Object A hit Object B that then hit Object C producing a change in Object C. We varied whether Objects A and B were involved in a direct launching or a delayed launching. This event was beyond the ability of 10-month-olds to process. They only noticed a change in Object A. Fifteen-month-olds, on the other hand, seemed to be able to handle the entire event. They tended to key on the causal agent, whether it was the first object (in the direct launching version) or the second object (in the delayed launching version). Then, we made the task even more complex by turning it into a category problem. Only the causality remained consistent. Individual objects could be involved in either causal or noncausal relationships (Cohen, Cashon, & Rundell, 2004). Now only 18-month-old infants seemed to understand the event.

So our study of infant causal perception has provided us with considerable evidence of the information processing principles stated earlier. Infants progressed through multiple levels, each constructed from the relationship among units at lower levels. At each of these levels, they also fell back to a simpler level when the information became too complex and the system became overloaded.

5. *Infant categorization.* For at least 30 years (e.g., Cohen & Caputo, 1978; Cohen & Strauss, 1977), researchers have known that infants can form concepts and categories. The minimal definition of such categorization is that infants

respond equivalently to discriminably different members of the category. In summarizing research on infant categorization, Cohen and Younger (1983) made a distinction that I believe still holds today. They divided such research into "demonstration" studies and "process" studies. Demonstration studies show that infants can respond on the basis of some category. There are now innumerable studies that indicate infants can respond to faces versus nonfaces, dogs versus cats; animals versus vehicles, items above a line versus items below a line etc. (e.g., Quinn, Adams, Kennedy, Shettler, & Wasnik, 2003; Quinn & Eimas, 2000; Quinn, Eimas, & Rosenkrantz, 1993).

One problem with many of these studies, particularly those that use natural categories, is that it is unknown to what extent infants learned these categories in the familiarization phase of the experiment and to what extent they knew something about these categories prior to entering into the experiment. A second problem is that most of these studies do not pay sufficient attention the information processing aspect of the task, that is how infants are processing individual exemplars and how that processing may change over age. Why do investigators often use simple two-dimensional shapes with infants under 6 months of age and more complex line drawings or photographs with infants later in their first year of life, and why do they tend to use moving animation or three-dimensional toys in the second year? These differences in types of stimuli employed at different ages seems to approximate those we discussed when referring to infant causal perception, but why certain types of stimuli are most appropriate at certain ages is rarely, if ever, given much emphasis in the infant categorization literature. Even when the most appropriate type of stimulus for a particular age is used, it often is unclear how the infant is processing that stimulus. Are they processing some subset of the features of the exemplars shown such as only the internal or external features? Are they really processing animals versus vehicles or legs versus wheels (Rakison & Butterworth, 1998)? To what extent do functional characteristics, as opposed to structural characteristics play a role in category assignment (Madole & Oakes, 1999)? These are just some of the questions whose answers require "process" studies.

In order to examine the processes underlying category acquisition one must (1) employ artificial categories the infant has not experienced previously and (2) manipulate the category exemplars to determine how the infant is processing and organizing them. Barbara Younger and I reported several such studies back in the 1980s (Younger & Cohen, 1983, 1986). These studies also provided some of the earliest evidence for the constructivist information processing principles stated above. The studies presented infants with line drawings of artificial animals. Several features varied from animal to animal, such as the type of ears, tail, body, and number and type of legs. In one set of experiments (Younger & Cohen, 1986) these feature values were tightly correlated with one another so that one animal always had fluffy ears, a horse tail, a giraffe-like body, and four long legs, while another animal always had antlers, a bunny tail, a bear-like body, and two short legs. Using the switch design with these animal stimuli, we showed that 4-month-old infants appeared to process the separate features or parts, but both 7- and 10-month-old infants were sensitive to the relationship among the parts. This developmental pattern fit nicely with our constructivist viewpoint.

Then we made the task more difficult. We designed animals in which only a subset of the features were correlated with one another. The remaining features varied randomly. This change essentially converted the task from requiring processing of two separate animals to processing two different animal categories. As before, 4-month-olds just processed the separate features, and 10-month-olds processed the relationship among features (i.e., in this case the categories). It was the 7-month-olds who were the most interesting. In the two-object task, they had responded like 10-month-olds. Now in the two-category task, they responded like 4-month-olds. Apparently turning it into a category task overloaded the system for 7-month-olds and they fell back to a simpler level of processing.

6. *Early word learning.* One of the greatest accomplishments during the 12- to 18-month age period is the ability to comprehend and then produce meaningful words. Most experimental studies of infant word learning are of relatively recent origin (Schafer & Plunkett, 1998; Werker, Cohen, Lloyd, Casasola, & Stager, 1998). In one set of studies, we used the switch design to see at what age infants would learn to associate a word with an object in a short period of time. Infants from 8 to 14 months of age were habituated to two different objects (i.e., a toy truck and a toy dog) each paired with its own nonsense label (i.e., "lif" and "neem"). The critical item in the test phase included both an object and label that were familiar, but the pairing between them was switched. Only the 14-month-old infants responded to this switch as novel, thereby demonstrating they had learned the association between the word and object. Additional control studies indicated that the younger infants could indeed discriminate between the two objects or between the two labels. They just were not forming the association between a label and an object. Thus, even infant early word learning appears to follow the bottom-up pattern predicted by the constructivist principles. Infants first learn the lower-order units (the labels and the object). Only later do they learn the relationship between them.

But that is not the entire story with respect to infant word learning. When the labels used are minimal pairs (e.g., "bih" vs. "dih"), 14-month-olds can no longer form the association with the objects. They can discriminate between the labels, however, when no objects are used, it is just that the word learning task seems to be beyond their capacity (Stager & Werker, 1997). By 17 to 20 months of age, though, they do solve this minimal pairs word-learning task as shown by the switch design (Werker et al., 2002). However, 14-month-old infants can solve minimal pairs word-learning task using the switch design when both words and objects are familiar (e.g., "ball" vs. "doll"; Fennell & Werker, 1997).

Fennell and Werker argue that this entire pattern of results can be explained by a "resource limitation" hypothesis. According to their hypothesis, by 14 months of age, the switch design becomes more than a simple association task for the infant. Infants are attempting to learn that specific words refer to specific objects and that adds additional meaningfulness to the task. Making the task more difficult by testing with minimal pairs exceeds their processing resources and infants revert to a simpler way of processing the information. By 17 to 20 months of age, infants have overcome this limitation and can now solve minimal pair word-learning tasks. One prediction from the resource limitation hypothesis, which Fennell and Werker found to be correct, was that if the required resources were reduced by use of familiar word–object pairs (e.g., ball and doll), then even 14-month-olds would succeed on the switch design task. From our point of view, this resource hypothesis view of early word learning is entirely consistent with our constructivist principles including the bottom-up forming of an association, the fallback to a simpler level when the task becomes overloaded, and the reconstruction to a higher level at an older age.

What can we conclude so far?

I hope this limited presentation of evidence, and similar evidence exists on additional topics as well, is persuasive that many aspects of infant perceptual, cognitive, and even early language development can be described in terms of the constructivist principles mentioned in this chapter. If that supposition is correct, then we can reach a number of conclusions.

1. *These principles are domain general.* They apply to the development of many different abilities from simple angle and form perception to more abstract cognitive abilities such as categorization, the understanding of causal events, and even some aspects of linguistic reference.

2. *These principles apply across a wide age range.* Examples have been provided from birth through 18 months. So it would be inaccurate to argue that infants process simple units at one age and more complex relations among those units at a specified later age. What counts as a unit is itself relative and depends upon the ability or task that is to be mastered.

3. *The bottom-up aspect of these principles applies more to initial acquisition than to subsequent use.* Once infants have acquired an advanced level of processing, they will tend to operate at that level unless something overloads the system. In that case, they will temporarily drop to a lower level. So one could argue this aspect of the principles is really top-down rather than bottom-up.

4. *The operation of these principles blurs the distinction between development and learning.* Assuming the domain generality of these principles and their applicability even to adult skills or abilities, the mechanisms of developmental change and those of learning or acquisition of expertise seem to overlap. These principles highlight some of the processes involved but they do not really specify the underlying mechanisms of change. An understanding of these mechanisms requires models that actually produce developmental changes consonant with the empirical evidence. Hopefully, these models will also be consistent with the constructionist principles outlined earlier in this chapter.

Connectionist Modeling to the Rescue?

One approach to explanation that has shown some promise in infant perception and cognition is called connectionist or neural-net modeling. (For examples, see the chapters by Christiansen, Dale, and Reali and by Mareschal and Westermann in this volume.) Many types of connectionist models have been proposed, but they all simulate a neural network to some degree in that they have input nodes that feed to intermediate networks that reorganize with experience and lead to some type of output. A few connectionist models have been described in detail in other chapters of this volume. Many of the early models related to infancy dealt with language acquisition and were a reaction to nativist assertions that the most important aspects of language were innate (Elman et al., 1996). Today, more and more of these models are presented as explanations for some topic within infant perception and cognition, including most of the topics described earlier in this chapter (see Cohen & Cashon, 2006). Connectionist models have several appealing characteristics:

1. *The models are explicit as to the nature of the input and the architecture.* The input nodes are usually numerical codings of a set of simple features and the internal architecture usually includes a network of weighted interrelationships produced by the input. Thus, in this sense at least, many of these models are consistent with our constructivist principles.

2. *The models tend to include actual mechanisms of change (or parameters of learning).* In fact, they are designed to change and reorganize as a function of repeated inputs and often feedback about the errors being made.

3. *They tend to simulate the behavior they were designed to explain.* Several of these models were designed to simulate specific results from specific experiments on topics such as object unity, categorization, or causal perception. They usually do a reasonable job in reproducing those results.

The models also have had some serious limitations:

1. Some suffer from architectural problems such as catastrophic interference. The model might gradually learn but then that learning can be undone by one negative instance.
2. Some might question whether too much of the work is built into the input nodes. Certainly one does not have to be a complete reductionist and assume input nodes must reflect biochemical changes in sensory receptors. On the other hand, one does not want to put too much explanatory power into sophisticated inputs. In that case, the actual learning of the model may be relatively trivial compared to what the inputs are assumed to be processing.
3. Some people question the neurological reality of certain types of models. One common learning mechanism used in models is backward propagation, which some argue does not occur neurologically in the brain. Of course, the reasonableness of this criticism depends upon the goal of the modeler. If the modeler is trying to provide an accurate

representation of the brain, the criticism is valid. However, if the modeler is just trying to reproduce the behavior of the infant given certain inputs, then the criticism may not hold.

4. Finally, most models of infant perception or cognition deal with performance at one particular age. Those that do look at developmental change tend to do so in a rather superficial way. Often the modeler will assume that development can be predicted from number of epochs the model has experienced with the training stimuli. Certainly actual developmental change involves much more than the amount of training including perhaps changes in the structure of the model itself (e.g., Shultz, 2003).

Recent Approaches to Modeling Infant Cognitive Development

Recently, I have taken two different approaches to foster connectionist modeling of infant cognitive development. The first has been to challenge modelers from three different laboratories, with somewhat different theoretical approaches, to model the same developmental data. These data came from the Younger and Cohen (1983, 1986) experiments on infant categorization mentioned earlier in this chapter. To recall, the experiments presented line drawings of animals to 4-, 7-, and 10-month-old infants. The 4-month-olds processed the separate features. Ten-month-olds processed the correlation among the features, and 7-month-olds processed the correlation when the task was simple involving only two animals. However, when the task was more complex involving two categories of animals, rather than just two animals, the 7-month-olds reverted to a lower level and processed separate features, as had the 4-month-olds.

Three different models (Gureckis & Love, 2004; Shultz & Cohen, 2004; Westermann & Mareschal, 2004) attempted to reproduce the developmental changes reported by Younger and Cohen. All three models were able to simulate the transition from independent features (shown at 4 months) to correlated features (shown at 10 months), but each model made somewhat different assumptions. Westermann and Mareschal's model assumed a decrease over age in the size of infants' cortical receptive fields; Shultz and Cohen's (2004) model assumed the addition of a hidden unit and an increase in depth of learning; and Gureckis and Love's (2004) model assumed an increase in perceptual and/or memory ability with age.

However, the model accomplished the change, each had to propose some additional mechanism to account for the developmental change in infant categorization. Each also made specific testable predictions, which generally were supported. Finally, although all three models predicted the transition from processing independent features at 4 months of age to processing correlations among features at 10 months of age, none was able to reproduce the 7-month-olds fallback to independent features when the task became too difficult for them.

These models were not presented to show that the task is done regarding modeling the development of infant categorization. I mentioned them simply to illustrate two points. The first is that each model had to add something or modify its architecture in some way in order to represent developmental change. The second is that it can be fruitful to compare and contrast multiple models on the same basic phenomenon. Each of those models made predictions that could have been tested empirically to distinguish between them. Unfortunately, in this case, with one exception, the modelers did not go on to conduct these empirical studies. Too often modelers stop after successfully simulating some previous empirical evidence. The true potential power of these models, however, is if they make future predictions that are shown to hold empirically.

The second approach has been to develop our own model, on the development of infants' perception of simple causal events that incorporates all of the constructivist principles mentioned earlier (Cohen, Chaput, & Cashon, 2002). Our model is a hierarchical, self-organizing system that processes simple direct launching and similar types of events in which one ball moves across a screen and either does or does not make contact with a second object that then moves the remaining distance across the screen. At one level, the model organizes two types of information separately, temporal information about the movement of the two balls and spatial information about the distance between the two balls. At a higher level, the model integrates the movement information with the spatial information. In so doing, it also sets up a causal continuum with the most causal event at one end, the least causal at the other end, and the somewhat causal events in the middle. This is just what infants eventually seem to do (Leslie and Keeble, 1987). Finally, we increased the complexity of the task by adding noise to the events and the model fell back to a simpler level, once again processing the movement and spatial information separately. Thus, the model clearly operated according to the constructivist principles outlined in this chapter.

Concluding comments

As the title of this chapter (and of this conference) implies, I have presented a bottom-up approach to infant perception and cognition. I have provided evidence from topics as wide ranging as infant angle perception to infant categorization and early word learning that a constructivist, building block type of system seems to capture much of the acquisition process. The system, which is domain-general, and occurs at many different ages, uses correlational, conditional, and perhaps other types of relations to construct higher-older units from combinations of lower-order units.

But this only describes the acquisition process, since whenever infants are confronted with information, they do not automatically start their processing at the bottom or most elementary level and then move on to higher levels. They operate at a high, more efficient level, unless the system becomes overloaded, in which case they may fall back to a lower level. That part of the process, obviously, is top-down, so one should consider the entire system as much more dynamic system with repeating cycles in which infants build up new levels of information, temporarily fall back to lower levels, and then rebuild once again.

Even though this system describes how changes may occur in many aspects of infant perception and cognition, it still is only a description of behavior and behavioral change. A more complete explanation requires models that are explicit about the mechanisms underlying that change. Connectionist models may be one vehicle for doing that, but most of the ones designed so far for infant perception and cognition are limited to a single area of application and do not deal adequately with underlying and repeated developmental changes. The models are a good first step, however, and they do highlight an interesting and important issue. Fundamentally, they are models of learning, some that do require feedback and others that just self-organize from the inputs they receive. But they do raise the issue of similarities and differences between mechanisms underlying learning and mechanisms underlying development. Perhaps the two are not so different after all. Perhaps neither is evolutionary change although, of course, it occurs across generations rather than within one generation. Investigators of infant development, and of development more generally, have been very good at demonstrating some ability at one age and showing that this ability differs at one or more later ages. But, the Achilles' heel of developmental research has been an inability to account for the actual changes that occur. Perhaps a new interdisciplinary field is needed, one that brings together those who study learning, development, adaptation, and evolution, a field dedicated to understanding various types of behavioral change. Each could learn from the others, and perhaps a more sophisticated understanding of the mechanisms of change would result. In the present volume on neoconstructive approaches to development, along with a couple of other books to have appeared recently on neuroconstructive approaches to cognition, Mareschal, Johnson, et al. (2007) and Mareschal, Sirois, and Westermann (2007) show that constructive approaches to development once again are on the ascendancy and they are becoming more and more interdisciplinary.

Acknowledgments

Much of the research presented in this chapter was supported by NIH Grants HD 15035 and HD 23397.

References

Cashon, C. H., & Cohen, L. B. (2003). The construction, deconstruction, and reconstruction of infant face perception. In A. Slater & O. Pascalis (Eds.), *The development of face processing in infancy and early childhood* (pp. 55–68). New York: NOVA Science.

Cashon, C. H., & Cohen, L. B. (2004). Beyond u-shaped development in infants' processing of faces [Special issue]. *Journal of Cognition and Development, 5,* 59–80.

Cohen, L. B., & Amsel, G. (1998). Precursors to infants' perception of the causality of a simple event. *Infant Behavior and Development, 21*(4), 713–731.

Cohen, L. B., Amsel, G., Redford, M. A., & Casasola, M. (1998). The development of infant causal perception. In A. Slater (ed.), *Perceptual development: Visual, auditory, and speech perception in infancy* (pp. 167–209). East Sussex, UK: Psychology Press Ltd.

Cohen, L.B., & Caputo, N.F. (May, 1978). *Instructing infants to respond to perceptual categories.* Paper presented at Midwestern Psychological Association Convention, Chicago.

Cohen, L. B., & Cashon, C. H. (2001). Do 7-month-old infants process independent features or facial configurations? *Infant and Child Development, 10,* 83–92.

Cohen, L. B., & Cashon, C. H. (2003). Infant perception and cognition. In R. Lerner, A. Easterbrooks, & J. Mistry (Eds.), *Comprehensive handbook of psychology. Vol. 6, Developmental Psychology. II. Infancy.* (pp. 65–89), New York: Wiley and Sons.

Cohen, L. B. & Cashon, C. H. (2006). Infant cognition. In D. Kuhn & R. S. Siegler (Eds.), *Handbook of child psychology: Vol. 2. Cognition, perception, and language* (6th ed., pp. 214–251) New York: Wiley.

Cohen, L. B., Cashon, C. H., & Rundell, L. (2004, May). *Infants' developing knowledge of a causal agent.* Poster presented at International Conference on Infant Studies, Chicago.

Cohen, L. B., Chaput, H. H., & Cashon, C. H. (2002). A constructivist model of infant cognition. *Cognitive Development, 17*(3/4), 1323–1343.

Cohen, L. B., & Oakes, L. M. (1993). How infants perceive simple causality. *Developmental Psychology, 29,* 421–433.

Cohen, L. B., Rundell, L. J., Spellman, B. A., & Cashon, C. H. (1999). Infants' perception of causal chains. *Psychological Science, 10,* 412–418.

Cohen, L. B., & Strauss, M. S. (1977). Concept acquisition in the human infant. *Child Development, 50,* 419–424.

Cohen, L. B., & Younger, B. A. (1983). Perceptual categorization in the infant. In E. Scholnick (Ed.), *New trends in conceptual representation* (pp. 197–220). Hillsdale, NJ: Lawrence Erlbaum Associates.

Cohen, L. B., & Younger, B. A. (1984). Infant perception of angular relations. *Infant Behavior and Development, 7,* 37–47.

Eizenman, D. R., & Bertenthal, B. I. (1998). Infants' perception of object unity in translating and rotating displays. *Developmental Psychology, 34*(3), 426–434.

Elman, J., Bates, E., Johnson, M. H., Karmiloff-Smith, A., Parisi, D., & Plunkett, K. (1996). *Rethinking innateness: A connectionist perspective on development.* Cambridge, MA: MIT Press.

Fennell, C. T., & Werker, J. F. (2003). Early word learners' ability to access phonetic detail in well-known words. *Language and Speech, 46*(2), 245–264.

Gureckis, T. M., & Love, B. C. (2004). Common mechanisms in infant and adult category learning. *Infancy, 5,* 173–198.

Johnson, S. P. (2000). The development of visual surface perception: Insights into the ontogeny of knowledge. In C. Rovee-Collier, L. P. Lipsitt, & H. Hayne (Eds.), *Progress in infancy research* (Vol. 1, pp. 113–154). Mahwah, NJ: Erlbaum.

Karmiloff-Smith, A. (1992, reprinted 1995) *Beyond modularity: A developmental perspective on cognitive science.* Cambridge, MA: MIT Press/ Bradford Books.

Kellman, P. J., & Spelke, E. S. (1983). Perception of partly occluded objects in infancy. *Cognitive Psychology, 15,* 483–524.

Leslie, A. M. (1982). The perception of causality in infants. *Perception, 11,* 15–30.

Leslie, A. M. (1986). Getting development off the ground: Modularity and the infant's perception of causality. In P. van Geert (Ed.), *Theory building in developmental psychology* (pp. 406–437). Amsterdam: North Holland.

Leslie, A. M., & Keeble, S. (1987). Do 6-month-olds perceive causality? *Cognition, 25,* 265–288.

Madole, K. L., & Oakes, L. M. (1999). Making sense of infant categorization: Stable processes and changing representations. *Developmental Review, 19,* 263–296.

Mareschal, D., Johnson, M.H., Sirois, S., Spratling, M., Thomas, M., & Westermann, G. (2007). *Neuroconstructivism, Vol. I: How the brain constructs cognition.* Oxford: Oxford University Press.

Mareschal, D., Sirois, S., & Westermann, G. (2007). *Neuroconstructivism, Vol. II: Perspectives and Prospects.* Oxford: Oxford University Press.

Michotte, A. (1963). *The perception of causality.* NewYork: BasicBooks.

Quinn, P. C., Adams, A., Kennedy, E., Shettler, L., & Wasnik, A. (2003). Development of an abstract category representation for the spatial relation between 6- to 10-month-old infants. *Developmental Psychology, 39*(1), 151–163.

Quinn, P. C., & Eimas, P. D. (2000). The emergence of category representations during infancy: Are separate perceptual and conceptual processes required? *Journal of Cognition and Development, 1,* 55–61.

Quinn, P. C., Eimas, P. D., & Rosenkrantz, S. L. (1993). Evidence for representations of perceptually similar natural categories by 3-month-old and 4-month-old infants. *Perception, 22,* 463–475.

Rakison, D. H., & Butterworth, G. E. (1998). Infants' use of object parts in early categorization. *Developmental Psychology, 34*(1), 49–62.

Schafer, G., & Plunkett, K. (1998). Rapid word learning by fifteen-month-olds under tightly controlled conditions. *Child Development* *69*(2): 309–320.

Shultz, T. R. (2003). *Computational developmental psychology.* Cambridge, MA: MIT Press.

Shultz, T. R., & Cohen, L. B. (2004). Modeling age differences in infant category learning. *Infancy, 5,* 153–171.

Slater, A. (1995). Visual perception and memory at birth. In C. Rovee-Collier and L. P. Lipsitt (Eds.), *Advances in infancy research* (Vol. 9, pp. 107–162). Norwood, NJ: Ablex.

Slater, A., Johnson, S. P., Brown, E., & Badenoch, M. (1996). Newborn infants' perception of partly occluded objects. *Infant Behavior and Development, 19,* 145–148.

Slater, A., Johnson, S. P., Kellman, P. J., & Spelke, E. S. (1994). The role of three-dimensional depth cues in infants' perception of partly occluded objects. *Early Development and Parenting, 3,* 187–191.

Slater, A. M., Mattock, A., Brown, E., & Bremner, J. G. (1991). Form perception at birth: Cohen and Younger revisited. *Journal of Experimental Child Psychology, 51,* 395–405.

Stager, C.L., & Werker, J.F. (1997). Infants listen for more phonetic detail in speech perception than in word learning tasks. *Nature, 388*(6640), 381–382.

Werker, J. F., Cohen, L. B., Lloyd, V. L., Casasola, M., & Stager, C. L. (1998). Acquisition of word–object associations by 14-month-old infants. *Developmental Psychology, 34*(6), 1289–1309.

Werler. J. F., Fennell, C. T., Corcoran, K. M., & Stager, C. L. (2002). Infants' ability to learn phonetically similar words: Effects of age and vocabulary. *Infancy, 3.* 1–30.

Westermann, G., & Mareschal, D. (2004). From parts to wholes: Mechanisms of development in infant visual object processing. *Infancy, 5,* 131–151.

Younger, B. A., & Cohen, L. B. (1983). Infant perception of correlations among attributes. *Child Development, 54,* 858–867.

Younger, B. A., & Cohen, L. B. (1986). Developmental change in infants' perception of correlations among attributes. *Child Development, 57,* 803–815.

AUTHOR INDEX

SUBJECT INDEX